Thieme

Masters of Cosmetic Surgery—The Video Atlas

The Dallas Cosmetic Model

Rod J. Rohrich, MD, FACS
Founding Partner
Dallas Plastic Surgery Institute;
Clinical Professor of Plastic Surgery
Baylor College of Medicine
Dallas, Texas, USA

Sammy Sinno, MD
Plastic Surgeon
TLKM Plastic Surgery;
Clinical Professor of Plastic Surgery
Northwestern University Feinberg School of Medicine
Chicago, Illinois, USA

Paul N. Afrooz, MD
Plastic Surgeon
Private Practice
Miami, Florida, USA

741 illustrations

Thieme
New York • Stuttgart • Delhi • Rio de Janeiro

Library of Congress Cataloging-in-Publication Data
is available from the publisher.

Important note: Medicine is an ever-changing science undergoing continual development. Research and clinical experience are continually expanding our knowledge, in particular our knowledge of proper treatment and drug therapy. Insofar as this book mentions any dosage or application, readers may rest assured that the authors, editors, and publishers have made every effort to ensure that such references are in accordance with **the state of knowledge at the time of production of the book.**

Nevertheless, this does not involve, imply, or express any guarantee or responsibility on the part of the publishers in respect to any dosage instructions and forms of applications stated in the book. **Every user is requested to examine carefully** the manufacturers' leaflets accompanying each drug and to check, if necessary in consultation with a physician or specialist, whether the dosage schedules mentioned therein or the contraindications stated by the manufacturers differ from the statements made in the present book. Such examination is particularly important with drugs that are either rarely used or have been newly released on the market. Every dosage schedule or every form of application used is entirely at the user's own risk and responsibility. The authors and publishers request every user to report to the publishers any discrepancies or inaccuracies noticed. If errors in this work are found after publication, errata will be posted at www.thieme.com on the product description page.

Some of the product names, patents, and registered designs referred to in this book are in fact registered trademarks or proprietary names even though specific reference to this fact is not always made in the text. Therefore, the appearance of a name without designation as proprietary is not to be construed as a representation by the publisher that it is in the public domain.

Thieme Medical Publishers, Inc.
333 Seventh Avenue, New York, NY 10001 USA
+1 800 782 3488, customerservice@thieme.com

Cover design: Thieme Publishing Group
Cover images: Courtesy of Alfredo E. Hoyos, MD and Daniel A. Del Vecchio, MD

Typesetting by TNQ Technologies, India

Printed in USA by King Printing Company, Inc. 5432

ISBN 978-1-68420-217-1

Also available as an e-book:
eISBN 978-1-68420-218-8

Contents

Videos

Video 27.1 Alar base surgery. Understanding the various morphologies of the alar base will allow the surgeon to appropriately determine the type of excision required to correct the flare morphologies. This video reviews a systematic approach to marking the patient and performing alar flare reduction.

Video 28.1 Revision rhinoplasty. This 41-year-old woman presented for a revision rhinoplasty. This video demonstrates the key technical components of this procedure as outlined in the chapter.

Video 29.1 Periorbital evaluation. This video demonstrates a systematic approach for performing the periorbital evaluation in preparation for upper and/or lower eyelid blepharoplasty.

Video 30.1 Upper eyelid blepharoplasty. This is a review of the five-step upper eyelid blepharoplasty as described by the senior author.

Video 31.1 The five-step lower blepharoplasty technique. This 58-year-old woman presented for an improvement in her lower eyelids. This video demonstrates the key technical components of this procedure as outlined in the chapter.

Video 32.1 Upper eyelid fat grafting.

Video 33.1 Forehead rejuvenation.

Video 34.1 Endoscopic temporal brow lift.

Video 35.1 Forehead and temple fat augmentation.

Video 36.1 Simplified lateral brow lift.

Video 37.1 Subcutaneous temporal brow lift.

Video 38.1 Otoplasty.

Video 39.1 Surgical correction of prominent ears. This video demonstrates the senior author's surgical technique for evaluating and correcting prominent ear deformity.

Video 40.1 Lip lift.

Video 40.2 Lip lift.

Video 41.1 Lip fillers.

Video 41.2 Lip injection.

Video 42.1 Technique for fat harvest. Usually, the senior author harvests autologous fat from the inner thigh and then prepares it for injection using centrifugation.

Video 42.2 Technique for perioral augmentation. In this video, the senior author first volumizes the lateral hollowing followed by augmentation of the upper and lower perioral regions.

Video 43.1 Perioral neuromodulation.

Video 44.1 Jawline filler technique. Recorded demonstration of a cannula filler treatment for the filler treatment of a patient's cheeks, administered by facial plastic surgeon K. Kay Durairaj, MD, FACS.

Video 45.1 Chin augmentation with permanent silicone implant.

Video 46.1 General fat harvest technique.

Video 46.2 Chin augmentation with autologous fat grafting.

Video 47.1 Anatomy dissection and operative examples of buccal fat excision.

Video 48.1 Neuromodulation injection: Forehead and glabella.

Video 49.1 Botulinum toxin injection to crow's feet.

Video 50.1 Microbotox of the face and neck.

Video 51.1 Neck bands. This 63-year-old woman presented for an improvement in her neck bands. This video demonstrates the key technical components of this procedure as outlined in the chapter.

Video 52.1 Neurotoxin use for masseter hypertrophy.

Video 53.1 Filler finesse: Forehead and temple.

Video 54.1 Temple injection with hyaluronic acid. A 45-year-old woman with hollow temples seen 4 months after injection. Note the apparent saline overfill which absorbs quickly.

Video 55A.1 Malar augmentation. This 42-year-old woman presented for increased cheek volume. This video demonstrates the key technical components of this procedure as outlined in the chapter.

Video 55B.1 Filler finesse: Cheek injection technique.

Video 56.1 Filler finesse: Tear trough and upper eyelid.

Video 57A.1 Filler finesse: Nose. This 39-year-old woman presented for nasal augmentation using filler. This video demonstrates the key technical components of this procedure as outlined in the chapter.

Video 57B.1 Structural approach to nonsurgical rhinoplasty.

Video 58.1 Filler finesse: Upper eyelid sulcus. A 48-year-old female 2 weeks after brow injections and 5 days after temple fill.

Video 59.1 Filler finesse: Hands—Cannula technique with Radiesse.

Video 59.2 The five-step hand rejuvenation: Filling with hyaluronic acid.

Video 60.1 TCA peel.

Video 61.1 Dermabrasion of the face.

Video 62.1 Laser resurfacing. Ablative fractional CO_2 resurfacing for acne scarring: Consultation, treatment, and post-treatment considerations.

Video 63.1 Microneedling. Pretreatment and post-treatment set-up with clinical demonstration of microneedling treatment of perioral rhytides, striae distensae, acne, and surgical scars.

Video 64.1 Breast augmentation. Video of a four-part, dual-plane breast augmentation on a 34-year-old female. Herein we illustrate tissue-based planning, preoperative markings, refine surgical techniques, and postoperative photos.

Video 65.1 Surgical technique for performing subfascial breast augmentation.

Video 66.1 Surgical technique for performing vertical scar mastopexy with autoaugmentation flap.

Video 67.1 A step-by-step guide to mastopexy via superior pedicle, top down, minus-plus technique with auto-augmentation and fat grafting.

Video 68.1 The author's surgical pearls in augmentation mastopexy.

Video 69.1 This video shows preoperative markings and surgical maneuvers from start to finish for a typical mastopexy augmentation. The patient presented with ptosis and deflation after breast feeding. The approach was a classic vertical mastopexy with the T added at the end to accommodate the implant height after augmentation. In our practice we refer to this pattern as the "owl-shaped" incision, as the outline appears as an owl with feet. The "feet" is represented by the adjustable horizontal incision to correct the inferior breast length at the end of the procedure.

Video 70.1 Augmentation mastopexy.

Video 71.1 Surgical technique for performing vertical scar breast reduction.

Video 72.1 Wise pattern breast reduction markings and key operative steps.

Video 73.1 Video showing a four-part, dual-plane breast augmentation on a 25-year-old female with constricted lower pole of the breast. This includes tissue-based planning, preoperative markings, refine surgical technique, and postoperative photos.

Video 74.1 Circumferential SAFE lipoplasty with gluteal augmentation.

Video 75.1 This 36-year-old man presented for high-definition abdominal liposculpture with BodyBanking. This video demonstrates the key technical components of this procedure as outlined in the chapter.

Video 76.1 High-definition lipoplasty.

Video 77.1 Male high-definition liposculpture.

Video 78.1 This 27-year-old man presented for gynecomastia excision with BodyBanking. He complained of gynecomastia. This video demonstrates the key technical components of gynecomastia excision with BodyBanking as outlined in the chapter.

Video 79.1 Mommy makeover finesse.

Video 80.1 Brachioplasty refinements.

Video 81.1 Medial thigh lift.

Video 82.1 Postbariatric brachioplasty markings and key operative steps.

Video 83.1 Lower body lift. The patient is a 46-year-old female with a history of 100-lb weight loss with lifestyle modification. Preoperative BMI was 26.7 kg/m^2. She desired a lower body lift with autoaugmentation.

Video 84.1 Step-by-step execution of vertical thigh lift using the avulsion thighplasty technique.

Video 85.1 Bra-line back lift.

Video 86.1 Buttock augmentation: S-curve.

Video 87.1 This 32-year-old woman presented for Brazilian butt lift (BBL). She complained of inadequate projection and excess fat in the waist, abdomen, and back. This video demonstrates the key technical components of SSBA as outlined in the chapter.

Video 88.1 Labiaplasty with Aviva.

Video 89.1 Bipolar radiofrequency treatment of labia majora and minora.

Video 89.2 Fractional radiofrequency treatment of mons and labia majora.

Video 90.1 Cryolipolysis.

Video 91.1 Marking for lower face and neck bipolar radiofrequency.

Video 91.2 Fractional radiofrequency using Morpheus8.

Video 91.3 An intraoperative example of fractional radiofrequency.

Video 92.1 Minimally invasive upper arm contouring with bipolar radiofrequency assisted liposuction.

Video 93.1 Demonstration of the submental markings used to identify the six regions of the expanded safe zone (ESZ).

Preface

Do we need another book on cosmetic surgery? The answer to that is absolutely not! However, this is not just a book but an amazing new way to learn and master all of cosmetic surgery and cosmetic medicine. This is a didactic video atlas by world experts on the most commonly performed techniques today. We selected the top global authorities who are not just superb surgeons and dermatologists but also top educators focused on excellence in all they do. In this procedure- and video-rich guide, we wanted to make sure that every technique described in the chapters would come to life with the expert "whispering in your ear" as you perform and perfect each of the techniques.

The guiding principles for each chapter had to be succinct. This meant that each chapter must have the five key principles for maximizing technical success, which are brought to life by key video segments with narration to expound on how to perform the procedure in a safe and efficient manner that results in optimal outcomes. This textbook has 90 procedures and more than 12 hours of video.

The unique aspect of this video atlas is your ability to read, see, and hear the expert and learn the key concepts of any procedure in minutes and then be able to perform the procedure with enhanced skill and safety.

Over the last decade, much has changed in the world of aesthetic surgery and cosmetic medicine. The rapid growth in global demand for aesthetic procedures comes with an increasing mandate for enhanced learning from videos to produce both excellent patient outcomes and patient safety.

This how and why guide will transform your technique and outcomes while enhancing patient safety. We will empower you to be your best as we will be guiding your mind and hand. We will show you how to perform a superb and safe cosmetic surgery consult in all areas. We cover what to know, what to do, when to say "no," and how to optimize results and minimize complications in cosmetic surgery.

The following key areas are covered:

- We feature the experts in face and neck lift surgery with all the modern technical details and finesse. You will see why it is so important to understand the science of aging and apply it to individualized facial analysis to optimize your facial rejuvenation results with key leaders in the field including Dr. Stuzin, Dr. Aston, Dr. Baker, Dr. Marten, Dr. Rohrich, Dr. Elyassnia, Dr. Sinno, and Dr. Afrooz.
- You will learn how to do an efficient rhinoplasty consult as well as the key maneuvers from the experts, namely, Dr. Rohrich, Dr. Toriumi, Dr. Ahmad, Dr. Afrooz, Dr. Sinno, Dr. Kosins, Dr. Cochran, Dr. Roostaeian, Dr. Guyuron, Dr. Ghavami, Dr. Albert, Dr. Aston, and Dr. Kurkjian, that will make you a better and more consistent rhinoplasty surgeon.
- Being an expert in periorbital rejuvenation is a challenge but you will be with the help of superb video sessions with Dr. Rohrich, Dr. Marten, Dr. Guyuron, Dr. Mustoe, Dr. Sinno, Dr. Afrooz, Dr. Trevidic, Dr. Thorne, and Dr. Elyassnia.
- How to become a finesse otoplasty surgeon with inputs from experts like Dr. Thorne, Dr. Byrd, Dr. Sinno, and Dr. Savetsky.
- There are many options to achieve spectacular results in perioral rejuvenation including lip lifts, fillers, and skin resurfacing. Experts like Dr. Rohrich, Dr. Afrooz, Dr. Surek, and Dr. Fagien will teach you the best techniques to achieve success in your patients.
- Learn fitness and safe chin augmentation with implants and fat with Dr. Rohrich, Dr. Dayan, and Dr. Durand.
- Neuromodulators have transformed aesthetic medicine. Learn the best of the best techniques with world-renowned experts, Dr. Fagien, Dr. Wu, Dr. Furnas, and Dr. Rohrich.
- We will teach you how to inject fillers with aesthetic artistry while staying safe and free of complications. You will understand the aesthetic implications and clinically relevant anatomy from the thought leaders in this area of cosmetic medicine—featuring Dr. Fagien, Dr. Rohrich, Dr. Devgan, Dr. Lambros, and Dr. Patel.
- There are several options available to resurface skin, but it must be done safely and effectively, no matter the technology. You will learn from masters of the skin including Dr. Levine, Dr. Rohrich, Dr. Dayan, Dr. Durand, and Dr. Savetsky.
- This video atlas will give you the tools necessary to be a better breast surgeon. The expert authors will show you their master techniques so that you will be able to analyze, mark, and operate in the same manner to provide safe and stellar results. Learn these cutting-edge techniques from world experts Dr. Adams, Dr. Sieber, Dr. Ahmad, Dr. Lista, Dr. Unger, Dr. Maxwell, Dr. Rohrich, Dr. Hammond, and Dr. Shestak.
- The field of body-contouring surgery has advanced tremendously over the past decade. We provide high-definition sculpting as taught by thought leaders including Dr. Hoyos, Dr. Wall, Dr. Del Vecchio, Dr. Ghavami, Dr. Lee, Dr. Steinbrech, Dr. Savetsky, Dr. Hunstad, Dr. Gusenoff, and Dr. Dayan. See the experts demonstrate their techniques and learn how to obtain better and safer results for your patients in procedures like liposuction and buttock augmentation.
- Vaginal rejuvenation is one of the most rapidly growing areas of aesthetic medicine. Learn the latest finesse

techniques from the experts like Dr. Hamori and Dr. Ahmad.

- Nonsurgical body contouring is one of the most popular treatments requested by aesthetic patients. Learn what techniques work and how to best administer with the experts like Dr. Stevens, Dr. Chia, Dr. Rohrich, Dr. Aston, Dr. Dayan, Dr. Theodorou, and Dr. Shridharani.

Our hope is that you enjoy this transformational cosmetic surgery/medicine video guide as much as we have enjoyed putting it together, and that it will help you in your cosmetic practice to improve your outcomes and above all to enhance patient safety.

Rod J. Rohrich, MD, FACS
Sammy Sinno, MD
Paul N. Afrooz, MD

Acknowledgments

We dedicate this amazingly unique educational book and interactive video atlas to our patients and to those who want to excel in delivering the best care and results to their patients with the most innovative techniques and latest technology in a safe outcome-driven manner. We have assembled the global experts to refine excellence in cosmetic surgery and cosmetic medicine. However, this time we did it with the maximal use of concise video to demonstrate the principles of excellence and show how to achieve superior results consistently in all cosmetic surgeries. This book will guide board-certified plastic surgeons, dermatologists, facial plastic surgeons, and oculoplastic surgeons to provide best care based upon the principles delineated in this book.

Cosmetic surgery today is all about putting patient safety and outcome first and foremost always. This unique video-integrated book brings the experts to you to see and hear them show you how to do a complex technique or procedure in a simplified, efficient, and safe and reproducible manner.

We acknowledge and appreciate all our patients and mentors who have helped each of us become better and more caring physicians throughout our practice of medicine.

Specifically, we want to thank our individual staff who have helped us complete this book, including Diane Sinn, my long-term assistant and administrator; Angela Martinez, my superb office manager; and our great Thieme staff, Judith Tomat and Sue Hodgson; as well as our illustrator Amanda Tomasikiewicz whose expertise is displayed in each page of this wonderful book.

Finally, we want to acknowledge our superb residents and fellows at Dallas Plastic Surgery Institute, especially this year's tremendous fellows, Dr. Ira L. Savetsky and Dr. Yash J. Avashia, for their tremendous work in completing so much of the finesse work of each chapter.

Enjoy, learn, give back, and always be the best you can for each of your patients. Now you can do so with this amazing new video atlas!

Rod J. Rohrich, MD, FACS
Sammy Sinno, MD
Paul N. Afrooz, MD

Contributors

William P. Adams Jr., MD, FACS
Program Director
Aesthetic Surgery Fellowship
University of Texas Southwestern Medical Center
Dallas, Texas, USA

Paul N. Afrooz, MD
Plastic Surgeon
Private Practice
Miami, Florida, USA

Nikhil A. Agrawal, MD
Fellow
Department of Plastic Surgery
Massachusetts General Hospital
Harvard Medical School
Boston, Massachusetts, USA

Jamil Ahmad, MD, FRCSC
Director of Research and Education
The Plastic Surgery Clinic
Mississauga, Ontario, Canada;
Assistant Professor
Department of Surgery
University of Toronto
Toronto, Ontario, Canada

Mark G. Albert, MD, FACS
Aesthetic Surgery Fellowship Program Director
Department of Plastic Surgery
Manhattan Eye, Ear, and Throat Hospital at Northwell Health
New York, New York, USA

Tina S. Alster, MD
Director
Washington Institute of Dermatologic Laser Surgery;
Clinical Professor of Dermatology
Georgetown University Medical Center
Washington, DC, USA

Sherrell J. Aston, MD, FACS
Professor of Plastic Surgery
New York University School of Medicine;
Associate Chairman
Department of Plastic Surgery
Manhattan Eye, Ear & Throat Hospital
New York, New York, USA

Ryan E. Austin, MD, FRCS(C)
Plastic Surgeon
The Plastic Surgery Clinic
Mississauga, Ontario, Canada

Yash J. Avashia, MD
Plastic Surgeon
Dallas Plastic Surgery Institute
Dallas, Texas, USA

Daniel C. Baker, MD
Plastic Surgeon
Private Practice
New York, New York, USA

Omer Baker, BS (pursuing)
Research Associate
University of Southern California
Los Angeles, California, USA

Jonathan P. Brower, MD
Body Contouring Fellow
Department of Plastic Surgery
University of Pittsburgh Medical Center
Pittsburgh, Pennsylvania, USA

H. Steve Byrd, MD
EarWell Centers
Dallas Plastic Surgery Institute
Dallas, Texas, USA

Christopher T. Chia, MD
Clinical Assistant Professor of Surgery
Zucker School of Medicine, Hofstra University
New York, New York, USA

Min-Jeong Cho, MD
Microvascular and Reconstructive Surgery Fellow
Department of Plastic Surgery
The University of Texas MD Anderson Cancer Center
Houston, Texas, USA

Jeffrey R. Claiborne, MD
Plastic Surgeon
Northshore Plastic Surgery
Mandeville, Louisiana, USA

C. Spencer Cochran, MD
Dallas Rhinoplasty Center
Dallas, Texas, USA

Joshua M. Cohen, MD
Resident
Hansjörg Wyss Department of Plastic Surgery
New York University Langone Health
New York, New York, USA

Rafael A. Couto, MD
Plastic & Reconstructive Surgeon
Couto Plastic Surgery
San Juan, Puerto Rico

Erez Dayan, MD
Plastic and Reconstructive Surgeon
Medical Director
Avance Plastic Surgery Institute
Reno, Nevada, USA

Daniel A. Del Vecchio, MD
Back Bay Plastic Surgery
Boston, Massachusetts, USA

Lara Devgan, MD, MPH, FACS, PLLC
Plastic Surgeon
Lara Devgan, MD, Plastic & Reconstructive Surgery
Lenox Hill Hospital
New York Presbyterian Hospital
New York, New York, USA

K. Kay Durairaj, MD, FACS
Chairman of Department of Head and Neck Surgery
Huntington Memorial Hospital
Los Angeles, California, USA

Paul Durand, MD
Plastic Surgeon
Private Practice
Miami, Florida, USA

Francesco M. Egro, MBChB, MSc, MRCS
Resident
Department of Plastic Surgery
University of Pittsburgh Medical Center
Pittsburgh, Pennsylvania, USA

Dino Elyassnia, MD, FACS
Plastic Surgeon
Marten Clinic of Plastic Surgery
San Francisco, California, USA

Steven Fagien, MD, FACS
Oculoplastic Surgeon
Aesthetic Oculoplastic Surgery (Private Practice)
Boca Raton, Florida, USA

Stephanie E. Farber, MD
Chief Resident Physician
Department of Plastic Surgery
University of Pittsburgh Medical Center
Pittsburgh, Pennsylvania, USA

Cory Felber, PA-C
Aesthetic Specialist
Marina Plastic Surgery
Marina Del Rey, California, USA

Paul M. Friedman, MD
Director
Dermatology and Laser Center;
Clinical Assistant Professor
Department of Dermatology
University of Texas Medical School;
Clinical Assistant Professor
Department of Dermatology
Weill Medical Center of Cornell University, The Methodist Hospital
Houston, Texas, USA

Heather J. Furnas, MD, FACS
Clinical Associate Professor
Division of Plastic & Reconstructive Surgery
Stanford University
Santa Rosa, California, USA

Palmyra Geissler, MD
Plastic Surgeon
Private Practice
Rio De Janeiro, Brazil

Ashkan Ghavami, MD
Assistant Clinical Professor
David Geffen UCLA School of Medicine and Private Practice
Ghavami Plastic Surgery
Beverly Hills, California, USA

Daniel J. Gould, MD, PhD
USC Trained Plastic Surgeon
Top Fellowship for Breast Surgery, Facelift and Rhinoplasty
Fellow of American Society of Aesthetic Plastic Surgery (ASAPS)
Marina Del Rey, California, USA
Beverly Hills, California, USA

Grace J. Graw, MD
Resident Physician
Division of Plastic and Reconstructive Surgery
Department of Surgery
Stanford Hospital and Clinics
Palo Alto, California, USA

Jeffrey A. Gusenoff, MD
Professor
Department of Plastic Surgery
University of Pittsburgh
Pittsburgh, Pennsylvania, USA

Bahman Guyuron, MD, FACS
Professor Emeritus
Department of Plastic Surgery
Case School of Medicine
Cleveland, Ohio, USA

Kristy L. Hamilton, MD
Plastic Surgeon
Private Practice
Houston, Texas, USA

Christine A. Hamori, MD, FACS
Director
Cosmetic Surgery & Skin Spa
Duxbury, Massachusetts, USA

Alfredo E. Hoyos, MD
Plastic and Aesthetic Surgeon
Department of Plastic Surgery
Dhara Clinic (Private Practice);
Scientific Director
Plastic Surgery & Professional Education
Total Definer
Bogota, Colombia

Joseph P. Hunstad, MD, FACS
Plastic Surgeon
Hunstad Kortesis Bharti Cosmetic Plastic Surgery;
Associate Consulting Professor
University of North Carolina
Chapel Hill Division of Plastic Surgery
Charlotte, North Carolina, USA

Matthew H. Isakson, MD
Plastic Surgeon
Department of Aesthetic Surgery
Private Practice
Augusta, Georgia, USA

Annette K. Kaminaka, BA
Medical Student
Albany Medical College
Albany, New York, USA

Roy Kim, MD
Private Practice
San Francisco, California, USA

Elizabeth Klein, MS
Medical Student
New York University Grossman School of Medicine
New York, New York, USA

Aaron M. Kosins, MD
Private Practice
Newport Beach, California, USA

David M. Kowalczyk, MD, MBA
Fellow
Department of Otolaryngology—Head & Neck Surgery
University of Illinois at Chicago
Chicago, Illinois, USA

Jon Kurkjian, MD
Private Practice
Fort Worth, Texas, USA;
Clinical Assistant Professor
University of Texas Southwestern Medical Center
Dallas, Texas, USA

Val Lambros, MD
Clinical Professor of Plastic Surgery
University of California, Irvine
Irvine, California, USA

Steven M. Levine, MD
Assistant Professor of Plastic Surgery
Donald and Barbara Zucker School of Medicine at Hofstra/Northwell
New York, New York, USA

Frank Lista, MD, FRCSC
Assistant Professor
Department of Surgery
University of Toronto
Toronto, Ontario, Canada

Timothy Marten, MD, FACS
Plastic Surgeon
Marten Clinic of Plastic Surgery
San Francisco, California, USA

G. Patrick Maxwell, MD
Maxwell Aesthetics
Nashville, Tennessee, USA

Raja Mohan, MD
Plastic Surgeon
Private Practice
Irving, Texas, USA

Thomas A. Mustoe, MD
Plastic Surgeon
TLKM Plastic Surgery;
Former Professor
Division of Plastic Surgery
Northwestern University Feinberg School of Medicine
Chicago, Illinois, USA

Vivian N. Nguyen, BS
Research Associate
Physiology and Neuroscience
University of California, San Diego
San Diego, California, USA

Eugene Park, MD
Resident
Division of Plastic Surgery
Northwestern University Feinberg School of Medicine
Chicago, Illinois, USA

Anup Patel, MD, MBA, FACS
Plastic and Reconstructive Surgeon
Orlando Plastic Surgery Institute
Orlando, Florida, USA

Mauricio E. Perez, MD
Medical Doctor and Surgeon
Department of Plastic Surgery
Total Definer Research Group
Dallas, Texas, USA

Abigail M. Rodriguez, MD
Plastic Surgeon
Houston, Texas, USA

Rod J. Rohrich, MD, FACS
Founding Partner
Dallas Plastic Surgery Institute;
Clinical Professor of Plastic Surgery
Baylor College of Medicine
Dallas, Texas, USA

Jason Roostaeian, MD
Division of Plastic and Reconstructive Surgery
University of California, Los Angeles
Los Angeles, California, USA

J. Peter Rubin, MD, MBA, FACS
UPMC Endowed Professor and Chair of Plastic Surgery
Director of UPMC Wound Healing Services
Department of Plastic Surgery
University of Pittsburgh Medical Center;
Professor of Bioengineering
University of Pittsburgh
Pittsburgh, Pennsylvania, USA

Sean Saadat, MD
Resident Physician
Plastic & Reconstructive Surgery
UCLA Health
Los Angeles, California, USA

Kyle Sanniec, MD
Department of Plastic Surgery
University of Texas Southwestern Medical Center
Dallas, Texas, USA

Elizabeth B. Savetsky, MS
Digital Influencer
Dallas, Texas, USA

Ira L. Savetsky, MD
Plastic Surgeon
Dallas Plastic Surgery Institute
Dallas, Texas, USA

Matthew Schulman, MD
Plastic Surgeon
Schulman Plastic Surgery
New York, New York, USA

Kenneth C. Shestak, MD
Professor
Department of Plastic Surgery
University of Pittsburgh Medical Center
Pittsburgh, Pennsylvania, USA

Sachin M. Shridharani, MD, FACS
Plastic Surgeon
Department of Plastic Surgery
Luxurgery
New York, New York, USA

Simranjit Sidhu, BS
Research Associate
Ecology and Evolution
University of California, Santa Barbara
Pasadena, California, USA

David Sieber, MD, FACS
Sieber Plastic Surgery
Sam Francisco, California, USA

Sammy Sinno, MD
Plastic Surgeon
TLKM Plastic Surgery;
Clinical Professor of Plastic Surgery
Northwestern University Feinberg School of Medicine
Chicago, Illinois, USA

Pooja Sodha, MD
Director
Center for Laser and Cosmetic Dermatology;
Assistant Professor of Dermatology
George Washington University School of Medicine and Health Sciences
Washington, DC, USA

Douglas S. Steinbrech, MD, FACS
Gotham Plastic Surgery
New York, New York, USA

W. Grant Stevens, MD, FACS
Clinical Professor of Surgery
Keck School of Medicine of the University of Southern California
Division of Plastic Surgery;
Director
USC Aesthetic Surgery Fellowship
American Society of Aesthetic Plastic Surgery
Los Angeles, California, USA

James M. Stuzin, MD
Plastic Surgeon
Institute of Aesthetic Medicine;
Chair of the Baker-Gordon Cosmetic Surgery Meeting
Professor of Plastic Surgery (Voluntary)
University of Miami School of Medicine
Miami, Florida, USA

Christopher C. Surek, DO
Clinical Assistant Professor
Department of Plastic Surgery
University of Kansas Medical Center;
Assistant Professor of Anatomy
Department of Anatomy
Kansas City University
Kansas City, Missouri, USA

Spero J. Theodorou, MD
BodySCULPT
New York, New York, USA

Charles H. Thorne, MD
Plastic Surgeon
Private Practice
New York, New York, USA

Grace M. Tisch, BA
Department of Plastic Surgery
Luxurgery
New York, New York, USA

Dean M. Toriumi, MD
Plastic Surgeon
Toriumi Facial Plastics (Private Practice)
Chicago, Illinois, USA

Shahryar Tork, MD
Plastic Surgeon
The Plastic Surgery Group
Cincinnati, Ohio, USA

Patrick Trevidic, MD
Plastic Surgeon
Expert2 Expert (Private Practice)
Paris, France

Jacob G. Unger, MD
Plastic Surgeon
Maxwell Aesthetics
Nashville Plastic Surgery Institute
Nashville, Tennessee, USA

Christina R. Vargas, MD
Chief Resident
Plastic and Reconstructive Surgery
University Hospitals Cleveland Medical Center
Case Western Reserve University
Cleveland, Ohio, USA

Vasileios Vasilakis, MD
Plastic Surgeon
Memorial Plastic Surgery
Houston, Texas, USA

Nathaniel L. Villanueva, MD
Plastic Surgeon
The Plastic Surgery Institute (Private Practice)
Beverly Hills, California, USA

Heidi A. Waldorf, MD
Waldorf Dermatology Aesthetics
Nanuet, New York, USA

Simeon Wall, Jr., MD, FACS
Board Certified Plastic Surgeon
The Wall Center for Plastic Surgery & Jade Medispa
Shreveport, Louisiana, USA

Dinah Wan, MD
Southlake Plastic Surgery
Southlake, Texas, USA

Woffles T. L. Wu, MBBS, FRCS (Edin), FAMS (Plastic Surg)
Woffles Wu Aesthetic Surgery and Laser Centre
Singapore

Introduction: Addressing the Most Common Procedures in Cosmetic Surgery: Why This Book Is Different

1 The Consult: What to Know, What to Do, and When to Say "No"

Rod J. Rohrich, Abigail M. Rodriguez, and Ira L. Savetsky

Abstract
The initial consultation is an important event in deciding if a patient is suitable for surgery. Listening to the patient and determining if a patient has realistic expectations are crucial for predicting surgical success. Patients who are rude to staff or active smokers may require careful consideration prior to becoming your surgical patients.

Keywords: Cosmetic surgery, aesthetic surgery, cosmetic consultation, aesthetic consultation, expectations, red flag

Key Points

- More than ever, patients are arriving to the initial consultation equipped with information from online sources with strong ideas regarding their self-diagnosis and the indicated surgery.
- Listening to the patient, forming a clear plan with distinct goals, performing a nasofacial analysis, obtaining preoperative photographs, and setting realistic expectations are paramount to embarking on a successful surgery.
- Special consideration should be given before agreeing to operate on teenage patients.
- Active smokers, rude patients, and patients with unrealistic or vague goals for surgery are not appropriate candidates for elective procedures.

1.1 Before the Consultation

- Though word-of-mouth referrals are still common in cosmetic surgery, "digital referrals" are becoming increasingly common.
- Much before the consultation, most patients already have an idea of what you (the plastic surgeon) may be like after reading your website and online reviews, as well as viewing social media platforms.
- Set the consultation up for success by providing prospective patients with educational information in the form of concise text and, preferably, videos and graphic illustrations on a mobile-friendly website and on social media.
- Some patients may have attended consultations with other plastic surgeons and may introduce the diagnosis and plan from other consultation(s) into the discussion.
- The clinic scheduler should arrange consultations as promptly as possible, as a new patient is often not willing to wait for months and will opt to find a different plastic surgeon instead.

1.2 Listen to the Patient

- Take the time to listen to the patients and learn their occupation, hobbies, lifestyle, and social support system.
- Careful attention should be paid to understand the patient's motivation for the consultation, the surgery, and the timing of the surgery (i.e., why now?).
- The patient should be asked to list *any* and *all* prior related treatments, including injections, laser treatment, and surgery.
- Although a patient may complain about a prior experience with a different plastic surgeon, always refrain from passing any judgment or speaking unfavorably about the other surgeon.
- Let the patients describe their concerns and encourage them to *prioritize* the top three areas of concern.

1.3 Nasofacial Analysis

- A thorough, standardized nasofacial analysis should be performed, using a mirror to facilitate the discussion with the patient to identify specific areas of concern.
- Gently guide the patient to view the face in its totality, thereby improving his or her understanding of the importance of facial proportions and relationships (e.g., the lip–chin relationship for a rhinoplasty patient).
- For FaceTime or Skype consultations, request the patient's photographs to be sent beforehand to review in preparation.

1.4 Setting Expectations

- Incorrect self-diagnosis and unreasonable expectations, if not corrected by the plastic surgeon preoperatively, can result in significant dissatisfaction postoperatively.
- Be honest and forthright with yourself and your patients with regard to what you can and cannot do.
- Pre-emptively dispel common misconceptions, such as "liposuction will make you lose weight" or "a facelift will last forever."
- Patients will retain only a fraction of what they are told during the consultation. Reinforce expectations set during the consultation by providing written materials with the same information.
- Remember, "You are a surgeon, not a magician." Never guarantee a result. Rather, always under-promise and over-deliver.

1.5 What to Do

- Both static and dynamic standardized photographs should be obtained preoperatively. These photographs are critical postoperatively to remind the patient of the significant improvements gained with surgery, particularly when the patient is preoccupied with a less significant feature.
- Computer imaging can be helpful to provide the patient with a general idea of the postoperative result but there is certainly no guarantee.

Table 1.1 Recommended age for common plastic surgery interventions

Procedure	Recommended age (year)
Otoplasty	5–7
Cosmetic rhinoplasty	Females: 15–17 Males: 16–18
Retin A Laser for acne scars	16–18
Breast augmentation Breast reduction Chemical peels Laser for cosmetic reasons Botulinum toxin Filler	≥18
Liposuction	≥18 (when unresponsive to diet/exercise)

Source: Adapted from Rohrich RJ, Cho MJ. When Is Teenage Plastic Surgery versus Cosmetic Surgery Okay? Reality versus Hype: A Systematic Review. Plast Reconstr Surg. 2018;142(3):293e–302e.

- As always, the risks and potential complications of surgery should be reviewed in detail and informed consent obtained preoperatively.
- If the patient is amenable, obtain a specific informed consent for posting the patient's photographs and videos on your social media account and website. Realistic images of patients taken preoperatively, intraoperatively, and postoperatively may help future patients develop realistic expectations.
- With the patient, define clear goals for the surgery and reiterate these on the morning of the surgery.

1.6 When to Say No

- Teenage patients must be of adequate physical and emotional maturity, with clear, valid motivations for surgery. ▶ Table 1.1 lists general suggestions (*not* necessarily strict guidelines) for teenage patient candidacy for plastic surgery based on age. Importantly, the patient's desire for surgery should not be dictated by other social media users or by the desire to look like celebrities.
- The debate over whether or not to operate on smokers for certain plastic surgery procedures is ongoing. Some plastic surgeons rationalize doing a less aggressive surgery on smokers with the hope that this will decrease the risk of complications. By operating on a person who smokes, you are subjecting that patient not only to a lesser procedure but also to a lesser result. Now both the procedure and the result are compromised. To be considered a candidate for elective plastic surgery, patients must stop smoking *at least* 4 weeks preoperatively.
- Tried and true guidelines for patient selection, originally coined by Dr. Gorney, can be easily remembered with two acronyms. Patients with potential problem can be predicted with the acronym SIMON: Single, Immature Male who is Overly expectant and Narcissistic (▶ Table 1.2). Patients who tend to do well can be predicted with the acronym SYLVIA: Secure, Young Listener who is Verbal, Intelligent, and Attractive (▶ Table 1.2).
- According to Dr. Goldwyn and Dr. Rohrich, you should not operate if:
  - You don't like an individual patient.

Table 1.2 Red flag and Green flag patient types

Red flag patient type = SIMON	Green flag patient type = SYLVIA
Single Immature Male Overly expectant Narcissistic	Secure Young Listen Verbal Intelligent Attractive

Source: Adapted from Rohrich RJ. Streamlining Cosmetic Surgery Patient Selection—Just Say No! Plast Reconstr Surg. 1999;104(1):220–221.

  - The patient asks you to do something you can't deliver.
  - The patient asks you to do something that is outside your aesthetic sense of what the result should be.
  - The patient is critical of previous surgeons or praises you excessively.
  - The patient is rude to you or your staff.
  - The patient lies to you or gives you a false history or information.
  - The patient refuses to be examined, to disrobe for examination, or to be photographed.
  - The patient is a perfectionist and wants a guarantee of results.
  - The patient is paranoid, delusional, or depressed.
  - The patient fails to communicate or is unable to understand what informed consent entails.
- The following features are not necessarily contraindications to cosmetic surgery, but they are high-risk. Proceed with great caution with:
  - The secretive patient who doesn't want anyone to know he or she is having surgery.
  - The "VIP" patient who is (or believes he or she is) famous or wealthy.
  - The patient in a hurry to have surgery.
  - The surgiholic patient who has had multiple, previous operative procedures.
  - The out-of-town patient who cannot stay long for postoperative care.
  - The recurrent, plastic surgery shopper patient.
  - The unkempt or unclean patient.
  - The patient who sees you in consultation multiple times preoperatively asking the same questions.
  - The patient who is vague or indecisive.
- In essence, when in doubt, don't!

1.7 Conclusion

Consultation is an integral component when deciding if a patient is suitable for surgery.

Listening to the patient and determining if a patient has realistic expectations is crucial for predicting surgical success.

Patients who are rude to your staff or active smokers are examples of red flags and these patients should not be operated.

See **Video 1.1.**

Further Readings

Rohrich RJ, Weinstein A. Paging Dr. Google: the changing face of plastic surgery. Plast Reconstr Surg. 2016; 138(5):1133–1136

Rohrich RJ, Timberlake AT, Afrooz PN. Revisiting the fundamental operative principles of plastic surgery. Plast Reconstr Surg. 2017; 140(6):1315–1318

Rohrich RJ, Cho MJ. When is teenage plastic surgery versus cosmetic surgery okay? Reality versus hype: a systematic review. Plast Reconstr Surg. 2018; 142(3): 293e–302e

Rohrich RJ. Cosmetic surgery and patients who smoke: should we operate? Plast Reconstr Surg. 2000; 106(1):137–138

Rohrich RJ. Streamlining cosmetic surgery patient selection—just say no! Plast Reconstr Surg. 1999; 104(1):220–221

2 How to Optimize Results and Minimize Complications in Cosmetic Surgery

Rod J. Rohrich and Yash J. Avashia

Abstract

Success in cosmetic surgery involves preoperative, intraoperative, and postoperative attention. Developing a rapport and understanding with the patient is a critical part of the initial patient visit and builds a foundation for all future interactions throughout the perioperative period. Proper patient selection is the first step in optimizing results. Setting patient expectations is a critical aspect to the preoperative process and directly influences patient's experience and satisfaction. A detailed preoperative analysis will set the surgeon up to perform the right operation. Inadequate patient assessment can lead to performing the wrong operation and result in complications and revision surgery.

Keywords: Safety, surgical complications, preoperative analysis, patient selection, imaging, patient expectations

Key Points

- Success in cosmetic surgery involves preoperative, intraoperative, and postoperative attention.
- Developing a rapport and understanding with the patient is a critical part of the initial patient visit and builds a foundation for all future interactions throughout the perioperative period.
- Proper patient selection is the first step in optimizing results.
- Setting patient expectations is a critical aspect to the preoperative process and directly influences patient's experience and satisfaction.
- A detailed preoperative analysis will set the surgeon up to perform the right operation. Inadequate patient assessment can lead to performing the wrong operation and result in complications and revision surgery.
- Safe technique is a principle in cosmetic surgery.

2.1 Initial Patient Experience

- There are three groups of new patients:
  - Patients who know about the surgeon's practice.
  - Patients who are referred by another patient.
  - Patients who are completely unknown.
- The surgeon typically has 60 seconds to develop a connection with the patient that sets the tone for the remainder of the patient visit.
- It is important for the surgeon to make a serious effort to connect with the patient during this time period. Engaging the patients in talking about themselves allows the surgeon to identify a potential connection.
- Following the patient visit, there is normally a 2 to 3 days window to seek a second contact with the patient by email or phone to follow-up. Lack of connecting with the patient during this period often leads to the patient not proceeding with surgery.
- Patient's experience is truly the intangible aspect that governs the patient's response to both good and bad surgical outcomes. This is an aspect that includes not only the surgeon, but every staff member. The patient interacts with everyone and all the interactions comprise the "patient's experience."

2.2 Patient Selection

- The major determinant of a successful cosmetic surgery is patient selection.
- Most patient dissatisfaction in aesthetic surgery is based on failure of communication and adhering to patient selection criteria.
  - Patient selection criteria: The following medical criteria deem patients as poor candidates and at risk for complications:
    - Smokers.
    - High body mass index (BMI) (>35).
    - Active cardiovascular disease (metabolic equivalents [METS] <4).
    - Anticoagulation and/or antiplatelet therapy.
    - Chronic inflammatory disease with steroid use.
    - Connective tissue disease (Ehlers–Danlos syndrome).
- Through trial-and-error, the aesthetic surgeon improves his or her sense of identifying patients who are poor candidates for aesthetic surgery.
- The practicing surgeon learns to identify certain patient characteristics or personality traits which predict a low level of postoperative satisfaction.
- Sarwer et al showed that individuals who seek cosmetic improvement have a higher rate of body dysmorphic disorder (BDD) and other psychiatric conditions than the general population.
- The rate of BDD may be as high as 15% in aesthetic surgery patients.
- Implicit in patient selection is performing a detailed preoperative evaluation that seeks to uncover both the patient's physical concerns and psychological perspective.
- Gorney described a set of guidelines for patient selection that was based on correlating the severity of deformity with the patient's level of concern.
  - Patients with a low level of concern for a severe deformity were considered good candidates for surgery.
  - Patients with a high level of concern for a minor deformity were considered poor candidates for surgery.

2.3 Setting Expectations

- Understanding the patient's postoperative expectation is a crucial aspect to the preoperative assessment.
- It is important for the surgeon to be able to see what the patient is seeing (vice versa is important as well).

- Begin by requesting the patients to define their three primary concerns. Patients who are unable to clearly define their concerns or who use generic descriptors require further questioning and education to better help them understand their physical or psychological disharmony.
- After defining their concerns, the patients should also be able to provide a realistic expectation of what they hope to achieve from surgery. Unrealistic expectations are a set up for an unhappy patient.
- It is the surgeon's responsibility to calibrate the patient's expectations and provide a realistic idea of what type of postoperative result is achievable.

2.4 Right Surgical Plan

- A detailed preoperative assessment is the prerequisite to developing a surgical plan.
- Preoperative imaging is a necessary aspect of every cosmetic surgery procedure. Proper imaging technique allows for preoperative planning, patient discussion, and comparing results during the postoperative follow-up.
- A thorough understanding of the anatomic basis of the patient's concern is critical, which is obtained through a detailed physical examination.
- There is a finesse in balancing the patient's and surgeon's perspectives on the physical deformity at hand and agreeing on a surgical plan.

2.5 Safe Technique

- Safe technique is identifying "what can go wrong" at each step in the surgery and taking the measures to prevent them. The opposite of safe technique is overconfidence, ignorance, and haste.
- Universal to safe technique is adhering to principles in plastic surgery that govern wound healing: tension free closure and preserving vascularity. Unique to cosmetic surgery is respecting the functional anatomy while achieving the aesthetic improvement. This is particularly important in periorbital rejuvenation, rhytidectomy, and rhinoplasty, but is also relevant in other aspects of cosmetic surgery such as breast and body.
- The purpose of this chapter is not to expunge the safe techniques in cosmetic surgery. The purpose of this book is to provide a safe guide of proven techniques in cosmetic surgery.

2.6 Conclusion

From the initial consultation to the final postoperative visit, the surgeon–patient relationship is continuously evolving. Setting patient expectations and patient selection are as important as the actual technique used. Senior surgeons often build upon their experience to navigate patient interactions. Junior surgeons can use these guidelines to help avoid early pitfalls.

Further Readings

Goldwyn RM. The patient and the plastic surgeon. 2nd ed. Boston: Little, Brown; 1991

Gorney M, Martello J. Patient selection criteria. Clin Plast Surg. 1999; 26(1):37–40, vi

Rohrich RJ. Streamlining cosmetic surgery patient selection—just say no! Plast Reconstr Surg. 1999; 104(1):220–221

Sarwer DB, Wadden TA, Pertschuk MJ, Whitaker LA. The psychology of cosmetic surgery: a review and reconceptualization. Clin Psychol Rev. 1998;18(1):1–22

3 How Social Media Has Changed All of Plastic Surgery

Rod J. Rohrich, Ashkan Ghavami, and Daniel J. Gould

Abstract

Social media is a rapidly growing mature platform for potential patients and surgeons from diverse locations to interact and communicate. This includes an opportunity for daily impressions, and not simply promotional marketing but also the delivery of educational content. In this chapter we will discuss the ethical use of this media to grow followers, improve practice exposure, and safeguard the fiduciary relationship between the surgeons and patients.

Keywords: Social media, Instagram, Snapchat, Twitter, Facebook

Key Points

- Social media encompasses all platforms for online social interaction, and is one of the most powerful and exciting new arenas for plastic surgical practices. Previous efforts have focused on methods to determine the return on investment (ROI) for certain social networks.
- The greatest ROI comes from Instagram, Snapchat, Realself, and Facebook, in roughly that order. Strengths are video and photo contents and ease of access.
- Surgeons should be aware of their appearance on platforms and should maintain high moral and ethical standards. Recent studies have proposed guidelines at least for residents in training.
- Social media is a powerful marketing tool, but with great power comes great responsibility.
- Avoid paying for followers; be careful with "influencers"; organic growth is sustainable and real.

3.1 Deciding on Your Platform: Which Is Best for You and Why?

3.1.1 Instagram (established 2010)

- Total number of daily active Instagram users: 500 million +.
- The number of Instagram likes per day: 4.2 billion.
- The number of photos and videos uploaded per day: 100 million +.
- Instagram demographics:
  - 110 million Instagram users are from the US.
  - Instagram is used by 43% of American women and 31% of men.
  - 31% of internet users between the ages of 18 and 24 use Instagram and 32% of internet users between the ages of 25 and 34 use Instagram.

Instagram for Business

- An estimated 71% of US businesses were on Instagram in 2018.
- Instagram now has more than 2 million monthly advertisers and 25 million business profiles.
- There are more than 500,000 influencers on Instagram.
- Instagram's mobile ad revenue is expected to hit $7 billion in 2018. In 2019, the revenue was $9.45 billion. In 2020, it grew to $13.86 billion, and is projected to reach $18.16 billion in 2021.
- One-third of the most viewed stories are from businesses.
- 78% of influencers prefer Instagram for brand collaboration.
- User-generated content has a 4.5% higher conversion rate.
- 55.4% of influencers use Instagram stories for sponsored campaigns.
- The potential reach of advertising on Instagram is 802 million.

Facts

- Posts with a location get 79% more engagement.
- 7 out of 10 hashtags on Instagram are branded.
- 60% of people say they discover new products on Instagram.
- Photos with faces get 38% more likes.
- Posts with at least one hashtag average 12.6% more engagement.
- Most used Giphy sticker in stories is Heart Love Sticker by Arata.
- Instagram users engage more on weekdays, with Tuesday and Thursday showing most engagement.
- Instagram videos get two times the engagement of photos in any other social media platform.
- The most popular hashtags on Instagram are #Love, #Instagood, #Me, #Cute, and #Follow.

3.1.2 Snapchat (established 2011)

- Total number of daily active Snapchat users: 190 million.
- Percentage of US social media users that use Snapchat: 24%.
- Number of Snaps created everyday (photos and videos): 3 billion.
- Average time spent per user on a daily basis: 30 + minutes.
- Percentage of users (18–24 years old) in the US: 73%.
- Snapchat demographics:
  - 75% of Snapchat users are under 34 years old.
  - 90% of Snapchat users are from 13 to 24 years old.
  - Roughly 61% of Snapchat users are female and 38% are male.
  - 30% of US Millennial internet users use Snapchat regularly.

Facts

- Active Snapchatters open the app 20 times every day.
- More than 400 million Snapchat stories are created per day.
- More than 60% of active Snapchatters create new content on a daily basis.
- It would take you 10 years to view all the photos shared on Snapchat in the last hour.
- 95% of Snapchat users say the app makes them feel happy.
- 528,000 snaps are sent every minute.

3.1.3 Facebook (Established 2004)

- Total number of mobile daily active users: 1.57 billion.
- Facebook stories daily viewers: 150 million.
- Facebook demographics:
  - Facebook users are 53% females and 47% males.
  - Average Facebook user has 155 "friends."
  - 62% of online seniors aged 65 + are on Facebook and 72% are between the age of 50 and 64.
  - 88% of online users of age 18 to 29 are on Facebook, 84% of those are 30 to 49.

Facebook Advertising Statistics

- In first quarter of 2020, Facebook had over 8 million monthly advertisers; in second quarter, it increased to 9 million; and by third quarter, it reached 10 million monthly active advertisers. The rise has been historic and may certainly be related to increased user interaction during the Covid-19 pandemic.
- 93% of marketers use Facebook advertising regularly.
- Images account for 75 to 90% of Facebook advertising effectivity/performance.
- The average cost per click (CPC) for Facebook ads is $1.72, average click-through rate (CTR) is 0.9%, and average cost per 1,000 impressions (CPM) is $7.92.
- Facebook's share in the global digital advertising market is 19.7%.

Facts

- Facebook accounts for over 42% of monthly social media visits.
- 42% of customer service responses happen during the first 60 minutes.
- The Facebook like button has been pressed 1.13 trillion times.
- Facebook gets over 8 billion average daily video views.
- 85% of Facebook users watch videos with the sound off.
- Captioned video ads can increase video view time by an average of 12%.
- 80% of users are annoyed when videos auto-play sound, and it gives them a negative impression of your brand.
- 20% of videos are live broadcasts.
- Twitter: Less important for practice building; this is a location for physicians to communicate and share ideas; very busy during conferences.

3.2 Ethics

- All surgeons should have accurate and unedited before and after surgery photos.
- Look for and provide good video content, which cannot be altered.
- Know the difference between engagement and entertainment.
- Be very cautious with intraoperative and immediate post-op content as late results and long-term follow-up are preferred.
- The core principle for all posts should be education.
- Authenticity is key.
- Surgeons should first "pay their dues." Do not falsely claim to be an expert. First contribute to the literature and to the specialty. The content is evidence of true expertise and can not only help your social media but also it shows you are a legitimate expert. Achieve board certification and stay involved in your society before creating those types of impressions on your social media platforms.

3.3 Pearls

- Challenges in social media include the fact that some patients do not "like" their surgeons. There are many that search but are not open about their interests—as such there are many false impressions. So don't judge early reach by "likes" alone.
- Slow and low: Organic slow steady growth is the key; only collaborate with real patients; avoid SOME marketing companies. Do not use auto like or auto followers; you will wind up with many failures. FOLLOW and LIKE your followers and fans!

3.4 Planning and Delivering Your Content

3.4.1 Instagram: These Recommendations Are Based on Observations from Current Trends

- *Accounts:* Divide into practice account and surgical account. Keep private accounts separate. Some advocate mixing but this can blur the lines of the office and personal life. Avoid gory photos on practice account; save those and intraoperative photos for the surgeon's account.
- *Stories versus posts:*
  - *Stories:* Should be updated daily with approximately seven posts. Each story should have a link or a swipe-up function with link to action. A good mix is two to three reposts from patients, two to three links back to posts on the main or surgical account, and two to three with a call to action to schedule or link back to the website or educational content. If on the surgery account, always precede the operative images with a warning. In general, these posts generate views but not patients. So, if the goal is growth then post, but if the goal is conversion and maintenance don't post as many surgical anatomic images; potential patients don't want to see bloody photos, especially on the primary practice account.
  - *Posts:* Should have a total of two to three per day, with consistent imaging and branding, and consistent filters and well composed. The wording should be short and sweet. Try to avoid very long multiparagraph posts. Include contact info and all the emojis after the first paragraph. BE SURE TO TAG THESE APPROPRIATELY; utilize local (geographically) tags and do this at the time of post for algorithm to work. Before and afters are of highest value for patient interaction. Awards and talks are also good and generate positive feedback and establish expertise. Stories or posts with family or on vacation are borderline, meaning they may help in certain practices to connect with patients, or make them feel like they already know you but too much can dilute your brand. Remember: These are consumers and they want to

see your aesthetic and your product. Develop your own hashtags and branding and avoid imitation as this will not help differentiate yourself.

- *Snaps:* Similar rules as stories; OK to post nudity and can show more of surgery. There should be many more of these posted every day in the order of 10 to 15, and these can be less well composed. Tagging is not as crucial; the patients here are a younger demographic.
- *Videos versus still photos/music:* Video content generates much more interaction; post movies which demonstrate a concept. Videos show results in a much more honest light. There is no way to fake the results—shadowing and angles are key to show contour and better demonstrate expectations. Utilize music and other options like picture in picture for before imagery to create the best content.
- *Timing of your posts:* Use an application to determine when your followers are online and then post accordingly, but in general peak times are 9 am, 12:30–1:30 pm, and 7–9 pm. Post accordingly, but also post with a purpose. 9 am can show your preop assessment, 1 pm can show your results, and 7 pm can show how to reach the office or a special.
- *Influencers:*
  - They are never free—get a contract for all of them.
  - Develop a curated selection of collaborators and friends of the practice.
  - Verify their followers and impressions before agreeing to get involved.
  - Do not try and fake influence here because savvy followers and celebrities know how to spot fake social media presence—they all do it and pay for it.

3.5 Metrics for Success

- *Impressions:* Target impressions but interaction is also very important.
- *Followers (location and impact):* Real followers will interact with organic content. Any Instagram account should have 10% of its followers like its posts for good interaction—these are "real" followers. Do not pay for bots or fake followers as they dilute your message and they give an impression of expertise without bringing new patients to your purview.
- *Conversion to Operating Room:* Patients should have an option to book or to swipe in every post. If they "like" a result you should have a strategy to reach out—DM. If they swipe on your contact or call in from Instagram, they will have a high rate of conversion and will likely convert with someone within hours or days. Do not lose your social patients!
- *Influence:* Influence can be measured in different ways and currently there are several companies and researchers looking at ways to quantify this. Do not get caught up in numbers as it is more about who is following you, not how many.

3.6 Problems in SOME

- "If they do it I should too"—do not get pulled into this sort of mentality; generate your own content and follow your own pace.
- Review pages like Yelp and other outlets have fake reviews, both positive and negative, and so none of them are reliable.
- Many of the early problems with search engine optimization and review page manipulations have actually been countered by SOME platforms, where ultimately followers and patients speak their message.

3.7 Conclusion

Social media is a valuable new tool for marketing and patient interaction. The modern plastic surgeon should utilize social media. Social media should be executed with finesse and class.

See **Video 3.1.**

Further Readings

Annual Instagram advertising revenues in the United States from 2018 to 2021. https://www.statista.com/statistics/1104447/instagram-ad-revenues-usa/. Accessed on 2/18/2021.

Branford OA, Kamali P, Rohrich RJ, et al. #PlasticSurgery. Plast Reconstr Surg. 2016; 138(6):1354–1365

Chandawarkar AA, Gould DJ, Stevens WG. Insta-grated plastic surgery residencies: the rise of social media use by trainees and responsible guidelines for use. Aesthet Surg J. 2018; 38(10):1145–1152

Gould DJ, Grant Stevens W, Nazarian S. A primer on social media for plastic surgeons: what do I need to know about social media and how can it help my practice? Aesthet Surg J. 2017; 37(5):614–619

Rohrich RJ, Weinstein AG. Connect with plastic surgery: social media for good. Plast Reconstr Surg. 2012; 129(3):789–792

Wheeler CK, Said H, Prucz R, Rodrich RJ, Mathes DW. Social media in plastic surgery practices: emerging trends in North America. Aesthet Surg J. 2011; 31(4):435–441

4 Social Media; The Dos and Don'ts

Rod J. Rohrich, Elizabeth B. Savetsky, and Ira L. Savetsky

Abstract
Social media is an invaluable tool for marketing, education, and communication. It allows our potential patients to become familiar with our skillset, visualize our artistry, and get to know us in person without ever entering our offices. There are multiple social media platforms available and each has its own advantages and disadvantages. Here we discuss the various platforms and give examples of the types of content that users post on each.

Keywords: Social media, Instagram, Facebook, Snapchat, Twitter

Key Points

- Social media is an invaluable tool for marketing, education, and communication.
- It allows our potential patients to become familiar with our skill set, visualize our artistry, and get to know us in person without ever entering our offices.
- There are multiple social media platforms available; each has its advantages and disadvantages.

4.1 Power of Social Media

- Provides today's most relevant form of branding.
- Provides plastic surgery practitioners the opportunity to reach greater number of patients.
- There are no shortages of tools (e.g., Facebook Insights) to analyze the demographics of your followers.
- Social media networks like Facebook and Twitter have tools that let you send out posts to certain demographics.
- Eliminates the need to hire marketers and publicists.
- Boosts exposure of one's practice not only locally and regionally, but globally.
- Opens the door for new patient referrals with easy access to contact information.
- Increases effectiveness as patient educator.
- Social media is a powerful tool for cosmetic practitioners to engage and build relationships with potential patients.
- Highlights positive feedback from patients.

4.2 General Tips

- Engage.
- Be positive.
- Educate.
- Comment.
- Post high-quality content consistently.
- More videos than static photos.
- Grow audience organically.
- Tag influencers.
- Use strategic hashtags.

4.3 Social Media Platforms

4.3.1 Facebook

- Gear posts to a more mature audience as users tend to be older.
- Post videos and links to news as well as interesting external content, like news stories and interviews, to help drive traffic to one's page.
- Eye-catching visuals generate more traffic than simply text-based posts.
- Evolve posts based on Facebook's algorithm, which is constantly changing, by keeping tabs on which content performs well and which does not.

4.3.2 Twitter

- Use as a tool for search engine optimization, as Google indexes every tweet.
- Post trending news to increase visibility.
- Link original content, like one's own blogs, but limit other links, as tweets without links perform better.
- Select hashtags strategically.
- Tag relevant profiles.
- Acknowledge everyone that mentions you.

4.3.3 Instagram

- Use high-resolution images and videos.
- Be creative. Unique posts or posts with shock-factor perform best (▶ Fig. 4.1).

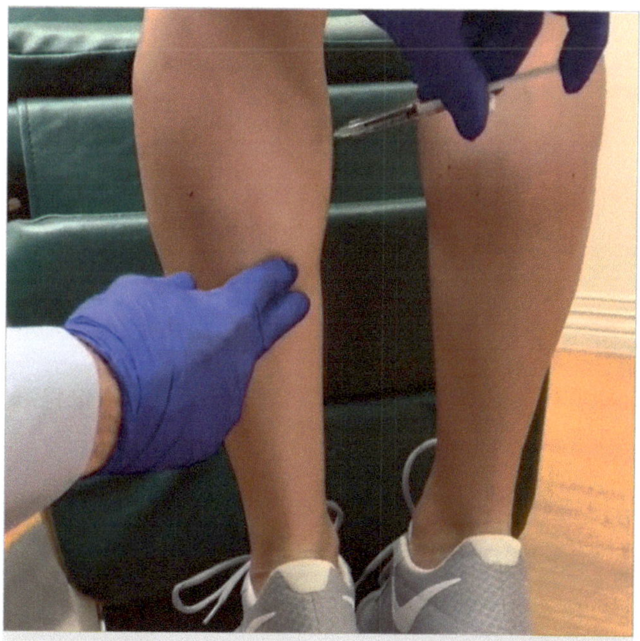

Fig. 4.1 Example of a unique post (neurotoxin for calf shaping) that performed well.

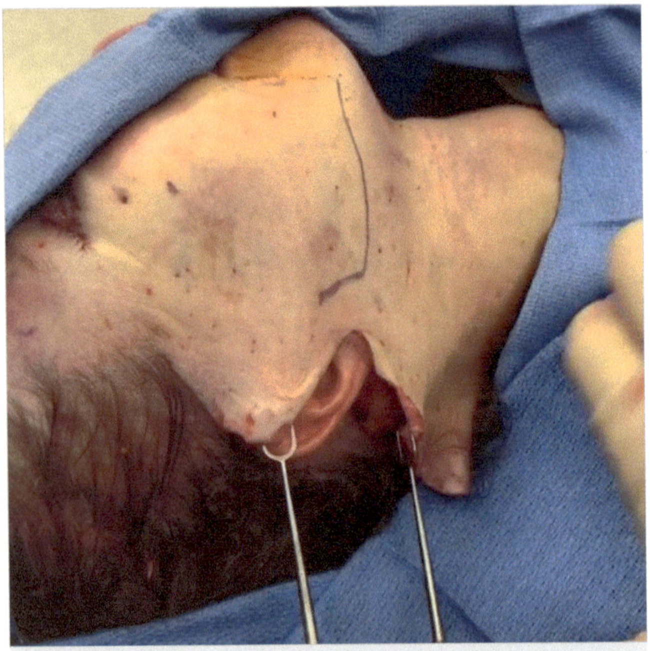

Fig. 4.2 Example of a post that some individuals may find to be overly graphic.

- Avoid overly graphic posts (▶ Fig. 4.2).
- Videos and arrows perform better than static images (▶ Fig. 4.3).
- Showcase personality and bedside manner to provide potential patients with an intimate look into one's practice.
- Post Instagram stories frequently.
- Select strategic hashtags.
- Tag relevant profiles and influencers.
- Interact with followers in the form of a conversation. Actively respond to questions and comments.
- Avoid selling anything.
- Convert to a business account to access analytics to monitor and improve results.

4.3.4 Snapchat

- Gear posts to a younger audience.
- Use attention-grabbing images and intriguing conversation starters.

4.3.5 Pinterest

- Post infographics and educational do-it-yourself (DIY) guides for best results.
- Provide tips for better self-care and advice on personal aesthetics.

4.3.6 YouTube

- House all of your videos here.
- Use as a tool for search engine optimization.

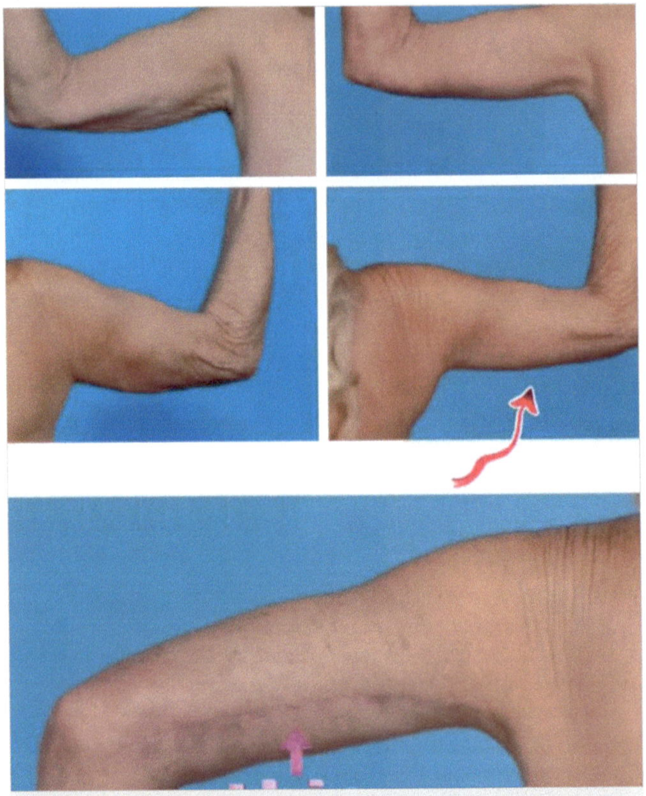

Fig. 4.3 The use of videos and arrows perform better than static images without symbols.

- Start a weekly vlog and create monthly roundup of your procedures.

4.4 Conclusion

Social media is an invaluable tool for marketing, education, and communication.

It allows our potential patients to become familiar with our skill set, visualize our artistry, and get to know us in person without ever entering our offices.

There are multiple social media platforms available, and each has its advantages and disadvantages.

See **Video 4.1**.

Further Readings

Cho MJ, Furnas HJ, Rohrich RJ. A primer on social media use by young plastic surgeons. Plast Reconstr Surg. 2019; 143(5):1533–1539

Mess SA, Bharti G, Newcott B, et al. To post or not to post: plastic surgery practice marketing, websites, and social media? Plast Reconstr Surg Glob Open. 2019; 7 (7):e2331

Rohrich RJ, Dayan E. Improving communication with millennial patients. Plast Reconstr Surg. 2019; 144(2):533–535

Rohrich RJ. So, do you want to be Facebook friends? How social media have changed plastic surgery and medicine forever. Plast Reconstr Surg. 2017; 139 (4):1021–1026

Vardanian AJ, Kusnezov N, Im DD, Lee JC, Jarrahy R. Social media use and impact on plastic surgery practice. Plast Reconstr Surg. 2013; 131(5):1184–1193

Part I

Face and Neck Lift

I

5 The Facial Aging Face Consultation

Rod J. Rohrich and Yash J. Avashia

Abstract
The anatomical components of facial aging include the skin, fat compartments, mimetic muscles, ligamentous support, and bony skeleton. Understanding the underlying processes that govern facial aging is important to be able to properly examine the patient. A detailed preoperative facial analysis requires both a gross overview of the face and its asymmetries, along with a focused examination of the various parts of the face: forehead, periorbital, midface, nose, perioral, chin, and neck. Surgical and nonsurgical options are available to treat the aging face. Skin care is a universal aspect in plastic surgery and is particularly important for the aging face.

Keywords: Facial aging, fat compartments, radial expansion, facial analysis, facial rejuvenation, fillers, neurotoxin, resurfacing, retinoids

Key Points

- The anatomical components to facial aging include the skin, fat compartments, mimetic muscles, ligamentous support, and bony skeleton.
- Understanding the underlying processes that govern facial aging is important to be able to properly examine the patient.
- A detailed preoperative facial analysis requires both a gross overview of the face and its asymmetries, along with a focused examination of the various parts of the face: forehead, midface, periorbital, perioral, and neck.
- Surgical and nonsurgical options are available to treat the aging face.
- Skin care is a universal aspect to facial plastic surgery and is particularly important for the aging face.

5.1 Components of Aging

The combination of facial fat descent, attenuation of retaining ligaments, and diminished fat volume and skeletal support produces the characteristic changes associated with the aging face.

5.1.1 Fat

- Gravity is a constant force applied to the structural fat compartments and bony contours of the face.
- Changes in facial fat during facial aging can be understood as either (1) volume loss, or (2) change in volume distribution.
- Landmark studies by Rohrich and Pessa described anatomical units of deep and superficial fat compartments of the face, separated by distinct septae.[3] These fibrous septae of connective tissue extend from the fascial layer to the dermis (▶ Fig. 5.1).
- There are 22 superficial facial fat compartments:
  - Forehead: Central, middle temporal, lateral temporal-cheek.
  - Periorbital: One supraorbital fat compartment and two infraorbital fat compartments.
  - Midface: Nasolabial, medial cheek, middle cheek, lateral temporal-cheek (same as above).
  - Lower face: Two jowl fat compartments and submental fat compartment.
- Three key fat compartments that influence midface volume loss are the nasolabial, deep medial, and deep lateral fat compartments. The deep midfacial fat compartment is medial to the zygomaticus major muscle (▶ Fig. 5.2).
- Change in volume distribution is attributed to the decline in the structural supportive function of the facial ligaments. Lambros described "radial expansion" of the soft tissues of the face as a result of weakening of the fibrous attachments between skin, fat, and deep fascia resulting in an outward expansion from the bony skeleton.

5.1.2 Skeletal

- The morphologic changes of the facial bony skeleton impact the soft tissues of the face.
- Prior studies have demonstrated skeletal changes in orbit, maxilla, and mandible influencing the relative prominence and position of facial soft tissues.

5.1.3 Muscle

- Volumetric changes in the facial bones and fat compartments impact the facial mimetic muscles with changes in laxity and muscle tension.

5.1.4 Skin

- The aging skin reflects the effect of a series of factors that influence the appearance of skin. These include speech and animation, sun and environmental exposure, weight changes, medical health, and other insults including smoking.
- Collagen and elastin are the primary components of the skin. Toxic injury to these components lead to the process of aging. Atrophy of skin appendages and decreased extracellular matrix of the skin further influence the overall thinning of skin with age.

5.2 Consultation

- An individualized approach to facial rejuvenation allows maximal patient satisfaction.
- The surgeon should spend the initial minutes of the consultation listening to the patient's concerns about his or her appearance. Common concerns with facial aging focus on the periorbital and neck regions.

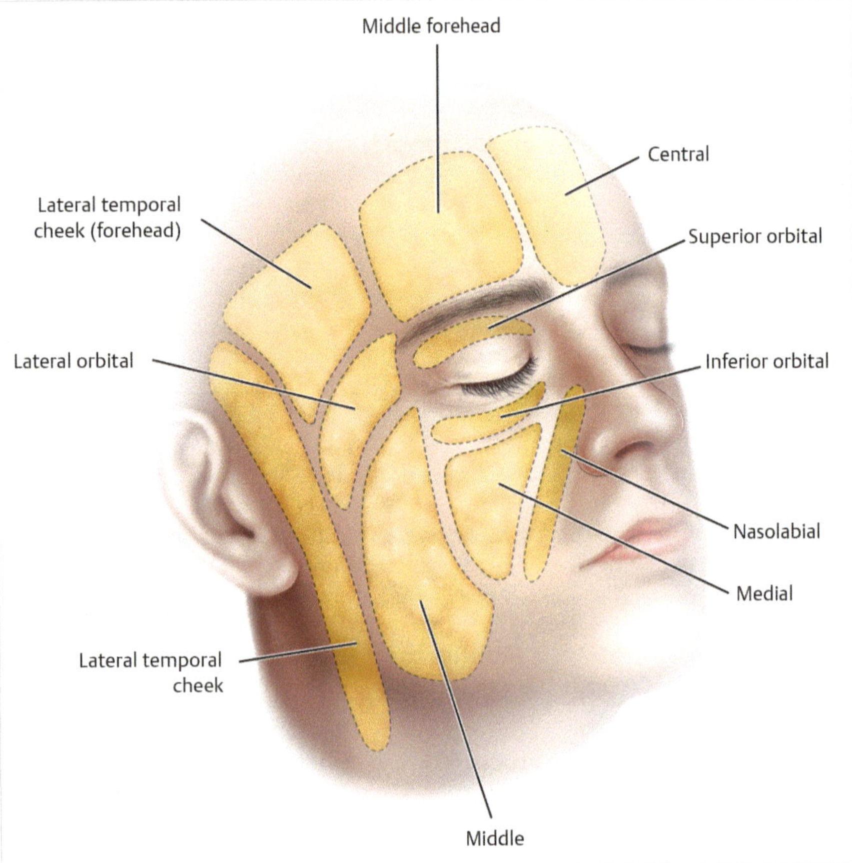

Fig. 5.1 Superficial fat compartments of the face. (Reproduced with permission from Leatherbarrow B, ed. Oculoplastic Surgery. 3rd ed. Thieme; 2019.)

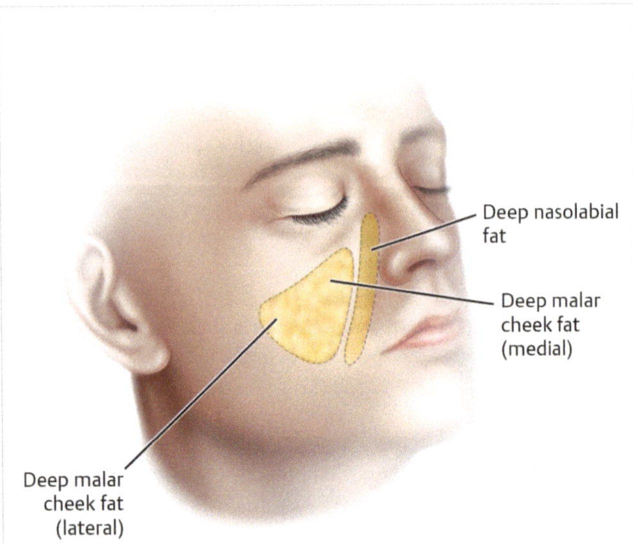

Fig. 5.2 Key fat compartments relevant to facial rejuvenation. (Reproduced with permission from Rohrich R, Ahmad J, eds. The Dallas Rhinoplasty and Dallas Cosmetic Surgery Dissection Guide. 1st ed. Thieme; 2018.)

5.2.1 Medical History

- Medical and surgical history should be taken to identify any potential reasons for delayed wound healing or bleeding.
- A complete list of medications should be obtained. This includes both prescribed and over-the-counter medications that can cause bleeding during a procedure (anticoagulant, antiplatelet, antihypertensives, immunosuppressive, hormone replacement medications).
- Herbal medications may cause bleeding. Patients should be specifically asked if they are taking any herbal supplements (*Remember the four G's: Ginger, Ginkgo biloba, Garlic, or Ginseng*).
- Smoking history.

5.2.2 Facial Analysis

- Understanding the anatomical basis for facial aging is essential to achieving a natural, predictable, and long-lasting outcome.
- General appearance and facial proportions:
  - The aging face analysis begins with gaining an understanding of the overall appearance of the face.
  - The facial proportions are divided into horizontal thirds and vertical fifths (▶ Fig. 5.3).
  - All patients have some degree of asymmetry in their faces (e.g., a wide side and a narrow side, one eye larger than the other eye, etc.).
  - Fitzpatrick skin type.
- Hairline and forehead:
  - Analysis of the face should proceed in a top-down fashion, beginning with the forehead.

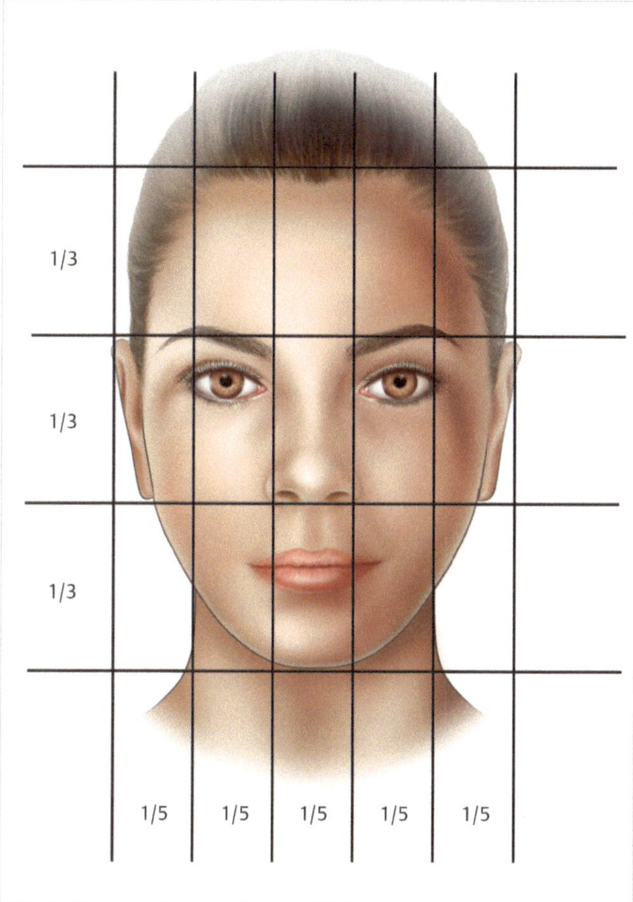

Fig. 5.3 Facial analysis begins by dividing the face into vertical thirds by horizontal lines. The upper third extends from the hairline to the glabella, the middle third from the glabella to the subnasale, and the lower third from the subnasale to the menton. The face may be divided by vertical lines into the facial fifths, with the nasal base width equal to the intercanthal distance and the width of the palpebral fissure. (Reproduced with permission from Papel I, Frodel J, Holt R et al, eds. Facial Plastic and Reconstructive Surgery. 4th ed. Thieme; 2016.)

- ○ The hairline should be examined for definition, color and quality of hair, and temporal recession.
- ○ Forehead length should be examined from the anterior hairline to the eyebrow position.
- ○ Quality and depth of forehead rhytides should be noted.
- ○ Presence of supraorbital and temporal hollowing due to fat atrophy.
- Periorbital:
  - ○ Shape and position of the eyebrow relative to the supraorbital rim.
  - ○ Excess skin of the upper and lower eyelids (dermatochalasis).
  - ○ Eyelid position (ptosis or inferior scleral show).
  - ○ Lateral canthal laxity or lower eyelid horizontal excess.
  - ○ Fat prominence in the upper eyelid fat compartments (particularly medial) and the lower eyelids (central, middle, and lateral).
  - ○ Tear trough deformity.
  - ○ Orbit-malar vector.
- Midface:
  - ○ Central facial fat atrophy as demonstrated by nasojugal folds.
  - ○ Central fat atrophy and periapical hypoplasia as demonstrated by the nasolabial fold.
  - ○ Overall flattened and square appearance of the face.
- Perioral:
  - ○ Perioral rhytides secondary to deflation and excessive use of the orbicularis oris.
  - ○ Upper lip hypoplasia and increased upper lip length.
  - ○ Oral commissures downturned.
  - ○ Nasolabial folds and jowls.
  - ○ Labiomental crease.
  - ○ Marionette lines.
- Neck and chin:
  - ○ The ideal chin and neck should have the following characteristics:
    - Chin should be at the same level or up to 2 mm anterior to the vertical facial plane from the upper lip.
    - Well-defined mandibular border.
    - Thyroid cartilage prominence.
    - Hyoid depression.
    - Cervicomental angle (105 to 120 degrees).
  - ○ All necks should be noted for any:
    - Submental adiposity.
    - Platysmal banding.

5.3 Managing the Aging Face

Understanding the anatomic changes through a detailed facial analysis will help tailor the right management options for the patient. Surgical and nonsurgical modalities are available.

5.3.1 Surgical

- The following chapters in this book will describe a variety of surgical options and techniques for correcting facial aging:
  - ○ Facelift.
  - ○ Necklift.
  - ○ Facial fat augmentation.
  - ○ Browlift.
  - ○ Upper and lower eyelid blepharoplasty.
  - ○ Rhinoplasty.

5.3.2 Nonsurgical

- Volume restoration with facial fillers:
  - ○ There are two types of fillers currently approved by the FDA:
    - Temporary: Hyaluronic acid (HA), calcium hydroxyapatite (CaHA), and poly-L lactic acid (PLLA).
    - Permanent: Poly methyl methacrylate (PMMA).
  - ○ An understanding of the differences between filler types, and aesthetic advantages and disadvantages, is important in selecting the appropriate filler.
  - ○ Knowledge of the vascular and musculature anatomy of the face helps to minimize intravascular injection and bruising along with maximizing efficacy.
- Muscle modulation with injectable neurotoxin:
  - ○ Botulinum toxin injection for treatment for facial wrinkles is one of the most frequently performed cosmetic procedures.

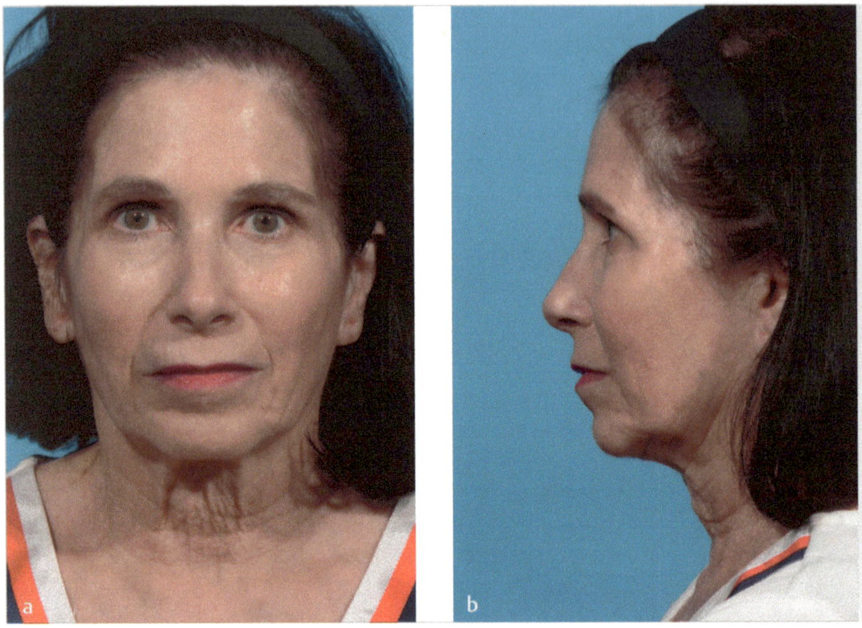

Fig. 5.4 (a, b) A 65-year-old female age-appropriate facial aging. On facial analysis, the patient demonstrates Fitzpatrick type II skin and mildfacial asymmetry.

- There are currently four FDA approved brands of botulinum toxin available for facial aesthetics:
  - Onabotulinum toxin (Botox).
  - Abobotulinum toxin (Dysport).
  - Incobotulinum toxin (Xeomin).
  - Prabotulinum toxin (Jeuveau).
- Facial resurfacing:
  - Indications for facial resurfacing include superficial or deep rhytides, dyschromias, skin disease such as acne, preneoplastic lesions (actinic keratoses and lentigines), and evidence of photodamage.
    - Laser resurfacing.
    - Chemical peel.
    - Dermabrasion.
- Skin care:
  - Skin care is a universal aspect to facial rejuvenation. One of the cornerstones to skin care is retinoids.
  - Retinoids are a family of compounds composed of vitamin A, its derivates, and synthetic molecules acting through the same pathway.
  - Topical tretinoin has shown to reduce collagen degradation, increase procollagen biosynthesis, increase smoothness of skin, efface wrinkle, and increase epidermal and dermal glycosaminoglycan deposition.
  - Sides effects include retinoid reaction such as erythema, scaling, xerosis, or pruritis.
  - Daily use will result in maximal benefit. The first 6 months of therapy should include nightly application at concentrations of 0.025 to 0.05%.
  - Maintenance therapy after 1 year includes application three times in a week.

5.4 Case Example

A 65-year-old female age-appropriate facial aging. On facial analysis, the patient demonstrates Fitzpatrick type II skin and mild facial asymmetry (left face is wide and short, right face is narrow and long); forehead length is slightly long with a well-defined anterior hairline with bilateral temporal hollowing; periorbital findings are notable for upper and lower eyelid dermatochalasis, mild lateral canthal laxity, and minimal fat compartment prominence; midfacial findings are notable for central facial atrophy on the right greater than the left, particularly the deep medial and nasolabial compartments; perioral findings show fine rhytides with increased upper lip length and marionette lines. The neck and chin show an irregular mandibular border with prominent jowl fat pads, mild platysmal banding, and excess skin with an obtuse cervicomental angle (▶ Fig. 5.4a, b).

5.5 Conclusion

Facial aging is a natural phenomenon of the various components of the face: skin, fat, mimetic muscles, and bony skeleton. Detailed preoperative analysis directs appropriate surgical and/or nonsurgical treatment.

See **Video 5.1**.

Further Readings

Ellenbogen R, Karlin JV. Visual criteria for success in restoring the youthful neck. Plast Reconstr Surg. 1980; 66(6):826–837

Hubbard BA, Unger JG, Rohrich RJ. Reversal of skin aging with topical retinoids. Plast Reconstr Surg. 2014; 133(4):481e–490e

Lambros V, Amos G. Facial shape, size, and gender. Plast Reconstr Surg. 2020 Nov;146(5):1012–1014

Rohrich RJ, Pessa JE. The retaining system of the face: histologic evaluation of the septal boundaries of the subcutaneous fat compartments. Plast Reconstr Surg. 2008; 121(5):1804–1809

Rohrich RJ, Pessa JE, Ristow B. The youthful cheek and the deep medial fat compartment. Plast Reconstr Surg. 2008; 121(6):2107–2112

Stuzin JM. MOC-PSSM CME article: face lifting. Plast Reconstr Surg. 2008; 121(1) Suppl:1–19

Wan D, Amirlak B, Rohrich R, Davis K. The clinical importance of the fat compartments in midfacial aging. Plast Reconstr Surg Glob Open. 2014; 1(9):e92

6 Facelift and Necklift: Incision Planning

Yash J. Avashia and James M. Stuzin

Abstract
Facelift and necklift incision planning is a critical aspect of the facelift and necklift operation. It directly influences the final aesthetic result. Detailed preoperative assessment and proper incision design will influence both scar placement and quality. Proper scar placement should highlight regional anatomic proportions and subunits, rather than the scar itself. Understanding the anatomic subunits of the preauricular incision will guide the surgeon during incision design and preserve the intricacies of this anatomy. Tension free closure is an important requirement for optimal wound healing. A systematic approach to skin excision and closure helps to provide consistency in results.

Keywords: Facelift, necklift, preauricular incision, scar

Key Points

- A detailed analysis must be performed prior to incision planning to minimize secondary deformities in the facelift and necklift patient.
- Proper scar placement should highlight regional anatomic proportions and subunits, rather than the scar itself.
- Incision design and tension free closure are primary factors for optimal scar quality and location.

6.1 Preoperative Steps

The facelift and necklift incisions are comprised of four segments: Temporal, preauricular, retroauricular, and occipital. Additionally, the necklift operation has a separate submental incision.

6.1.1 Temporal Incision (▸ Fig. 6.1)

- Options for incision placement include (1) within hair-bearing region, posterior to temporal hairline, or (2) anteriorly, along the temporal hairline.
- Youthful individuals have approximately 4 cm of distance between lateral canthus and anterior temporal hairline.
- In patients with minimal skin redundancy, the incision may be placed behind the temporal hairline without a noticeable change in hairline position.
  - Connell described a prehelical flap that serves as a "rescue flap." This avoids a hairless notch above the root of the helix when performing this temporal incision (▸ Fig. 6.1).
  - Appropriate rotation of the facial skin in a lateral vector will avoid vertical displacement of temporal hair and side burn elevation.
- The anterior temporal hairline is an alternative approach but can result in a visible scar in some patients with an abrupt transition between the cheek and the temporal hair.

6.1.2 Preauricular Incision (▸ Fig. 6.2)

- There are five subunits in the preauricular aesthetic: helix width, pretragal hollow, tragal height, superior and inferior intertragal notches, and earlobe–cheek junction. They should be carefully respected when designing the preauricular portion of the incision.
- The preauricular incision can be divided into three segments: helix, tragus, and lobule.
  - Helix:
    - This portion is a parallel curve to the posterior helical margin.
    - It should mimic the visual transverse width (X) of the helical cartilage (▸ Fig. 6.2).
    - The hypopigmented scar will help create a normal appearing helical margin of anatomic proportion.
  - Tragus:
    - The tragal cartilage is a rectangular structure. Close attention to its anatomical subunits will allow for precise incision placement.
    - After the helical segment, the incision follows the depression of the superior intertragal notch.
    - The incision is then carried along the tragal rim to the inferior intertragal notch.
    - The intratragal incision is preferred in men as they provide a better disguise for the color difference between the whiter ear skin and the blush colored cheek skin.

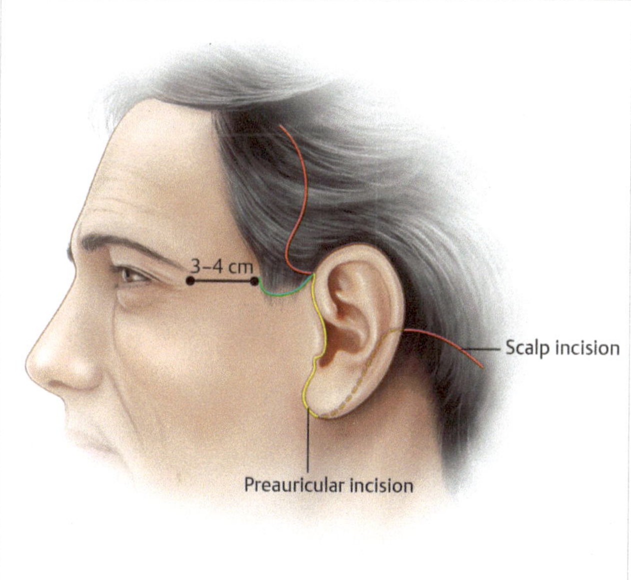

Fig. 6.1 Facelift incision planning. Preauricular and retroauricular incision planning (*Yellow*). Hairline incision planning (*Green*). Hair-bearing region incision planning (*Red*). The average distance between the lateral canthus and temporal hairline should be 3 to 4 cm to maintain a youthful appearance. (Reproduced with permission from Connell B, Sundine M, eds. Aesthetic Rejuvenation of the Face and Neck. 1st ed. Thieme; 2016.)

- From here, the incision turns anteriorly before turning again inferiorly at a 90-degree angle, anterior to the lobular-facial sulcus. This preserves the inferior intertragal notch, which would otherwise be blunted (▶ Fig. 6.2).
  - Lobule:
    - The incision at the perilobular region should preserve 2 mm of natural sulcus between the earlobe and cheek.
- Secondary deformity in the preauricular segment is seen when the incision does not properly follow the helical or tragal cartilages as detailed. An anteriorly placed incision results in a conspicuous scar.
- In males, more so than females, the preauricular region may have varied color gradient and surface irregularity. An incision placed in the preauricular crease may still risk the potential for a visible scar.

6.1.3 Retroauricular Incision

- This portion of the incision is made along the auriculomastoid groove.
- The incision transitions posteriorly onto the occipital segment at the level of the anterior crus of the antihelix, which also coincides with the superior extent of the conchal–mastoid junction (▶ Fig. 6.1).

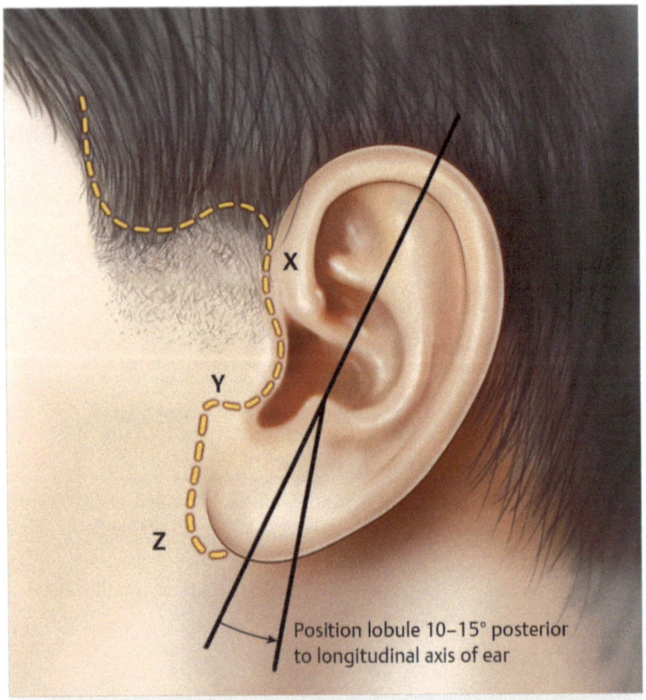

Fig. 6.2 Preauricular incision details. The helical portion of the preauricular incision should parallel the posterior helical border and result in creating a single helical width (X). Note the preserved infratragal flap (Y) as a part of the tragal incision. This preserves the inferior intertragal notch subunit which is otherwise blunted if the incision is placed into it. At the time of inset, the lobule should be positioned 10 to 15 degrees posterior to the longitudinal axis of the ear. (Reproduced with permission from Connell B, Sundine M, eds. Aesthetic Rejuvenation of the Face and Neck. 1st ed. Thieme; 2016.)

6.1.4 Occipital Incision (▶ Fig. 6.3)

- This portion is analogous to the temporal portion (▶ Fig. 6.1).
- Deciding between an incision along the hairline versus within the hair-bearing region depends on the degree of skin redundancy.
- To avoid a visible elevation in the hairline with an unnatural step-off from the remaining hairline, the incision is kept along the hairline in patients anticipated for large skin resection (massive weight loss patient).
- In most patients, the incision can be safely carried into the hair-bearing region.

6.1.5 Submental Incision

- In addition to approaching the neck laterally from the incision detailed above, the neck should be approached from a submental incision to address submental lipodystrophy and platysmal bands.
- The incision is placed posterior to the submental chin crease and is 3 to 4 cm in length.
- This incision allows direct access for both preplatysmal and deep submental fat compartment excision. Furthermore, it allows the surgeon to manipulate the platysma with midline plication and a distal myotomy to achieve a well contoured neck and cervicomental angle.

6.2 Operative Steps

See **Video 6.1**.

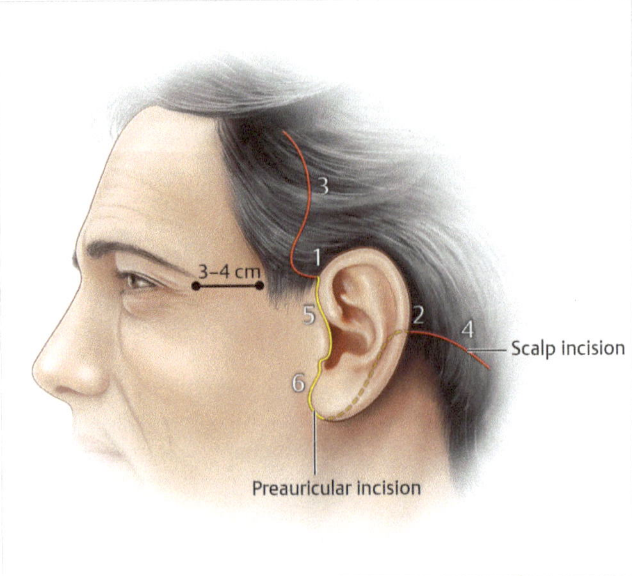

Fig. 6.3 Six key alignment points as described by Bruce Connell. These points allow for tension free closure in the temporal, preauricular, retroauricular, and occipital regions. (Reproduced with permission from Connell B, Sundine M, eds. Aesthetic Rejuvenation of the Face and Neck. 1st ed. Thieme; 2016.)

6.2.1 Incision

- After marking the incision line, certain maneuvers allow easier visualization of the incision markings in hair-bearing regions. This includes shaving hair and surgical lubricants or rubber bands to part the hair.
- The incision is made with a #15 scalpel blade and is perpendicular to the skin plane. In regions of hair, the scalpel is beveled parallel with the hair follicles to minimize postoperative scar alopecia.

6.2.2 Closure

- Skin excision is made by advancing the face and neck skin in the appropriate superior/posterior vector.
- Skin excision is performed to allow 2 to 3 mm of redundancy along the closure line. Tension free closure is a crucial aspect of minimizing scar visibility.
- Key alignment sutures are placed to provide tension free closure (▶ Fig. 6.3). This is performed with buried interrupted 4–0 Vicryl.
- The hair-bearing region of the occipital incision is closed with staples. It is important to properly appose and evert the skin when stapling to provide the best scar.
- The retroauricular incision is then closed with a running 5–0 fast absorbing suture.
- The remaining portions of the incision (temporal, preauricular, lobular) are closed with interrupted 5–0 nylon sutures.
- Proper skin apposition with mild edge-to-edge eversion should be achieved. The nylon sutures should be spaced 1 cm apart. Sutures should not be placed tightly as this will cause visible dimpling along the closure line and not accommodate postoperative swelling.

6.3 Postoperative Care

Permanent sutures are removed between 5 and 7 days after surgery.

6.4 Conclusion

Preoperative analysis is critical to designing appropriate facelift and necklift incisions. The final scar placement should highlight the anatomic proportions and subunits while allowing the scar to be adequately concealed. Tension-free closure is a primary factor for scar quality.

Further Readings

Hamilton S, Connell B. Fifty years of progression in face and neck lifting. In: Connell B, Sundine M, eds. Aesthetic Rejuvenation of the Face. 1st ed. Thieme; 2016

Marten TJ. High SMAS facelift: combined single flap lifting of the jawline, cheek, and midface. Clin Plast Surg. 2008; 35(4):569–603, vi–vii

Stuzin JM. MOC-PSSM CME article: face lifting. Plast Reconstr Surg. 2008; 121(1) Suppl:1–19

7 Extended Superficial Musculoaponeurotic System Technique

Ira L. Savetsky and James M. Stuzin

Abstract

Modern facelift techniques utilize the superficial musculoaponeurotic system (SMAS) to reposition facial fat from the anterior cheek into regions of lateral cheek and malar deflation, restoring the volumetric highlights noted in youth. In this chapter, we discuss the extended SMAS technique and methods to avoid inadvertent injury to the motor branches of the facial nerve.

Keywords: Facial aging, facelift, necklift, SMAS, extended SMAS

Key Points

- Facial aging is due to intrinsic and extrinsic changes in skin, loss of ligamentous support, and volume deflation due to fat atrophy.
- The extended superficial musculoaponeurotic system (SMAS) technique for facelifting repositions facial fat from the anterior cheek into regions of deflation in the lateral cheek and malar region, restoring the volumetric highlights noted in youth.

7.1 Preoperative Planning

7.1.1 Analysis

- A comprehensive and systematic facial analysis is the most critical initial step in establishing goals and formulating a precise surgical plan for facial rejuvenation.
- Areas of volume deflation are noted and marked preoperatively in the dependent position.

7.1.2 Standardized Photography and Digital Imaging

- Standardized photographs including frontal, lateral, oblique, and basal views should be obtained for every patient.
- Digital imaging is an excellent tool for communicating with the patient and evaluating patient's expectations.

7.1.3 Managing Expectations

- Review all photographic views with the patient.
- It is extremely important to discuss with the patient what can and cannot be achieved with surgery.

7.2 Anatomy

7.2.1 Facial Soft Tissue Layers

- From the superficial to the deep, the layers of the facial soft tissue are: (1) Skin, (2) subcutaneous fat, (3) superficial musculoaponeurotic system (SMAS), (4) mimetic muscle, (5) parotidomasseteric fascia (deep facial fascia), (6) plane of facial nerve, (7) parotid duct, and (8) buccal fat pad.

7.2.2 Superficial Musculoaponeurotic System

- The SMAS represents a discrete fascial layer that separates the overlying subcutaneous fat from the underlying parotidomasseteric fascia (deep fascia) and facial nerve branches.
- The SMAS represents a continuation of the superficial cervical fascia cephalad into the face; the corresponding deeper layer of cervical fascia (the superficial layer of the deep cervical fascia) continues into the face and has been termed the parotidomasseteric fascia or deep facial fascia.
- Within the cheek, the facial nerve branches, and the parotid duct, lie deep to the parotidomasseteric fascia after exiting the parotid. Therefore, when performing sub-SMAS dissection, if deep facial fascia is not violated, facial nerve injury will be prevented. The exceptions to this anatomic rule are along the lateral malar eminence and along the caudal masseter, both locations where facial nerve branches penetrate the deep fascia and lie within the plane between the SMAS and the deep fascia (see Staying Safe).

7.2.3 Retaining Ligaments

- Zygomatic and mandibular ligaments are examples of osteocutaneous ligaments that originate from periosteum and insert directly into the dermis.
- The masseteric cutaneous ligaments and parotid cutaneous ligaments are formed as a condensation between the superficial and deep fascia.
- Attenuation of the retaining ligaments is responsible for many of the stigmata that occur with aging.

7.3 Staying Safe to Prevent Injury to the Facial Nerve during Subcutaneous Undermining

7.3.1 Frontal Branch

- Must stay superficial to the temporoparietal fascia in the subcutaneous fat when dissecting inferior to superior.
- The sentinel vein, noted when dissecting from the forehead toward the superior orbital rim, can be used as a landmark indicating proximity to the nerve while dissecting within the temporal region.
- When using a lateral or superior approach, staying right on the superficial leaf of the deep temporal fascia is a safe plane of dissection.

7.3.2 Zygomatic and Buccal Branches

- Be aware of the relative danger zones adjacent to retaining ligaments along the lateral malar eminence.
- It is helpful to dissect both cephalad and caudal to the retaining ligaments to establish the proper plane of dissection superficial to the SMAS.

- The zygomatic and upper masseteric retaining ligaments just lateral to the zygoma can then be safely divided in the subcutaneous plane superficial to the SMAS.
- Some of the zygomatic and buccal branches can be less than 1 mm deep to the SMAS in the region adjacent to the upper masseteric ligaments, and therefore this region must be approached with extreme caution.
- A relatively safe area of dissection is directly over the zygomatic eminence, an area that is relatively free of facial nerve branches.

7.3.3 Marginal Mandibular Branch

- Always stay superficial to the platysma-SMAS.
- It is important to note that the platysma can be particularly atrophic, thin, and lax, making the dissection at times difficult as the proper plane is not clear when dissecting in the lower cheek.
- When transitioning from the preplatysmal plane caudally in the neck and along the jaw line, careful dissection is necessary to avoid getting deep to the platysma along the caudal border of the masseter.
- Caution should be taken around the region where the facial vessels cross the mandible anterior to the mandibular tuberosity as the marginal mandibular nerve becomes more superficial while crossing over the vessels.

7.3.4 Cervical Branch

- Staying superficial to the platysma will protect the cervical branches.

7.4 Staying Safe to Prevent Injury to the Facial Nerve during SMAS Elevation

- The majority of SMAS elevation occurs overlying the parotid, the accessory lobe of the parotid, and the lateral zygoma, all regions where facial nerve branches are protected.
- Anterior to the parotid and along the region lateral to the zygomatic eminence are the areas where the facial nerve branches are susceptible.
- Limiting the dissection within the mobile region of the SMAS minimizes the risk to motor nerve injury, which are more exposed in the anterior region of the cheek.
- Directly lateral to the zygoma, the SMAS requiring dissection tends to become thin as it transits from the lateral cheek superiorly along the superficial surface of the zygomaticus major.
- Accurate plane identification is essential in this region of the dissection, for both motor branch protection as well as to not tear the SMAS flap as it is dissected from the upper masseteric ligaments.
- Once the SMAS is dissected from the upper masseteric ligaments, the mobile region of the SMAS is encountered, and dissection should be terminated. This limits the dissection just cephalad to the juxtaposed zygomatic nerve branches, which are commonly found in the plane between the SMAS and the deep fascia in this region.
- Dissection anteriorly along the superior malar eminence, superficial to the zygomaticus major, is critical for malar pad repositioning. Facial nerve branches are protected (deep to the zygomaticus major) in the region directly overlying the zygoma.
- The inferior SMAS dissection should extend along the lateral boarder of the platysma and free the lateral platysma from its ligamentous attachments to the anterior border of the sternocleidomastoid muscle (SCM) to ensure adequate flap mobility. Once the SMAS/platysma is free from the SCM, an areolar plane is encountered, which can dissected bluntly, minimizing risk to the underlying cervical and marginal branches.

7.5 Markings

- The subcutaneous dissection of the cheek is preformed prior to the SMAS dissection. The medial extent of the dissection should proceed into the mobile anterior cheek and transit from the middle to the malar and jowl fat compartments. This carries the subcutaneous dissection anterior to the lateral malar eminence and anterior to the masseter. The junction between the fixed and mobile cheek can be marked on the skin at the start of the procedure.
- A line is then drawn within the hair-bearing scalp of the temporal region extending inferiorly, anterior to the ear, within the tragus. This line is carried under the lobule, postauricular, in the vertical direction within the junction of the posterior concha, and the postauricular skin (▶ Fig. 7.1).
- This line takes a right-angle turn posteriorly, where the helix meets the hairline, and the line extends into the hair-bearing scalp of the occipital region, taking a gentle curve posteroinferiorly within the hair-bearing scalp (▶ Fig. 7.2).

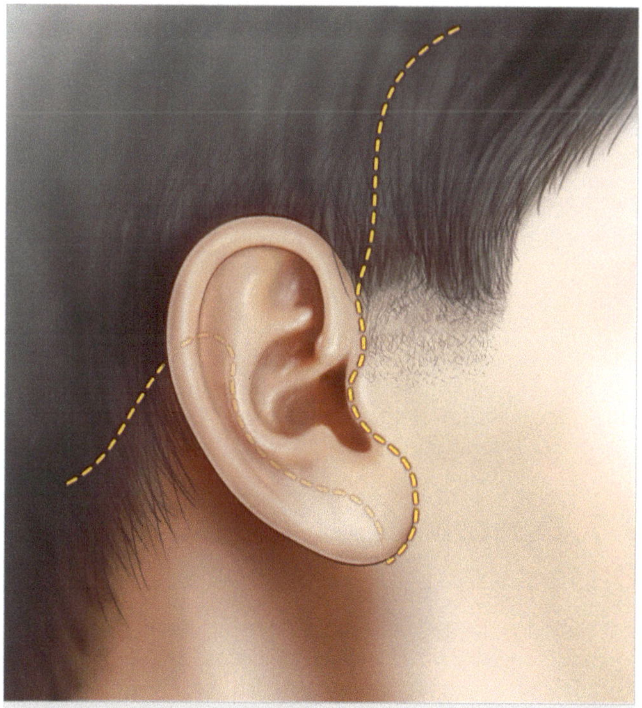

Fig. 7.1 Retrotragal facelift incision.

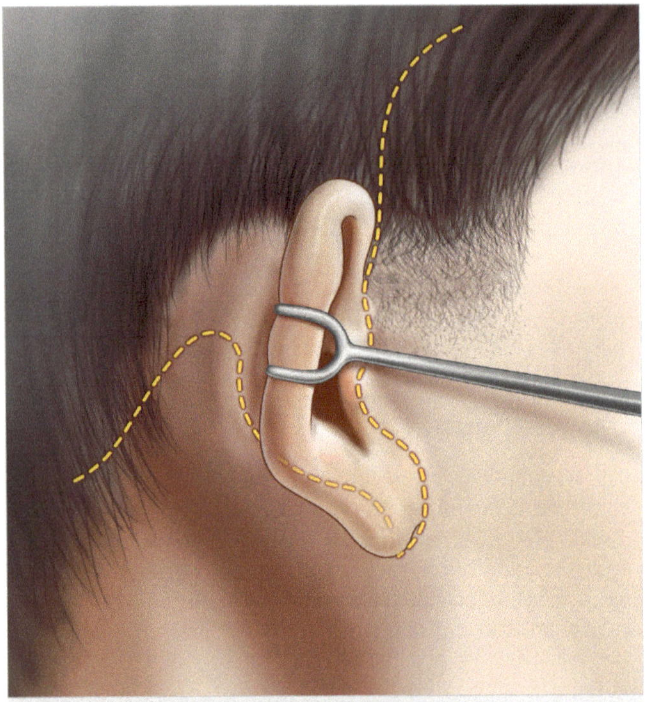

Fig. 7.2 Postauricular extension of facelift incision.

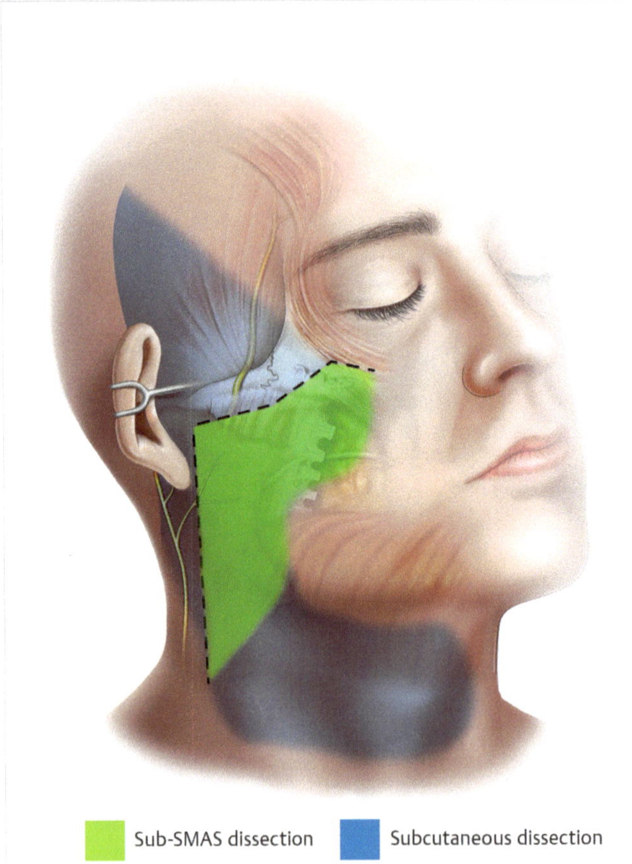

Fig. 7.3 The incision for an extended superficial musculoaponeurotic system (SMAS) dissection is shown in this illustration. The limits of sub-SMAS dissection required to release the SMAS from fixed structures are also noted. This incision design allows release of the SMAS of the lateral cheek and malar pad from the restraint of the retaining ligaments and provides the opportunity to reposition anterior facial fat into regions of deflation in the upper lateral cheek, restoring the volumetric highlights noted in youth. (Reproduced with permission from Rohrich RJ, Stuzin JM, Dayan E, Ross EV. Facial Danger Zones. Thieme; 2019.)

7.6 Operative Details—Skin Flap Dissection

- Lidocaine 0.5% with epinephrine is instilled along the incision lines and the planes of subcutaneous dissection.
- Transillumination is helpful in accurate skin flap dissection.
- The skin is incised with care to preserve the incisura of the tragus, the junction of the inferior-most aspect of the tragus with the cephalad-most portion of the ear lobe.
- Dissection is initially performed with a #10 blade followed by sharp scissor dissection.
- The temporal dissection is carried directly superficial to the deep temporal fascia.
- The subcutaneous dissection is carried toward the neck. This dissection is continued over the angle of the mandible and into the neck, superficial to the platysma.
- The dissection is continued medially into the anterior neck forward through the submental incision.
- The subcutaneous dissection in the cheek continues until the skin is released from the zygomatic ligaments along the lateral zygoma and anterior to the masseter to free the skin from the masseteric ligaments.

7.7 Operative Details—SMAS Dissection

- The incision design for an extended SMAS dissection laterally parallels the zygomatic arch, which places the SMAS incision caudal to the path of the frontal branch (▶ Fig. 7.3).
- Anteriorly, in the region where the zygomatic arch joins the lateral zygoma, the SMAS incision courses superiorly along the superior border of the malar fat pad. The junction between the superior malar fat and the lateral orbicularis oculi marks the superior or "high" segment of the extended SMAS dissection.
- The lateral/inferior SMAS incision follows the lateral border of the platysma inferiorly in the neck, extending several centimeters caudal to the earlobe.
- The SMAS is infiltrated with local anesthesia to help with hydrodissection.
- The SMAS elevation begins sharply overlying the parotid gland, identifying the interface between the parotid capsule and the SMAS.
- The dissection is continued along the lateral border of the platysma inferiorly into the neck, several centimeters below the earlobe.
- The dissection is then carried along the undersurface of the platysma, freeing the platysma from attachments to the SCM.
- The SMAS is elevated just anterior to the tail of the parotid and anterior to the retaining ligaments along the anterior

border of the SCM, where an areolar plane is identified. At this point, the mobilization of the lower SMAS/platysma is completed with blunt dissection.

- Anterior to the tail of the parotid, sub-SMAS fat is identified, which is an important landmark, as this is the region where the marginal mandibular branch exits the parotid.
- Dissection in this region should proceed bluntly, with care to dissect superficial to the deep fascia.
- Dissection superiorly along the main body of the parotid is carried toward its anterior border to ensure ligamentous release. Scissors, scalpel, or electrocautery can be used to elevate the superficial fascia from its attachments to the parotid.
- Once the anterior border of the parotid is reached, sub-SMAS fat typically becomes visible, the mobile region of the SMAS is encountered, and the dissection terminated.
- Anterior to the parotid, sub-SMAS dissection becomes less fibrous as the SMAS has been released from the retaining ligaments. When the dissection becomes easy, it is advisable to stop the dissection. Further dissection provides negligible flap mobility and significantly increases the morbidity of the surgery.
- The facial nerve branches are more exposed in the mobile region of the cheek, which is another reason to limit dissection once the SMAS flap has been mobilized.
- The malar extension of the SMAS dissection, to reposition the malar fat pad, carries the SMAS dissection over the lateral zygoma. The malar pad is then dissected free from its attachments to the zygoma, in the plane between the malar pad and the zygomaticus major (▶ Fig. 7.4).

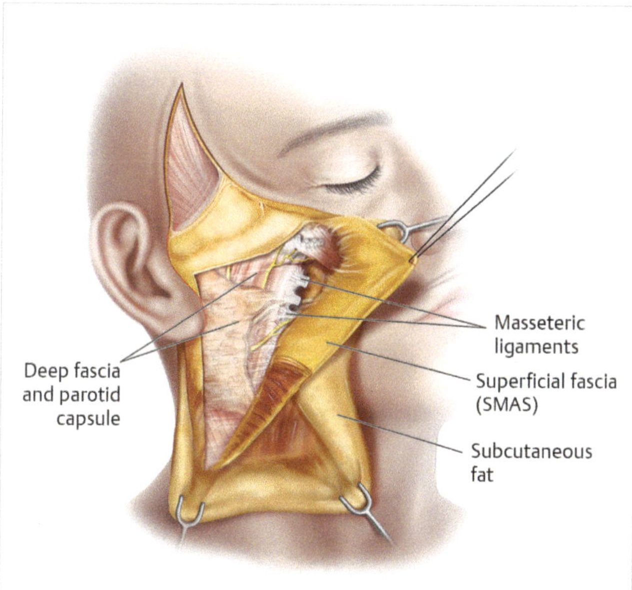

Fig. 7.4 The limits of an extended superficial musculoaponeurotic system (SMAS) dissection are reached when the SMAS is freed from the anterior border of the parotid, the accessory lobe of the parotid, the lateral zygomatic ligaments, the upper masseteric ligaments, and the anterior border of the sternocleidomastoid muscle (SCM). (Reproduced with permission from Rohrich RJ, Stuzin JM, Dayan E, Ross EV. Facial Danger Zones. Thieme; 2019.)

- When elevating the malar pad, the fibers of the zygomaticus major are visualized, which are innervated along their deep surfaces.
- The extended SMAS dissection is carried superficially to these muscles; therefore, motor branch injury will be prevented.
- The SMAS is elevated until the flap is freed from the underlying lateral zygomatic ligaments.
- During SMAS elevation, leaving sub-SMAS fat intact overlying the deep fascia provides increased protection against motor branch injury.
- Adequate mobilization of the SMAS can be determined by observing the effect of facial contouring when traction on the SMAS is applied.
- Freeing the SMAS past the restraint of the retaining ligaments provides the mobility necessary to obtain consistent facial contouring through SMAS redraping (▶ Fig. 7.5).
- The SMAS can be folded onto itself to augment the malar eminence if desired, otherwise excess SMAS can be incised and discarded.
- The SMAS is then split at the point where it overlaps the lobule, allowing some SMAS to be secured anterior and some SMAS to be secured posterior to the ear (▶ Fig. 7.6).
- A submental incision is made in a crease 5 mm caudal to the submandibular crease.
- Dissection is carried in a subcutaneous plane until the dissection from either side of the face is met.
- The platysma muscle can be sutured together in the midline if indicated. Any excess platysma should be resected.
- An incision to transect the medial portion of the platysma inferiorly allows the platysma to redrape itself (▶ Fig. 7.7).
- A drain is placed, and meticulous hemostasis is performed.
- The facial skin flaps are rotated and closed in the vector chosen based on preoperative evaluation.
- These skin flaps are inset with a minimum degree of tension and trimmed with a degree of redundancy between the key sutures to minimize tension along the incision sites, as facial

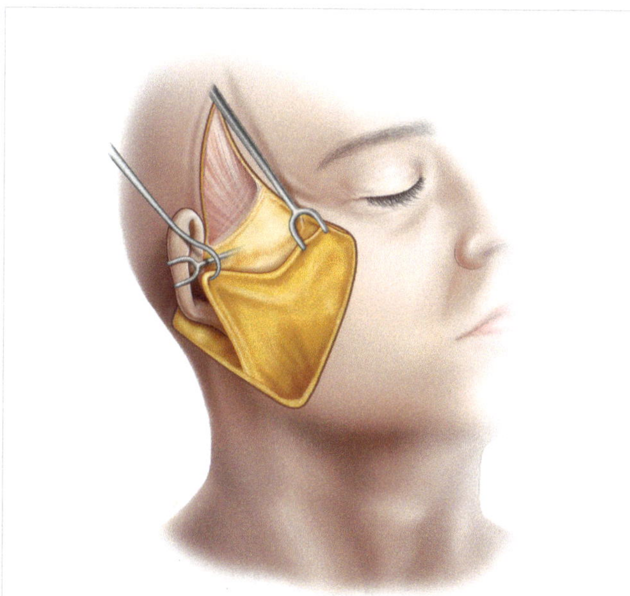

Fig. 7.5 Superficial musculoaponeurotic system (SMAS) redraping with vertical vector of pull.

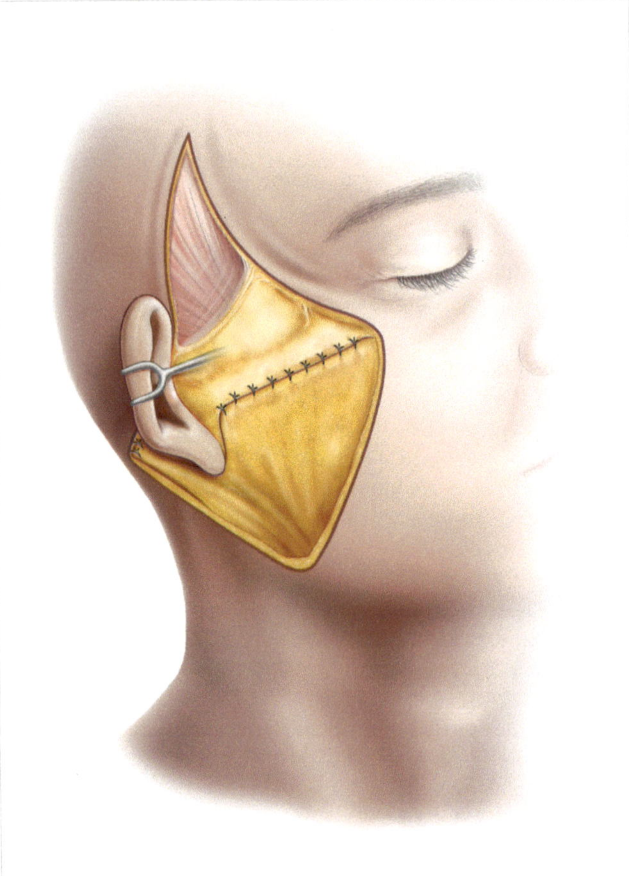

Fig. 7.6 Superficial musculoaponeurotic system (SMAS) suturing.

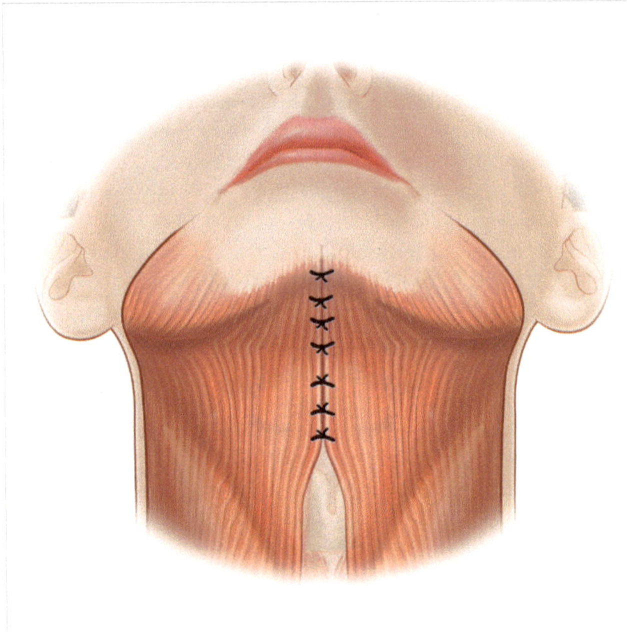

Fig. 7.7 Medial repositioning of the platysma and platysmal myotomy.

contouring is restored through deep layer support rather than through tension in skin flap redraping (▶ Fig. 7.8).

- Incisions are closed with 4–0 and 6–0 nylon sutures.
- Fat grafting can be performed at this time if indicated.

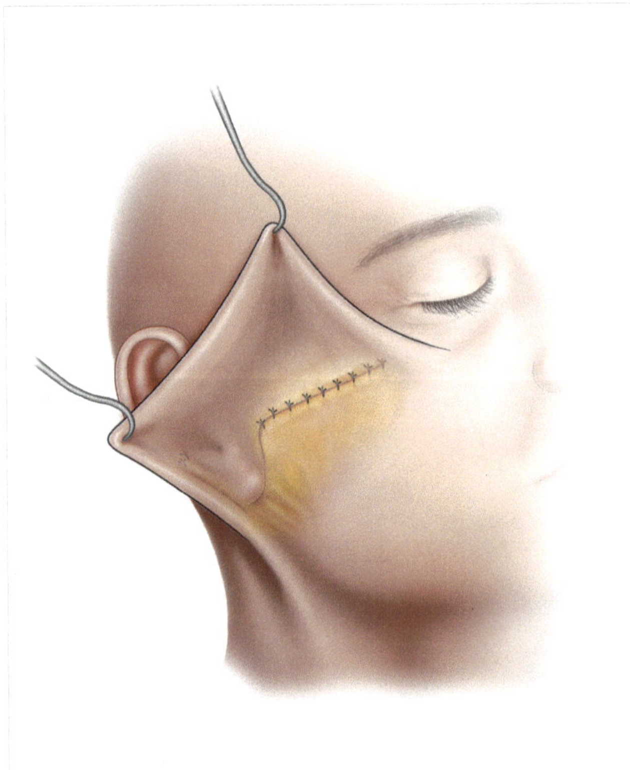

Fig. 7.8 Skin redraping with a horizontal vector of pull.

7.8 Postoperative Protocol

- Patients are initially observed in the postanesthesia care unit and then discharged if they are tolerating liquids and not nauseated.
- Head of bed elevation at all times, ice packs to the face, and pressure off of incisions are advised.
- Patients are seen on postoperative day 1 and the dressing is removed.
- The drains are removed on postoperative day 3 or 4.

7.9 Case Example

Facial aging involves deflation of both the superficial and deep malar fat compartments. As the deep malar compartment deflates, the vertical height of the lower eyelid increases, the anterior cheeks lose volume, and a sharp demarcation develops between the lateral and anterior cheek where the deep malar fat abuts the buccal fat pad. This patient is seen before and after an extended SMAS facelift with autologous fat grafting to the deep compartment to restore deep malar volume (▶ Fig. 7.9a, b).

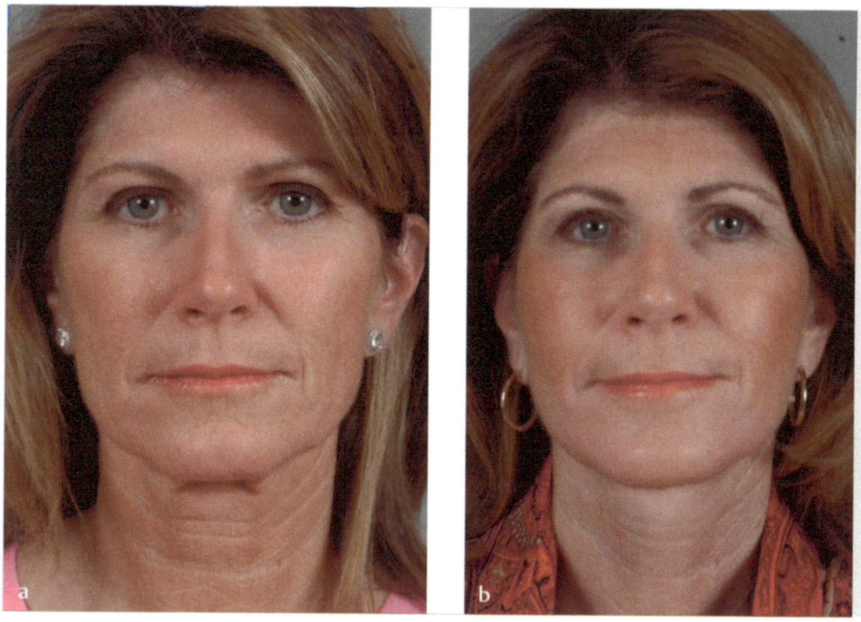

Fig. 7.9 (a, b) Facial aging involves deflation of both the superficial and deep malar fat compartments. As the deep malar compartment deflates, the vertical height of the lower eyelid increases, the anterior cheeks lose volume, and a sharp demarcation develops between the lateral and anterior cheek where the deep malar fat abuts the buccal fat pad. This patient is seen (a) before and (b) after an extended superficial musculoaponeurotic system (SMAS) facelift with autologous fat grafting to the deep compartment to restore deep malar volume.

7.10 Conclusion

Accurate preoperative systematic facial analysis is crucial for surgical success. The extended SMAS technique for facelifting repositions facial fat from the anterior cheek into regions of lateral cheek and malar deflation, restoring the volumetric highlights noted in youth.

See **Video 7.1**.

Further Readings

Farkas JP, Pessa JE, Hubbard B, Rohrich RJ. The science and theory behind facial aging. Plast Reconstr Surg Glob Open. 2013; 1(1):e8–e15

Hoschander AS, Stuzin JM. Extended SMAS rhytidectomy. In: Anh Tran T, Panthaki Z, Hoballah JJ, Thaller SR, eds. Operative Dictations in Plastic and Reconstructive Surgery. Springer; 2017:13–16

Narasimhan K, Stuzin JM, Rohrich RJ. Five-step neck lift: integrating anatomy with clinical practice to optimize results. Plast Reconstr Surg. 2013; 132(2): 339–350

Rohrich RJ, Pessa JE. The fat compartments of the face: anatomy and clinical implications for cosmetic surgery. Plast Reconstr Surg. 2007; 119(7):2219–2227, discussion 2228–2231

Rohrich RJ, Stuzin JM, Dayan E, Ross EV. Facial danger zones: staying safe with surgery, fillers, and non-invasive devices. Thieme Medical Publishers, Inc.; 2020

Roostaeian J, Rohrich RJ, Stuzin JM. Anatomical considerations to prevent facial nerve injury. Plast Reconstr Surg. 2015; 135(5):1318–1327

Stuzin JM, Baker TJ, Gordon HL, Baker TM. Extended SMAS dissection as an approach to midface rejuvenation. Clin Plast Surg. 1995; 22(2):295–311

8 SMASectomy

Daniel C. Baker, Palmyra Geissler, and Paul N. Afrooz

Abstract

In 1992, the senior author (Daniel C. Baker) discovered that an alternative to formally elevating the superficial musculoaponeurotic system (SMAS) flap was to perform a "lateral SMASectomy" by removing a portion of the SMAS in the region of its fixed and mobile junction. Excision and suturing of the superficial fascia in this region allow the surgeon to achieve results similar to a formal SMAS flap, but the technique is simpler and less invasive. The width of SMAS resection depends upon the fullness of the patient's face and whether debulking is advantageous. However, in order to preserve facial fat in thin patients, SMASectomy is not performed. Instead, SMAS plication is performed in these patients to augment and sculpt the face.

Keywords: Facelift, necklift, SMAS plication, SMASectomy

Key Points

- There are several advantages of lateral SMASectomy in comparison with traditional superficial musculoaponeurotic system (SMAS) elevation.
- The procedure does not require traditional SMAS flap elevation. There is less concern about tearing of the superficial fascia.
- The potential for facial nerve injury is less because most of the deep dissection is over the parotid gland.
- If SMAS flaps are not elevated, they tend to hold suture fixation more strongly, and the potential for postoperative dehiscence and relapse of contour is decreased.
- The design of the lateral SMASectomy is along the anterior border of the parotid.
- The SMASectomy is performed at the interface of the superficial fascia fixed by the retaining ligaments and the more mobile anterior superficial facial fascia. Upon closure, this brings the mobile SMAS up to the junction of the fixed SMAS producing a durable elevation of both superficial fascia and facial fat.

8.1 Preoperative Steps

8.1.1 Instructions for Patients to Reduce the Incidence of Infection

- Wash neck, behind the ears, and the external ear canal with Hibiclens soap twice daily for 5 days preoperatively. DO NOT USE ON FACE.
- Shampoo hair daily including morning of surgery.
- Use Bactroban ointment (mupirocin 2%—prescription). Swab the inside of each nostril and the external ear canal (DO NOT PUT DEEP INSIDE).

8.1.2 Anesthesia

- All facelifts are performed under monitored intravenous propofol sedation.
- Patients are given oral clonidine, 0.1 to 0.2 mg, 30 minutes prior to surgery to control their blood pressure.
- The face and neck are infiltrated with local anesthesia, 0.5% lidocaine with 1:200,000 epinephrine, through use of a 22-gauge spinal needle.
- The face is injected prior to scrubbing in order to provide the requisite 10 minutes for vasoconstriction.

8.2 Operative Steps

See **Video 8.1**.

8.2.1 Incisions

- If the temporal hairline shift is assessed as minimal, the preferred incision is within the temporal hair. In this incision, it is often necessary to excise a triangle of skin below the temporal sideburn at the level of the superior root of the helix to preserve the sideburn.
- When a larger skin shift is anticipated, if the distance between the lateral canthus and temporal hairline is greater than 5 cm, a beveled incision a few millimeters within the temporal hairline is preferable. This is an effort to avoid the alternative of a receding temporal hairline, which is usually never acceptable for a female patient.
- The choice of preauricular incision is up to the surgeon. When executed properly, all of these incisions heal well and are imperceptible. The senior author (Daniel C. Baker) prefers a curved incision anterior to the helix, which then continues inferiorly anterior to the tragus in a natural skin fold.
- Intratragal incisions are carried out in those patients whose cheek and tragal skin are similar, and the tragal cartilage is not sharp or prominent. Closure must be performed without tension, and the flap overlying the tragus is defatted to dermis.

8.2.2 Skin Flap Elevation

- All skin flap undermining is performed under direct vision (with scissors dissection) to minimize trauma of the subdermal plexus and preserve 5 mm of subcutaneous fat on the undersurface of the flap.
- Subcutaneous dissection in the temporal region is preferable because the skin seems to redrape better. Subcutaneous dissection in the temporal region must be performed carefully to avoid penetrating the superficial temporal fascia that protects the frontal branch of the facial nerve.

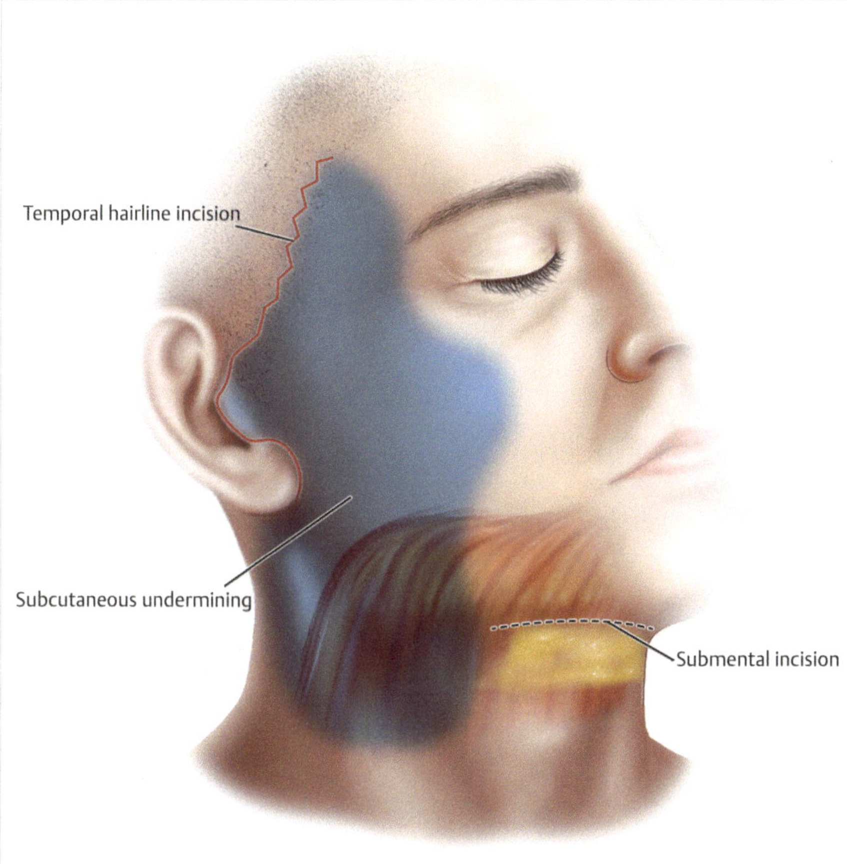

Fig. 8.1 Extent of subcutaneous undermining in temporal area, cheek, and lateral neck. If excess fat is present, closed or open liposuction, superficial to the platysma, is executed in submental and submandibular areas. When necessary, medial platysma approximation is performed via the submental incision.

- All dermal attachments between the orbicularis oculi muscle and the skin are separated up to the lateral canthus (▶ Fig. 8.1).
- Dissection extends across the zygoma to release zygomatic ligaments but stops several centimeters short of the nasolabial fold. The senior author does not believe that further dissection provides significant benefits; on the contrary, the only result is increased bleeding.
- In the cheek, dissection releases the masseteric-cutaneous ligaments and, if necessary, the mandibular ligaments.
- Subcutaneous dissection continues over the angle of the mandible and sternocleidomastoid for 5 to 6 cm into the neck, which exposes the posterior half of the platysma on muscle. If a submental incision has been made, the facial and lateral neck dissection is connected through and through to the submental dissection.

8.2.3 Defatting the Neck and Jowls

- When possible, closed suction-assisted lipoplasty is performed in the neck and jowls. A 2.4-mm Mercedes tip cannula is used under constant and steady motion in the subcutaneous space. A 5-mm layer of subcutaneous fat on the undersurface of the cervical skin is maintained.
- If the jowls are suctioned, this is always done conservatively.

8.2.4 Lateral SMASectomy Including Platysma Approximation

- The outline of the SMASectomy is marked on a tangent from the lateral malar eminence to the angle of the mandible, essentially in the region along the anterior edge of the parotid gland. In most patients, this involves a line for resection extending from the lateral aspect of the malar eminence toward the tale of the parotid gland. Usually, a 2 to 4 cm segment of superficial fascia is excised, depending on the degree of SMAS-platysma laxity.
- In SMAS resection, the superficial fascia is grasped in the region of the tale of the parotid, and the resection is carried out from inferior to superior in a controlled fashion.
- When SMAS resection is being performed, it is important to keep the dissection superficial to the deep fascia and avoid dissection into the parotid parenchyma (▶ Fig. 8.2).
- Note that the size of the parotid gland varies from patient to patient; consequently, the amount of protection for the underlying facial nerve branches also varies. Despite this, as long as one carries the dissection superficial to the deep facial fascia, ensuring that only the superficial fascia is resected, facial nerve injury and parotid injury will be prevented.

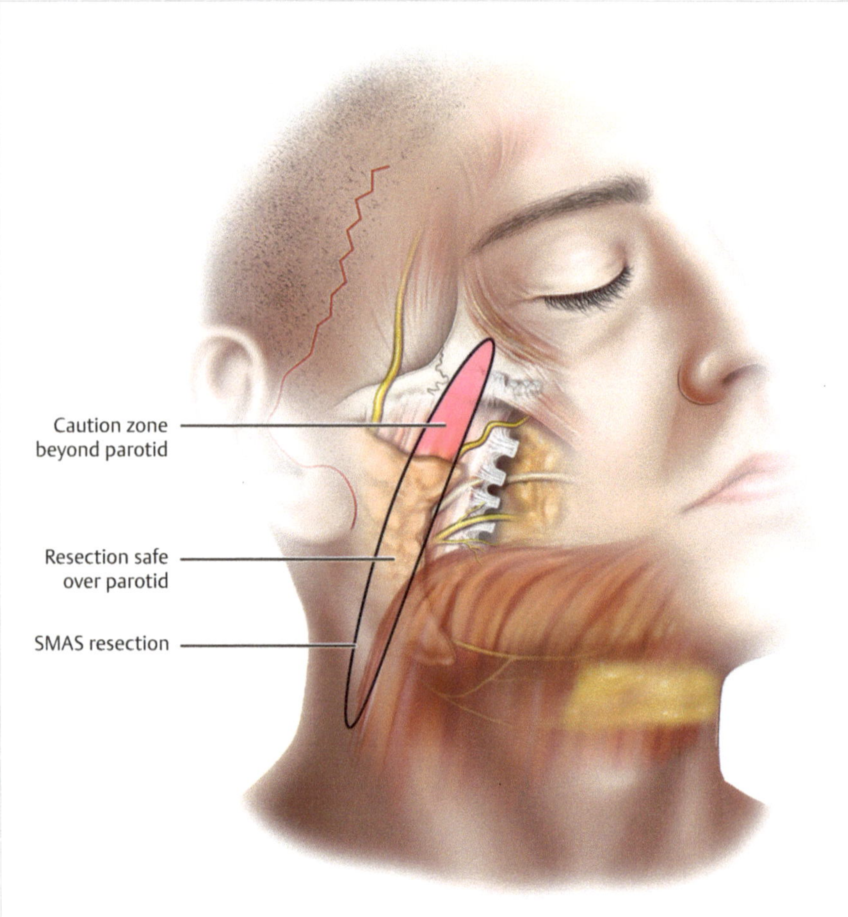

Fig. 8.2 Design of superficial musculoaponeurotic system (SMAS)-platysma resection. The level of resection is superficial to the parotid masseteric fascia that overlies the facial nerve branches.

- In essence, this is a resection of the superficial fascia in the same plane of dissection in which one would normally raise a SMAS flap.
- After SMAS resection, interrupted 3–0 PDS buried sutures are used to close the SMASectomy.
- The fixed lateral SMAS is evenly sutured to the more mobile anterior superficial fascia.
- Vectors are usually perpendicular to the nasolabial fold.
- The last suture lifts the malar fat pad, securing it to the malar fascia.
- It is important to obtain a secure fixation to prevent postoperative dehiscence and relapse of facial contour.

8.2.5 Vectors of SMASectomy Closure

- The various vectors accomplish correction of the anterior neck, the cervicomental angle, the jowls, and the nasal labial fold.
- The first key suture grasps the platysma at the angle of the mandible and advances in a posterosuperior direction; it is secured with 2–0 Maxon to the fixed lateral SMAS overlying the parotid. This action lifts the cervical platysma and cervical skin.
- The vectors which produce the desired facial rejuvenation must be chosen by the surgeon and individualized for each patient (▶ Fig. 8.3).

8.2.6 Skin Closure; Temporal and Earlobe Dog-Ears

- A buried 3–0 PDS suture is placed through the temporal fascia with a generous bite of dermis on the skin flap. Closure is under minimal to moderate tension.
- A wedge is usually removed at the level of the sideburn to preserve the hairline.
- If an anterior hairline incision has been made, it is closed with buried 5–0 Monocryl (Ethicon, Inc) and 5–0 nylon sutures.
- Time and attention are required during this closure to eliminate dog-ears and obtain the finest scar.
- Excess skin is trimmed from the facial flap so that there is no tension on the preauricular closure. Wound edges should be "kissing" without sutures.

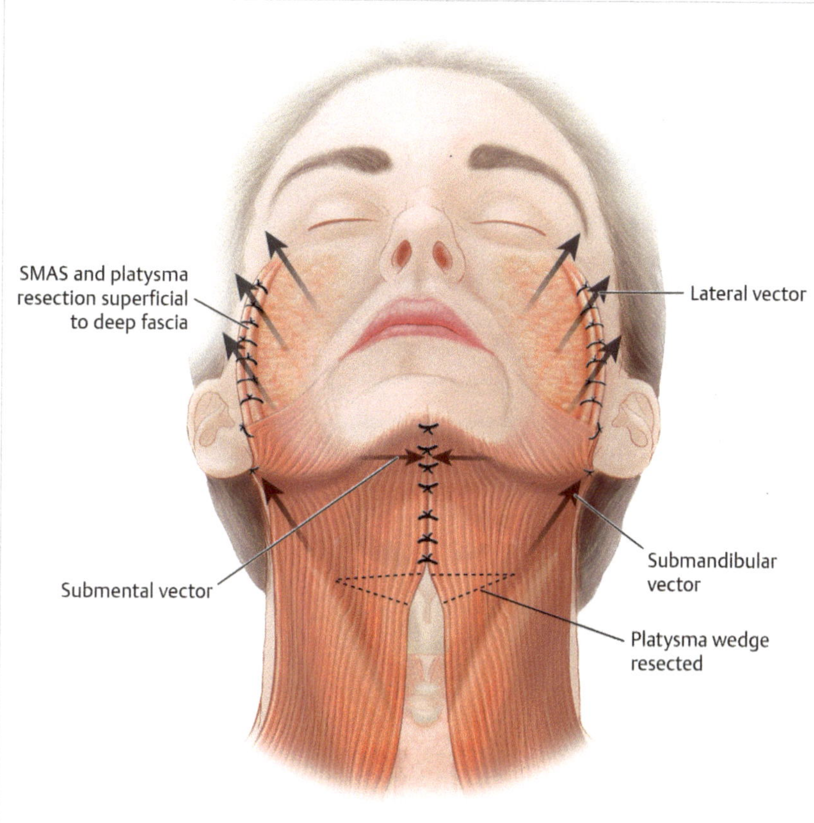

Fig. 8.3 Vectors of superolateral elevation of superficial musculoaponeurotic system (SMAS)-platysma and vectors of medial approximation of anterior platysma in the submental area above the hyoid.

- Trimming at the earlobe must also be without tension, and the skin flap is tucked under the earlobe with 4-0 PDS sutures, taking a bite of the earlobe dermis, cheek flap dermis, and conchal perichondrium to minimize any tension.
- If a short scar facelift is performed, a small dog-ear might be present behind the earlobe; this is easily trimmed and tailored into a short incision in the retroauricular sulcus.
- A closed suction drain is usually brought out through a separate stab in the retroauricular sulcus.

8.3 Case Example

(▶ Fig. 8.4a–c and ▶ Fig. 8.5a, b)

8.4 Conclusion

There are several advantages to the lateral SMASectomy when one compares it with formal SMAS elevation. Since the procedure does not require a formal SMAS flap elevation, there are fewer concerns about tearing of the superficial fascia. The potential for facial nerve injury is less because the majority of the dissection is carried over the parotid gland. If the SMASectomy is performed anterior to the parotid, the deep fascia similarly will provide protection for the facial nerve branches as long as the resection of the superficial fascia is done precisely and the deep facial fascia is not violated. When SMAS flaps are not elevated, they tend to be more substantial in terms of holding suture fixation, and the problems of developing postoperative dehiscence and relapse of contour are reduced.

Lateral SMASectomy offers similar advantages over simple SMAS plication. Because of the design of the lateral SMASectomy along the anterior border of the parotid, the SMASectomy is performed at the interface of the superficial fascia fixed by the retaining ligaments and the more mobile anterior superficial facial fascia. On closure, this brings the mobile SMAS up to the junction of the fixed SMAS, producing a durable elevation of both superficial fascia and facial fat.

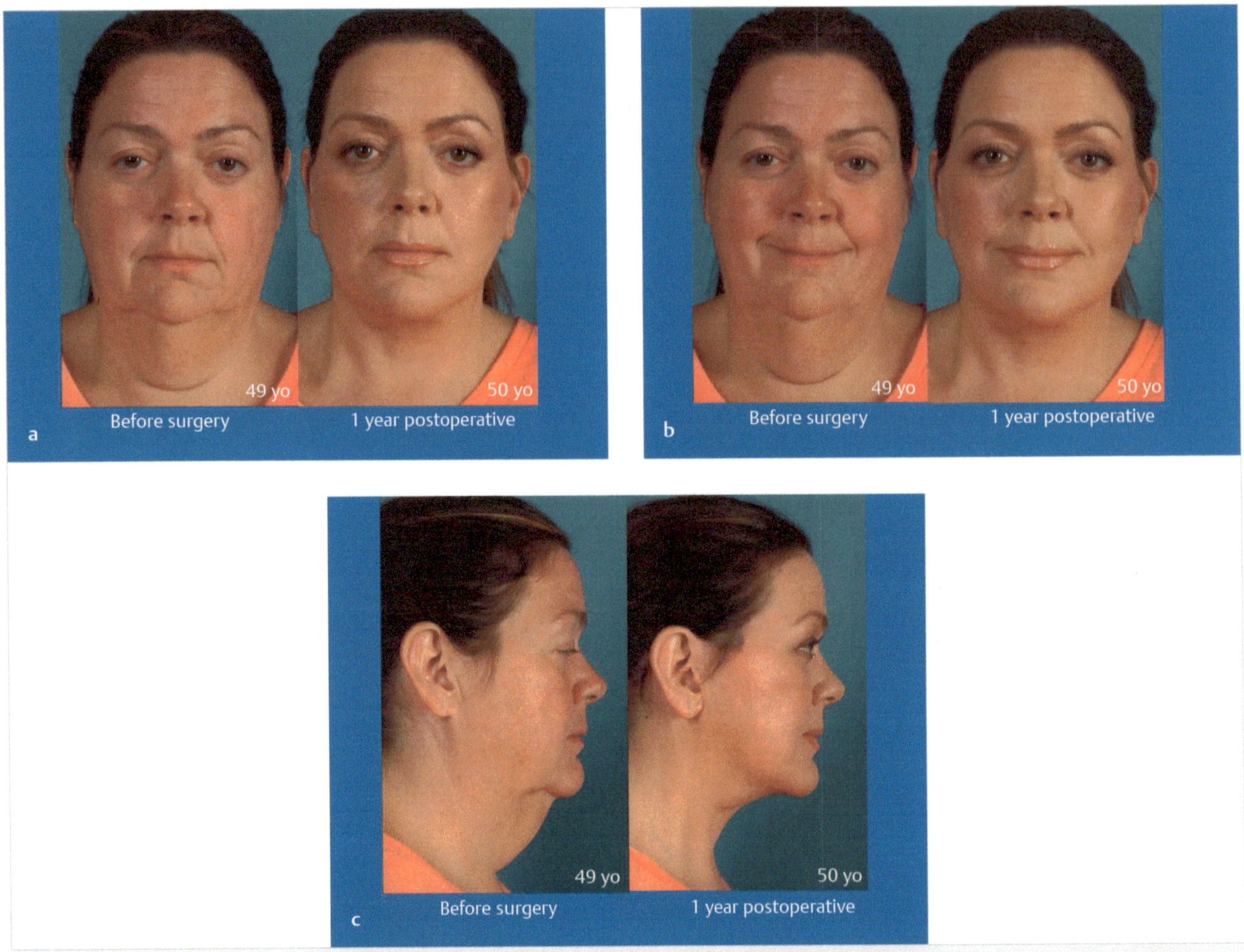

Fig. 8.4 (a–c) Female case example. Face and lateral SMASectomy; open neck with platysmaplasty; subplatysma fat excision; buccal fat excision; prejowl chin implant.

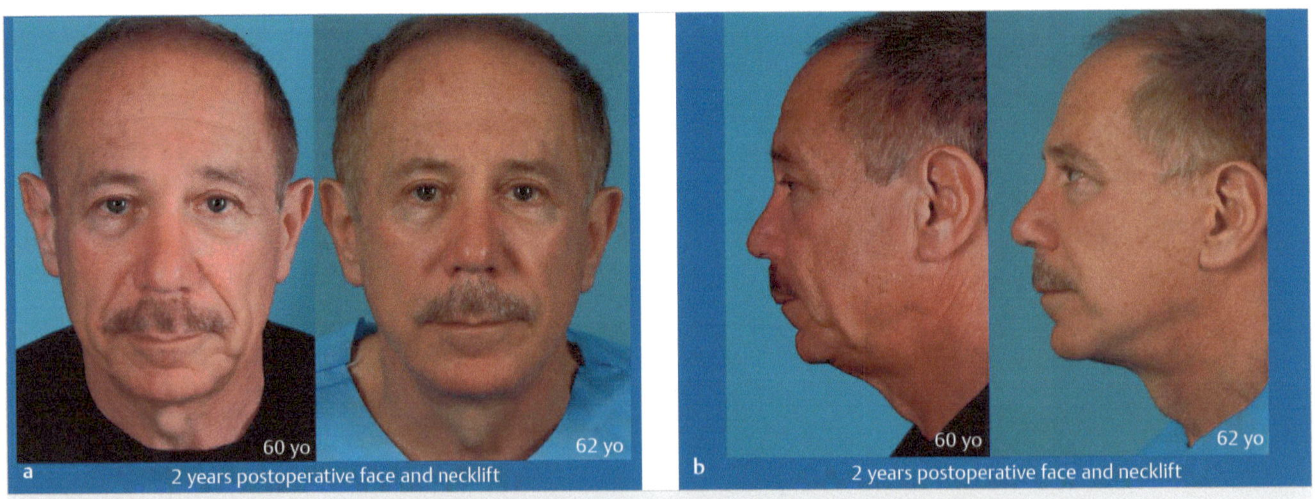

Fig. 8.5 (a, b) Male case example. Face with lateral SMASectomy; open neck with playsmaplasty; Bleph 4; chin implant.

Further Readings

Alpert BS, Baker DC, Hamra ST, Owsley JQ, Ramirez O. Identical twin face lifts with differing techniques: a 10-year follow-up. Plast Reconstr Surg. 2009; 123(3): 1025–1033, discussion 1034–1036

Baker DC. Lateral SMASectomy, plication and short scar facelifts: indications and techniques. Clin Plast Surg. 2008; 35(4):533–550, vi

Baker DC. Short scar facelift. In: Aston SJ, Steinbrech D, Walden J, eds. Advances in Aesthetic Surgery. London: Elsevier; 2009

Baker DC, Conley J. Avoiding facial nerve injuries in rhytidectomy: anatomical variations and pitfalls. Plast Reconstr Surg. 1979; 64(6):781–795

Baker DC. Complications of cervicofacial rhytidectomy. Clin Plast Surg. 1983; 10(3): 543–562

Baker DC. Lateral SMASectomy. Plast Reconstr Surg. 1997; 100(2):509–513

Baker D. Rhytidectomy with lateral SMASectomy. Facial Plast Surg. 2000; 16(3): 209–213

9 The Lift and Fill Facelift: Autologous Fat Grafting

Rod J. Rohrich and Paul N. Afrooz

Abstract
Much of facial aging can be attributed to volume deflation and tissue laxity. Successful surgical rejuvenation can be achieved through volume restoration with autologous fat grafting of the facial fat compartments. In conjunction with volume restoration, correction of tissue laxity and recontouring of the face and neck can be achieved. Current strategies for surgical correction of the face and neck involve superficial musculoaponeurotic system (SMAS) manipulation, medial platysma plication, and lateral platysma tightening through the lateral platysma window. These combined techniques facilitate optimal results in facial rejuvenation.

Keywords: Facelift, necklift, facial rejuvenation, SMAS facelift, SMAS plication, SMASectomy, fat grafting, fat compartments, facial rejuvenation

Key Points

- Much of facial aging can be attributed to volume deflation and soft tissue laxity.
- Surgical rejuvenation aims to address tissue laxity and volume restoration.

9.1 Preoperative Steps

9.1.1 Analysis

- The facial rejuvenation procedure begins with a thorough preoperative analysis to identify areas of volume deflation, rhytides, and tissue laxity.
- Areas of volume deflation as well as deep rhytides are marked preoperatively in the dependent position to facilitate intraoperative accuracy.

9.2 Operative Steps

See **Video 9.1**.

9.2.1 Fat Harvest and Facial Fat Compartment Augmentation

- Fat is typically harvested from the medial thighs with manual, low-pressure aspiration using a 10-cc syringe and a 3-mm multihole cannula.
- To optimize cell viability, no local anesthetic or epinephrine is used before aspiration.
- The aspirate is centrifuged for 1 minute at 2,250 rpm to remove cellular debris.
- Fat is then isolated and transferred to 1-cc syringes.
- Autologous fat transfer is performed at the beginning of the procedure to facilitate accurate volume restoration.
- Just lateral to the alar–cheek junction, a 14-gauge needle is used to introduce the Coleman cannula into the deep compartments.
- Fat is injected into the deep malar compartments bilaterally using 1-cc syringes.
- Approximately 10 to 12 cc of healthy yellow fat is distributed into the deep central facial compartments.
- This includes 2 cc into the deep nasolabial compartment and 2 to 4 cc in the deep malar compartments (▶ Fig. 9.1).
- Depending on the desired malar contour, the high superficial malar and middle superficial malar compartments are augmented with 1 to 2 cc of fat (▶ Fig. 9.1).

9.2.2 Skin Elevation

- Each hemiface is injected in the subcutaneous plane with 100 cc of a solution of 1:400,000 epinephrine.
- A curvilinear intratragal and preauricular incision is designed. Superiorly, the incision travels preauricularly, and at the level of the helical root, the incision extends anteriorly along the infratemporal hairline.
- The inferior incision extends along the root of the lobule and around the contour of the conchal cartilage.
- The postauricular incision is carried superiorly along the hairline, and depending on the extent of skin removal, the incision is carried into the hair-bearing scalp, or along the posterior hairline.
- Skin elevation is carried out strategically in zones 1, 2, and 3.

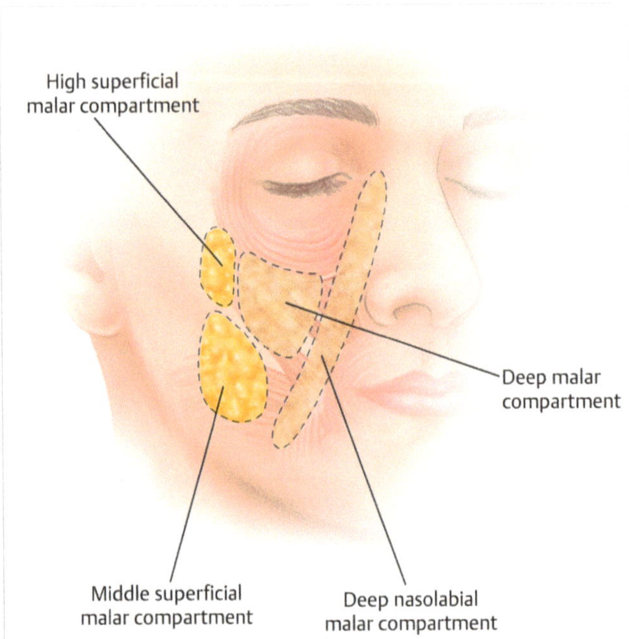

Fig. 9.1 Key fat compartments.

- The borders of zone 1 include a line drawn from the alar base to the tragus superiorly, and the anterior border of the sternocleidomastoid muscle inferolaterally.
- Zone 2 is the region posterior to the sternocleidomastoid toward the posterior hairline.
- Zone 3 is the region from the superior border of zone 2 extending superiorly to the lateral canthus.
- The submental incision is made approximately 3 to 4 mm posterior to the submental crease.
- Skin is elevated from the underlying platysma.

9.2.3 Neck Contouring

- Following elevation of skin from platysma through the submental incision, the medial borders of the platysma are identified.
- Medial platysma banding and diastasis are corrected with medial platysma plication.
- Beginning as inferiorly as possible and traveling superiorly, the medial borders of the platysma are plicated with buried, interrupted sutures.
- To prevent bowstringing of the medial platysma, and to accentuate the cervicomental angle, a wedge of platysma is excised inferiorly at the medial border.
- Care is taken to break through the posterior cervical fascia to ensure proper release and accentuation of the cervicomental angle.
- The lateral platysma window is initiated one fingerbreadth below the angle of the mandible and one fingerbreadth in front of the sternocleidomastoid muscle (▶ Fig. 9.2).
- The platysma is elevated carefully in a medial and inferior direction for 2 to 3 cm (▶ Fig. 9.2).
- The lateral platysma is tightened and secured to the mastoid fascia with two or three figure-of-eight sutures (▶ Fig. 9.2).

9.2.4 Superficial Musculoaponeurotic System (SMAS)

- Preoperative analysis of facial symmetry and shape dictates the application of the SMAS technique.
- In the case example, the long side of the face is treated with a horizontal SMASectomy.
- The SMASectomy is designed beginning medially along the zygomatic arch traveling toward the ear lobule (▶ Fig. 9.3).
- Approximately 1 cm of SMAS is excised followed by reapproximation with a running, locked suture.
- On the contralateral side, a SMAS stacking (modified imbrication) technique is used, imbricating the SMAS from the level of the superior portion of the zygomaticus major muscle to the angle of the mandible (▶ Fig. 9.4).

9.3 Postoperative Care

- Patients rest with head elevated to 45 degrees without the use of pillows to avoid flexion of the neck.
- Cold compresses are applied to the face intermittently for the first 72 hours postoperatively.

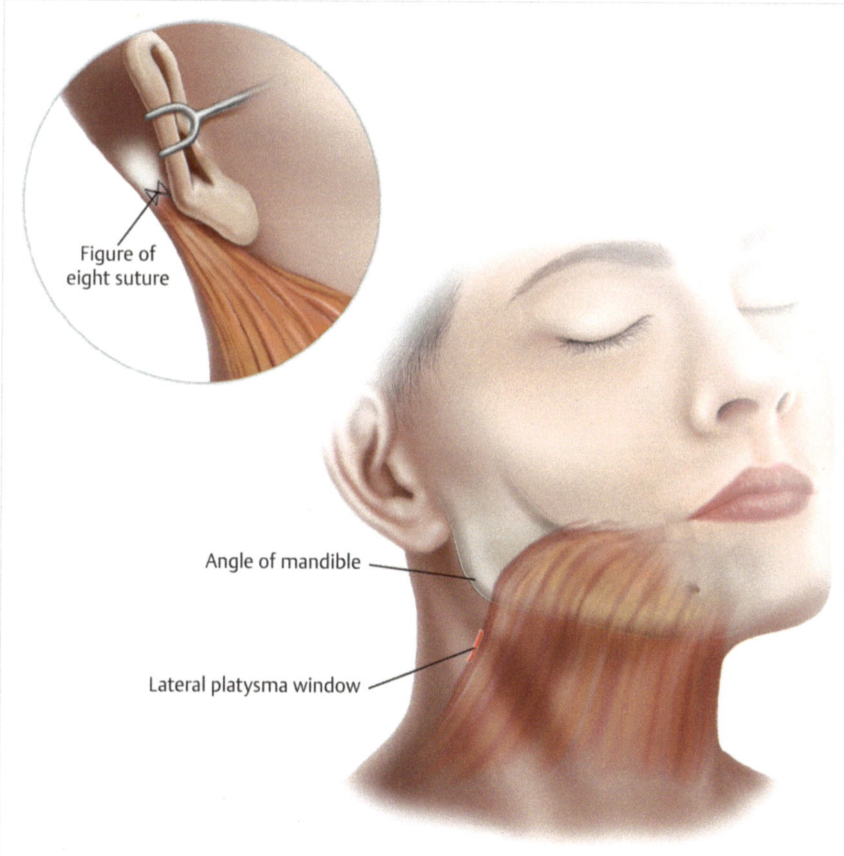

Fig. 9.2 Schematic illustration of the lateral platysmal window.

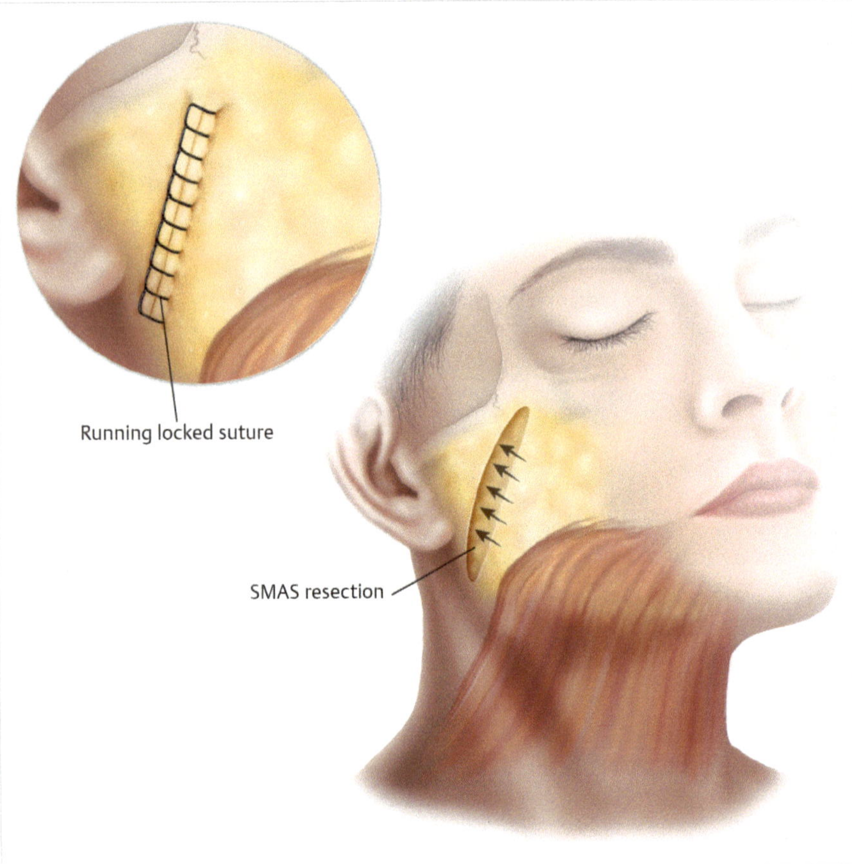

Fig. 9.3 Schematic illustration of the SMASectomy technique.

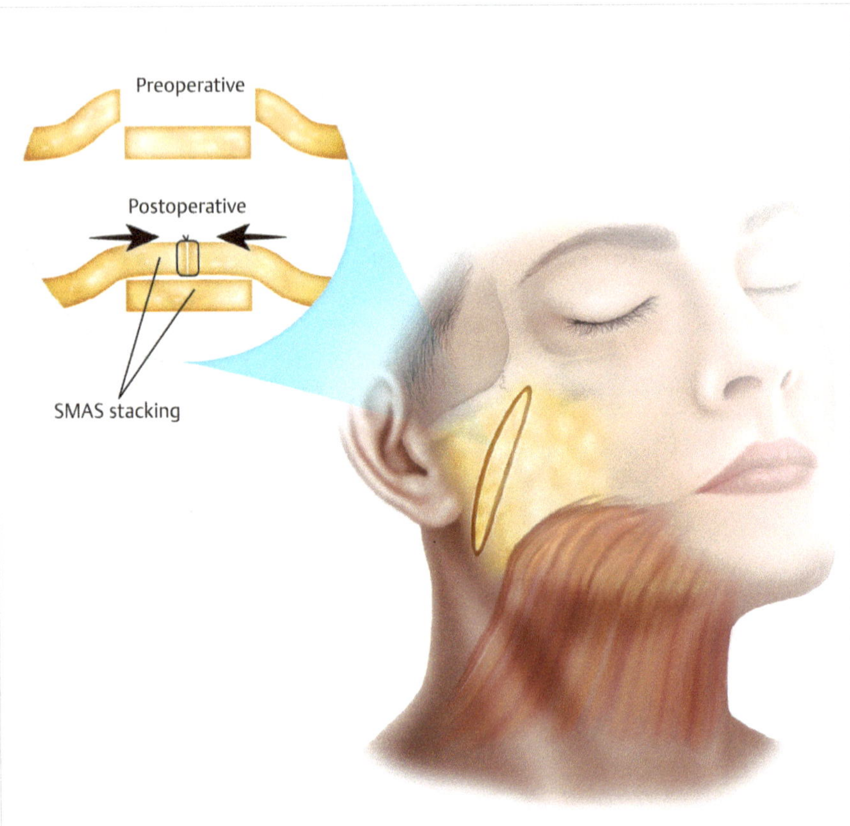

Fig. 9.4 Schematic illustration of the superficial musculoaponeurotic system (SMAS) stacking technique.

- Patients are started on a liquid diet and advanced slowly.
- Patients are encouraged to avoid head turning and limit facial movements for the first week.
- Sutures are removed between 7 and 10 days.

9.4 Case Examples

9.4.1 Case 1

This 45-year-old female had significant neck skin and desired contouring of her neck and face. Dr. Rohrich performed a lift and fill SMAS facelift and upper eyelid surgery. He did a central fat compartment fat augmentation in the deep and superficial fat compartments—a lift and fill facelift (▶ Fig. 9.5a–c).

9.4.2 Case 2

This 75-year-old desired facial rejuvenation procedures. He had a lift and fill SMAS face/neck lift as well as an upper and lower blepharoplasty. He had both deep and superficial fat compartment fat injections to his malar and nasolabial folds. The left photos are before surgery, and the right photos are 1 year and

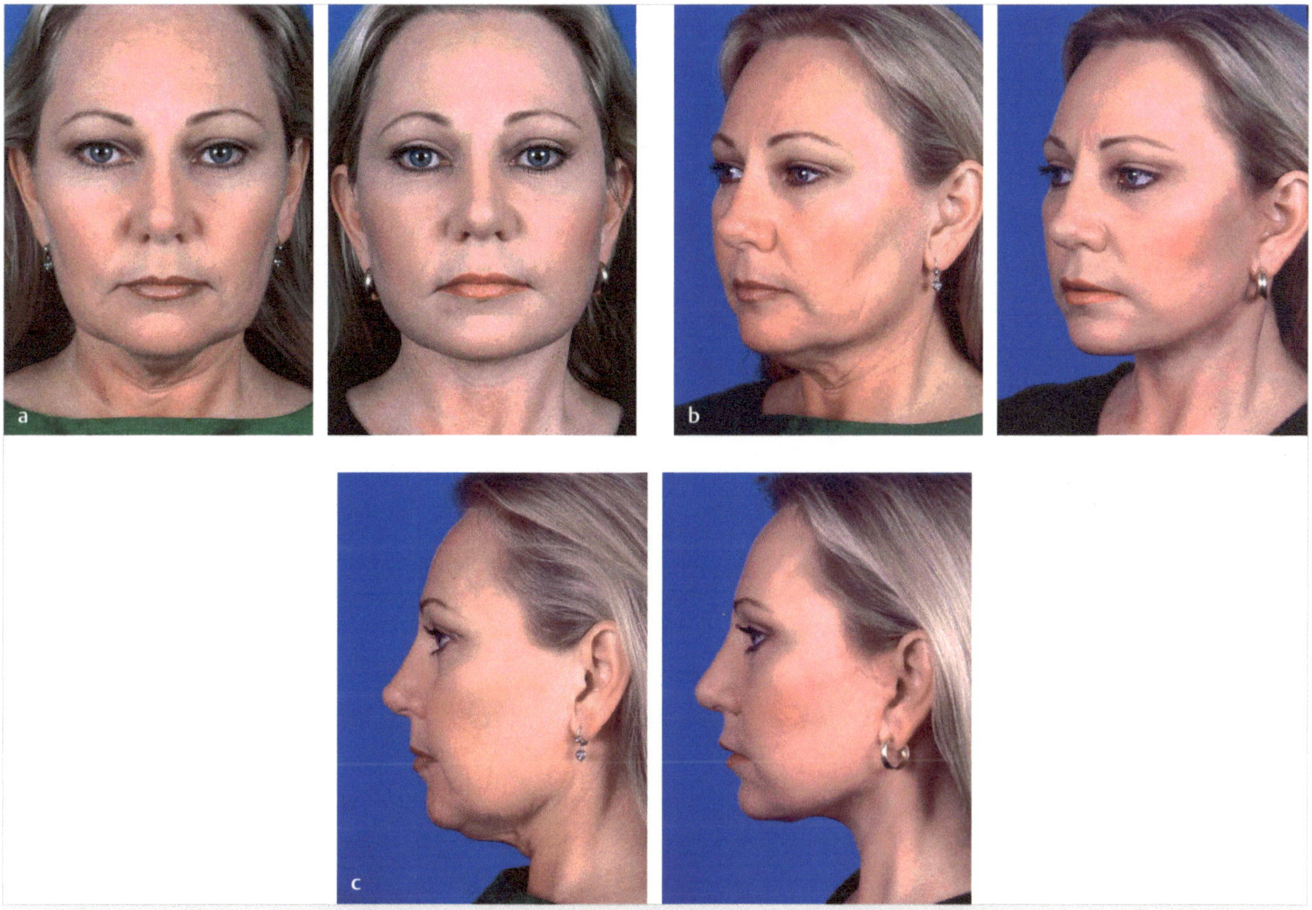

Fig. 9.5 (a–c) Case 1. This 45-year-old female had significant neck skin and desired contouring of her neck and face. Dr. Rohrich performed a lift and fill superficial musculoaponeurotic system (SMAS) facelift and upper eyelid surgery. He did a central fat compartment fat augmentation in the deep and superficial fat compartments—a lift and fill facelift.

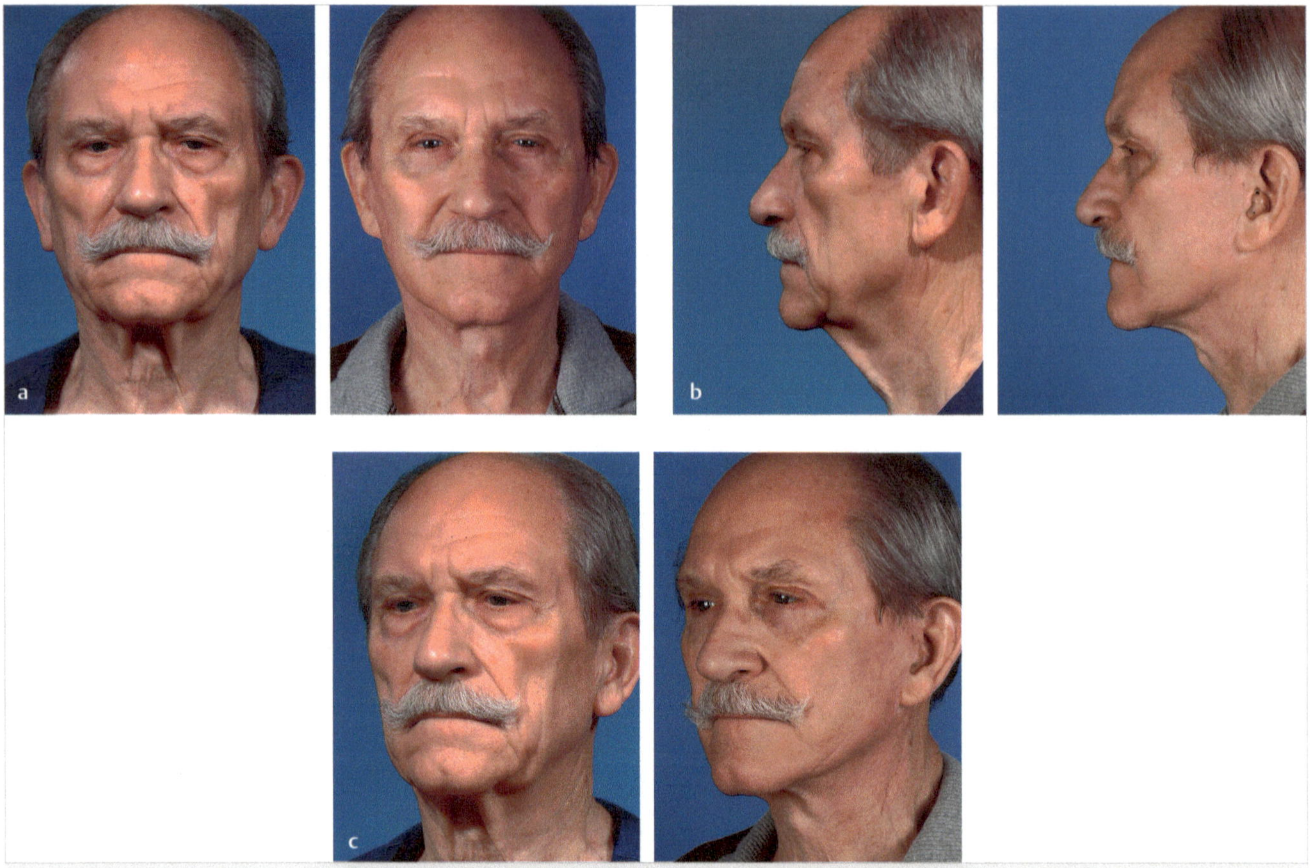

Fig. 9.6 (a–c) Case 2. This 75-year-old desired facial rejuvenation procedures. He had a lift and fill superficial musculoaponeurotic system (SMAS) face/neck lift as well as an upper and lower blepharoplasty. He had both deep and superficial fat compartment fat injections to his malar and nasolabial folds. The left photos are before surgery, and the right photos are 1 year and 6 months after surgery, revealing his amazing transformation with central restoration.

6 months after surgery, revealing his amazing transformation with central restoration (▶ Fig. 9.6a–c).

9.5 Conclusion

Facial rejuvenation can be achieved through the combination of volume restoration and face and neck contouring. Volumization is achieved with autologous fat grafting of the facial fat compartments. Neck contouring is achieved through medial platysma plication and the lateral platysma window. Lateral midface rejuvenation is achieved through SMAS stacking or SMASectomy techniques.

Further Readings

Farkas JP, Pessa JE, Hubbard B, Rohrich RJ. The science and theory behind facial aging. Plast Reconstr Surg Glob Open. 2013; 1(1):e8–e15

Pezeshk RA, Sieber DA, Rohrich RJ. Neck rejuvenation through the lateral platysma window: a key component of face-lift surgery. Plast Reconstr Surg. 2017; 139(4): 865–866

Rohrich RJ, Ghavami A, Constantine FC, Unger J, Mojallal A. Lift-and-fill face lift: integrating the fat compartments. Plast Reconstr Surg. 2014; 133(6):756e–767e

Rohrich RJ, Ghavami A, Lemmon JA, Brown SA. The individualized component face lift: developing a systematic approach to facial rejuvenation. Plast Reconstr Surg. 2009; 123(3):1050–1063

Rohrich RJ, Afrooz PN. Finesse in face lifting: the role of facial fat compartment augmentation in facial rejuvenation. Plast Reconstr Surg. 2019; 143(1):98–101

10 Deep Plane Facelift

Thomas A. Mustoe, Eugene Park, and Sammy Sinno

Abstract
Facial aging is caused by atrophy and attenuation of deep layers of the face, including the subcutaneous fat and the underlying superficial fascial layers that encompass the superficial facial muscles and the skin. The deep plane facelift recognizes that all layers must be addressed with complete release, even tension and redraping, and excess tension on the skin must be avoided to achieve a natural appearance and longevity of result.

Keywords: Facelift, deep plane, necklift, SMAS, retaining ligaments

Key Points

- Retaining ligaments must be released to allow for adequate mobilization of overlying tissues.
- The extent of inferior dissection is determined by the degree of neck mobilization aimed to be achieved.
- A superb understanding of facial anatomy is imperative to prevent damage to the branches of the facial nerve.

10.1 Preoperative Steps

10.1.1 Planning

- It is critical to understand that the superficial musculoaponeurotic system (SMAS), a thin fascia layer just under the subcutaneous fat, is contiguous with and encloses the platysma muscle and inferior surface of the orbicularis oculi muscle, respectively.
- The retaining ligaments are collagen attachments that pass through the skin to the SMAS and deeper tissues (▶ Fig. 10.1).
- The zygomatic retaining ligaments and masseteric retaining ligaments must be released in the face to allow adequate mobilization.
- In the neck, the retaining ligaments are along the posterior border of the platysma just anterior to the great auricular nerve. They also run obliquely down the neck where they have attachments to the sternocleidomastoid muscle (SCM) and attachments to the anteroinferior portion of the parotid gland (▶ Fig. 10.2). All of these attachments must be released for the neck to be mobile. The further inferiorly

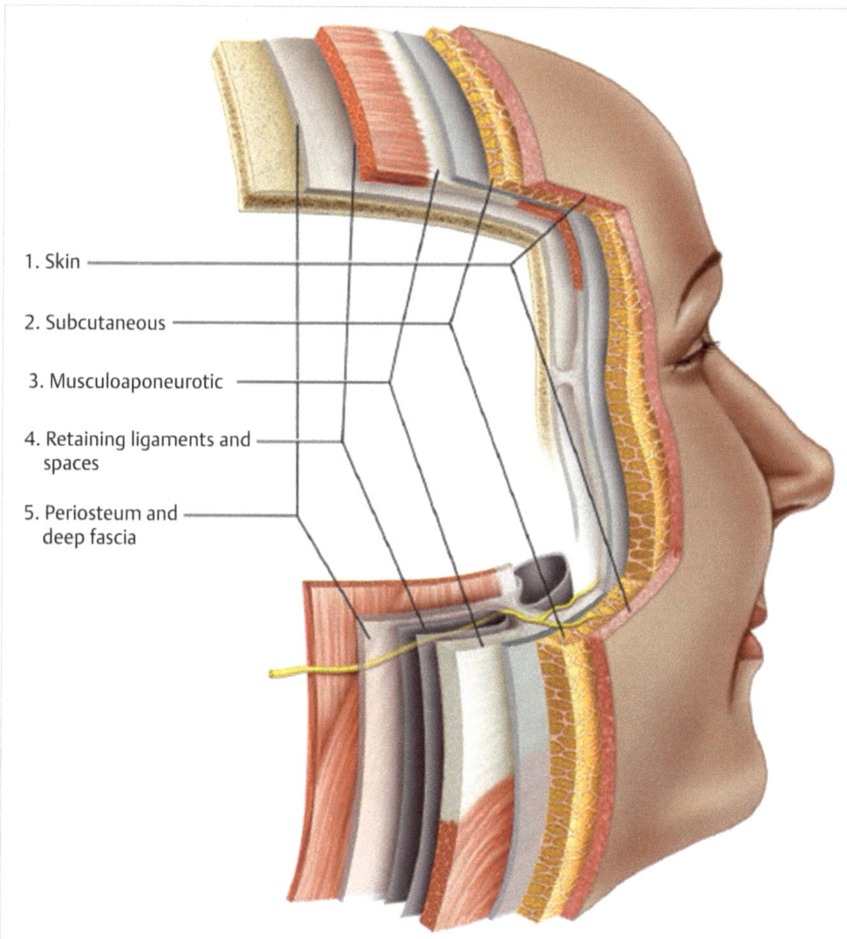

Fig. 10.1 Layers of the face. (Reproduced with permission from Watanabe K, Shoja M, Loukas M, et al, eds. Anatomy for Plastic Surgery of the Face, Head, and Neck. 1st ed. Thieme; 2016.)

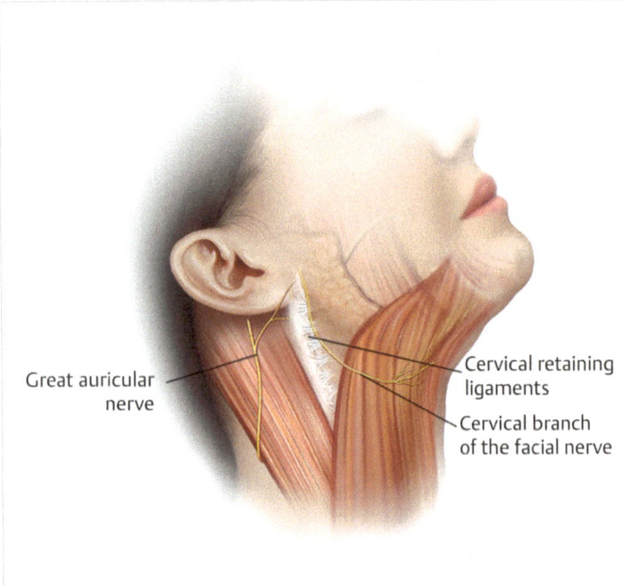

Fig. 10.2 Extent of neck dissection to allow adequate mobilization.

the attachments are released, the more inferior the pivot point, and the more the neck tissues (composite of SMAS-platysma and skin) can be mobilized and moved superiorly and posteriorly.

- The SMAS-platysma is directly above the branches of the facial nerve:
  - In the neck, the cervical branch enters the platysma anterior to the retaining ligaments.
  - The marginal mandibular branch is protected by the parotidomasseteric fascia (▶ Fig. 10.3).
  - The buccal branch runs just above Stensen's duct (▶ Fig. 10.4).
  - The zygomatic branch runs underneath the zygomaticus major muscle.
  - The frontal branch becomes more superficial above the zygomatic arch.
- Prior to surgery, routine labs and an electrocardiogram (EKG) should be obtained. Hypertension is managed with clonidine. Smoking must be stopped at least 3 weeks prior to surgery.
- Risks including hematoma, facial nerve injury, skin necrosis, and limitations of skin elasticity are discussed with the patient.

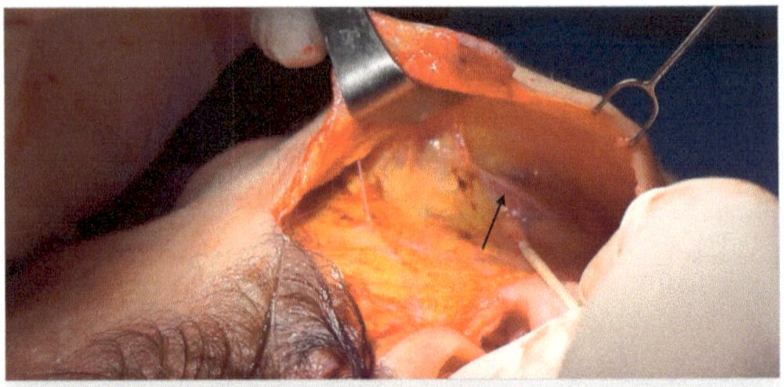

Fig. 10.3 Intraoperative view of the marginal mandibular branch of facial nerve (*black arrow*) beneath superficial musculoaponeurotic system (SMAS)-platysma flap.

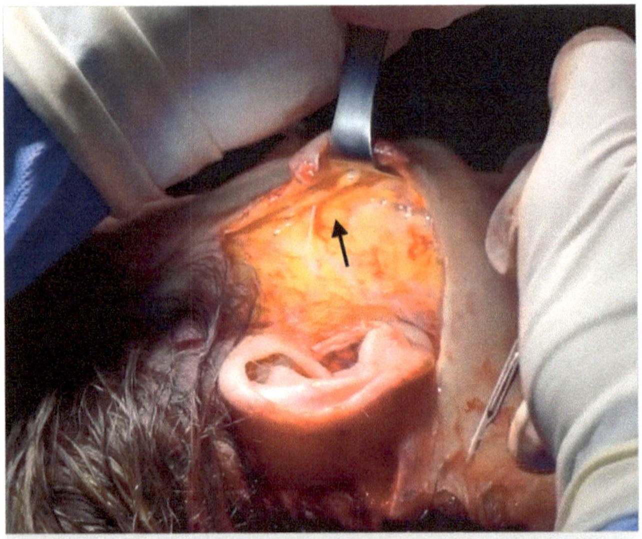

Fig. 10.4 Intraoperative view of the buccal branch of facial nerve (*black arrow*) beneath superficial musculoaponeurotic system (SMAS)-platysma flap.

10.2 Operative Steps

See **Video 10.1**.

10.2.1 Markings and Incision

- For a deep plane facelift, the typical facelift incision has an extension above the helix into the hair directly vertically, then a V-shaped extension into the sideburn, stopping at

a point anteriorly where the hair can no longer hide the incision.
- A retrotragal incision is preferred and sharp angles are used to define the superior and inferior endings of the tragus.
- The postauricular incision curves high on the mastoid and into the hairline at the level of the superior tragus.
- Using a #15 blade, incisions are made and then a subcutaneous flap is raised to the lateral edge of the orbicularis oculi muscle.

10.2.2 SMAS Elevation and Dissection

- The SMAS is elevated to the point of the previous subcutaneous dissection.
- The dissection behind the ear is started at the level of the superficial fascia and extends inferiorly with exposure of the posterior auricular muscle, great auricular nerve, and the entire investing fascia of the SCM.
- Sharp dissection is carried out around the ear lobule, connecting the anterior sub-SMAS dissection with the posterior dissection and taking care to elevate the entire SMAS, which extends to the great auricular nerve.
- The sub-SMAS dissection is then extended beyond the parotid gland anteriorly to expose the masseteric fascia. There is an occasional perforating vessel in this area.
- Midface dissection requires release of the zygomatic and masseteric ligaments, exposing the zygomaticus major muscle, and extending to the inferior edge of the orbicularis oculi to allow malar elevation.
- Inferiorly, the dissection extends just beyond the anteroinferior edge of the parotid with exposure of the external jugular vein and great auricular nerve. The extent of dissection depends on the degree of neck mobilization aimed to be achieved.

10.2.3 SMAS Fixation

- Two 3–0 PDS sutures are placed from the mid face (above zygomaticus major and at inferior edge of the orbicularis) to the temporal fascia.
- Next, the corner of the SMAS is sutured in a superolateral direction into the deep tissues just above the anterior helical rim.

10.2.4 Closure

- The skin is rotated superiorly, with a slightly more posterior vector than the SMAS.
- For patients with more skin relaxation, the skin flap may require further anterior elevation to allow separate vectors for the skin flap and SMAS flap.
- At the anterior edge of the sideburn, excess skin is excised which avoids a dog-ear but still allows for tensionless closure.
- Posteriorly, two or more sutures are placed from the SMAS-skin composite flap up to the mastoid.
- The periauricular skin is then trimmed and defatted along the tragus and posterior skin is excised.
- Staples are used in hair-bearing areas. Otherwise a subcuticular 4–0 Monocryl or simple running 4–0 Prolene is used.

10.2.5 Submental Liposuction

- This is carried out using a handheld fine cannula.
- The cannula is used to undermine the entire neck down to the sternal notch and separate skin-platysma attachments. This step is performed even if there is no submental fat.
- Selective fat removal of pre- and subplatysmal fat can be performed.
- In patients with heavier necks, it is important to perform liposuction below the platysma.
- Excessive bleeding from the vascular subplatysmal fat can be prevented by increasing the volume of local anesthetic infiltrated in the submental region.

10.3 Postoperative Care

- The senior author does not use drains. It is important to obtain hemostasis several times prior to closure.
- The head is wrapped overnight. Antibiotic ointment is applied to the incisions twice a day for 7 days.
- Staples and sutures are removed in 7 days.

10.4 Case Example

Pre- and postoperative photos of a 60-year-old patient, 6 months following a deep plane facelift technique in (a) anteroposterior (AP), (b) oblique, and (c) lateral views (▶ Fig. 10.5a–c).

10.5 Conclusion

The deep plane facelift is a comprehensive technique for facial and neck rejuvenation that addresses all anatomic components that contribute to facial aging.

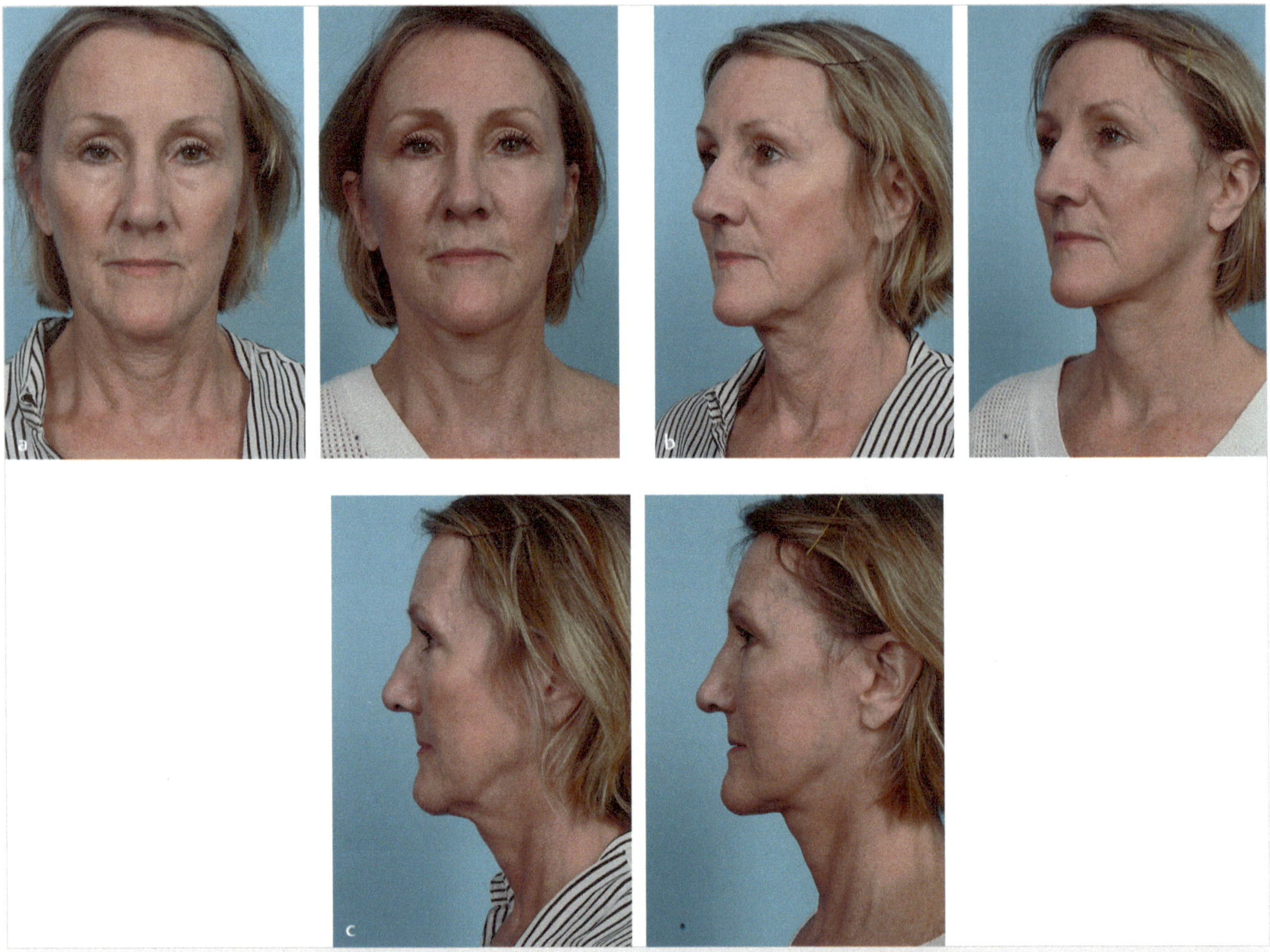

Fig. 10.5 **(a–c)** Pre- and postoperative photos of a 60-year-old patient, 6 months following a deep plane facelift technique in **(a)** anteroposterior (AP), **(b)** oblique, and **(c)** lateral views.

Further Readings

Mendelson BC. Surgery of the superficial musculoaponeurotic system: principles of release, vectors, and fixation. Plast Reconstr Surg. 2001; 107(6):1545–1552, discussion 1553–1555, 1556–1557, 1558–1561

Mustoe TA, Park E. Evidence-based medicine: facelift. Plast Reconstr Surg. 2014; 133 (5):1206–1213

Mustoe TA, Rawlani V, Zimmerman H. Modified deep plane rhytidectomy with a lateral approach to the neck: an alternative to submental incision and dissection. Plast Reconstr Surg. 2011; 127(1):357–370

Rohrich RJ, Sinno S, Vaca EE. Getting better results in facelifting. Plast Reconstr Surg Glob Open. 2019; 7(6):e2270

Swanson E. Outcome analysis in 93 facial rejuvenation patients treated with a deep-plane facelift. Plast Reconstr Surg. 2011; 127(2):823–834

11 SMAS Plication with Extended Platysma–SMAS Flap

Sherrell J. Aston, Joshua M. Cohen, and Sammy Sinno

Abstract

Modern facelift techniques have advanced in terms of better understanding of anatomy and maneuvers that produce the longest-lasting results. What was once a skin-only procedure has now evolved into surgery that addresses deeper tissues (superficial musculoaponeurotic system [SMAS] and platysma) independent of the skin, with a high degree of safety and a relatively short recovery period.

Keywords: Facelift, SMAS, Plication, extended platysma-SMAS

Key Points

- The superficial musculoaponeurotic system (SMAS) plication must be planned and executed meticulously.
- Adequate SMAS plication can achieve improvement in the volume over the zygoma, restore malar deflation, and correct lower facial laxity.
- Release of the submental crease, mandibular retaining ligaments, and platysma retaining ligaments allows for effective skin redraping and smooth chin and jawline contour.

11.1 Preoperative Steps

11.1.1 Planning

- Patients are encouraged to bring their youth photographs.
- Although limitations are discussed, a similar shape and greatly improved appearance can be obtained reliably.
- Almost always, the two sides of the face will be noticeably asymmetric. For instance, there will be a dominant cheek, wider palpebral aperture, long and short side, asymmetric brows, etc. These differences should be noted preoperatively.
- Skin quality, elasticity, extent of soft tissue descent (i.e., jowling), and underlying bony support are evaluated, as these qualities will all influence the final result.
- The neck is evaluated at rest and by having the patient tense the platysma muscle (i.e., grimace). Significant banding, an obtuse cervicomental angle, indistinct thyroid cartilage bulge, noticeable pre- and subplatysmal fat, and excess skin are all signs of neck aging (▶ Fig. 11.1).
- If patients exhibit significant signs of deflation in addition to descent of facial soft tissues, then autologous fat grafting should be considered.

11.2 Operative Steps

See **Video 11.1**.

11.2.1 Preparation

- The patient is marked preliminarily in the preoperative holding area and then brought to the operating room.
- After administration of general anesthesia, a neurosurgical headrest is used to allow proper head positioning and to allow the surgeon to operate slightly closer to the patient.
- A solution consisting of 150 cc of normal saline, 50 cc of 1% lidocaine, and 1 ampule of epinephrine is injected into the neck and the first side of the face.

11.2.2 Open Neck Treatment

- A #10 blade is used to open the submental incision and undermine the flap for 1 or 2 cm.
- Facelift scissors are then used to elevate the subcutaneous flap above the platysma muscle down to the level past the thyroid cartilage, commonly caudal to the first cervical crease.
- A single port liposuction cannula is used to remove fat off the medial borders of the left and right platysma muscle for better visualization.
- Interrupted 3–0 buried Mersilene sutures are placed to approximate the platysma in the midline (starting at the thyroid cartilage and working up), followed by a running layer on top of this repair (with 3–0 or 4–0 Mersilene).
- Commonly at this point, a several centimeter wedge of platysma is resected caudal to the repair if significant banding is present; this maneuver breaks the continuity of the band (▶ Fig. 11.2).
- Hemostasis is achieved; then a temporary gauze is placed.

11.2.3 Lateral Approach

- Either a pretragal or retrotragal incision is used. With the exception of secondary cases, an incision hidden in the temporal hair is also used. A full retrotragal incision is used in an S-shaped pattern, with a small non-hair bearing segment of incision in the retroauricular sulcus, which is covered by the ear.
- After making the preauricular stab incisions, the cheek flap is preliminarily undermined by suctioning with a 2.4-mm cannula. This facilitates flap dissection.

11.2.4 Flap Elevation

- The incisions are opened with a #10 blade and then undermined for several centimeters before switching to facelift scissors.
- In the cheek, precise flap elevation is paramount to balance flap vascularity while leaving enough tissue on the SMAS (▶ Fig. 11.3).
- In the temporal region, the flap is raised in a consistent subcutaneous plane to allow greater versatility in flap redraping.
- A transverse cut is made at an acceptable location along the sideburn, and two staples are placed at the medial extent of this incision to avoid flap tearing.
- Retroauricular flaps are kept thick to avoid flap ischemia, though great care is taken to avoid injury to the great auricular nerve, which can be identified 6.5 cm below the tragus.
- Once significant flap elevation has been achieved, a lighted retractor is used.

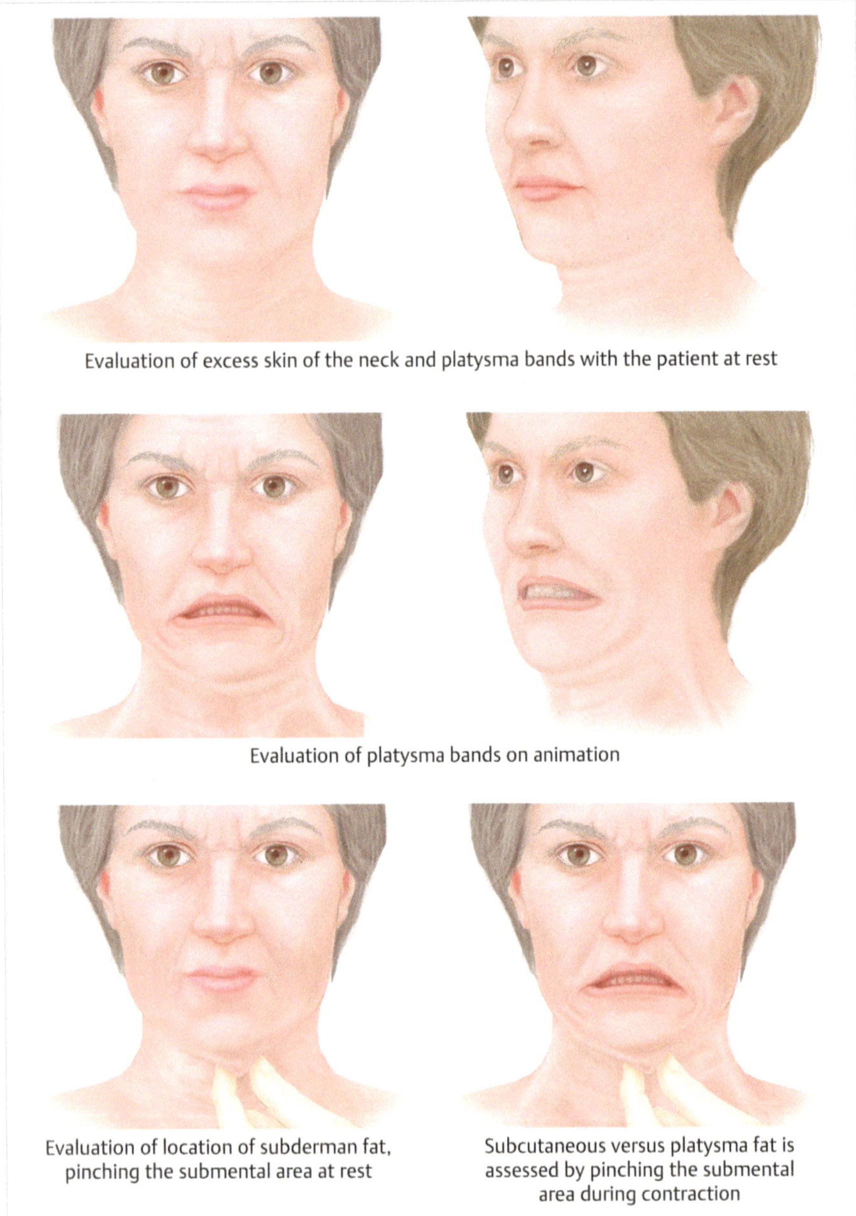

Fig. 11.1 Evaluation of the neck preoperatively.

- The subcutaneous flap is dissected caudally, releasing the mandibular ligament, and is then connected to the submental incision (▶ Fig. 11.4).
- It is critical to keep the platysma muscle down in this region as injury to a cervicomandibular branch can occur if dissection is deep to the muscle.

11.2.5 Lateral Platysma/SMAS Flap

- At the completion of subcutaneous flap undermining, where the endpoint is determined based on mobility and "feel," the angle of the mandible is marked.
- Below this mark, the lateral border of the platysma is briefly suctioned with the single port liposuction cannula and is then grasped with long smooth forceps, lifted, and elevated bluntly with vertical scissor spreads.
- Great care is taken to stay on the immediate undersurface of the muscle (and subsequent SMAS superiorly) to avoid facial nerve injury and injury to external jugular vein.
- Blunt spreading can be used, and the platysma retaining ligaments are released.
- The platysma-SMAS flap is secured to the mastoid fascia with 3–0 PDS.

11.2.6 SMAS Plication

- The zygomatic arch is palpated and marked (▶ Fig. 11.5).
- Using a pair of smooth forceps, the SMAS below the zygoma is grasped and brought superiorly to assess the amount of SMAS that can be plicated. The goal is to build volume over the zygoma, restore malar deflation, and correct lower facial laxity.

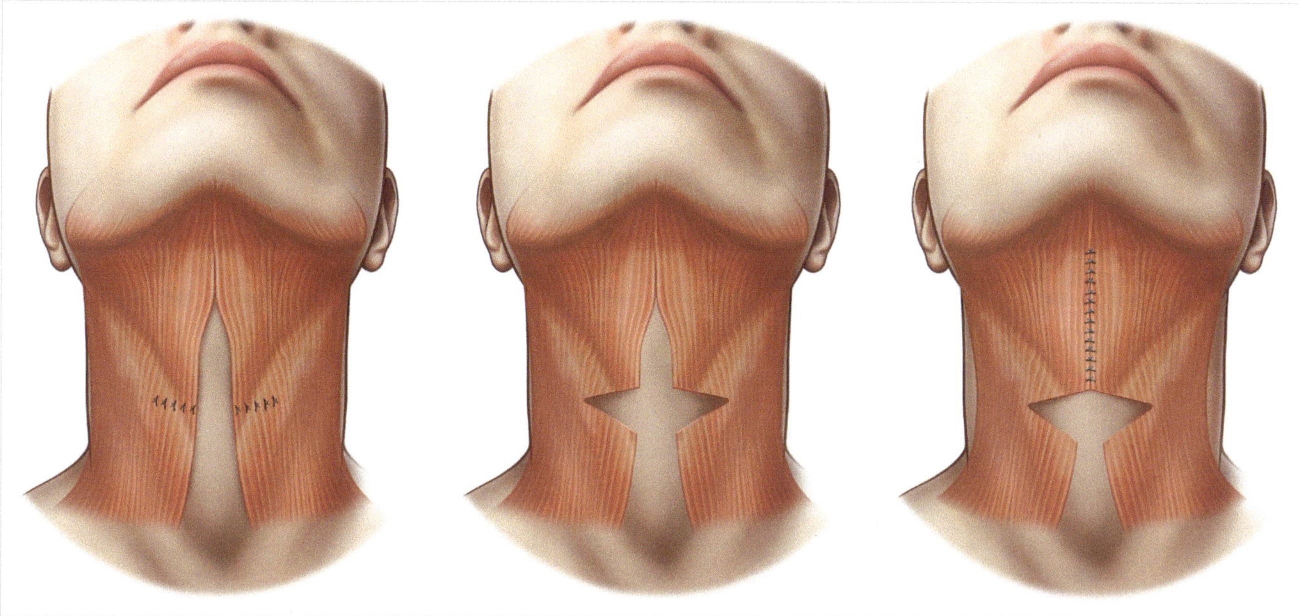

Fig. 11.2 Approximation of midline platysma and wedge resection of platysma caudal to repair, if banding is present.

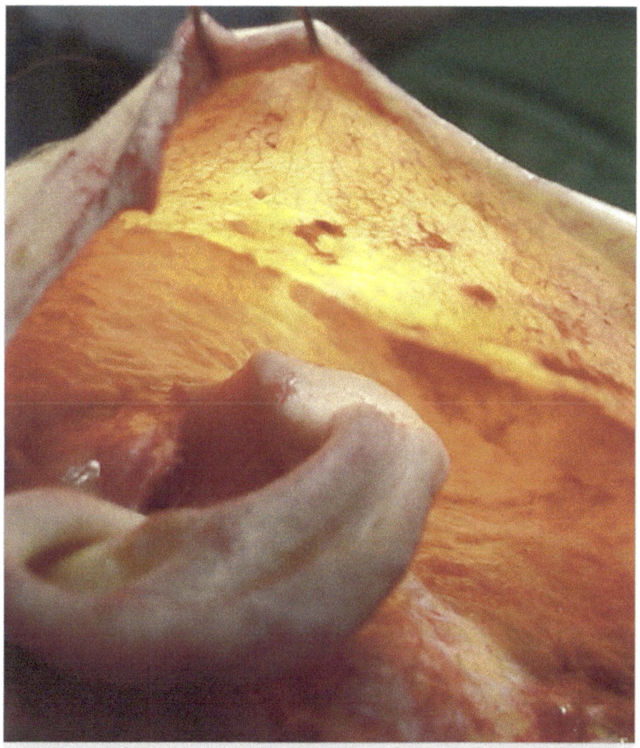

Fig. 11.3 Appearance of a transilluminated skin flap in the cheek. If dissection is in the proper plane, the fat on the undersurface of the flap will have a rough "cobblestone" appearance to it.

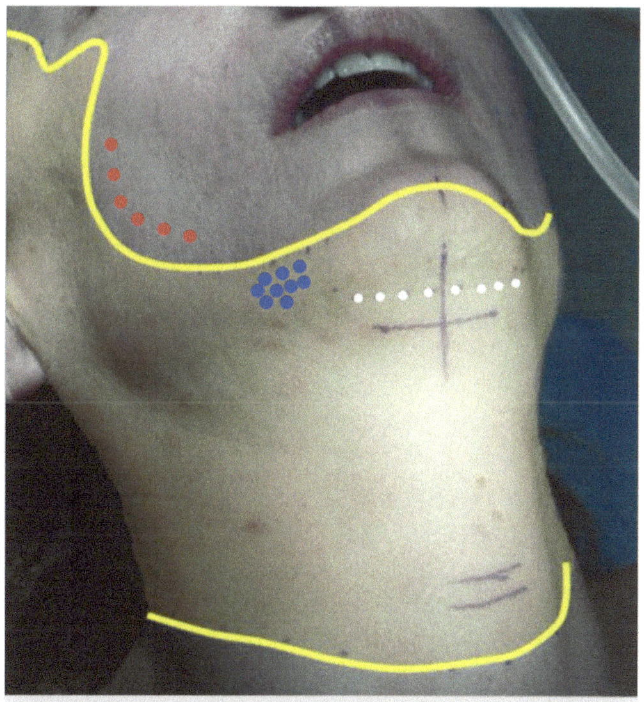

Fig. 11.4 Area of undermining subcutaneous flap and release of mandibular ligaments (*blue*) and submental crease (*white*).

- The SMAS is plicated medially starting at the level of the lateral canthus with interrupted 3–0 PDS sutures.
- The malar fat pad is anchored to periosteal soft tissue, but care is taken to avoid deep bites medially as injury to a facial nerve branch can occur.
- A second running 3–0 PDS layer is performed to smooth and even the plication.
- At this point, meticulous hemostasis is achieved, while removing any irregularities directly and dissecting any tethering points.
- The contralateral side can be injected with local anesthesia at this time.

11.2.7 Closure

- The skin is redraped and 3–0 Monocryl is placed in the deep dermis at the retroauricular apices as well as in the cheek at the level of the root of the helix.
- Excess skin is trimmed conservatively with care taken not to place undue tension.
- All the incisions in the hair are stapled, while the preauricular skin is closed with 5–0 nylon.
- The retroauricular skin is closed with a running 4–0 plain suture.
- A drain is placed in the retroauricular incision and secured with a plain suture.

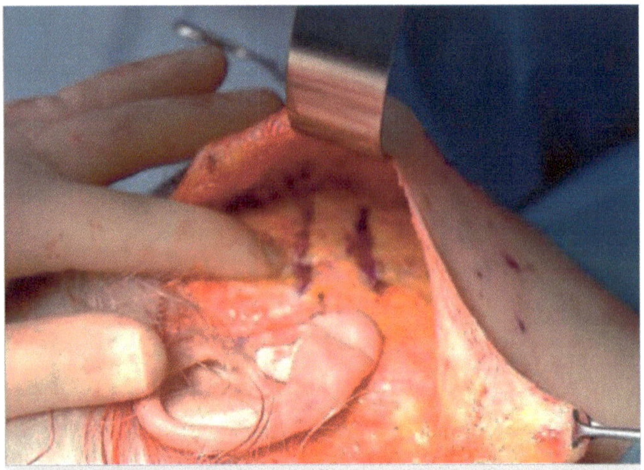

Fig. 11.5 Marking of the zygomatic arch for the upper extent of the superficial musculoaponeurotic system (SMAS) plication.

- At the conclusion of the second side, hemostasis is obtained in the neck, and the submental incision is closed with a running 5–0 nylon suture.
- The patient is placed in a multilayered head dressing.

11.3 Postoperative Care

- It is critical that blood pressure is strictly controlled in the perioperative period. Clonidine is frequently used.
- Patients are discharged from the recovery area with a private nurse to a nearby hotel and monitored overnight.
- Drains are commonly removed the next morning but if significant drainage occurs, they can be left longer.
- The dressings are removed in 1 or 2 days postoperatively.
- Patients can shower 1 day after drains and dressings are removed.
- Nylon sutures are removed on day 5 while all staples are removed on day 8.

11.4 Case Example

Pre- and postoperative photos of a 55-year-old patient, 2 years following the SMAS plication with extended platysma-SMAS flap technique, 4-lid blepharoplasty, and chin implant, in (a) anteroposterior (AP) and (b) oblique views (▶ Fig. 11.6a, b).

11.5 Conclusion

Significant jawline contouring can be achieved with formal elevation of the lateral platysma-SMAS. SMAS plication is a powerful procedure for building volume over the zygomatic highlights.

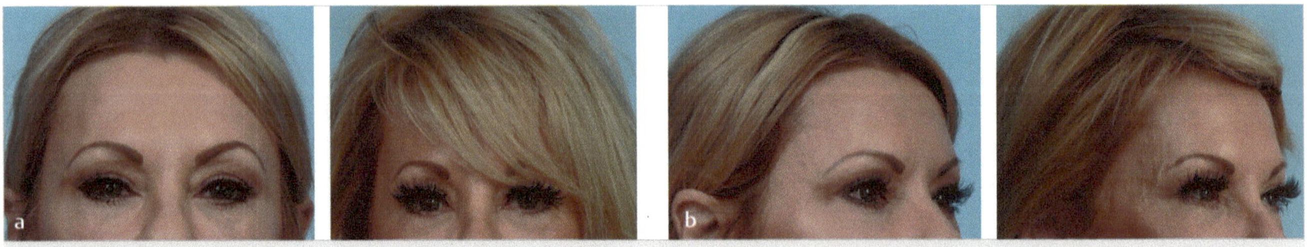

Fig. 11.6 Pre- and postoperative photos of a 55-year-old patient, 2 years following the SMAS plication with extended platysma–superficial musculoaponeurotic system (SMAS) flap technique, 4-lid blepharoplasty, and chin implant, in **(a)** anteroposterior (AP) and **(b)** oblique views.

Further Readings

Aston SJ. Platysma-SMAS cervicofacial rhytidoplasty. Clin Plast Surg. 1983; 10(3): 507–520

Baker DC, Stefani WA, Chiu ES. Reducing the incidence of hematoma requiring surgical evacuation following male rhytidectomy: a 30-year review of 985 cases. Plast Reconstr Surg. 2005; 116(7):1973–1985, discussion 1986–1987

Baker DC, Aston SJ, Guy CL, Rees TD. The male rhytidectomy. Plast Reconstr Surg. 1977; 60(4):514–522

Feldman JJ. Neck lift my way: an update. Plast Reconstr Surg. 2014; 134(6):1173–1183

Warren RJ, Aston SJ, Mendelson BC. Face lift. Plast Reconstr Surg. 2011; 128(6): 747e–764e

12 High SMAS Facelift and Necklift with Fat Grafting

Timothy Marten, Kristy L. Hamilton, and Dino Elyassnia

Abstract

Modern-day facial rejuvenation surgery has evolved significantly from simplistic lifting to advanced contouring techniques that re-establish a youthful, three-dimensional shape to the face and neck. Proper treatment of sagging facial tissue requires emphasis on superficial musculoaponeurotic system (SMAS) repositioning which allows only redundant skin to be excised and wound closure under no tension. This averts a tight, "pulled" appearance and produces high-quality scars. A high SMAS has the advantage of achieving a simultaneous lifting of the midface, lower cheek, and jowl. With the addition of volume, facial fat grafting allows surgeons to work in a different dimension of facial rejuvenation. This significantly amplifies the outcomes that can be obtained in comparison to traditional facelifting techniques alone. In the neck, the key principle is a reduction in volume. This is achieved by focusing on subplatysmal problems, which will allow precious subcutaneous fat to be preserved. This chapter will present analysis and technical considerations for performing a high SMAS flap, subplatysmal neck contouring, and comprehensive facial fat grafting.

Keywords: Facial fat grafting, facelift, necklift, high SMAS flap, subplatysmal fat, submandibular glands, digastric muscles, platysmaplasty

Key Points

- Proper treatment of sagging facial tissue requires emphasis on superficial musculoaponeurotic system (SMAS) repositioning which allows only redundant skin to be excised and wound closure under no tension. This averts a tight, "pulled" appearance and produces high-quality scars.
- A high SMAS flap planned along the upper border of the zygomatic arch has the advantage of achieving a simultaneous lifting of the midface, lower cheek, and jowl.
- In the neck, subplatysmal problems will contribute significantly to aging and require treatment in most cases if optimal results are to be obtained. Focus on the subplatysmal layer will allow precious subcutaneous fat to be preserved.
- With the addition of volume, fat grafting allows surgeons to work in a different dimension of facial rejuvenation which significantly amplifies the outcomes that can be obtained in comparison to traditional facelifting techniques alone.

12.1 Preoperative Steps

12.1.1 Analysis

- For the temporal portion of the facelift incision, each patient's cheek skin redundancy must be examined along with the location of temple and sideburn hair. If cheek skin redundancy is small and ample temple and sideburn hair is present, a temple incision can be placed within the temple scalp, otherwise a temple hairline incision should be used as is the case for most patients.
- Similar planning is performed for the occipital incision. If minimal excess neck skin is present, the incision can be placed transversely, high on the occipital scalp into the hair, otherwise the incision should be placed along the occipital hairline as is the case for most patients.
- The neck of each patient should be examined, noting the amount of preplatysmal and subplatysmal fat, size of submandibular glands, presence of static and dynamic platysmal bands, and visibility of prominent digastric muscles.
- Careful preoperative markings must be made in the sitting position to guide the precise location for fat grafting. These markings should be photographed and used intraoperatively to help guide treatment.

12.2 Operative Steps

See **Video 12.1**.

12.2.1 Fat Harvest and Facial Fat Grafting

- Fat is typically harvested from the hip or lateral thigh from both sides with the patient turned into a semilateral decubitus position with a limited prep and drape.
- Approximately 1 cc of a dilute 0.1% lidocaine with 1:1,000,000 epinephrine solution is injected into the harvest site for every 3 cc of anticipated fat removal. At least 120 cc of total fat is harvested for a typical case.
- Fat is harvested with manual, low-pressure aspiration using a 10-cc syringe and a 2.1 to 2.4 mm harvesting cannula.
- The unprocessed fat is then centrifuged for 1 to 3 minutes at 2,500 rpm.
- After discarding the oil and water components, fat is then transferred to 1-cc Luer lock syringes.
- The higher density fat or fat at the bottom of the syringe is considered better quality and used preferentially in the procedure.
- Fat grafting is performed at the beginning of the procedure as we believe it allows for more accurate placement of fat and overall improved outcomes.
- Injections are made using fine cannulas (0.7–1.2 mm) with multiple stab incisions throughout the face using a 20-gauge needle.
- Infiltration is made in a "spray painting" type fashion versus bolus injections to optimize the chance of graft viability. This requires rapid movement of a fine cannula with very slow movement of the plunger to disperse the fat in tiny aliquots.
- In most cases volume loss has occurred globally in the face and thus fat grafting must be performed in a fairly comprehensive manner as opposed to only treating a few limited regions.
- Ultimately this technique should be viewed as an artistic endeavor in terms of the volume and distribution of fat placement; however with time, a systematic approach to the face is developed, which requires separating the face into regions with a range of volumes used for each region (▶ Fig. 12.1).

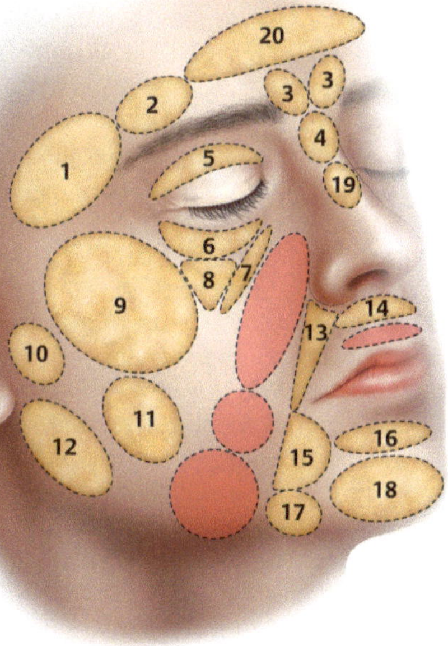

Anatomic region	Volume of fat
1) Temple	3–7 cc per side
2) Supra-brow	1–3 cc per side
3) Glabella	1–3 cc (total both sides)
4) Radix	1–3 cc (total both sides)
5) Supra-orbital	1–3 cc per side
6) Intra-orbital	1–3 cc per side
7) Naso-jugal groove ("tear trough")	0.5–1.5 cc per side
8) Mid-face	1–3 cc per side
9) Cheek	3–7 cc per side
10) Lateral face/pre-auricular	1–3 cc per side
11) Buccal recess	1–3 cc per side
12) Jaw line	3–9 cc per side
13) Nasolabial crease	0.5–1.5 cc per side
14) Pyriform	1–3 cc (total both sides)
15) Labiomandibular groove ("drool line")	1–3 cc per side
16) Labiomental sulcus ("chin crease")	2–4 cc (total both sides)
17) Geniomandibular groove ("GMG")	0.5–2 cc per side
18) Chin	1–3 cc per side
19) Nasal dorsum	1–3 cc (total both sides)
20) Forehead	2–4 cc per side

a

Area (region on illustration)	Cannula size/length	Tissue plane	Amount (per side) (except as noted)	Special considerations
Forehead	0.7 mm (20 ga) / 5 cm	Subcutaneous	2 to 4 cc	Most often treating depression in mid-central area and not entire forehead. (intermediate)
Supra-brow (2)	0.7 mm (20 ga) / 5 cm	Subcutaneous	1 to 3 cc	Goal is to blend prominent brow with forehead. (intermediate)
Glabella (3)	0.7 mm (20 ga) / 4 cm	Subcutaneous	1 to 3 cc* (total)	GF lines are not effectively treated with AFG unless neurotoxin also used. (intermediate)
Radix (4)	0.7 mm (20 ga) / 4 cm	Pre-periosteal to skin	1 to 3 cc* (total)	Can be continued on bridge of nose if inverted V or rhinoplasty irregularities present (19). (intermediate)
Temples (1)	0.9 mm (19 ga) / 5 cm	Subcutaneous	3 to 7 cc	Larger cannula less likely to perforate temporal veins. If vein perforated hold pressure on area for 3 to 5 minutes and may then resume injections. (intermediate)
Brow-supra-orbital ("upper eyelid") (5)	0.7 mm (20 ga) / 4 cm	Pre-periosteal/suborbicularis oculi	1 to 3 cc	Conceptualize as lowering the supra-orbital rim not filling the eyelid. Must protect ocular globe during fat infiltration. (advanced)
Infra-orbital ("lower eyelid") (6)	0.7 mm (20 ga) / 4 cm	Pre-periosteal/suborbicularis oculi	1 to 3 cc	Important to inject perpendicularly from below rather than parallel to defect. Must protect ocular globe during fat infiltration. (advanced)
Naso-jugal groove ("tear trough") (7)	0.7 mm (20 ga) / 4 cm	Pre-periosteal/suborbicularis oculi	0.5 to 1.5 cc	Important to inject perpendicularly from below rather than parallel to defect. (advanced)
Cheeks (9)	0.7 mm (20 ga) / 5 cm	Pre-periosteal to skin	3 to 7 cc	Must consider shape of forehead, prominence of chin, and width of mandible. If temples are hollow and not treated filling cheeks will look unnatural. Some of this fat will typically be encountered during subsequent SMAS dissection. (beginner)
Mid-face (8)	0.7 mm (20 ga) / 4 cm	Pre-periosteal to skin	1 to 3 cc	Overlaps infra-orbital, tear trough and cheek areas. (beginner)
Buccal recess (11)	0.7 mm (20 ga) / 5 cm	Subcutaneous	1 to 3 cc	(intermediate)
Lateral face / pre-auricular (10)	0.7 mm (20 ga) / 5 cm	Subcutaneous and sub-SMAS	1 to 3 cc	Carefully placed in pre-parotid sub-SMAS location, this fat will not be encountered during skin and SMAS flap dissections. (intermediate)
Nasolabial crease (13)	0.7 mm (20 ga) / 4 cm	Subcutaneous	0.5 to 1.5 cc	Inject superficially if treating NL crease – deep if treating maxillary recession. Injecting larger volumes won't improve results and can crease bizarre appearance. Over-filling NLC area can result in reduced dental show when smiling. (intermediate)
Pyriform (14)	0.7 mm (20 ga) / 4 cm	Pre-periosteal	1 to 3 cc* (total)	Project nasal tip. Over-filling can result in decreased upper dental show when smiling. (intermediate)
Columellar-labial junction	0.7 mm (20 ga) / 4 cm	Pre-periosteal to skin	0.5 to 1.5 cc	Improves columellar angle and projects tip of nose. (intermediate)
Upper lip	0.7 mm (20 ga) / 5 cm	Submucosal with emphasis on vermilion-cutaneous junction	0.5 to 1.5 cc	Injection should be made to create a central tubercle with a sulcus on each side of it. Upper lip should be distinctively smaller than lower lip (golden ratio). If upper lip the same size as lower lip the mouth will appear contrived and unnatural. (intermediate)
Lower lip	0.7 mm (20 ga) / 5 cm	Submucosal beneath vermilion	1 to 2.5 cc	Injection should be made to create a central sulcus with a tubercle on each side of it. Lower lip should be distinctively larger than lower lip (golden ratio). (intermediate)
Labiomental groove ("drool line") (15)	0.7 mm (20 ga) / 4 cm	Mucosa to skin	0.5 to 2 cc* (total)	Goal is to fill and add structure to entire region – not to spot fill crease. (intermediate)
Chin (18)	0.7 mm (20 ga) / 4 cm	Pre-periosteal to skin	1 to 3 cc	Exceeding 3 cc per side (6 cc total) can result in excessive vertical height and globular appearance of chin. (intermediate)
Labiomental sulcus ("chin crease") (16)	0.7 mm (20 ga) / 4 cm	Mucosa to skin	1 to 4 cc* (total)	Adds vertical height to chin. Useful with chin implant to avoid "implant look" (intermediate)
Geniomandibular groove (GMG) (17)	0.7 mm (20 ga) / 4 cm	Pre-periosteal to skin	1 to 3 cc	Goal is to integrate chin and jawline to create smooth, continuous aesthetic line. (beginner)
Jawline (12)	1.2 mm (18 ga) / 6 cm	Pre-periosteal/submasseteric	3 to 9 cc	Approached medial to lateral from puncture near corner of mouth – Injection made on face of bone, not subcutaneously, into muscle, or into parotid. (intermediate)

* **Important notes regarding recommended amounts:**

1) Amounts listed in table above are amount administered **per side** except where noted with asterisk and "(total)"
2) Amounts listed in table above are for fat harvested with a 2.1 to 2.4 mm harvesting cannula centrifuged for 1-3 min at 1,000 rpm administered to average sized female head in 0.5 cc aliquots as part of a facelift procedure. Larger amounts may be required for un-centrifuged or "tea strained" fat, larger female faces, male patients, and patients not undergoing facelift procedures.
3) A prudent and proven strategy for determining the amount of fat needed for a given site is to **rate the severity of the defect based on what is seen in the pre-operative photos, and then to use empirical data (above) to chose the amount to be administered.** As a practical matter this amounts to simply rating the severity of the problem at each proposed site of treatment as "small", "medium" and "large", and then using data above to determine the amount typically needed for treatment of each area. If the defect is "small" one would choose an amount from the low end of the recommended range. If the defect is "large" one would choose an amount from the high end, and if "medium" somewhere in between.

b

Fig. 12.1 (a, b) Marten clinic of plastic surgery: facial fat grafting reference guidelines.

- For most regions, multiple planes of injection are used. The major exception is around the eyes where one should adhere to a deep pre-periosteal plane.

12.2.2 Skin Elevation

- For sensory nerve blocks and for infiltrating the area marked for incision, 0.25% bupivacaine with epinephrine 1:200,000 is used.
- Areas of subcutaneous dissection are infiltrated with 0.1% lidocaine with epinephrine 1:1,000,000. A total of approximately 400 to 500 cc is used.
- In most cases, a temple hairline incision is used to prevent excessive hairline displacement.
- The prehelical portion of the preauricular incision should be made as a soft curve paralleling the curve of the anterior border of the helix. As the tragus is approached, the incision is carried into the depression superior to it and then into a retrotragal position.
- At the inferior portion of the tragus the incision must turn anteriorly and then again inferiorly into the crease between the anterior lobule and cheek. The incision will then continue around the lobule and precisely within the auriculomastoid crease.
- In most cases, the incision should be placed along the occipital hairline but then turned into the scalp at the junction of the thick and thin hair at the nape of the neck. This design will avoid notching of the occipital hairline.
- All skin flap elevation is carried out using a medium Metzenbaum scissors.
- Skin elevation begins with the postauricular skin flap at the most inferior point of the occipital hairline incision. At this point more subcutaneous fat is present and the proper plane is easier to identify. The dissection then continues anteriorly to release the postauricular skin and then over the lateral neck.
- In the cheek, it is easiest to begin skin flap elevation in front of the lobule.
- In order to avoid thinning of the SMAS, the cheek skin flap must be elevated in a slightly more superficial plane compared to the neck. If dissection is in the proper plane, transilluminated flaps will have a rough "cobblestone" appearance.
- A submental incision is made approximately 1 to 2 cm posterior to the submental crease and the crease along with the mandibular ligaments is released. The dissection of the anterior neck skin flap will be more easily performed through it rather than the postauricular incisions.
- The neck should be undermined completely in most cases. However, it should not arbitrarily include the entire face (▶ Fig. 12.2). Preservation of the anterior platysma-cutaneous ligaments in the perioral cheek will allow a better SMAS effect in this area that would otherwise be lost with wide undermining.

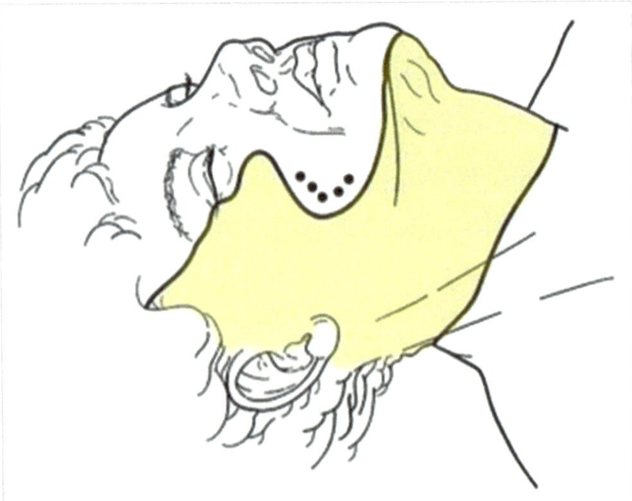

Fig. 12.2 Extent of subcutaneous undermining. *Shaded* area shows area of subcutaneous undermining. Note that the platysma-cutaneous ligaments (*black dots*) are not undermined and are preserved.

12.2.3 Neck Contouring

- Following neck skin elevation through the submental incision, the subplatysmal space is exposed by elevating platysmal muscle flaps.
- Hugging the underside of the platysma, the dissection is carried laterally over the anterior belly of the digastric, exposing the submandibular gland.
- Next, all subplatysmal fat lying superficial to a plane tangent to the anterior bellies of the digastric muscles should be theoretically removed, leaving interdigastric fat in place.
- The subplatysmal fat is typically triangular in shape with the base of the triangle over the hyoid and the two sides lying along the digastric muscles (▶ Fig. 12.3a, b).
- For patients in the typical facelift or necklift age group, little, if any, subcutaneous fat will need to be removed.
- Prominent submandibular glands will be encountered just lateral to the digastric muscle. Reduction is begun by incising the capsule overlying the gland and performing a thorough intracapsular mobilization of the gland.

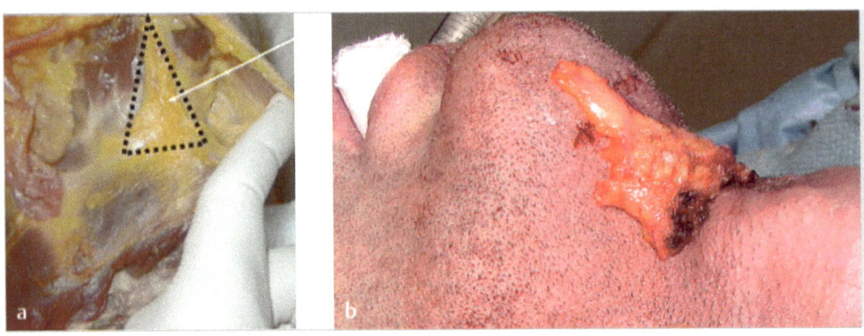

Fig. 12.3 **(a)** Cadaveric demonstration of subplatysmal fat (*arrow*). The right and left borders of the platysma have been elevated. The subplatysmal fat pad can be seen overlying the digastric muscles to the upper right and left of the *triangle* with the hyoid bone at the base of the triangle. **(b)** Intraoperative demonstration of the subplatysmal fat specimen lying over the submental space from which it was removed. The patient's chin is pointing superiorly with the neck to the right.

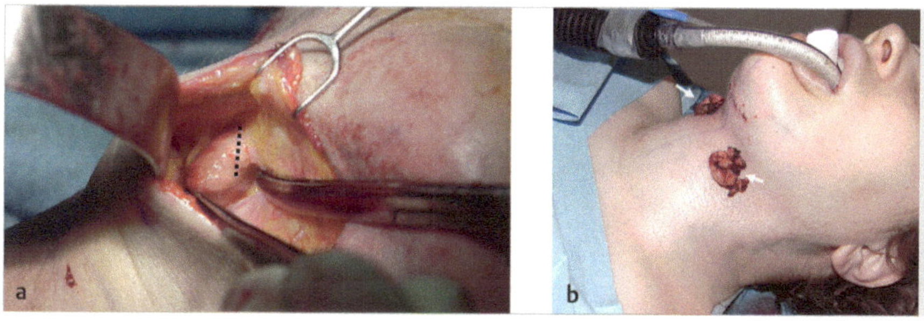

Fig. 12.4 **(a)** Intraoperative photo prior to resection of the excess portion of the gland. The gland has been mobilized and gently pulled inferiorly. The *dotted line* represents the level at which the inferior portion of the gland will be excised. **(b)** Patient seen immediately after necklift that included submandibular reduction. The excised portions of the glands are demonstrated on both the right and left sides (*arrows*).

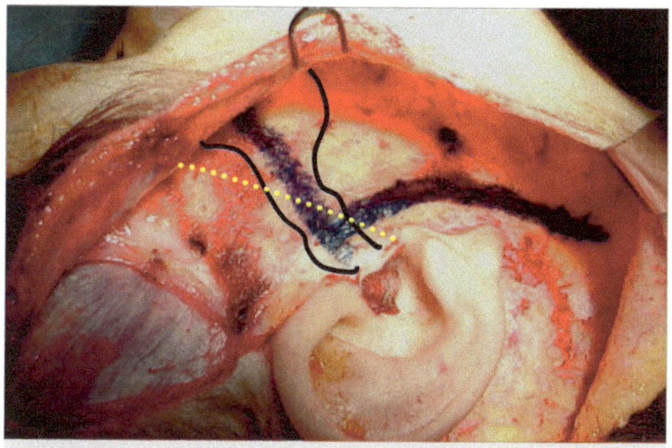

Fig. 12.5 Plan for "high superficial musculoaponeurotic system (SMAS)" flap. The superior margin of flap is planned over the zygomatic arch. The frontal branch of the facial nerve (*dashed line*) lies safely posterior and deep to the majority of the dissection.

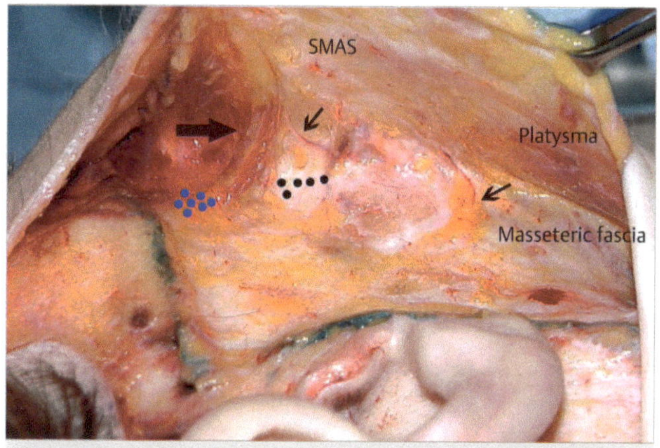

Fig. 12.6 Completed superficial musculoaponeurotic system (SMAS) flap elevation. Inferior to the origin of the zygomaticus major muscle (*large arrow*) lies the zone of transition between the zygomatic (*blue dots*) and masseteric-cutaneous ligaments (*black dots*) and the most potentially dangerous part of the SMAS dissection. Proper liberation and release of the SMAS flap usually require at least partial division of restraining attachments in this area, but moves the dissection into very close proximity to the zygomatic branch of the facial nerve (*small arrows*).

- Once mobilized, the redundant portion of the gland, which is defined as the portion protruding below a plane tangent to the ipsilateral mandibular border and the anterior belly of the digastric muscle, is incrementally removed (▶ Fig. 12.4a, b).
- After subplatysmal fat and submandibular gland reduction have been performed, superficial subtotal anterior digastric myectomy should be done using a tangential strip excision method.
- Once these maneuvers are completed, an anterior platysmaplasty is performed by first trimming the redundant portion of the medial platysmal borders followed by edge-to-edge approximation in one layer using interrupted sutures. Note that cheek SMAS flaps should be suspended prior to anterior platysmaplasty.
- Platysma myotomy should be performed after anterior platysmaplasty if indicated.
- Prior to skin closure, a drain should be placed in the subplatysmal space and a second drain placed subcutaneously.

12.2.4 SMAS Elevation and Suspension

- Markings for the SMAS flap include a line "high" over the mid portion of the zygomatic arch from the infraorbital rim to the superior tragus. It then turns inferiorly and posteriorly to the anterior border of the sternocleidomastoid. The frontal branch will be deep to and away from the majority of the dissection (▶ Fig. 12.5).
- SMAS dissection can be performed with Metzenbaum scissors or cautery set to low.
- In the lower cheek, SMAS dissection must be carried over the anterior border of the parotid to insure release of parotid-masseteric ligaments.
- In the upper cheek, dissection is more extensive and must include release of the zygomatic ligaments near the origin of the zygomaticus major muscle and at least partial division of masseteric-cutaneous ligaments inferiorly (▶ Fig. 12.6).
- The endpoint to the SMAS dissection is ultimately clinical and not anatomic. Gentle traction on the superior margin of the flap should produce motion at the nasal ala, philtrum, and stomal angle.
- Once released, the superior margin of the SMAS flap is secured in a posterior-superior vector parallel to the long axis of the zygomaticus major muscle.
- To provide additional support to the anterior neck, the excess tissue along the posterior margin of the SMAS flap is used as a postauricular transposition flap and secured to the mastoid fascia but only after completion of the anterior platysmaplasty.

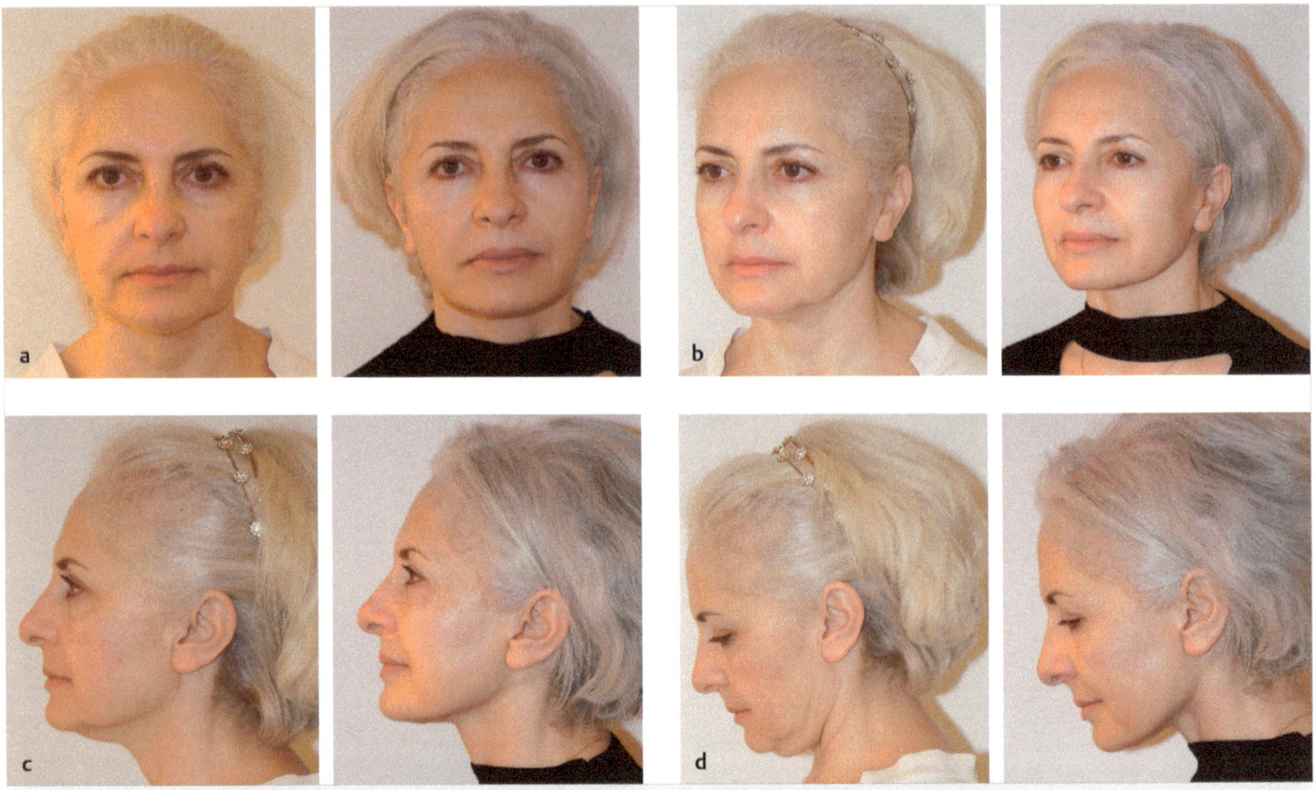

Fig. 12.7 Pre- and postoperative photos of a patient 2 years following facelift, necklift, and temple lift, comprehensive facial fat grafting, and laser resurfacing to the lower eyelids and perioral area in **(a)** anteroposterior (AP), **(b)** oblique, **(c)** lateral, and **(d)** Connell views. (Courtesy of Dino Elyassnia MD, FACS.)

12.2.5 Skin Flap Repositioning, Trimming, and Closure

- Skin flaps should be shifted in a slightly more posterior direction than that of the SMAS to avoid unnatural appearances.
- Cheek skin flaps should be shifted along a vector roughly perpendicular to the nasolabial fold while neck skin should be shifted along a vector parallel to the mandibular border.
- It is critical to remember that the goal of skin excision is to remove redundancy and not tighten the skin flap.
- The earlobe must be inset in a superior position and slightly posterior compared to the long axis of the ear to avoid a tell-tale abnormal earlobe position or frank pixie ear.

12.3 Postoperative Care

- All patients are instructed to sleep flat on their backs without a pillow or with a small cylindrical neck roll. This posture averts folding of the neck skin flap.
- Most patients are discharged to an aftercare specialist for the first night with specific instructions. Patients are asked to rest quietly and apply cool compresses to their eyes for the first 3 days.
- Drains are usually left in the neck until the first postoperative visit 4 to 5 days after surgery. Sutures are removed in two visits over a period of 7 days.
- Patients begin a daily routine of showering and shampooing no later than 3 days after their procedure.
- Patients are asked to set aside 2 to 3 weeks to recover from surgery and are advised to avoid all strenuous activity during the first 2 weeks after surgery.

12.4 Case Example

Pre- and postoperative photos of a patient 2 years following facelift, necklift, temple lift, comprehensive facial fat grafting, and laser resurfacing to the lower eyelids and perioral area in (a) anteroposterior (AP), (b) oblique, (c) lateral, and (d) Connell views (▶ Fig. 12.7a–d).

12.5 Conclusion

Facial rejuvenation can be achieved through the combination of lifting of sagging facial tissue, volume addition in the face, and volume reduction in the neck.

A high SMAS flap planned along the upper border of the zygomatic arch achieves a simultaneous lifting of the midface, lower cheek, and jowl.

Autologous fat grafting is an excellent tool for comprehensive facial volume restoration.

For neck contouring, subplatysmal problems will contribute significantly to aging and will require proper volume reduction in most cases.

Further Readings

Marten TJ. Simultaneous facelift and fat grafting: combined lifting and filling of the face. In: Nahai F, ed. The Art of Aesthetic Surgery. 2nd ed. Thieme; 2011

Marten T, Elyassnia D. Neck lift: defining anatomic problems and choosing appropriate treatment strategies. Clin Plast Surg. 2018; 45(4):455–484

Marten T, Elyassnia D. Facial fat grafting: why, where, how, and how much. Aesthetic Plast Surg. 2018; 42(5):1278–1297

Marten TJ. Elyassnia D. Simultaneous facelift and fat grafting: combined lifting and filling of the aging face. In: Coleman SR, Mazzola R, Pu L, eds. Fat Injection: From Filling to Regeneration. 2nd ed. Thieme; 2018

Marten TJ, Elyassnia D. Simultaneous facelift and fat grafting. In: Connell BF, ed. Aesthetic Rejuvenation of the Face and Neck. Thieme; 2016

13 Fat Grafting to the Face as an Isolated Procedure

Rod J. Rohrich, Erez Dayan, and Ira L. Savetsky

Abstract

The discovery of facial fat compartments and loss of volume in these compartments with aging has been well described. Both deep and superficial fat compartments lose volume, which contributes significantly to facial aging. The purpose of this chapter is to describe the authors' approach to full facial revolumization and restoration of fat compartment volume using autologous fat.

Keywords: Fat grafting, facial fat compartments, autologous fat, facial revolumization

Key Points

- Detailed preoperative facial analysis is critical to accurately identify and correct facial asymmetry.
- Key deep compartments include nasolabial and deep malar compartments. More superficial compartments include middle malar, superior cheek, temporal, perioral, and submental (▶ Fig. 13.1 and ▶ Fig. 13.2).
- Deep facial compartments are always restored first because they are the foundation of facial volumization (▶ Fig. 13.3). Preoperative bony contour and distribution of fullness dictate the contour and volume of grafting.

13.1 Preoperative Steps

- The facial rejuvenation procedure begins with a thorough preoperative analysis to identify areas of volume deflation and rhytides.
- Areas of volume deflation as well as deep rhytides are marked preoperatively in the dependent position to facilitate intraoperative accuracy.
- Careful donor site assessment and estimation of volume needed for volume restoration are key to a well-planned operation.
- Discussion with the patient is important to manage expectations of donor site incision placement.
- Fat is generally harvested from the medial thigh as this area contains the highest concentration of stromal vascular cells and is associated with the least amount of pain.

13.2 Operative Steps

See **Video 13.1**.

13.2.1 Fat Harvest

- Fat is typically harvested from the medial thighs with manual, low-pressure aspiration using a 10-cc syringe and a 3-mm multihole cannula.
- To optimize cell viability, no local anesthetic or epinephrine is used before aspiration.
- The aspirate is centrifuged for 1 minute at 2,250 rpm to remove cellular debris.
- The supernatant and infranatant are discarded before transferring the fat graft into 1-cc syringes.
- Fractionated fat is developed by emulsification of centrifuged fat between two 10-cc syringes through a 2-mm filter 60 to 80 times. Fractionated fat is primarily used for periorbital injections.
- Fat is then isolated and transferred to 1-cc syringes.

13.2.2 Facial Fat Augmentation

- The cheek is approached with a 14-gauge needle allowing access for a 2-mm blunt-tip Coleman cannula. Single entry point adjacent to the alar base provides access to deep and superficial cheek compartments. Antegrade/retrograde injections always begin deep, addressing nasolabial and deep medial compartments first, followed by superficial fat compartments.
- Augmentation of the mandibular border can greatly aid in creating a more aesthetic jawline. Up to 2 mm of chin projection can be achieved with fat grafting to correct mild microgenia.
- Temporal injection is performed using a single-port access within the temporal hairline. The key principle is disruption of the temporal fusion line to allow uniform fill in a radial fashion just lateral to the lateral brow.
- Central forehead injections must correct three distinct compartments—the glabella and the two superior brow regions. Injection is performed in the subcutaneous plane using an access point either in a mid-forehead crease (for those with long forehead) or in the hairline (for those with a shorter forehead).
- Perioral rejuvenation focuses small aliquots around the commissures in a cross-radial fashion, and into the philtral columns, providing subtle but vital restoration of youthful features. The senior author does not recommend injection into the vermilion of the lips due to the unpredictable nature of fat graft take within the lip.
- Fractionated fat is ideal for the periorbital region. Injection is performed through three separate access points in an

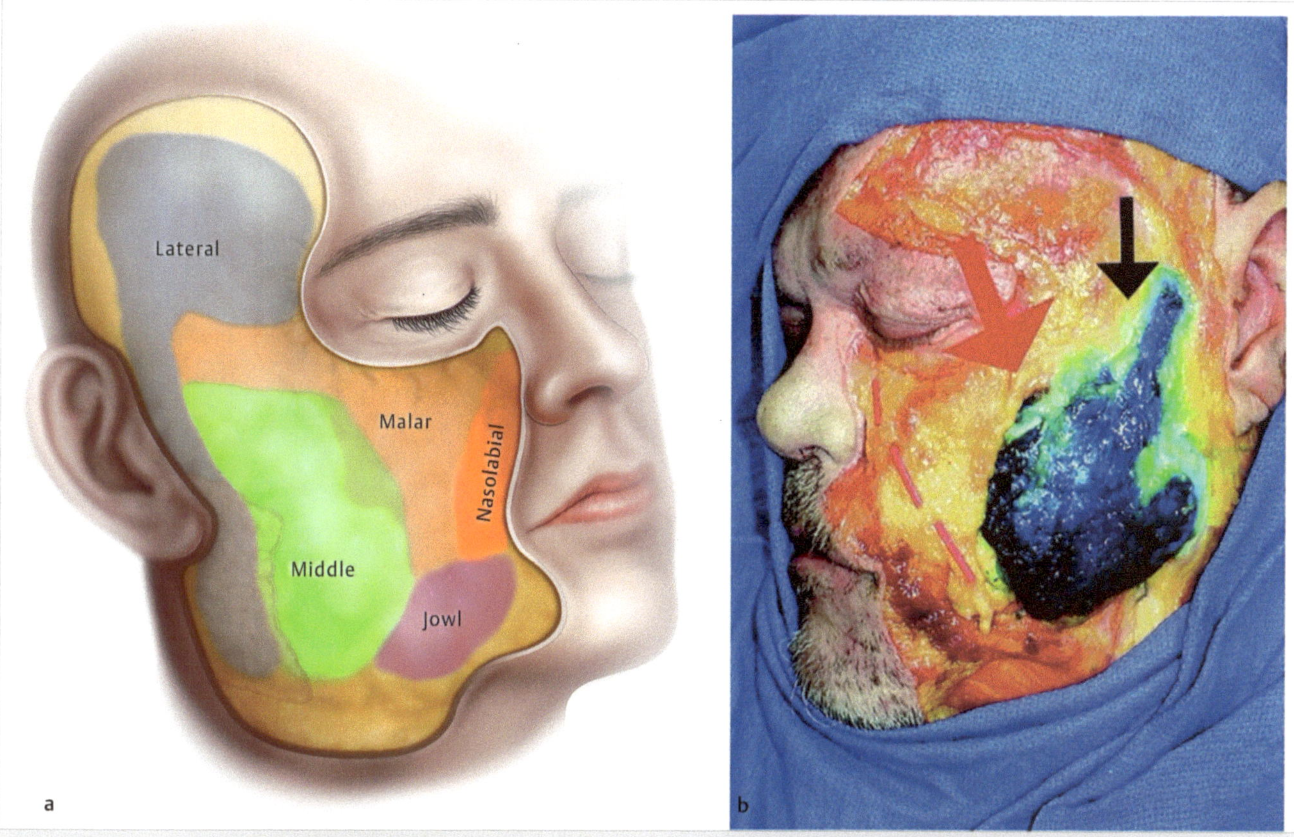

Fig. 13.1 **(a)** The superficial facial fat compartments are situated in the subcutaneous plane, partitioned by the terminal extensions of the retaining ligaments. The five superficial compartments of the cheek from lateral to medial are (1) lateral, (2) middle, (3) malar, (4) jowl, and (5) nasolabial. Each compartment has its own septal boundaries, a separate perforator blood supply, and its own tendency to deflation on aging. **(b)** Cadaver dissection of the facial fat compartments of the cheek. The inked compartment shown is the middle compartment. The *red arrow* marks the transition between the middle and malar compartments, which are separated by a high density of zygomatic ligaments along the lateral zygoma. (Reproduced with permission from Rohrich R, Stuzin J, Dayan E, Ross E. Facial Danger Zones. New York: Thieme; 2019.)

equilateral triangle configuration using a blunt cannula. The sequence of injection commences inferiorly into the cheek–orbital rim junction disrupting orbital retaining ligament in the suborbicularis plane, superiorly along medial superior orbital rim in a supraperiosteal plane, and along the lateral orbital rim and canthus.

- Fat augmentation is the ideal method for correction of deflated ear lobes. A 21-gauge needle is used for direct injection into the lobule with correction of the deformity as the end point.

13.3 Postoperative Care

- Patients rest with head elevated to 45 degrees.
- Cold compresses are applied to the face intermittently for the first 72 hours postoperatively.
- Patients are instructed to avoid strenuous activity for 2 to 4 weeks post facial fat grafting and use caution when applying glasses to avoid compression over grafted areas.

13.4 Case Example

A 57-year-old female who underwent facial fat augmentation. Autologous fat was harvested from the medial thigh and then prepared with centrifugation (2,250 rpm for 3 minutes). Facial fat compartments focused on were the deep nasolabial, deep medial malar, along with the lateral cheek compartments. Fractionated fat was used for periorbital augmentation and blending of the lower eyelid–cheek junction (▶ Fig. 13.4a–d).

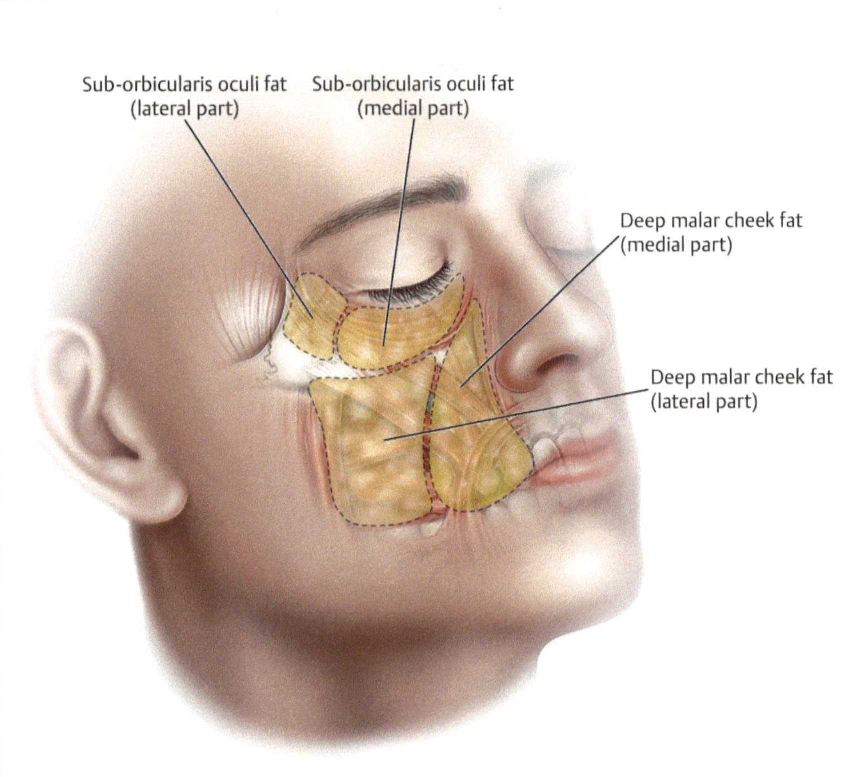

Fig. 13.2 The deep facial fat compartments are situated deep to the mimetic muscles and superficial to the periosteum of the midface. The deep fat of the lower eyelid is located just deep to the orbicularis oculi and is divided into medial and lateral components. The deep malar fat similarly is situated deep to the elevators of the upper lip and is separated into medial and lateral components. In youth, the deep periorbital fat blends with the deep malar fat to volumetrically support the lower eyelid and cheek. Aging causes deflation of deep fat resulting in the loss of anterior cheek volume and an abrupt demarcation along the eyelid–cheek junction, and it contributes to the formation of the infraorbital V-deformity. (Reproduced with permission from Rohrich R, Stuzin J, Dayan E, Ross E. Facial Danger Zones. New York: Thieme; 2019.)

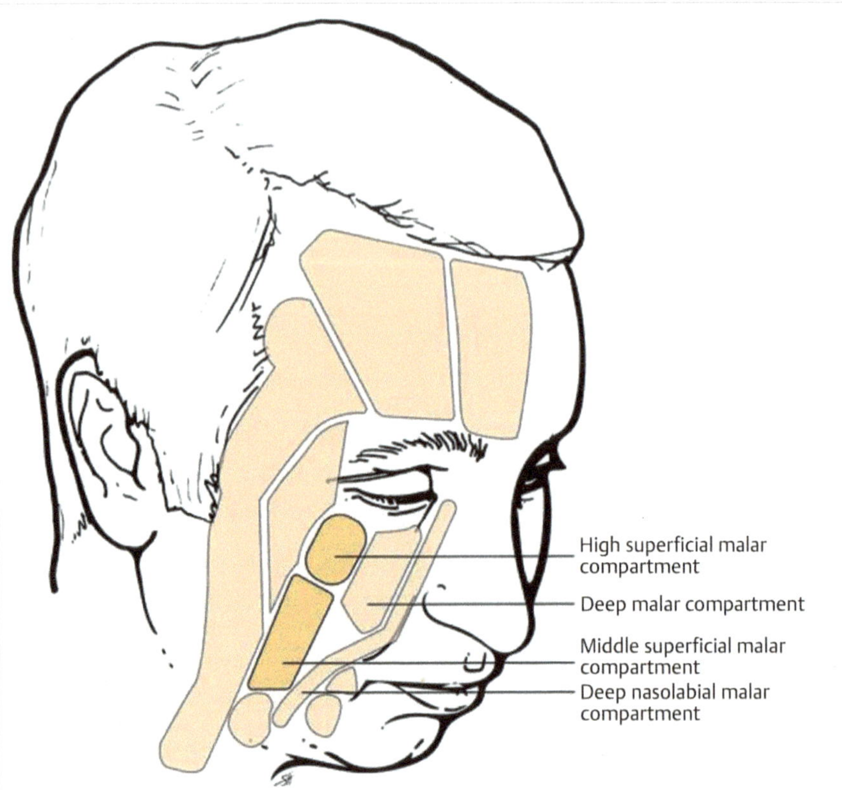

Fig. 13.3 Four key midfacial fat compartments to address with fat grafting in facial rejuvenation procedures. (Reproduced with permission from Schultz K, Raghuram A, Davis M, et al. Fat grafting for facial rejuvenation. Semin Plast Surg 2020;34(1):30–37.)

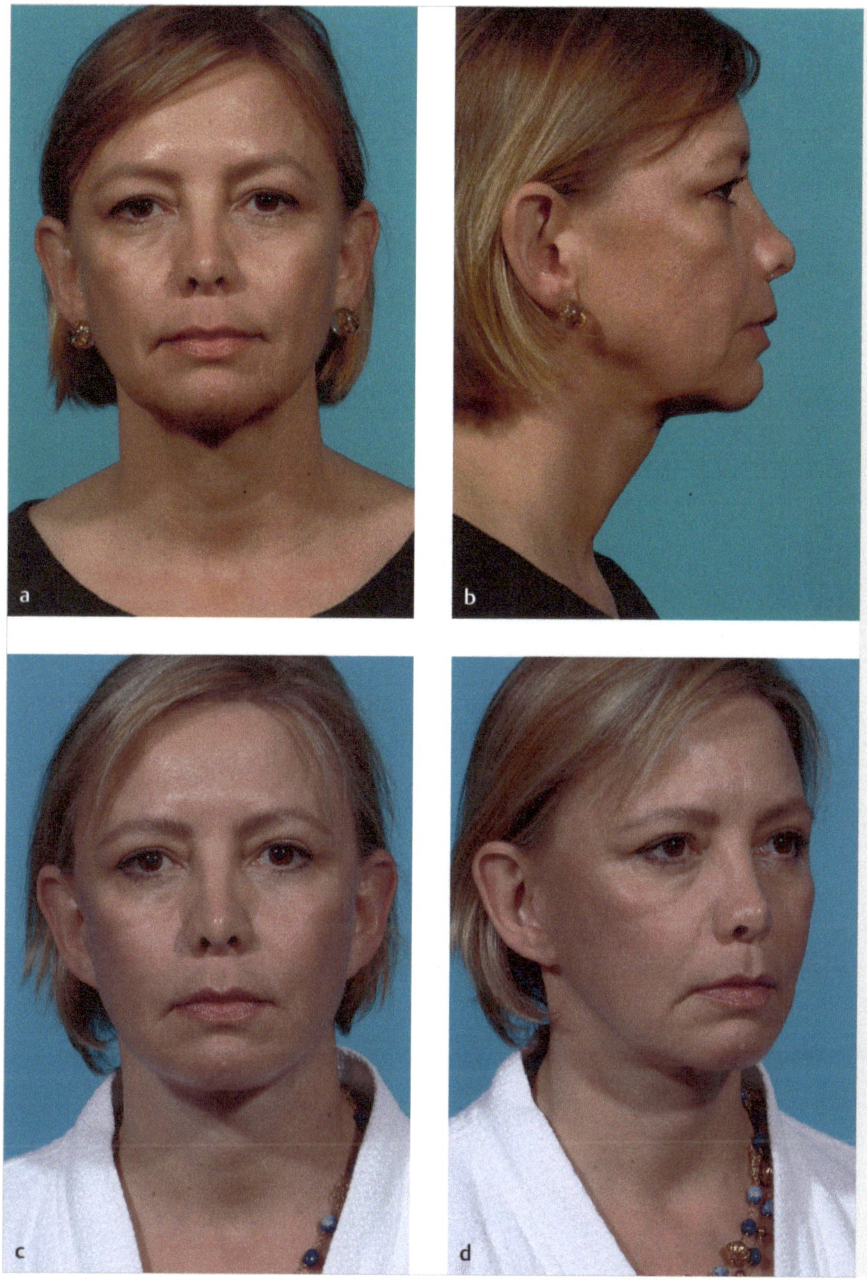

Fig. 13.4 (a–d) A 57-year-old female who underwent facial fat augmentation. Autologous fat was harvested from the medial thigh and then prepared with centrifugation (2,250 rpm for 3 minutes). Facial fat compartments focused on were the deep nasolabial, deep medial malar, along with the lateral cheek compartments. Fractionated fat was used for periorbital augmentation and blending of the lower eyelid–cheek junction.

13.5 Conclusion

Volume restoration with autologous fat of the facial fat compartments is essential to facial rejuvenation. It can be used independently or as an adjunct to rhytidectomy and blepharoplasty. Accurate preoperative facial analysis, knowledge of fat compartment anatomy, and precise intraoperative techniques are needed for successful outcomes.

Further Readings

Coleman SR. Facial augmentation with structural fat grafting. Clin Plast Surg. 2006; 33(4):567–577

Lambros V. Observations on periorbital and midface aging. Plast Reconstr Surg. 2007; 120(5):1367–1376, discussion 1377

Owsley JQ. Lifting the malar fat pad for correction of prominent nasolabial folds. Plast Reconstr Surg. 1993; 91(3):463–474, discussion 475–476

Rohrich RJ, Ghavami A, Constantine FC, Unger J, Mojallal A. Lift-and-fill face lift: integrating the fat compartments. Plast Reconstr Surg. 2014; 133(6):756e–767e

Rohrich RJ, Pessa JE. The fat compartments of the face: anatomy and clinical implications for cosmetic surgery. Plast Reconstr Surg. 2007; 119(7):2219–2227, discussion 2228–2231

Stuzin JM. Restoring facial shape in face lifting: the role of skeletal support in facial analysis and midface soft-tissue repositioning. Plast Reconstr Surg. 2007; 119(1):362–376, discussion 377–378

Part II

Rhinoplasty

II

14 The Rhinoplasty Consult

Rod J. Rohrich and Ira L. Savetsky

Abstract

The initial consultation is an integral component when deciding if a patient is suitable for surgery. The patient should identify their top three nasal aesthetic and/or functional concerns and record them precisely. The surgeon's goals and patient's expectations must be aligned. Caution should be taken in any patients that exhibit unrealistic expectations or signs of underlying psychosocial issues.

Keywords: Rhinoplasty, rhinoplasty consult, nasofacial analysis, expectations, red flag

Key Points

- A comprehensive and systematic nasofacial analysis is the most critical initial step in establishing goals and formulating a precise surgical plan for aesthetic nasal surgery.
- Setting realistic expectations with the patient is critical in achieving high postoperative patient satisfaction.

14.1 Preoperative Planning

14.1.1 Defining Rhinoplasty Goals

- Have the patient list their top three nasal aesthetic and/or functional concerns and record them precisely.

14.1.2 Focused Nasal History

- The patient should be asked about a history of allergic or inflammatory disorders such as hay fever, asthma, rhinitis, and sinusitis.
- Patients with long-standing allergic rhinitis typically have nasal obstruction due to inferior turbinate hypertrophy.
- Prior nasal trauma and operations including rhinoplasty, septal reconstruction/septoplasty, and sinus surgery should be noted and, when possible, prior operative reports should be reviewed.
- A review of smoking status, alcohol consumption, and use of illicit drugs, particularly cocaine, is essential as these behaviors can affect outcomes.
- Medications and dietary supplements such as acetylsalicylic acid, nonsteroidal anti-inflammatory drugs, and fish oil should be reviewed as they can increase bleeding and ecchymosis.

14.1.3 Nasofacial Proportions and Systematic Nasal Analysis

- See ▶ Table 14.1.

"10–7–5" Nasal Analysis

- On the front view, evaluation should include 10 key areas: Facial proportions, skin type/quality, symmetry/nasal deviation, dorsal aesthetic lines, bony vault, midvault, nasal tip, alar rims, alar base, and upper lip.
  - Facial proportions: Evaluation of the patient should include static and dynamic views to identify possible dynamic changes of the nose and upper lip while smiling. Examples of application of nasofacial analysis are the facial golden proportions (three similar distances: trichion-to-eye, nose-to-chin, and eye-to-mouth) and ratios (equivalent horizontal thirds: hairline-to-brows, brows-to-nasal base, and nasal base-to-menton; vertical fifths: limits adjacent to the most lateral projection of the head, the lateral canthi, and the medial canthi).
  - Skin type/quality: Skin thickness can be a major factor affecting rhinoplasty outcomes. Thin skin may show reconstructed nasal frame imperfections; however, nasal shape definition is more easily achieved. A thicker skin can camouflage minor imperfections, but reduces the surface contour definition due to prolonged edema and inflammation that can lead to scaring and unfavorable aesthetics. Nasal skin is thickest at the radix and nasal tip and thinner at the rhinion and columella.
  - Symmetry/nasal deviation—three basic types: Caudal septal deviations (septal tilt, C-shaped and S-shaped), concave dorsal deformities (C-shaped, reverse C-shaped), and concave/convex dorsal deformities (S-shaped with bony pyramid deviation).
  - Dorsal aesthetic lines: Dorsal aesthetic lines were defined as originating on the supraorbital ridges, traversing medially along the glabellar area, converging at the medial canthal ligaments, diverging at the keystone area, and ending at the nasal tip. Dorsal aesthetic lines width should match either the interphiltral distance or the tip-defining points width. Male dorsum is wider and straighter, with less concavity at the superciliary ridges compared with women.
  - Bony vault: The bony vault is composed of three distinct structures, the paired nasal bones and the perpendicular plate of the ethmoid. Bony vault width, symmetry, and length of nasal bones are analyzed in frontal view. Bony base width should be 70 to 80% of the alar base, typically equal to the intercanthal distance.
  - Midvault: The cartilaginous midvault includes the paired upper lateral cartilages and the cartilaginous septum. The keystone area represents a triangular region, union of the six distinct anatomical structures between the bony vault and the cartilaginous midvault. Midvault width and deformities like the inverted-V or saddle-nose are identified.
  - Nasal tip: The normal tip configuration (triangular and well-defined) should be distinguished from the bulbous tip (rounded and ill-defined) and the boxy tip (square and wide).

Table 14.1 Systematic nasofacial analysis

Nasal view	Analysis
Frontal	
1. Facial proportions	Height (thirds), width (fifths), symmetry
2. Skin type/quality	Fitzpatrick type, thin or thick, sebacious
3. Symmetry/nasal deviation	Midline, dorsal deviation, C-, reverse C, or S-shaped deviation
4. Dorsal aesthetic lines	Straight, symmetric or asymmetric, well- or ill-defined, narrow or wide
5. Bony vault	Narrow or wide, asymmetric, short or long nasal bones
6. Midvault	Narrow or wide, collapse, inverted-V, saddle deformity
7. Nasal tip	Ideal/bulbous/boxy/pinched, supratip, tip-defining points, infratip lobule
8. Alar rims	Gull-shaped, facets, notching, retraction
9. Alar base	Width
10. Upper lip	Long or short, dynamic depressor septi, upper lip crease
Lateral	
1. Nasofrontal angle and radix	Acute or obtuse, high or low radix, prominent or low nasion
2. Nasal length, dorsum, and supratip	Length: long or short; dorsum: smooth, hump, scooped out; supratip: break, fullness, pollybeak
3. Top projection	Over- or underprojected
4. Tip rotation	Over- or underrotated
5. Alar–columellar relationship	Hanging or retracted ala, hanging or retracted columella
6. Periapical hypoplasia	Maxillary or soft tissue deficiency
7. Lip–chin relationship	Normal, over- or underprojected chin
Basal	
1. Nasal projection	Over- or underprojected, well- or ill-defined tip-defining points, columellar-to-lobule ratio
2. Nostril	Symmetry, long/narrow or short/wide nostril, nostril–tip ratio, concave or convex ala
3. Columella	Caudal septal deviation, flaring of medial crura
4. Alar base	Width
5. Alar flaring	Type I, II, III, or IV

Anatomically, the nasal tip has an angle of divergence of 30 degrees, the domal arc a width of 4 mm or less, and a distance between the tip-defining points of 5 to 6 mm. It can be broad and less defined in men. The boxy tip may result of an increased angle of divergence (>30 degrees), a widened domal arc (>4 mm), or a combination of the two.

   - Alar rims: The alar rim's ideal shape resembles a gull in flight. Alar rim deformities, such as retraction, notching, collapse, and asymmetry, are common problems in rhinoplasty patients.
   - Alar base: Alar base width ideally approximates the intercanthal distance, one-fifth of the face width, or 70% of nasal height. Alar base surgery is performed to address excessive width of the nasal base, alar flaring, large nostril size, and alar base or nostril asymmetries.
   - Upper lip: Ideal upper lip position is considered 1 to 2 mm of gingival show on maximum smile (slightly less in males). A hyperactive depressor septi muscle is associated with a deformity during animation (particularly with smiling) characterized by a drooping nasal tip, shortened upper lip, and a transverse crease in the midphiltral area. Resection and release/transposition techniques were proposed to correct this deformity and enhance the tip–lip relationship.
- The profile view includes 7 areas: Nasofrontal angle and radix, nasal length, dorsum and supratip, tip projection (▶ Fig. 14.1), tip rotation, alar–columellar relationship, periapical hypoplasia, and lip–chin relationship.
   - Nasofrontal angle and radix: Two lines tangent to the glabella and to the nasal dorsum, intersecting at nasion, define the nasofrontal angle. The nasofrontal angle (radix) should lie between the superior lash line and the supratarsal crease, with the nasion approximately 15 mm anterior to the medial canthus. The ideal nasofrontal angle varies by gender, with 130 degrees considered acceptable in White men versus 134 degrees in women.
   - Nasal length, dorsum, and supratip: The ideal nasal length (nasofrontal angle to the tip-defining points) is equivalent to two-thirds of midfacial height, the stomion-to-menton distance, or to chin vertical. The nasal dorsum should be smooth, with a slight supratip break in women, roughly 2 to 3 mm above the tip-defining points. In male patients, the dorsum should follow a line drawn from the radix to the tip-defining points, while in women, it should be along a parallel line approximately 2 mm more posterior. The nasal dorsum should be smooth, with a slight supratip break in women, roughly 2 to 3 mm above the tip-defining points. In male patients, the dorsum should follow a line drawn from the radix to the tip-defining points, while in women, it should be along a parallel line approximately 2 mm more posterior. A supratip break is accomplished through creating tip-defining points with good projection and reducing the dorsum to the desired effect.
   - Tip projection: Projection is considered ideal when 50 to 60% of the tip lies anterior to a vertical line adjacent to the upper lip or represents 0.67 times the ideal nasal length.

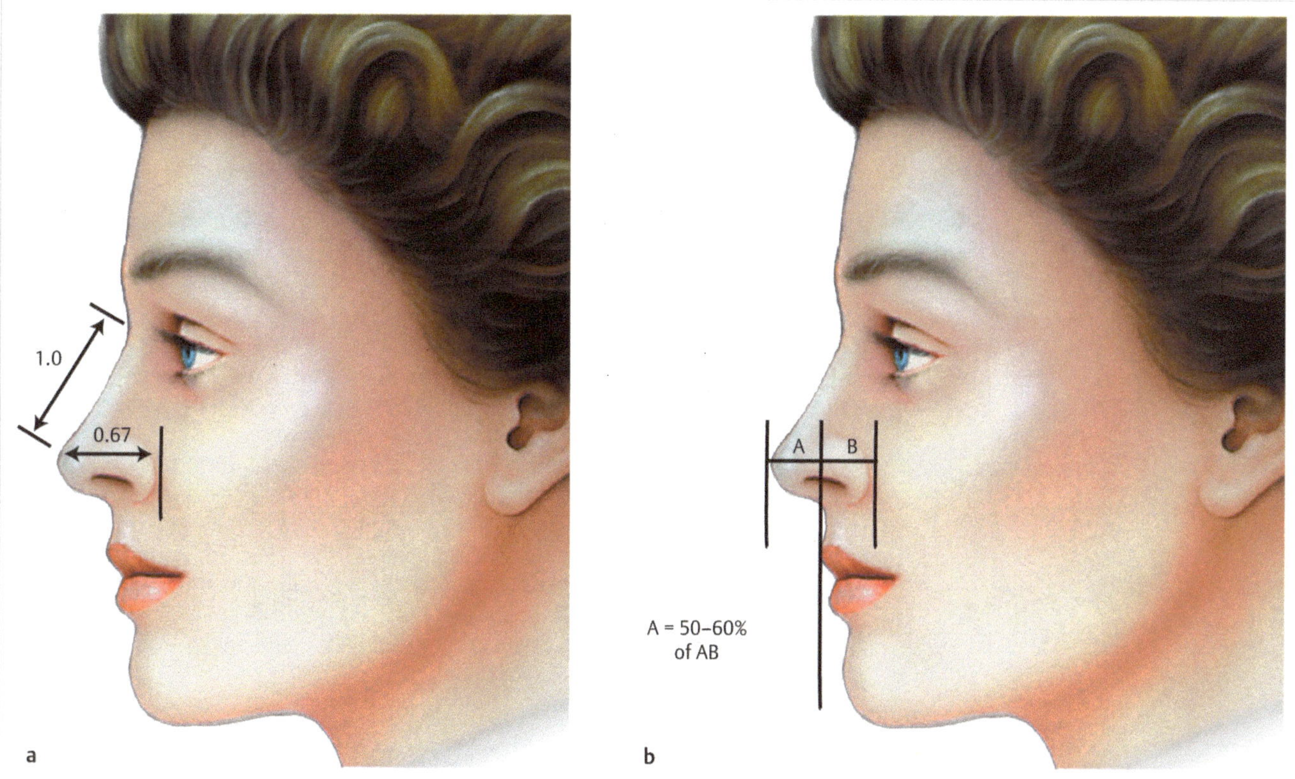

Fig. 14.1 (a, b) Ideal nasal projection on the lateral view. About 50 to 60% of the tip should lie anterior to a vertical line drawn adjacent to the most projecting part of the upper lip and can also be measured as 0.67 times the ideal nasal length. (Reproduced with permission from Rohrich R, Adams W, Ahmad J, eds. Dallas Rhinoplasty: Nasal Surgery by the Masters. 1st ed. Thieme; 2014.)

  - Tip rotation: Tip rotation is determined by the nasolabial angle and should equal approximately 90 to 95 degrees in men and 95 to 100–110 degrees in women.
  - Alar–columellar relationship: The ideal alar–columellar relationship is 2 to 3 mm of columellar show in the lateral view. Excess columellar show is associated with a hanging columella or a retracted ala.
  - Periapical hypoplasia: Skeletal (maxillary) or soft tissue deficiency may produce periapical hypoplasia. Augmentation of the pyriform aperture can decrease the apparent size of the nose, increase the nasal tip and base projection, and widen the nasolabial angle.
  - Lip–chin relationship: Chin projecting surface should lie approximately at (preferred in men) or up to 3 mm posterior (in women) to a vertical line drawn from the half-distance point of the ideal nasal length and tangential to the upper lip vermilion anterior-most point.
- Use the base view to assess 5 areas: Nasal projection (▸ Fig. 14.2), nostril shape/symmetry, columella symmetry/width, alar base, and alar flaring (▸ Fig. 14.3).
  - Nasal projection: On basal view, the nose should create an equilateral triangle with a columella-to-lobule ratio of 2:1.
  - Nostril shape/symmetry: The nostrils should be symmetric and have a teardrop shape with a long axis extending from the base to apex. The ideal nostril–tip relationship should be approximately 2:1.

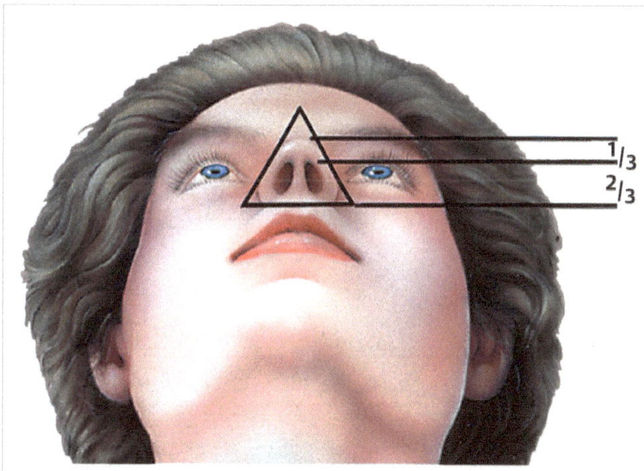

Fig. 14.2 Ideal nostril–tip relationship should be approximately 2:1 on the basal view. (Reproduced with permission from Rohrich R, Adams W, Ahmad J, eds. Dallas Rhinoplasty: Nasal Surgery by the Masters. 1st ed. Thieme; 2014.)

  - Columella symmetry/width: The ideal columella requires a smooth concave shape bridging the nasal tip and nasolabial junction. Primary (intrinsic) deformities of columella originate from malpositioned medial crura or excessive soft tissue. Most commonly, a widened or asymmetric

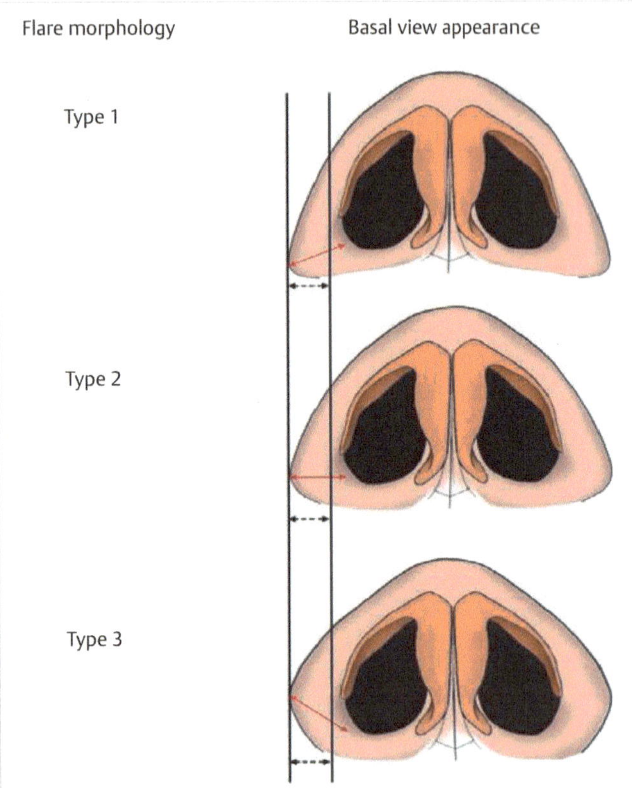

Fig. 14.3 Classification of alar flare.

columella results from premature or excessive medial crura flaring.
  - Alar base and flaring: Proper assessment of nasal base width requires a clear distinction between the width of the alar base and the degree of alar flare. Ideal nasal width approximates the intercanthal distance (normal, 31–33 mm). Alar flare is defined as the greatest width of the ala, whose convexity should not exceed 2 to 3 mm lateral to the alar-facial crease.

14.1.4 Focused Nasal Examination

- Palpation of the nose is also important to assess the length of the nasal bones and strength of the lower lateral cartilages.
- The following are key structures that affect nasal airway and should be evaluated in all patients:
  - External nasal valve—examine for collapse on deep inspiration.
  - Internal nasal valve—perform a Cottle test to evaluate patency.
  - Septum—examine for deviation, tilt, spurs, and perforations.
  - Inferior turbinate—examine for hypertrophy, which typically occurs contralateral to the septal deviation.

14.1.5 Standardized Photography and Digital Imaging

- Standardized photographs including frontal, lateral, oblique, and basal views should be obtained for every patient.
- Additional dynamic views including a smiling view and inspiratory view are recommended.
- Digital imaging is an excellent tool for communicating with the patient and evaluating patient's expectations.

14.1.6 Managing Expectations

- Review all photographic views with the patient.
- It is extremely important to discuss with the patient what can and cannot be achieved with surgery.
- A patient who is focused on minor or uncorrectable problems or with unrealistic expectations despite extensive discussion will likely be disappointed postoperatively regardless of the aesthetic improvement.
- Preoperative identification of unhealthy motivating factors such as feelings of inadequacy, immaturity, family conflicts, divorce, and other major life changes may predict postoperative dissatisfaction.

14.2 Perioperative Preparation

- Prepare the patient for what to expect on the day of surgery and during recovery.
- Provide the patient with written preoperative and postoperative instructions.

14.3 Conclusion

Accurate preoperative systematic nasal analysis and evaluation of the nasal airway are crucial for surgical success. All three top concerns of the patient must be addressed. The surgeon's goals and patient's expectations must be aligned. Caution should be taken when operating on any patient who exhibits unrealistic expectations or signs of underlying psychosocial issues.

See **Video 14.1**.

Further Readings

Rohrich RJ, Afrooz PN. Primary open rhinoplasty. Plast Reconstr Surg. 2019; 144(1): 102e–117e

Rohrich RJ, Ahmad J. A practical approach to rhinoplasty. Plast Reconstr Surg. 2016; 137(4):725e–746e

Rohrich RJ, Villanueva NL, Small KH, Pezeshk RA. Implications of facial asymmetry in rhinoplasty. Plast Reconstr Surg. 2017; 140(3):510–516

Tanna N, Nguyen KT, Ghavami A, et al. Evidence-based medicine: current practices in rhinoplasty. Plast Reconstr Surg. 2018; 141(1):137e–151e

Villanueva NL, Afrooz PN, Carboy JA, Rohrich RJ. Nasal analysis: considerations for ethnic variation. Plast Reconstr Surg. 2019; 143(6):1179e–1188e

15 Open Rhinoplasty Finesse

Rod J. Rohrich, Erez Dayan, and Kristy L. Hamilton

Abstract
Rhinoplasty remains a technically and conceptually challenging procedure for plastic surgeons. Over the past 25 years, nasal analysis and strategies for correction of functional and aesthetic nasal deformities have evolved considerably. According to the American Society of Plastic Surgeons, rhinoplasty was among the top five most popular cosmetic surgical procedure in 2017, with 218,924 procedures performed. This chapter describes preoperative considerations, nasal analysis, and technical maneuvers that allow the plastic surgeon to obtain consistent results in rhinoplasty.

Keywords: Rhinoplasty, open rhinoplasty, revision rhinoplasty

Key Points

- The open approach allows for optimal visualization and correction of nasal aesthetic and functional issues.
- Functional assessment including examination of the internal and external nasal valve patency, septal deviation, and relevant history (i.e., recurrent sinusitis, rhinitis, allergies) is important.

15.1 Preoperative Steps

- Comprehensive and systematic preoperative nasofacial analysis is requisite to define surgical goals and achieve satisfactory results. However, aesthetic ideals should be approached cautiously as there is significant variability among different ethnicities.
- The senior author (Rod J. Rohrich) approaches the nasofacial examination in a systematic fashion, from three different views—frontal, lateral, and basal (**Video 15.1**).
- Prior to prepping and draping, a 27-gauge needle is used to infiltrate 1% lidocaine containing 1:100,000 epinephrine into the columella, along the infracartilaginous incision, the dorsum, and soft tissues medial and lateral to the nasal bones. The nose is then packed bilaterally with oxymetazoline-soaked pledgets. A moist 3-inch gauze throat pack is placed by the surgeon. This sequence allows ample timing for the vasoconstrictive effect of the local anesthesia to take effect.

15.2 Operative Steps

- A stair-step transcolumellar incision is designed at the narrowest part of the columella and carried into the vestibule 2 to 3 mm laterally. In revision rhinoplasty, the location of the transcolumellar incision is placed in the preferred location regardless of the presence of previous scars.
- Next, a wide double hook is placed to evert the alar rim over the fourth finger. This maneuver allows for reliable identification of the caudal margin of the lateral crus upon which an infracartilaginous incision is made in a lateral to medial direction toward the nostril apex. This incision sequence leaves a vestibular tissue bridge under the soft triangle, which is incised last (**Video 15.2**).
- A wide double hook is placed at the nostril apices and retracted caudally. The nasal soft tissues are elevated off the cartilaginous framework with fine dissecting scissors. When the caudal portion of the nasal bones is reached, a Joseph periosteal elevator is used to achieve a limited subperiosteal dissection over the areas of planned bony work.
- The oxymetazoline-soaked pledgets are removed from the vestibules bilaterally and a long heavy Vienna nasal speculum is used to microfracture the inferior turbinates through a closed approach from posterior to anterior while pushing the speculum laterally onto the inferior turbinate (**Video 15.3**).
- The five-step component dorsal hump reduction (CDHR) serves to reduce the dorsum in a precise and graduated fashion while maintaining the upper lateral cartilages (ULCs). CDHR begins with (1) separation of the ULCs from the septum (▶ Fig. 15.1), (2) incremental reduction of the septum proper, (3) dorsal bony reduction, (4) verification by palpation, and (5) final modifications (spreader grafts [▶ Fig. 15.2a], autospreader flaps [▶ Fig. 15.2b], suturing techniques, osteotomies) (**Videos 15.4** and **15.5**).
- The ULC tension spanning suture functions to stabilize the ULC to the septum while establishing symmetric dorsal aesthetic lines (▶ Fig. 15.2c).
- Autospreader flaps can be performed when there is excess horizontal dimension to the ULCs, typically after reduction of a dorsal hump. The anterior edge of the ULCs is folded inward and a 5–0 PDS suture is secured in a horizontal mattress fashion (▶ Fig. 15.2b).
- Additional sutures can be placed cephalically along the ULCs and septum, as needed, for support or improved contour.
- Septoplasty may be required in cases of nasal obstruction and/or deviation (septal tilt, anterior posterior deviation, craniocaudal deviation, or septal spurs) or in cases where donor cartilage is required.
- Nasal osteotomies are primarily used to narrow a widened bony vault, close an open roof deformity, or straighten deviated nasal bones. The authors prefer a low-to-low percutaneous perforated lateral discontinuous osteotomy (▶ Fig. 15.3a–c). A sharp 2-mm osteotome is introduced percutaneously at the level of the inferior orbital rim and nasofacial junction parallel to the horizontal surface of the maxilla (**Video 15.6**).

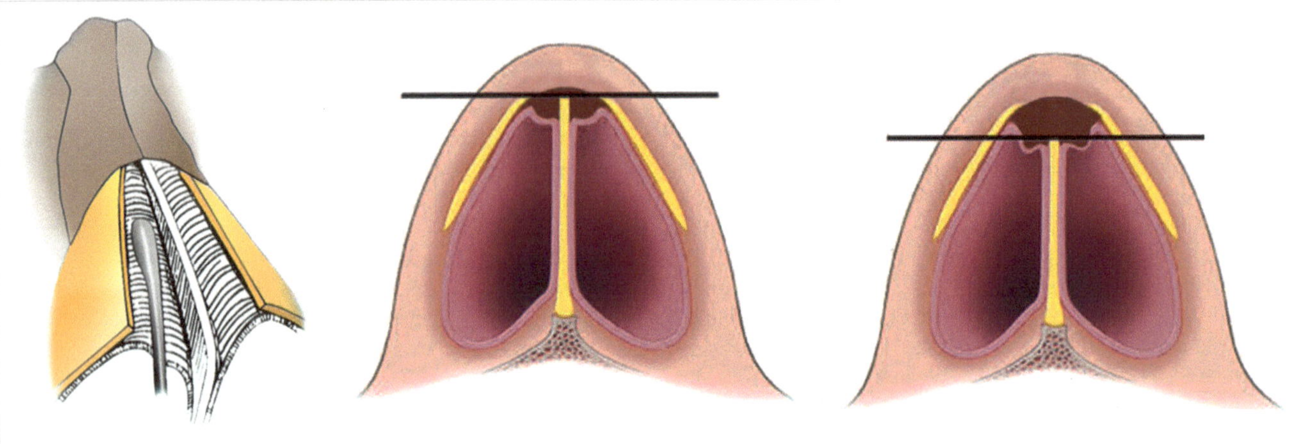

Fig. 15.1 Component dorsum. Surgical approach to the dorsum: separation of the upper lateral cartilages (ULCs) from the septum. The mucoperichondrium of the dorsal septum is elevated, from caudal to cephalad, until the elevator reaches the nasal bones. (Reproduced with permission from Rohrich R, Adams W, Ahmad J, et al. Dallas Rhinoplasty: Nasal Surgery by the Masters. 3rd ed. Thieme; 2014.)

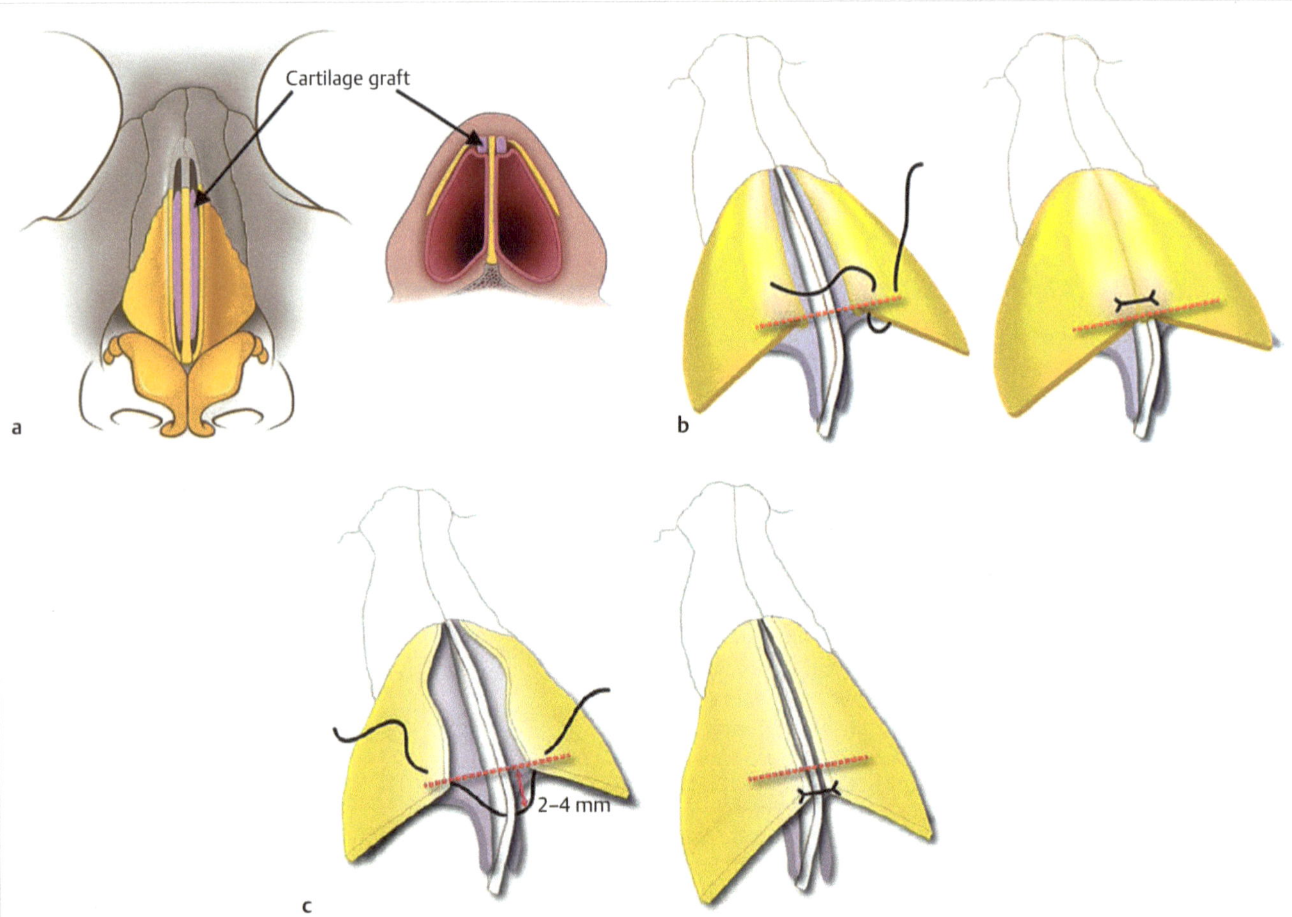

Fig. 15.2 (a) Spreader grafts. Reconstitution of the dorsum: spreader grafts. Spreader grafts may be positioned at or above the plane of the dorsal septum to be visible for aesthetic indications or below it as invisible grafts for purely functional indications. **(b)** Spreader flaps. Reconstitution of the dorsum: type 3: midvault restoration with spreader flap modification. The 5–0 PDS sutures are placed caudal to the upper edge of the upper lateral cartilages (ULCs), thereby infolding the superior edge of the ULCs. This serves a spreader-type function. This technique should be employed when attempting to widen the midvault. **(c)** ULC tension spanning sutures. (Reproduced with permission from Rohrich R, Adams W, Ahmad J, et al. Dallas Rhinoplasty: Nasal Surgery by the Masters. 3rd ed. Thieme; 2014.)

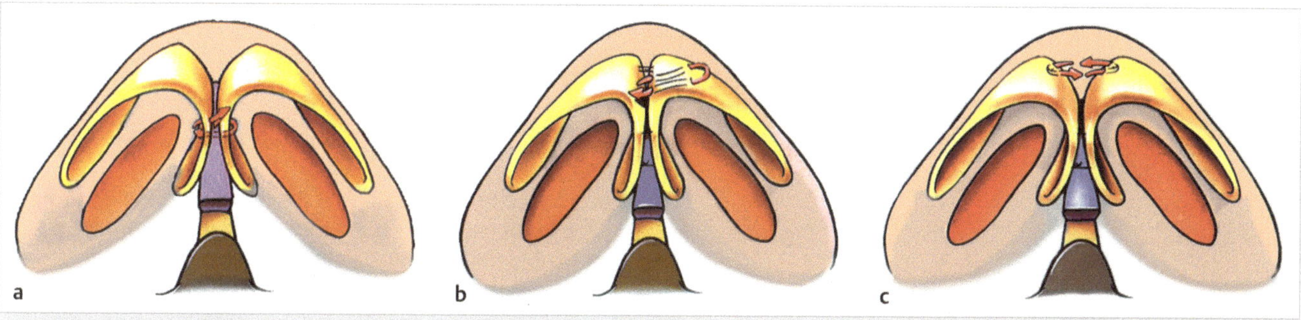

Fig. 15.3 Tip sutures. **(a)** Medial crural suture. The positioning of the medial crural suture is dictated by the underlying deformity and intended goal. **(b)** Transdomal sutures. This is a horizontal mattress suture that is placed through the lateral and medial aspects of the domes. **(c)** Interdomal suture. This is a horizontal mattress suture placed between the domal segments of the middle crura of the lower lateral cartilages (LLCs). (Reproduced with permission from Rohrich R, Adams W, Ahmad J, et al. Dallas Rhinoplasty: Nasal Surgery by the Masters. 3rd ed. Thieme; 2014.)

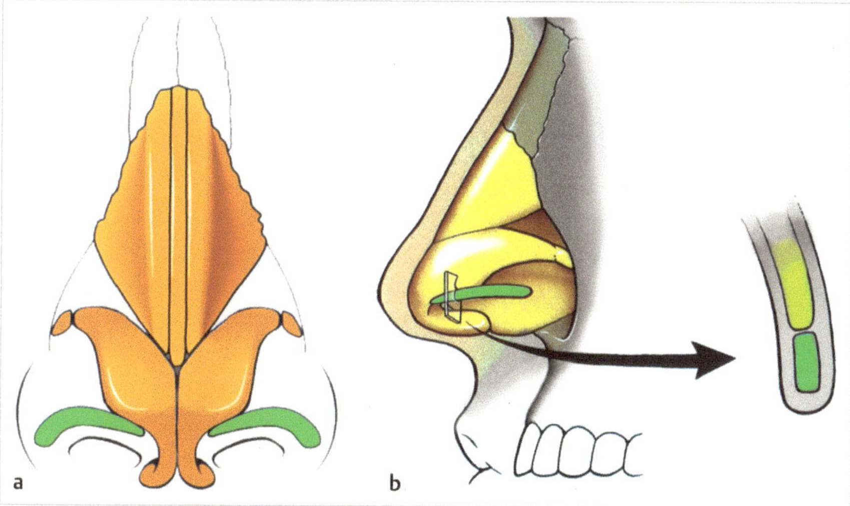

Fig. 15.4 (a, b) Alar contour grafts. Operative planning: alar rim grafts. The primary indications for the alar contour graft are as follows: Primary rhinoplasty patients with congenital alar rim notching, primary rhinoplasty patients with weak nasal alae/soft triangles with propensity for notching, primary or secondary rhinoplasty with mild to moderate external nasal valve collapse, primary or secondary rhinoplasty patients with malpositioned lower lateral crural cartilages, and secondary rhinoplasty patients with minimal vestibular lining loss and at least 3 mm of residual lower lateral cartilage (LLC) alar rim strips. (Reproduced with permission from Rohrich R, Adams W, Ahmad J, et al. Dallas Rhinoplasty: Nasal Surgery by the Masters. 3rd ed. Thieme; 2014.)

- The purpose of cephalic trim is to refine the nasal tip and decrease supratip fullness by reducing the vertical height of the lower lateral cartilages (LLCs). The LLC is separated from the ULC at the scroll area. The cephalic portion of the LLC is trimmed leaving 5 to 7 mm medially and 8 to 10 mm laterally.
- Three key tip-suturing techniques to improve position and shape include medial crural, transdomal, and interdomal sutures (▶ Fig. 15.4a, b) (**Video 15.7**).
- Alar rim grafts are frequently employed (>90% of cases) to prevent alar retraction (▶ Fig. 15.5).
- The transcolumellar incision is meticulously reapproximated with 6–0 nylon interrupted sutures. A double hook is used to slightly evert the alar rim to place interrupted chromic sutures in the lateral aspect of the infracartilaginous incision. The incision behind the soft triangle is left open and dressed with mupirocin-covered Surgicel (oxidized regenerated cellulose) to avoid suture-driven alar retraction or notching in this region.
- Although assessment of alar flare is part of the standard preoperative nasal analysis, the final decision to perform alar flare reduction occurs only after wound closure. The reason for this is because alar flare heavily depends on tip projection, rotation, and by the length/strength of the lateral crura and alar rims.

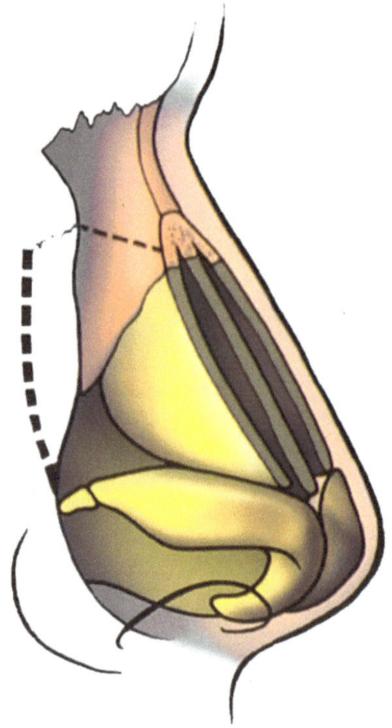

Fig. 15.5 Low-to-low osteotomies. Lateral osteotomy levels. Low-to-low: This osteotomy starts low along the piriform aperture and remains low along the base of the bony vault ending at a location near the intercanthal line. (Reproduced with permission from Rohrich R, Adams W, Ahmad J, et al. Dallas Rhinoplasty: Nasal Surgery by the Masters. 3rd ed. Thieme; 2014.)

15.3 Postoperative Care

- Keep head of bed elevated on two pillows for first 7 days postoperatively.
- Apply crushed ice for first 72 hours to minimize swelling/ bruising.
- Avoid pressure on nasal splint (i.e., avoid glasses).
- Keep inside edges of your nostrils clean with hydrogen peroxide saturated Q-tip followed by thin coating of Polysporin ointment. This will prevent crust from forming.
- Patients are instructed to avoid strenuous activity for 4 to 6 weeks.

15.4 Case Example

Frontal, basal, and lateral before and after views to correct a bulbous tip, excess tip projection, and dorsal hump are shown (▶ Fig. 15.6a–c).

15.5 Conclusion

Rhinoplasty continues to be among the most challenging procedures for plastic surgeons. However, with careful preoperative nasofacial analysis and functional assessment, the rhinoplasty surgeon can approach each nasal component systematically. The graduated approaches outlined in this article allow the rhinoplasty surgeon to achieve desired modifications and corrections to the nose while maintaining adequate nasal support and minimizing complications.

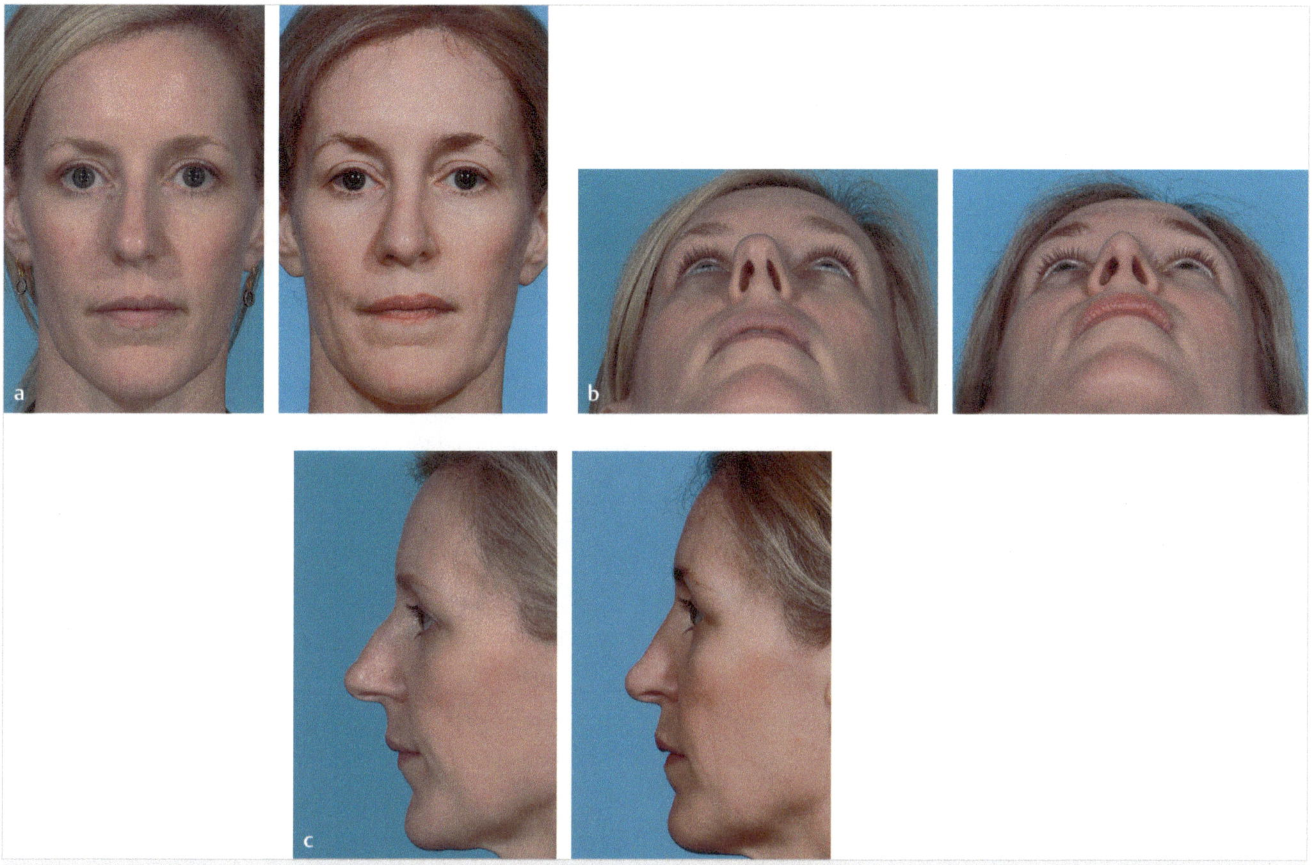

Fig. 15.6 **(a)** Frontal, **(b)** basal, and **(c)** lateral before and after views to correct a bulbous tip, excess tip projection, and dorsal hump.

Further Readings

Ghavami A, Janis JE, Acikel C, Rohrich RJ. Tip shaping in primary rhinoplasty: an algorithmic approach. Plast Reconstr Surg. 2008; 122(4):1229–1241

Gunter JP, Rohrich RJ. Management of the deviated nose: the importance of septal reconstruction. Clin Plast Surg. 1988; 15(1):43–55

Mojallal A, Ouyang D, Saint-Cyr M, Bui N, Brown SA, Rohrich RJ. Dorsal aesthetic lines in rhinoplasty: a quantitative outcome-based assessment of the component dorsal reduction technique. Plast Reconstr Surg. 2011; 128(1): 280–288

Rohrich RJ, Ahmad J. A practical approach to rhinoplasty. Plast Reconstr Surg. 2016; 137(4):725e–746e

Rohrich RJ, Afrooz PN. Rhinoplasty refinements: the role of the open approach. Plast Reconstr Surg. 2017; 140(4):716–719

16 The Closed Rhinoplasty

Mark G. Albert

Abstract

Closed rhinoplasty, or endonasal rhinoplasty, was the first approach used to surgically modify the nose in the 19th century. Since the open approach gained popularity in the 1970s, trainees have generally considered this technique easier to visualize anatomy and observe surgical maneuvers. Once a surgeon understands the basics of closed rhinoplasty, the unique benefits of this approach can be seen. This chapter provides a concise guide to the fundamentals of closed rhinoplasty.

Keywords: Endonasal, closed, rhinoplasty, delivery, cartilage

Key Points

- Closed rhinoplasty involves surgical maneuvers to alter the surface anatomy of the nose. By leaving the skin and soft tissue envelope down, the surgeon can see the immediate effect of these maneuvers.
- By leaving nasal soft tissue undisturbed, and avoiding external incisions, the risk of deformity and complications is minimized.
- Variations in closed techniques allow surgeons to make decisions based on the goals of each patient. Some closed rhinoplasty surgeons prefer to leave the cartilage within the nose and add grafts, others routinely perform intracartilaginous incisions to access the lower lateral cartilage, and others favor tip delivery.

16.1 Preoperative Steps

- Establish the primary concerns of the patient. Understand why the patient is seeking rhinoplasty. Determine whether he or she has breathing concerns.
- Inquire about prior surgery or trauma to the nose as well as medical history, smoking history, medications, and recreational drug use (i.e., cocaine).
- Perform an intranasal speculum examination and assess the septum, turbinates, and the internal and external nasal valves.
- Palpate the nose to determine the length of the nasal bones and stability of the upper and lower lateral cartilage.
- Assess for body dysmorphic disorder. If there is suspicion of the condition, one should use a screening questionnaire such as the Body Dysmorphic Disorder Questionnaire (BDDQ).

16.1.1 Analysis

- Begin by asking the patient what he would specifically like addressed during the rhinoplasty. Provide a mirror for patients to point out exactly their concerns and document this conversation thoroughly. Photo-editing software can be a useful tool to communicate with patients in the preoperative period as long as patient's expectations are appropriately managed.
- Tell the patient the maneuvers you plan to do and consider explaining step-by-step how you will achieve the goals. Not only does this satisfy part of the informed consent process, many patients appreciate having a thorough understanding of what will be happening on the day of surgery.
- While analyzing the nose in front, oblique, profile, and base views, examine the nose top-down by upper, middle, and lower one-thirds. This order is based on surgeon's preference. Rohrich's 10–7-5 rule provides guidelines for a thorough evaluation of anatomic features of each nose.
- Contact the patient by phone the day before surgery to summarize the plan, review nil per os (NPO) requirements, answer questions, and provide reassurance.

16.2 Operative Steps

See **Video 16.1**.

16.2.1 Opening the Nose

- Following skin prep and placement of a head drape, vibrissae are cut and collected with an ointment-coated cotton-tip applicator.
- The nose is infiltrated with 6 to 8 cc of 1% lidocaine with epinephrine 1:100,000 and 10 minutes are allowed for vasoconstriction. Afrin-soaked pledgets are then inserted until the procedure begins.
- A #15 blade is used to make an intercartilaginous incision on the left and right sides sequentially. The incisions are carried to the mucosa on the medial aspect of the nares (▶ Fig. 16.1).

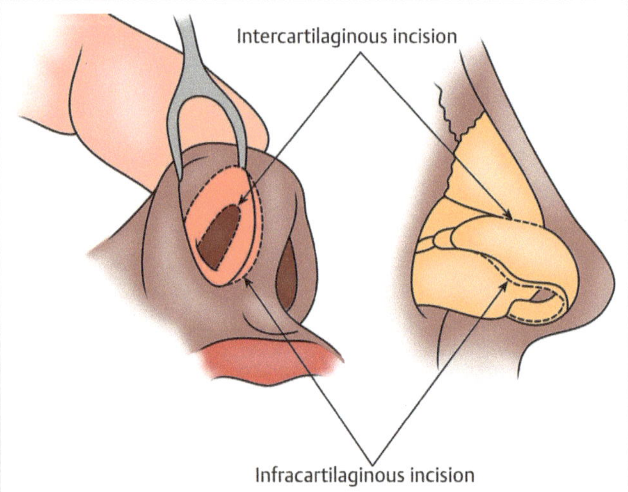

Fig. 16.1 Intercartilaginous and infracartilaginous incisions. Intercartilaginous incisions are made on the cephalic aspect of the lower lateral cartilages to avoid scarring and stricture of the internal valve. These incisions are often lengthened to join the full transfixion incision to allow for cartilage delivery. Infracartilaginous incisions closely follow the caudal margin of the lower lateral cartilages.

- Using a double hook for counter-traction, a full transfixion incision is made and is often connected with the intercartilaginous incisions for tip delivery.
- The depressor septi nasi muscle can be freed from the incisive foramen of the maxilla using a Joseph elevator as indicated.

16.2.2 Dorsum

- A periosteal elevator is then used to elevate periosteum and other soft tissue from the dorsum.
- A lighted Aufricht retractor and angled septal scissors are used remove excess cartilaginous septum and upper lateral cartilage. A headlight can be used if a lighted Aufricht is unavailable.
- The upper lateral cartilage does not need to be preserved for spreader flaps in closed rhinoplasty. Constantian demonstrated the important effect of spreader *grafts* on airflow in his 160 consecutive patient rhinomanometry series in 1996.
- A rasp is then used to lower the nasal bones to match the height of the septal cartilage. It is important to perform this step before harvesting septal cartilage in order to ensure at least 15 mm of strut is left behind.

16.2.3 Septum

- Septal cartilage harvest is performed through a Killian incision in the left nare for a right-handed surgeon. A freer elevator is used to dissect medially to the septal cartilage, and the perichondrium is then elevated along the length of the septum.
- Care is taken to leave the dorsal perichondrium intact and undisturbed so that spreader graft tunnels can later be dissected.
- The sharper end of a freer is used to make a vertical incision in the septal cartilage and the right perichondrium can be dissected from the left nare through this incision.
- A nasal speculum can be used to facilitate this dissection. Once all soft tissue is dissected from the septal cartilage, a Ballenger swivel knife (or septal scissor) is used to excise the graft material. Care is taken to preserve > 15mm of caudal and dorsal septum.
- The dead space left behind from the excised cartilage is closed with a 4–0 chromic quilting suture.

16.2.4 Midvault Reconstruction

- Spreader grafts are used for many reconstructive and cosmetic purposes, the most common of which is correction of nasal obstruction due to internal valve insufficiency.
- Each spreader graft is approximately 20 mm long × 4 mm wide and 1.5 mm thick and they are usually harvested from septal cartilage.
- In cases of secondary rhinoplasty where the nasal septum is depleted, conchal, rib, or fresh frozen cartilage may be used.
- Narrow spreader graft tunnels are dissected using a Cottle elevator in the subperichondrial plane on both side of the dorsal nasal septum. The tunnels are created so that the spreader grafts fit so tightly that no suture fixation is necessary.
- To correct asymmetry or septal deviation, spreader grafts of different thicknesses may be used. In such cases, it is preferable to use spreader grafts of different sizes rather than opting for a unilateral spreader graft only.

16.2.5 Tip Delivery and Refinement

- Using a thimble hook, bilateral infracartilaginous incisions are made and carried to the caudal aspect of the medial crura.
- An angled converse scissor is used to dissect soft tissue off the lower lateral cartilages.
- A blunt scissor or curved hemostat is inserted beneath the middle crus from lateral to medial to remove the dissected cartilage from the nare.
- This instrument remains in place if a cephalic trim is to be performed. The cephalic margin can be removed from the lower lateral cartilage using a #15 blade with care taken to preserve 8 to 10 mm of cartilage on each side (▶ Fig. 16.2).
- The incised cartilage is dissected free from the underlying mucosa with an angled converse scissor, and preserved on the mayo stand for possible use as a graft.
- Following bilateral cephalic trim, digital pressure is applied to the contralateral nare to deliver both lower lateral cartilages through the same nare. A single hook retracts the columella to the contralateral side to allow the lower lateral cartilages to remain in the midline for tip suturing.

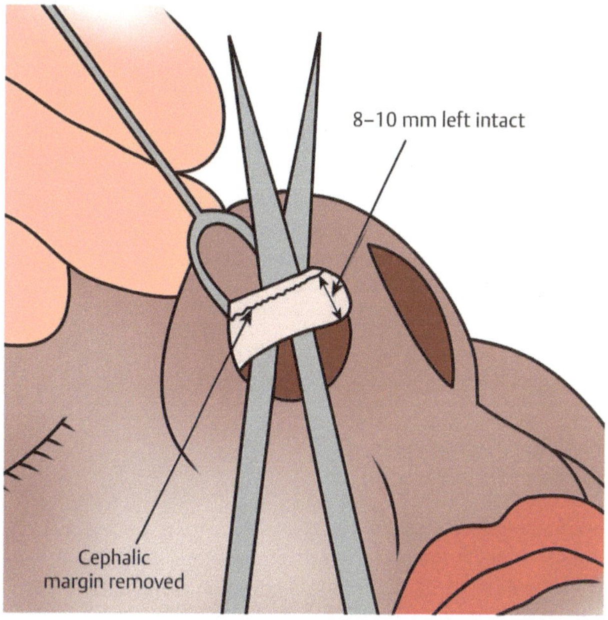

Fig. 16.2 Cephalic trim. Removal of the cephalic portion of the lower lateral cartilage is performed after cartilage delivery. At least 8 to 10 mm of cartilage should be left behind to maintain structural integrity and avoid a pinched tip deformity.

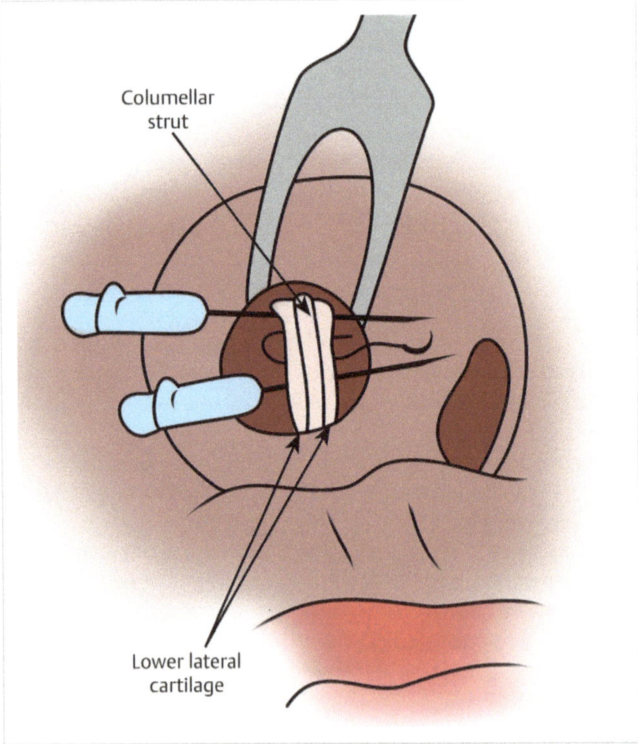

Fig. 16.3 Columellar strut. The columella is retracted to the contralateral side so that the lower lateral cartilages can remain midline for the sake of symmetry during tip suturing. A columellar strut can be placed on the nasal spine or floated between the medial crura of the lower lateral cartilage. Hypodermic needles are used to secure the graft while horizontal mattress sutures are placed.

- A columellar strut can be used to support the tip. It is inserted in a dissected pocket above the nasal spine, or can be floated in cases of a shorter cartilage graft.
- The superior aspect of the strut is placed at the level of the lower lateral cartilage domes and secured with 27-gauge hypodermic needles to the medial crura on either side.
- Multiple 4–0 chromic horizontal mattress sutures are placed in a transmucosal fashion to secure the strut to the medial crura on either side (▶ Fig. 16.3).
- Intradomal and interdomal sutures are placed with 5–0 PDS sutures. Cartilage grafts can be secured to the lower lateral cartilages with 5–0 PDS suture as needed.

16.2.6 Osteotomies

- A 1 to 2 mm vestibular stab incision is made at the base of the bony pyramid.
- A Joseph elevator is used to create a subperiosteal tunnel anterior and posterior to the nasal bones. This helps minimize edema and ecchymosis from excessive soft tissue trauma from the osteotome.
- Bilateral high-low-high osteotomies are performed using a 2 mm mini-Lambotte osteotome from the inferior aspect of the nasal bones stopping short of the medial canthal tendon.
- The stab incisions are closed with 5–0 chromic simple interrupted sutures, though some authors prefer to leave these open.

16.2.7 Closure

- Before closing, a thorough intranasal inspection is performed to confirm hemostasis.
- The infracartilaginous incisions are closed with simple interrupted 5–0 chromic suture. Closure of the intercartilaginous incisions are optional.
- Alcohol, Steri-Strips, liquid adhesive, and an aquaplast splint are placed. Nasal drip pads can be fabricated using liquid adhesive on the cheeks, Steri-Strips, a rubber band, and absorbent pads.

16.3 Postoperative Care

- Ice packs can be applied to the nose and eyes for 15 minutes every 2 hours. Strict head elevation is recommended for the first week.
- The nasal vestibule is gently cleansed three times a day with peroxide-soaked cotton swabs and antibacterial ointment is gently applied.
- Sterile saline sprays can be used as needed. Patients are advised to refrain from nose blowing or sneezing through the nose for at least 7 days.
- The splint is removed on postoperative day 7.

16.4 Case Example

Front, oblique, lateral, and basal before and after views of ethnic rhinoplasty is shown. This patient specifically requested to maintain the shape and ethnic features of her nose (▶ Fig. 16.4a–d).

16.5 Conclusion

Closed rhinoplasty allows the surgeon to visualize how changes to the framework directly affect the surface contour of the nose. By minimizing external incisions and the degree of soft tissue dissection, additional variables that could impact the final cosmetic and functional result can be avoided. Closed rhinoplasty generally results in minimal postoperative edema and a relatively predictable postoperative course. Surgeons who are considering adopting the closed approach can convert to an open approach intraoperatively, if needed, during the learning process.

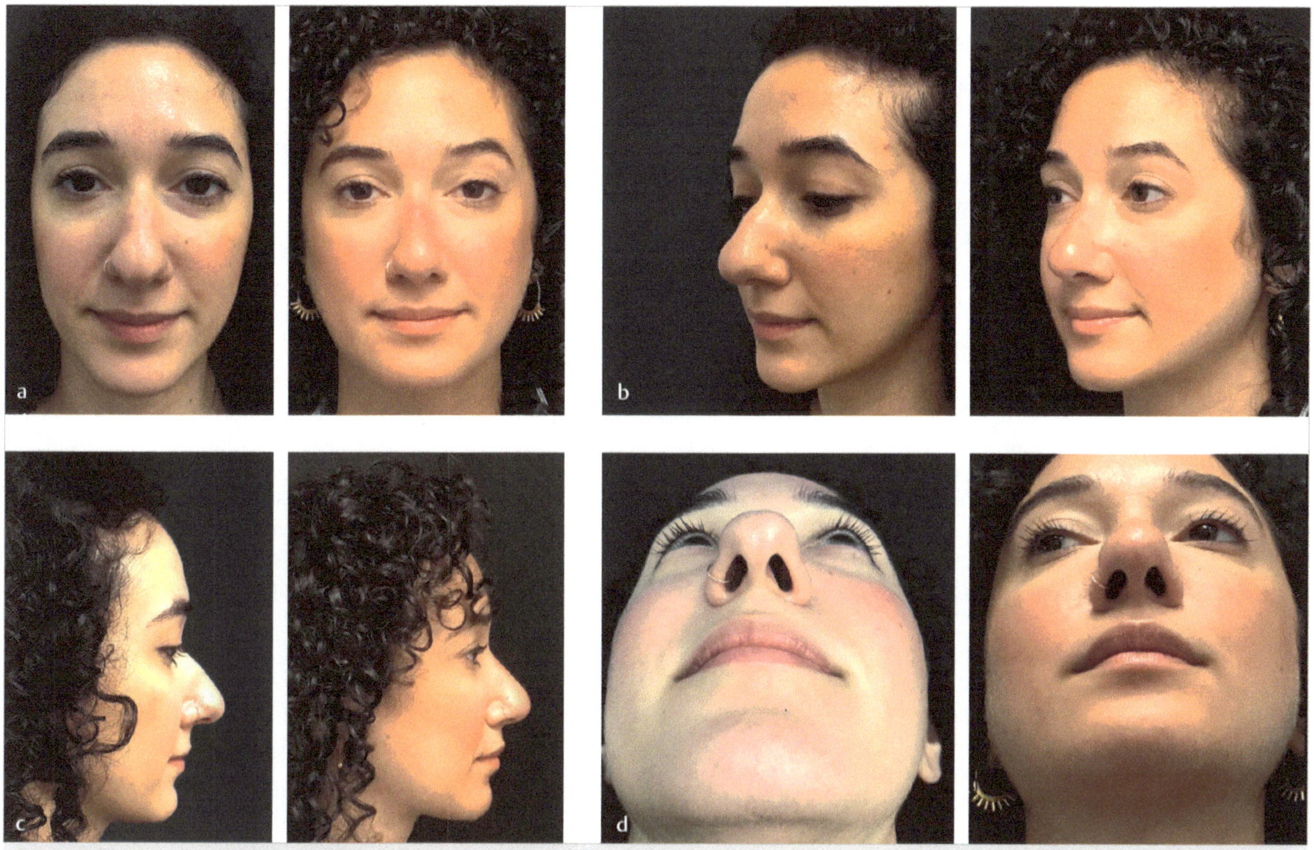

Fig. 16.4 Ethnic rhinoplasty: **(a)** Front, **(b)** oblique, **(c)** lateral, and **(d)** basal before and after views. This patient specifically requested to maintain the shape and ethnic features of her nose.

Further Readings

Barış Çakır. Aesthetic septorhinoplasty. New York, NY: Springer; 2016

Constantian MB, Clardy RB. The relative importance of septal and nasal valvular surgery in correcting airway obstruction in primary and secondary rhinoplasty. Plast Reconstr Surg. 1996; 98(1):38–54, discussion 55–58

Constantian MB. Rhinoplasty, Craft and Magic. St. Louis, MO: Quality Medical Publishing; 2009

Rohrich RJ, Adams WP, Jr., Ahmad J, Gunter JP, eds. Dallas rhinoplasty: nasal surgery by the Masters. 3rd ed. Boca Raton, FL: CRC Press; 2014

Sheen J, Sheen A. Aesthetic rhinoplasty. 2nd ed. St. Louis, MO: C.V. Mosby Company; 1987

17 Graduated Approach to Tip Projection

Rod J. Rohrich, Ira L. Savetsky, and Paul D. Durand

Abstract

The approach to the nasal tip requires a combination of techniques that will improve tip shape and establish proper support. Here, we provide a focused review of nasal tip analysis and surgical technique, with particular emphasis on tip sutures and cartilage grafts.

Keywords: Rhinoplasty, nasal tip, tip shaping, tip rotation, tip projection, tip sutures, septal extension graft

Key Points

- Understanding the underlying anatomic components that provide nasal tip support, and their effect on tip projection and shape is a prerequisite for successful tip shaping.
- A comprehensive and systematic nasofacial analysis is the most important initial step in establishing goals and formulating a precise surgical plan for nasal tip projection and shape.

17.1 Factors that Determine Tip Projection

- Length, width, and strength of the lower lateral cartilages.
- Length and stability of the medial crura.
- Suspensory ligament that spans the crura over the anterior septal angle.
- Fibrous connections between the upper and lower lateral cartilages.
- Abutment with the pyriform aperture.
- Anterior septal angle.
- Skin and soft tissue thickness.

17.2 Preoperative Planning

17.2.1 Nasofacial Proportions and Systematic Nasal Analysis: "10–7-5" Nasal Analysis

- On the front view, evaluation should include 10 key areas: Facial proportions, skin type/skin thickness, symmetry/nasal deviation, bony vault width, midvault asymmetry, dorsal aesthetic lines, tip shape/tip-defining points, alar rims/base, infratip lobular projection, and periapical hypoplasia/upper lip length.
- The profile view includes 7 areas: Radix height and position, dorsal convexity, nasal length, tip projection, tip rotation, alar-columellar relationship, and chin projection.
- The base view aids in the assessment of 5 areas: Nasal projection, nostril shape/symmetry, columella symmetry/width, alar base width, and alar rim flaring.

17.2.2 Nasal Tip Assessment

- Thick and sebaceous skin may camouflage the results of tip modification.
- Domal asymmetry, tip dysmorphology (boxy or bulbous tip), degree of nostril show, columellar excess, caudal septal deviation, and a plunging or hyperdynamic tip should be noted.
- Animated views should be obtained to diagnose depressor septi nasi hyperactivity resulting in hyperdynamic tip ptosis.
- On the lateral view, 50 to 60% of the tip should lie anterior to a vertical line drawn adjacent to the most projecting part of the upper lip and can also be measured as 0.67 times the ideal nasal length (▸ Fig. 17.1a, b).
- On the basal view, the ideal nostril–tip relationship should be approximately 2:1 (▸ Fig. 17.2).

17.3 Intraoperative Assessment

- The lateral crura are assessed for their degree of convexity/concavity, length/width dimensions, position, and symmetry.
- Analysis of the length and strength of the medial crura are critical for tip projection and definition:
  - Medial crura that are long and stable are less likely to contribute to loss of tip projection postoperatively.
  - Short and/or weak medial crura can lead to a loss of supratip definition as the differential between dorsal height and domal peak is diminished.
- The domes are characterized in terms of the domal arch width, angle of divergence, and degree of symmetry.
- Analyzing the relationship between the lateral crura, domes, and medial crura is important as modifications to one will often have an effect on the others.

17.4 Operative Technique

- Cephalic trim: It is performed in cases of bulbous or boxy domes by separating the lower lateral cartilages from the upper lateral cartilages at the scroll area and trimming them, leaving at least a 6-mm-wide rim strip. This reduces the length of the cartilaginous framework and facilitates passive cephalic rotation of the lower lateral cartilage (▸ Fig. 17.3).
- Septal extension graft: A versatile graft that effectively controls tip projection, shape, and rotation whereas a columellar strut graft is only effective for unifying the nasal tip and maintaining projection while lacking control over nasal tip rotation. The septal extension graft is keel-shaped to mimic the inferior margin of the middle crura. It is placed onto the anterior septal angle as a "fixed-floating" graft with extension beyond the anterior septal angle into the interdomal space with the most caudal and inferior portion of the graft placed on the cephalic border of the medial crus at the columellar-lobular angle.

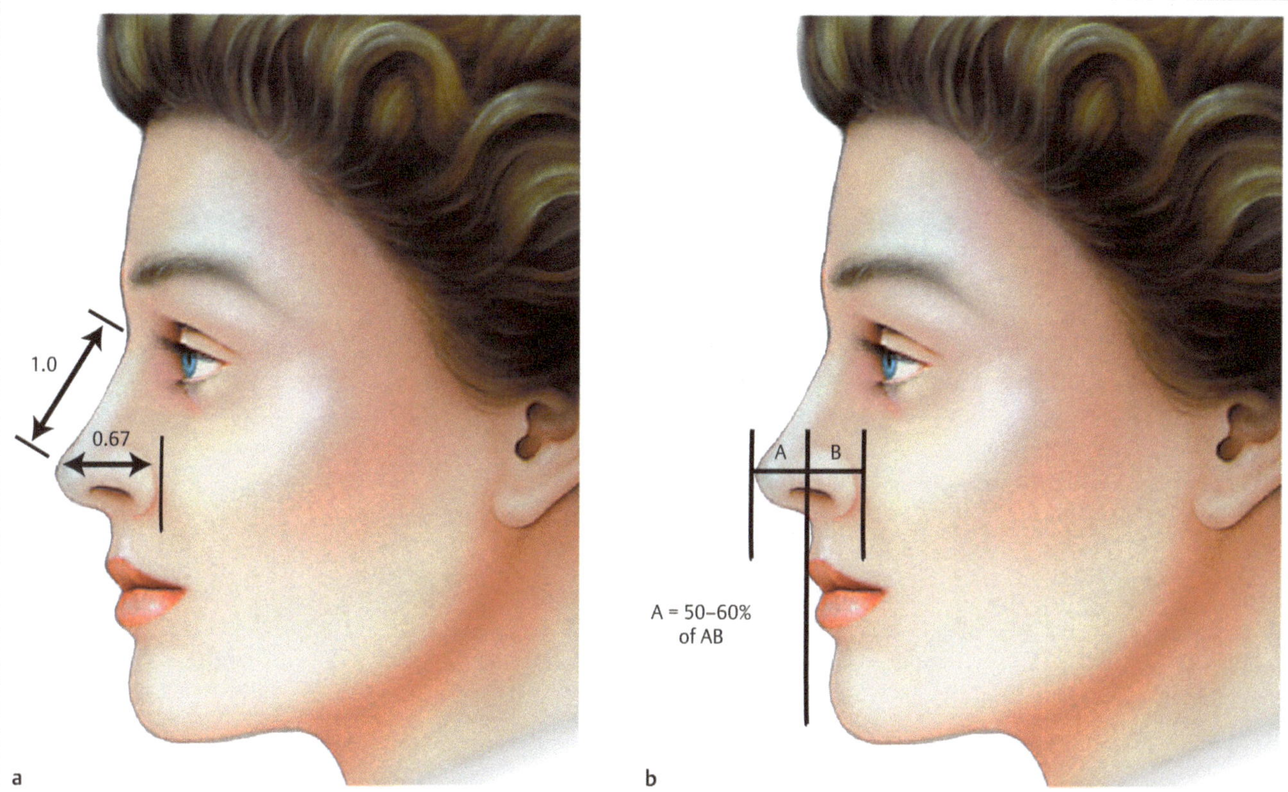

Fig. 17.1 (a, b) Ideal nasal projection on the lateral view. About 50 to 60% of the tip should lie anterior to a vertical line drawn adjacent to the most projecting part of the upper lip and can also be measured as 0.67 times the ideal nasal length. (Reproduced with permission from Rohrich R, Adams W, Ahmad J, eds. Dallas Rhinoplasty: Nasal Surgery by the Masters. 1st ed. Thieme; 2014.)

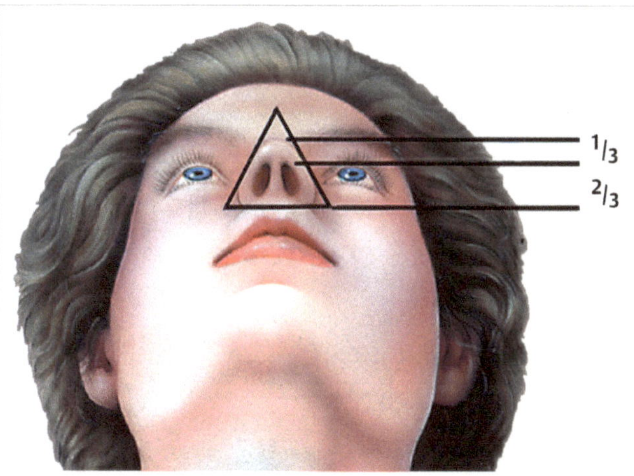

Fig. 17.2 Ideal nostril–tip relationship should be approximately 2:1 on the basal view. (Reproduced with permission from Rohrich R, Adams W, Ahmad J, eds. Dallas Rhinoplasty: Nasal Surgery by the Masters. 1st ed. Thieme; 2014.)

- ○ A four-step suture technique is performed (▶ Fig. 17.4):
  - Body fixation horizontal mattress suture.
  - Superior stabilization suture.
  - Inferior stabilization suture.
  - Body stabilization horizontal mattress suture.

17.4.1 Reshaping of the Nasal Tip Proceeds Using a Bottom-up Approach

- Medial crural footplate approximation corrects footplate deformities and asymmetries (▶ Fig. 17.5).
- "Low" medial crural approximation stabilizes the graft, corrects asymmetries, controls columellar width, and strengthens the medial crura (▶ Fig. 17.6).
- "High" medial crural approximation further stabilizes the medial crura to the graft and aids in establishing columellar width and proper symmetry (▶ Fig. 17.6).
- Transdomal suturing increases tip projection, corrects lateral crural convexities, and narrows and defines the tip (▶ Fig. 17.7).
- Interdomal approximation decreases the angle of divergence, narrows the tip-defining points, and corrects vertical asymmetries (▶ Fig. 17.8).
- Tip grafts are used to camouflage prominent and sharp angles of the underlying framework. Cap grafts, infratip lobular grafts, and morselized cartilage are examples of commonly used grafts (▶ Fig. 17.9).
  See **Video 17.1.**

17.5 Postoperative Care

- When sleeping, keep your head elevated on two pillows for the first 7 days after surgery.

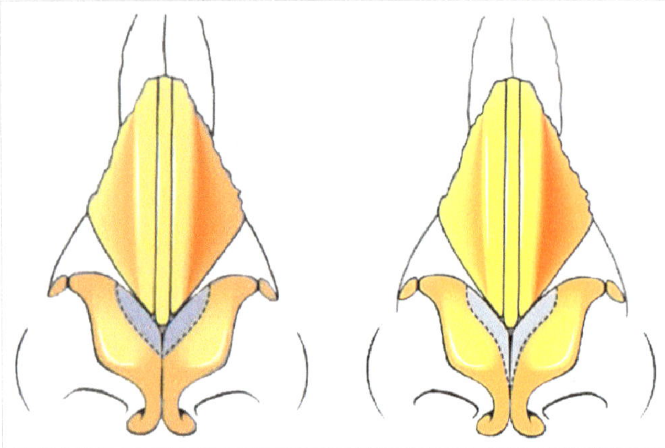

Fig. 17.3 Cephalic trim of the lateral crus of the lower lateral cartilages. (Reproduced with permission from Rohrich R, Ahmad J, eds. The Dallas Rhinoplasty and Dallas Cosmetic Surgery Dissection Guide. 1st ed. Thieme; 2018.)

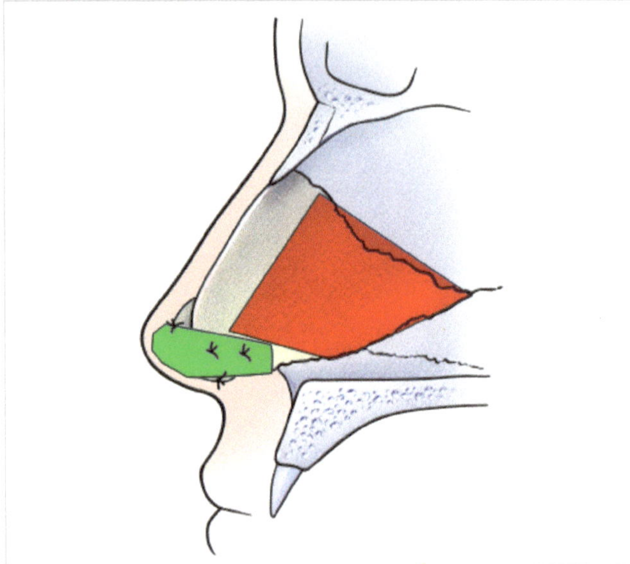

Fig. 17.4 Septal extension graft. Four-step suture technique.

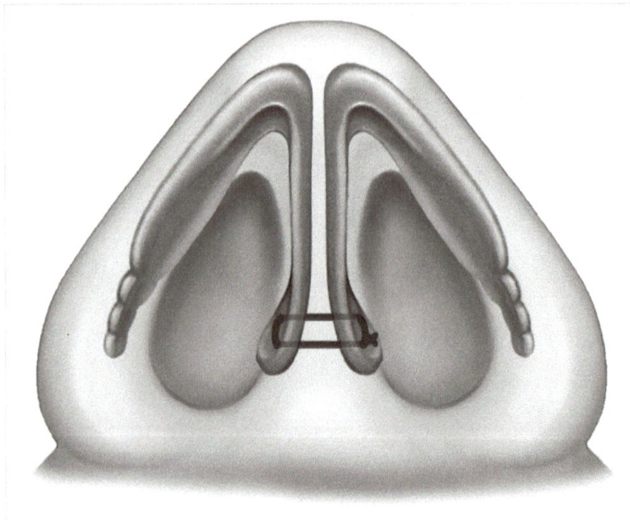

Fig. 17.5 Medial crural footplate suture. (Reproduced with permission from Janis J, ed. Essentials of Aesthetic Surgery. 1st ed. Thieme; 2018.)

- During the day for the first 72 hours after surgery, apply crushed ice in an ice bag or other forms of cold compress to minimize swelling and bruising. Do not put pressure on the nasal splint.
- It is normal to continue to swell after the first 48 hours. Swelling reaches its peak at 48 to 72 hours.
- If you have pain, take the pain medication every 4 to 6 hours.
- If you feel anxious, take the antianxiety medication (alprazolam) every 8 hours for the first 24 to 48 hours.
- Following surgery, begin with a light diet: liquids only. The next day you can begin a soft, regular diet but for 2 weeks avoid foods that require excessive lip movement.
- You will probably have a bloody nasal discharge for 3 to 4 days and may change the drip pad under your nose as often as needed. Do not rub or blot your nose, as this will tend to irritate it.
- To prevent bleeding, do not sniff or blow your nose for the first 4 weeks after surgery. Try not to sneeze, but if you do, sneeze through your mouth.
- While the nasal splint is on, you may have your hair washed in a beauty salon fashion. Take care to prevent the nasal splint from getting wet.
- Keep the inside edges of your nostrils and any stitches clean by using a Q-tip saturated with hydrogen peroxide followed by a thin coating of Polysporin, which is an over-the-counter antibiotic ointment. This is done in a circular manner. Please do this at least four to five times per day.
- Avoid hitting or getting bumped in your nose for 6 weeks after surgery.
- After the splint is removed, do not wear glasses or allow anything else to rest on your nose for 4 weeks.
- Protect the incision line from sun exposure for 12 months.
- The nasal splint will be removed in 6 to 7 days after surgery.
- After your sutures are removed and the internal/external splints are removed, it is recommended that you use two squirts of a saline solution (salt water), in each nostril, six to eight times daily, to gently remove crusty formation from inside your nose.
- You can use nasal spray (Afrin) intermittently ONLY after the first week postoperative for improved nasal breathing, and then stop it after 5 to 7 days.
- If you experience increased nasal bleeding with bright red blood (with a need to change nasal pad every 30–40 minutes) notify you doctor immediately. You should sit up and apply pressure to the end of your nose for 15 minutes and you can

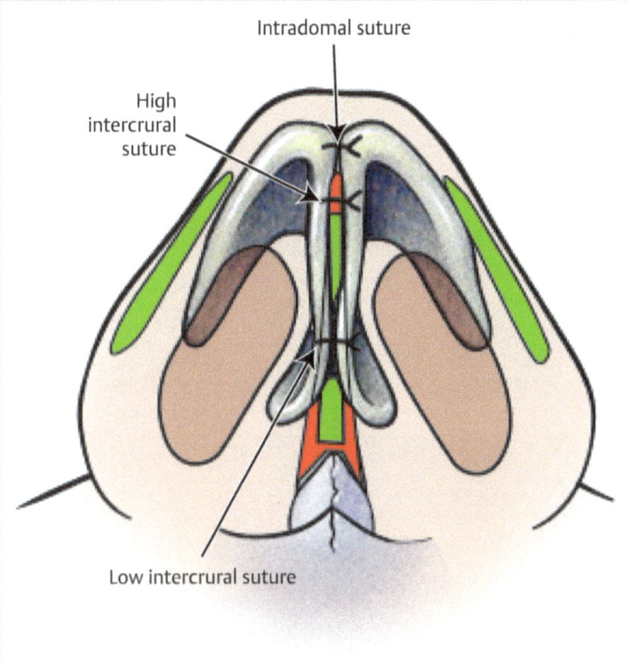

Fig. 17.6 Low and high intercrural sutures. (Reproduced with permission from Rohrich R, Ahmad J, eds. The Dallas Rhinoplasty and Dallas Cosmetic Surgery Dissection Guide. 1st ed. Thieme; 2018.)

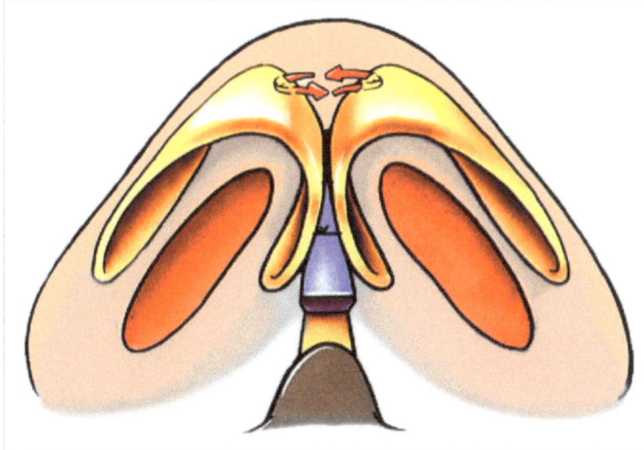

Fig. 17.8 Interdomal suture. (Reproduced with permission from Rohrich R, Ahmad J, eds. The Dallas Rhinoplasty and Dallas Cosmetic Surgery Dissection Guide. 1st ed. Thieme; 2018.)

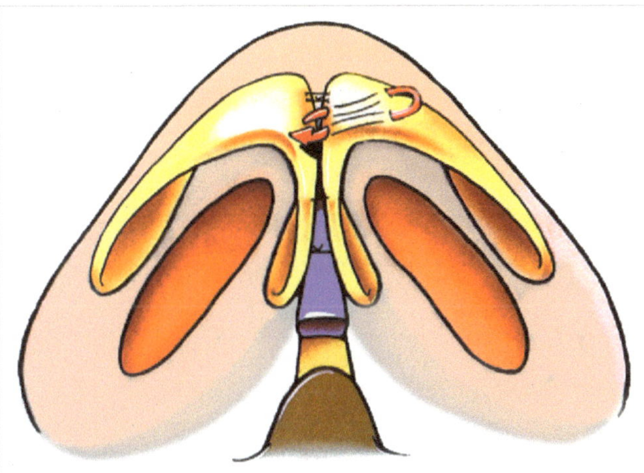

Fig. 17.7 Transdomal suture. (Reproduced with permission from Rohrich R, Ahmad J, eds. The Dallas Rhinoplasty and Dallas Cosmetic Surgery Dissection Guide. 1st ed. Thieme; 2018.)

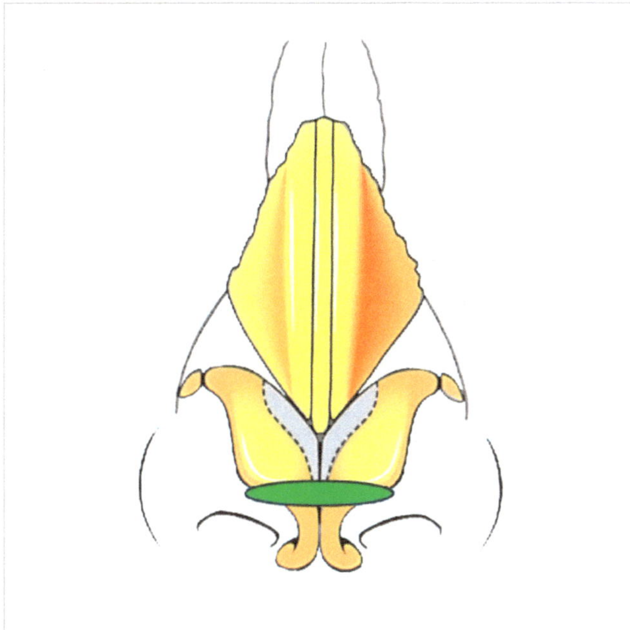

Fig. 17.9 Butterfly graft. (Reproduced with permission from Rohrich R, Ahmad J, eds. The Dallas Rhinoplasty and Dallas Cosmetic Surgery Dissection Guide. 1st ed. Thieme; 2018.)

use Afrin spray to stop the oozing in the interim. Bleeding usually stops with these maneuvers.

17.6 Case Example

Preoperative (left) and postoperative (right) views (12 months) of a 49-year-old male patient who underwent primary rhinoplasty with a septal extension graft reveals an improvement in nasal tip refinement and projection (▶ Fig. 17.10a–c).

17.7 Conclusion

Understanding the underlying anatomical components that provide nasal tip support and their effect on tip projection as

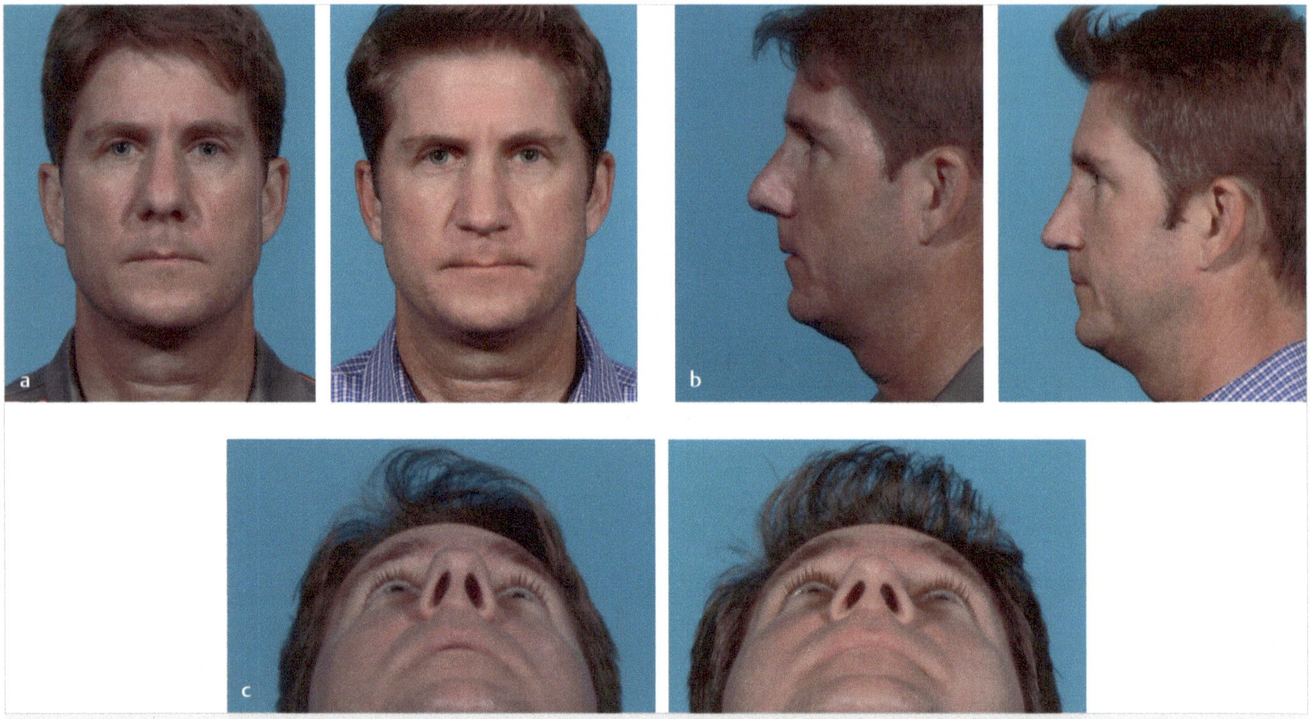

Fig. 17.10 (a–c) Preoperative (left) and postoperative (right) views (12 months) of a 49-year-old male patient who underwent primary rhinoplasty with a septal extension graft reveals an improvement in nasal tip refinement and projection.

well as a comprehensive and systematic nasofacial analysis is essential for success in nasal tip shaping.

Further Readings

Afrooz PN, Carboy JA, Mendez BM, Rohrich RJ. Cephalic rotation of the nasal tip. Plast Reconstr Surg. 2019; 143(4):734e–743e

Rohrich RJ, Afrooz PN. The infratip lobule butterfly graft: balancing the transition from the tip lobule to the alar lobule. Plast Reconstr Surg. 2018; 141(3): 651–654

Sieber DA, Rohrich RJ. Finesse in nasal tip refinement. Plast Reconstr Surg. 2017; 140 (2):277e–286e

Tanna N, Nguyen KT, Ghavami A, et al. Evidence-based medicine: current practices in rhinoplasty. Plast Reconstr Surg. 2018; 141(1):137e–151e

Villanueva NL, Afrooz PN, Carboy JA, Rohrich RJ. Nasal analysis: considerations for ethnic variation. Plast Reconstr Surg. 2019; 143(6):1179e–1188e

18 The Bulbous versus Boxy Tip

Rod J. Rohrich and Yash J. Avashia

Abstract

The bulbous and boxy tips are two common morphologies encountered in rhinoplasty. The management algorithms for both tips share various techniques. These techniques include but are not limited to cephalic trim, lateral crural turnover flaps, transdomal sutures, and interdomal sutures. A graduated approach to managing the bulbous and boxy tips will help in achieving consistent results. New concepts applied to the management include supporting alar rims with alar contour grafts, closing dead space through a series of techniques, and managing the soft tissue envelope.

Keywords: Tip shaping, bulbous, boxy, cephalic trim, dead space

Key Points

- Nasal tip reshaping is an important aspect of rhinoplasty.
- Two common tip morphologies are the bulbous and the boxy tip.
- Detailed preoperative analysis and intraoperative assessment aid in understanding the anatomic cause of the nasal tip morphology.
- A graduated approach to the tip with appropriate technique selection will provide consistent results in tip reshaping and minimize the risk of secondary deformity.

18.1 Preoperative Steps

- A detailed analysis of the nose is a critical prerequisite for understanding the anatomic framework underlying the shape abnormalities (▶ Fig. 18.1a, b).
- Bulbous tip:
  - The bulbous tip is described as having a wide, poorly defined shape.
  - The underlying anatomic causes include large lateral crura, dysmorphology of the lateral crura, and cephalically malpositioned lower lateral cartilages (LLCs).
  - The lateral crus may have one of the three morphologies:
    - Type I: Flat.
    - Type II: Convex.
    - Type III: Concave.
  - The cartilage may be strong or weak, which will also influence surgical technique.
  - Patients with bulbous nasal tips may often have external causes contributing to the tip volume, namely, thick, sebaceous skin.
- Boxy tip:
  - The boxy tip is best assessed from the basal view.
    - It is described as having a squared off shape.
  - Rohrich et al described a classification system based on intercrural angle of divergence and domal arch width (▶ Fig. 18.2a–c):
    - Type I: Intercrural angle >30 degrees with normal domal arch width (4mm).
    - Type II: Intercrural angle <30 degrees with wide domal arch width (>4mm).
    - Type III: Intercrural angle >30 degrees with wide domal arch width (>4mm).

18.2 Operative Steps

See **Video 18.1**.

18.2.1 Management

- The fundamental principles governing tip reshaping include cartilage preservation and suture techniques.
- Rohrich et al described a management algorithm that incorporates the techniques below for both classification systems for the boxy and bulbous tips.

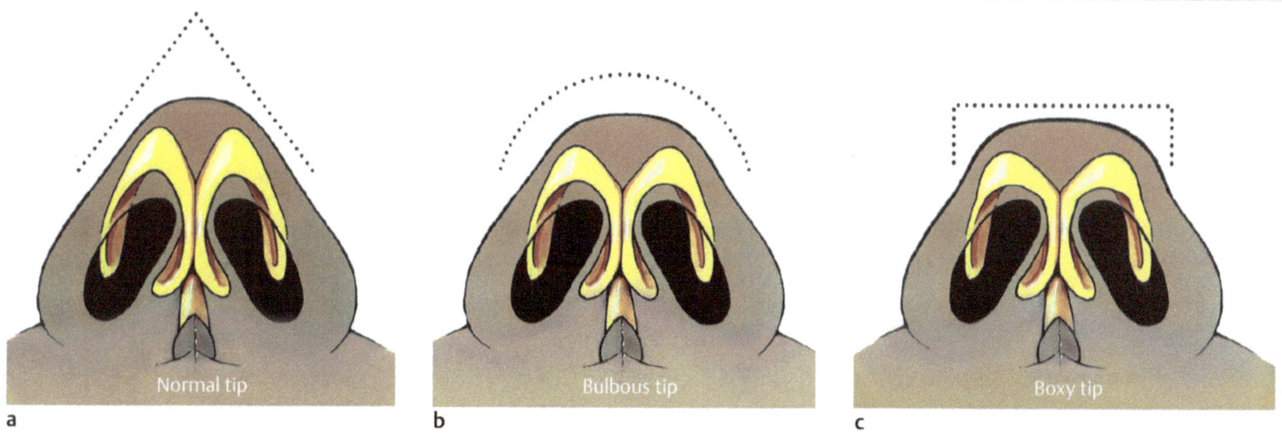

Fig. 18.1 (a–c) Morphology of normal, bulbous, and boxy tips. (Reproduced with permission from Rohrich R, Adams W, Ahmad J, et al, eds. Dallas Rhinoplasty: Nasal Surgery by the Masters. 3rd ed. Thieme; 2014.)

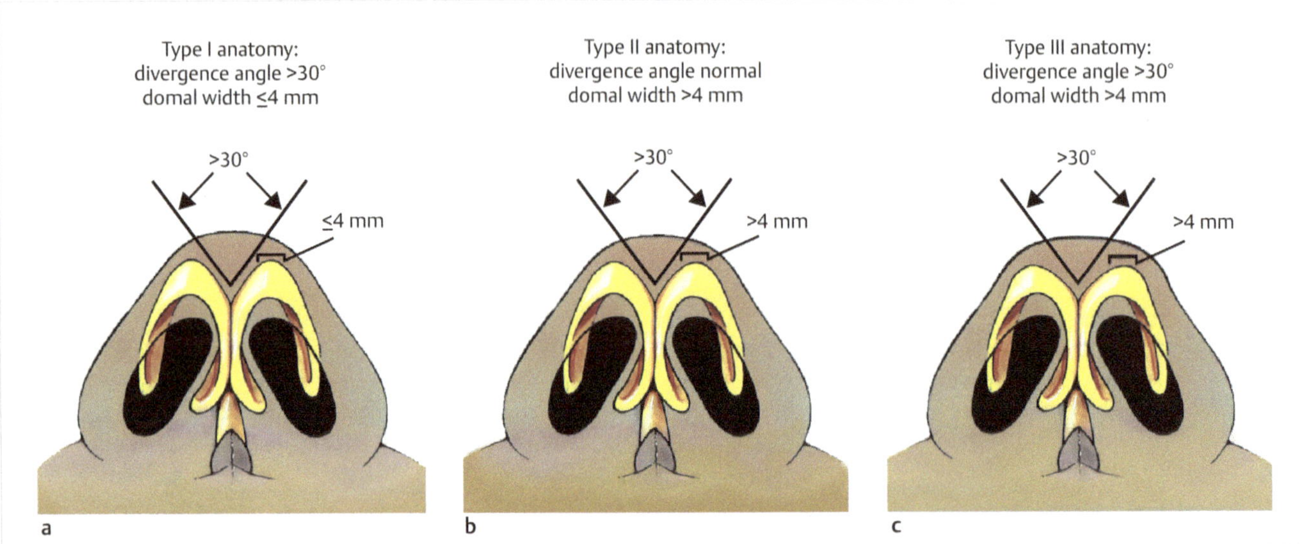

Fig. 18.2 (a–c) Classification of boxy tip based on domal arch width and interdomal angle of divergence. (Reproduced with permission from Rohrich R, Adams W, Ahmad J, et al, eds. Dallas Rhinoplasty: Nasal Surgery by the Masters. 3rd ed. Thieme; 2014.)

- Managing lower lateral cartilage cephalic excess:
  - Cephalic trim:
    - Separate the LLCs from the upper lateral cartilages at the scroll area.
    - LLC cephalic portion is undermined and excised to maintain at least 6 mm of LLC width to avoid excessive weakening of the lateral crura.
    - Cephalic trim may be applied to the lateral and/or middle crus depending on the tip morphology (see Algorithm Applied) (▶ Fig. 18.3).
  - Lateral crural turnover flap:
    - Lateral crus is partially incised, maintaining a 6-mm strip of cartilage caudally.
    - The cephalic cartilage is turned over and sutured to the caudal lateral crura.
    - This strengthens the lateral crura while reducing concavity.
- Tip sutures:
  - Transdomal suture:
    - The transdomal suture is a horizontal mattress suture placed through the medial and lateral aspects of the dome.
    - End points of this suture include (1) well-defined tip, (2) narrowing of the domal arch, (3) everted inferior margin of the lateral crus, and (4) straight and flat lateral crus.
    - The entry and exit points of this mattress suture dictate these end points.
  - Interdomal suture:
    - Horizontal mattress suture placed between the middle crura of the LLC.
    - The interdomal suture narrows the angle of domal divergence, narrows distance between tip-defining points, increases tip projection, and provides camouflage to the columellar strut or septal extension grafts.

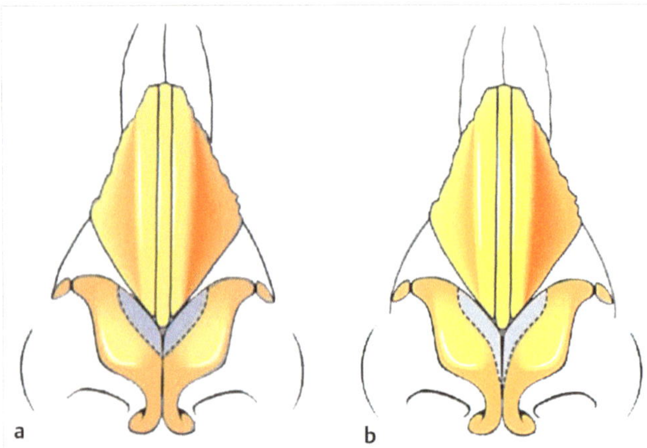

Fig. 18.3 Incremental approach to cephalic trim. **(a)** Shows limited cephalic trim. **(b)** Shows middle and lateral crural cephalic trim. (Reproduced with permission from Rohrich R, Ahmad J, eds. The Dallas Rhinoplasty and Dallas Cosmetic Surgery Dissection Guide. 1st ed. Thieme, 2018.)

- Current concepts for improved outcomes:
  - Septal extension graft (SEG):
    - In the bulbous or boxy tip, the SEG provides a stable point of fixation at the tip complex to aid in correcting lateral crural concavities. It allows superior control for change in projection and rotation.
    - Technical details of the SEG are discussed in Chapters 13 and 22.
  - Supporting alar rims with extended alar contour grafts (ACGs) and dual ACG:
    - Patients with bulbous or boxy tips often have weak alar rims.
    - Cephalic trim techniques inherently weaken the LLC.
    - To provide improved shape and structural support to the alar rims, nonanatomic extended alar contour

grafts are placed in pockets created along the alar margin.
  - 15 × 2 mm beveled cartilage grafts (septal or costal cartilage) are fashioned and placed in pretunneled pockets at the inferior alar margin.
  - After placement of extended ACG, any focal notching or contour irregularity along the inferior alar rim can be addressed by placing a dual ACG.
  - A small stab incision inferior to the irregularity is created with a #11 blade and a short 5-mm graft is placed in retrograde fashion to obliterate the residual notching.
- Dead space closure:
  - Dead space secondary to excess soft tissue envelope in a reduced framework needs to be addressed. This is most notable at the tip.
  - The infratip lobular butterfly graft provides additional infratip lobule definition with filling of the soft tissue triangles bilaterally. This helps in preventing soft tissue triangle scarring and retraction.
  - The soft tissue triangles may also be packed with crushed cartilage.
  - Splinting the soft tissue triangle can be done with Surgicel® coated with antibiotic ointment. These small antibiotic-covered pledgets are packed into the soft triangle to ensure tissue apposition and dead space closure.
  - Horizontal mattress sutures of 5–0 chromic gut at the columella and caudal septum at the end of rhinoplasty provide additional dead space closure and internal splinting.
  - Meticulous closure of the transcolumellar incision and infracartilaginous incisions additionally aids in reducing dead space.
- Skin management: In patients with thick nasal tip skin, incremental defatting of the skin envelope is performed with reassessment.

18.2.2 Algorithm Applied (▶ Fig. 18.4)

- Rohrich et al have provided an algorithm for management of the boxy tip along with an algorithm for cephalic trim that incorporates managing both the bulbous and boxy tips.
- The degree of cephalic trim depends on underlying anatomy of the LLC, its quality, and the aesthetic goals.
- Transdomal and interdomal sutures are applicable to all groups, and may be used incrementally to achieve the desired aesthetic outcome.

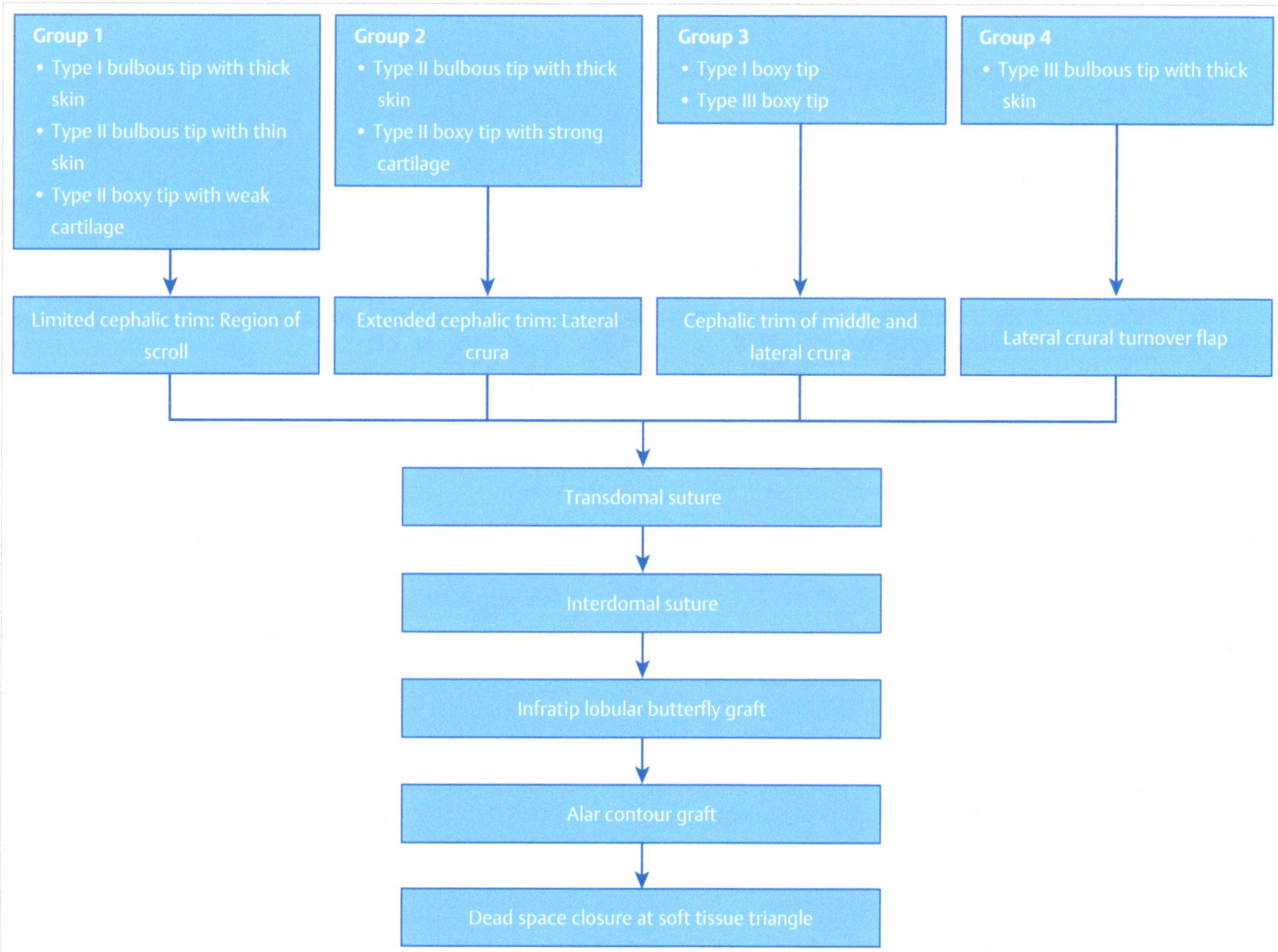

Fig. 18.4 Management algorithm for bulbous and boxy tip morphology.

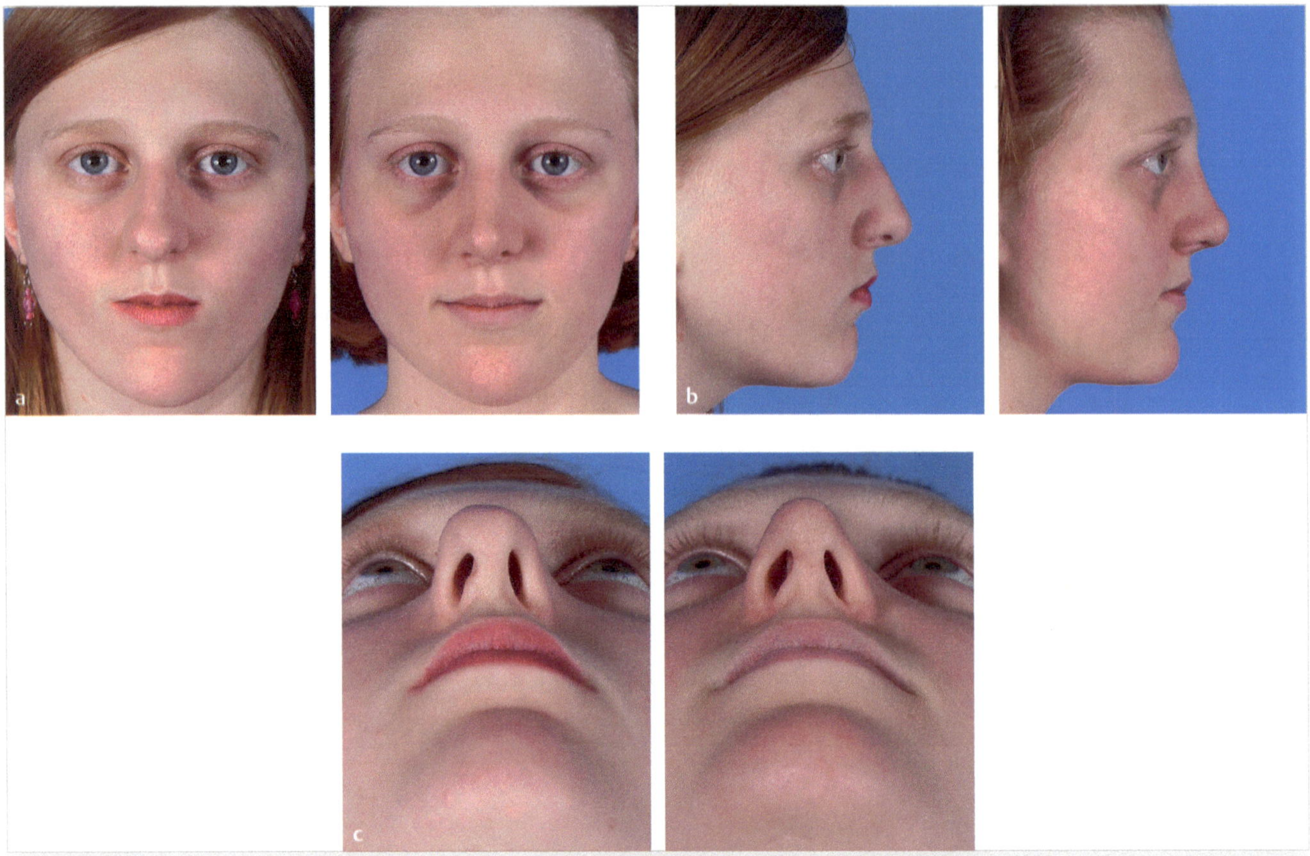

Fig. 18.5 (a–c) This is a 17-year-old female with physical examination findings of a Type II boxy nasal tip (upper row images). She underwent an open rhinoplasty with cephalic trim of her middle and lateral crura, leaving a lateral crural width which is greater than 6 mm. High intercrural sutures helped to stabilize the medial crura of the lower lateral cartilage (LLC). Oblique, transdomal, and interdomal sutures were applied to correct the boxy tip and to straighten the lateral crura, evert the LLC, and refine the tip by accentuating the caudal tip point. Extended bilateral alar contour grafts were used to support the alar rims and correct alar notching. Postoperative images are seen in the lower row.

- Finishing steps in the rhinoplasty include the use of infratip lobule butterfly graft, placement of extended alar contour grafts, and closure of dead space at the soft tissue triangle.

18.3 Case Example

This is a 17-year-old female with physical examination findings of a Type II boxy nasal tip (▶ Fig. 18.5a, b). She underwent an open rhinoplasty with cephalic trim of her middle and lateral crura, leaving a lateral crural width which is greater than 6 mm. High intercrural sutures helped to stabilize the medial crura of the LLC. Oblique, transdomal, and interdomal sutures were applied to correct the boxy tip and to straighten the lateral crura, evert the LLC, and refine the tip by accentuating the caudal tip point. Extended bilateral alar contour grafts were used to support the alar rims and correct alar notching. Postoperative images are seen in the (▶ Fig. 18.5c).

18.4 Conclusion

Correction of the bulbous and boxy tips includes a detailed preoperative analysis, intraoperative assessment, and selection of appropriate techniques described to achieve optimal nasal tip shape.

Further Readings

Nagarkar P, Stark RY, Pezeshk RA, Amirlak B, Rohrich RJ. Role of the cephalic trim in modern rhinoplasty. Plast Reconstr Surg. 2016; 137(1):89–96

Rohrich RJ, Adams WP, Jr. The boxy nasal tip: classification and management based on alar cartilage suturing techniques. Plast Reconstr Surg. 2001; 107(7):1849–1863, discussion 1864–1868

Rohrich RJ, Afrooz PN. The infratip lobule butterfly graft: balancing the transition from the tip lobule to the alar lobule. Plast Reconstr Surg. 2018; 141(3):651–654

Sieber DA, Rohrich RJ. Finesse in nasal tip refinement. Plast Reconstr Surg. 2017; 140(2):277e–286e

Unger JG, Roostaeian J, Small KH, et al. Alar contour grafts in rhinoplasty: a safe and reproducible way to refine alar contour aesthetics. Plast Reconstr Surg. 2016; 137(1):52–61

19 The Crooked Nose

Christina R. Vargas and Bahman Guyuron

Abstract

The approach to the crooked nose is determined by thoughtful analysis of the face in its entirety, including all of the components of the nasal structure and function. Attention to correction of deviated nasal bones, septum, dorsum, and base, as well as associated turbinate hypertrophy is critical to successful outcomes.

Keywords: Rhinoplasty, deviated, correction, turbinectomy, septum, bone, cartilage

Key Points

- A deviated nose is almost invariably associated with some degree of nasal dysfunction.
- Circumspect examination of the entire face, the external nasal frame, and internal nasal structures is crucial in avoiding residual or persistent deviations, which may be multifaceted.
- The intersecting point of the eyebrows should not be used for judging the nose alignment since often this is altered by the patients differentially to place the deviated nose in the center of the eyebrows.

19.1 Preoperative Steps

19.1.1 Analysis

- A detailed patient history including nasal trauma, prior surgery, airway complaints, and allergies is obtained.
- Thorough preoperative analysis is performed, including the external nose and face, oral or nasal breathing, overall symmetry, occlusal plane canting, nose alignment with other facial structures, chin position, intercanthal midline, palatal arch, and facial nerve function.
- The nose is observed zone by zone for deviated structures, including the nasal bones, anterior septum, and upper and lower cartilages with basilar and overhead views. The presence of nasal valve incompetence, internal septal deviation, turbinate hypertrophy, synechia, perforation, spurs, contact points, ulceration, and polyps is assessed.
- Examination is repeated after vasoconstriction of the nasal mucosa using phenylephrine or ephedrine sulfate.
- Review of a computed tomography scan may be performed in patients reporting frequent sinus headaches, infections, or migraine headaches to detect underlying sinusitis, concha bullosa, septa bullosa, and contact points.

19.2 Operative Steps

See **Video 19.1**.

19.2.1 Correction of Deviated Nasal Bones

Onlay Grafting

- Under general anesthesia, the face is prepped and nasal vasoconstriction achieved.
- An intercartilaginous incision is made or an open approach is used and the target nasal bone is exposed. The periosteum is elevated in limited fashion.
- A septal or conchal cartilage graft in the form of a single or double layer is gently crushed. Depending on the degree of the nasal bone shift, diced cartilage or a layer of soft tissue, such as dermis or fascia graft, is applied in the subperiosteal plane and molded in place.
- The incision is repaired loosely to allow for drainage.

Unilateral Out-fracture

- Through a small vestibular incision at the pyriform aperture, the periosteum is elevated using a Joseph's periosteal elevator.
- A low-to-low osteotomy is made and the nasal bone is out-fractured.
- A spreader graft is placed via a 3-mm incision in the mucoperichondrium immediately caudal to the junction of the upper lateral cartilage and the septum anteroposteriorly. A septal elevator is used to create a pocket and the graft is inserted between the septum and the upper lateral cartilage.
- A piece of folded Adaptic or Surgicel saturated in Bacitracin ointment is placed between the nasal bone and the septum and kept in place for at least 1 week. The patient is maintained on systemic antibiotics during this period.

19.2.2 Correction of Deviated Septum

- An open technique is employed with concomitant rhinoplasty, or an L-shaped (Killian) incision is used for a closed approach.
- Mucoperichondrium of the left side of the septum is elevated beginning with the caudal septal angle.
- Once the correct, glistening, greyish cartilage plane is exposed, the blunt end of a periosteal elevator is used to raise the mucoperichondrial flap posteriorly, cephalically, and caudally.

- An L-shaped incision is carried through the quadrangular cartilage using the sharp end of a septal elevator, leaving at least a 15 mm wide L-strut anteriorly and 10 mm caudally.
- The caudal portion of the septal cartilage is gently separated from the maxillary crest of the vomer bone using the sharp end of the septal elevator. Cartilage is separated from the perpendicular plate of the ethmoid bone in similar fashion and subsequently removed.
- Deviated portions of the vomer bone and perpendicular plate are removed as extensively as necessary to eliminate the internal deviations and the spur posteriorly.
- Any midvault deviation is the consequence of septal deviation and five out of six classes of septal deviations described by the senior author could be involved in nasal deviations.

Septal Tilt (▸ Fig. 19.1)

- The septal tilt is corrected initially by removing the posterocaudal portion of the septum, leaving an L-strut septum anteriorly and caudally.
- It is crucial to disengage the dislodged caudal and posterior portions of the retained L-strut from the vomerine groove and anterior nasal spine.
- Overlapping redundant caudal portions of the septal cartilage are removed to provide a "swinging door" type free movement of this cartilage.
- The anterior nasal spine is palpated between the right thumb and index finger to ensure it is in midline position. If it is deviated, a greenstick fracture is performed to allow repositioning.
- The septum is repositioned and fixed to the periosteum of the anterior nasal spine using a figure-of-eight 5–0 PDS suture.

Correction of Anteroposterior C-Shaped Deviation (▸ Fig. 19.2)

- Resection of the posterocaudal portion of the septum is performed as described previously. Osteotomy of the anterior nasal spine and residual vomer plate is often necessary in order to reposition this structure in the midline.
- Release of tension by removal of the posterior and caudal portion of the cartilage and creation of a swinging door-type movement will often eliminate the C-shaped cartilage deformity.
- Otherwise, cephalocaudal-oriented scoring of the concave surface of the L-shaped frame is performed, although this is seldom necessary.
- Bilateral extramucosal stents are placed and fixed in position with a through-and-through suture to mold the cartilage during healing. These are left in place for at least 2, preferably 3, weeks.
- Anterior deviation of the nose is corrected by separation of the upper lateral cartilages from the septum, osteotomy, repositioning of the frame, differential trimming of the upper lateral cartilages, and placement of spreader grafts, often without scoring.

C-Shaped Cephalocaudal Deviation (▸ Fig. 19.3)

- The same approach is used as in anteroposterior C-shaped deviation, with the exception of the direction of scoring, if necessary. Cartilage should be scored in an anteroposterior direction on the concave side of the cartilage.
- Often, as above, release of tension is accomplished by resection of the posterior portion of the cartilage and removal of the redundant portion of the cartilage overlapping the vomer bone and the nasal spine.

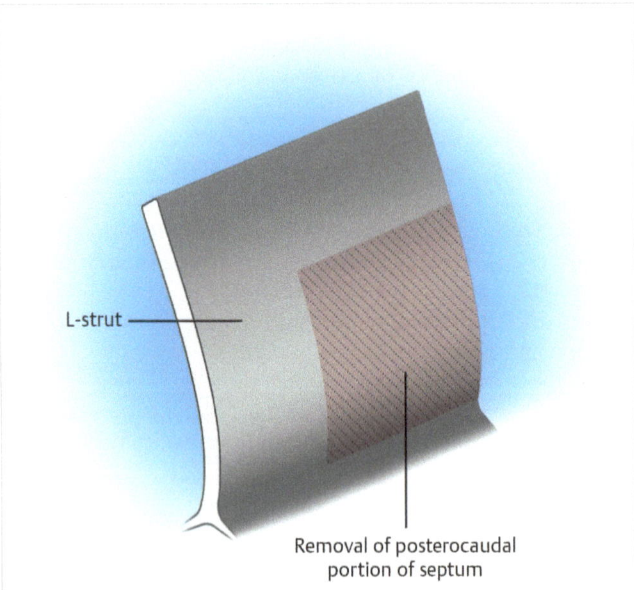

Fig. 19.1 Septal tilt.

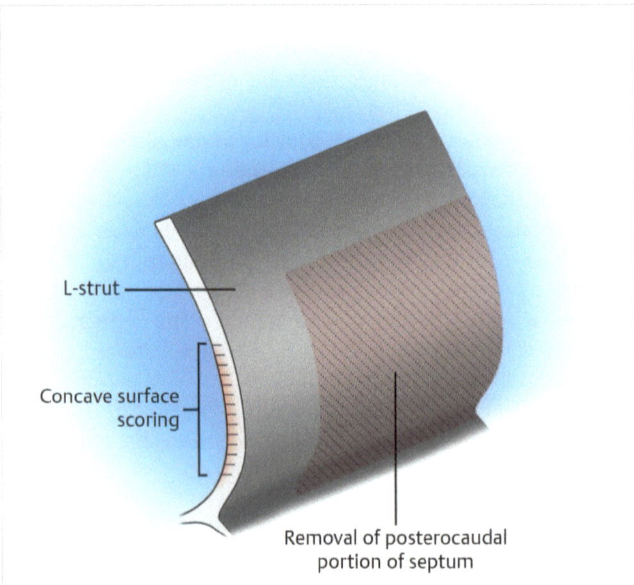

Fig. 19.2 Correction of anteroposterior C-shaped deviation.

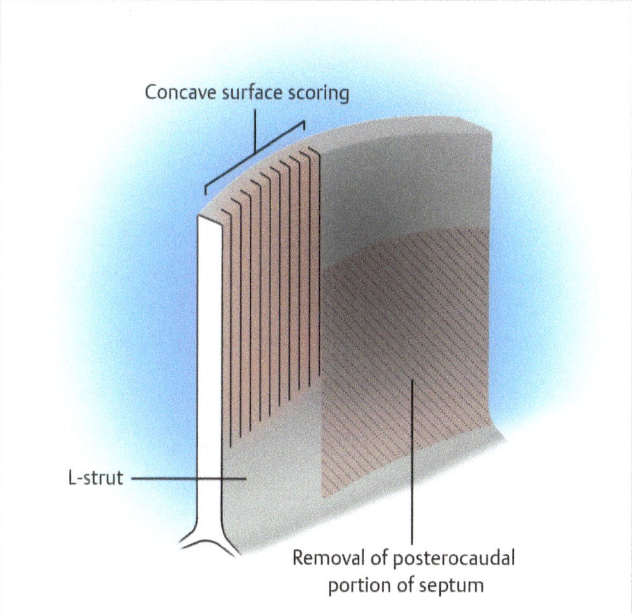

Fig. 19.3 C-shaped cephalocaudal deviation.

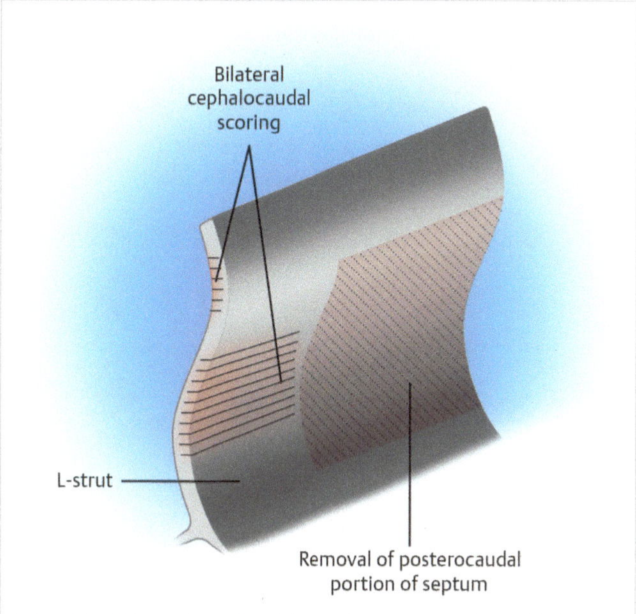

Fig. 19.4 S-shaped anteroposterior deviation.

- Extramucosal stents and spreader grafts help to keep the septum straight until there has been adequate healing.

S-Shaped Anteroposterior Deviation (▶ Fig. 19.4)

- Correction is achieved by removal of the posterior portion of the cartilage and bone, bilateral cephalocaudal scoring of the cartilage on both concave surfaces if necessary, and osteotomy with repositioning of the nasal spine and vomer bone when indicated.
- Commonly, elimination of tension and application of spreader grafts to direct the memory of the cartilage is sufficient to preclude scoring.
- Extramucosal stents and spreader grafts are applied if caudal scoring is performed.

S-Shaped Cephalocaudal Deviation (▶ Fig. 19.5)

- Correction is similar to that for S-shaped anteroposterior deviation with the exception of the direction of scoring, which is in the anteroposterior direction, if deemed necessary.
- Placement of bilateral spreader grafts is crucial.

Localized Deviation and Spurs (▶ Fig. 19.6)

- Posterocaudal resection of septal cartilage often results in correction of this deformity and elimination of spurs, which are often located at the junction of the vomer bone with the quadrangle cartilage and perpendicular plate of the ethmoid bone.

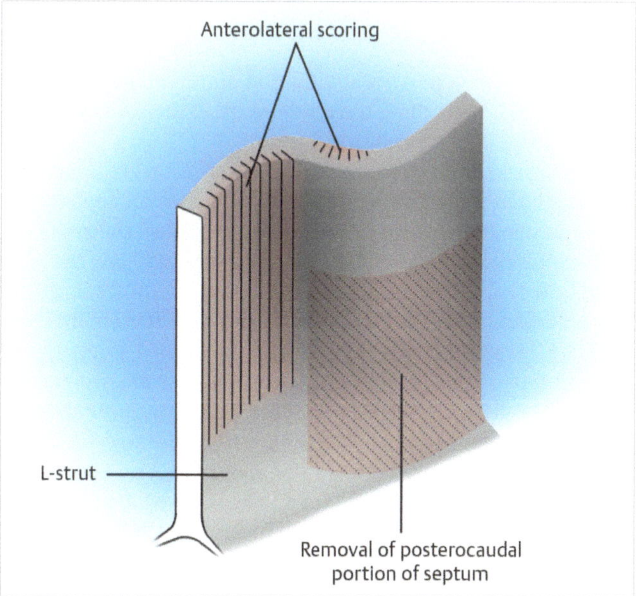

Fig. 19.5 S-shaped cephalocaudal deviation.

- Dissection of the mucoperichondrium on the concave side of the septum is essential to avoid inadvertent tearing.
- Unilateral mucoperichondrial tears are inconsequential. Bilateral nonapposing tears may also heal without persistent perforation. However, these, as well as bilateral apposing tears, are addressed using a straight piece of septal cartilage, perpendicular plate of the ethmoid bone, or a PDS plate placed in between the mucoperichondrial flaps spanning fully across the perforation site.

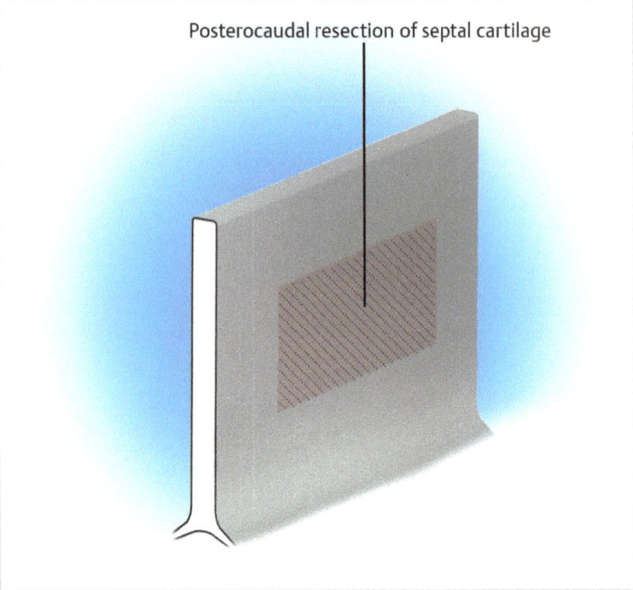

Fig. 19.6 Localized deviation and spurs.

19.2.3 Correction of Deviated Caudal Dorsum

- For correction of persistent deviation of the caudal portion of the dorsal L-strut along the caudal third of the anterior septum, a septal rotation suture is used.
- After spreader grafts are secured, a 5–0 PDS suture is passed through the caudal upper lateral cartilage further cephalically on the side toward which the septum should be shifted.
- The suture is passed through the spreader grafts and the septum, then through the opposite upper lateral cartilage relatively caudally on the side toward which the septum is currently deviated, and brought back to the side of its origin. This suture is tied incrementally until the septum becomes perfectly aligned along a line bisecting the intercanthal line and the upper incisor midline, as long as these structures are positioned centrally.
- A second suture may be required to avoid bowing of the upper lateral cartilage on the side toward which the septum is being rotated.

19.2.4 Correction of Deviated Nasal Base

- This deviation is the result of disparity in the length of the lower lateral cartilage and correction will require shortening of the lower lateral on one side or elongation of the other side governed by the aesthetics of the nasal tip.

Reduction in Projection of the Lower Lateral Cartilage

- If the caudal septum is displaced, it is straightened prior to adjusting the length of the lower lateral cartilage.
- Cartilage is exposed, transected, and overlapped laterally, medially, or both depending on the orientation of the lower lateral cartilage.
- A columellar strut is used for support.
- The domes are aligned at the midline and the segments sutured to avoid shifting.
- Under most circumstances bilateral Gunter lateral crura struts are placed.

Elongation of the Lower Lateral Cartilage

- The lower lateral cartilage is mobilized completely, advanced anteriorly, and fixed in position with the support of a columella and lateral crus strut, with or without the interruption of the lateral and medial crura.
- The segments are fixed in position securely to reposition the deviated nasal base.

19.2.5 Turbinectomy

- Partial resection of hypertrophic middle and inferior turbinates is performed evenly across the full length of the turbinate.
- The middle turbinate is out-fractured or partially or completely removed if indicated in the case of migraine headaches originating from the retrobulbar region.

19.3 Postoperative Care

- A dorsal splint is applied if an osteotomy is part of the procedure, otherwise Steri-Strips are applied.
- Doyle splints are placed on either side of the septum in an extramucosal fashion and fixed in position using 4–0 Prolene sutures.
- The external splint is removed after 8 days; the internal Doyle stent is removed in 3 to 8 days, depending on the condition.
- The extramucosal internal splints that are placed after septal scoring are maintained for 2 to 3 weeks.
- The patient is kept on antibiotics for the duration of time that the Doyle internal splints are used.
- If a nasal bone osteotomy is part of the procedure, a Medrol dose pack is also prescribed to minimize edema and bruising, unless the patient has active or severe acne.
- Heavy physical activity is curtailed for 3 weeks.
- The patient is instructed to avoid wearing any kind of glasses for 5 weeks after nasal bone osteotomy.

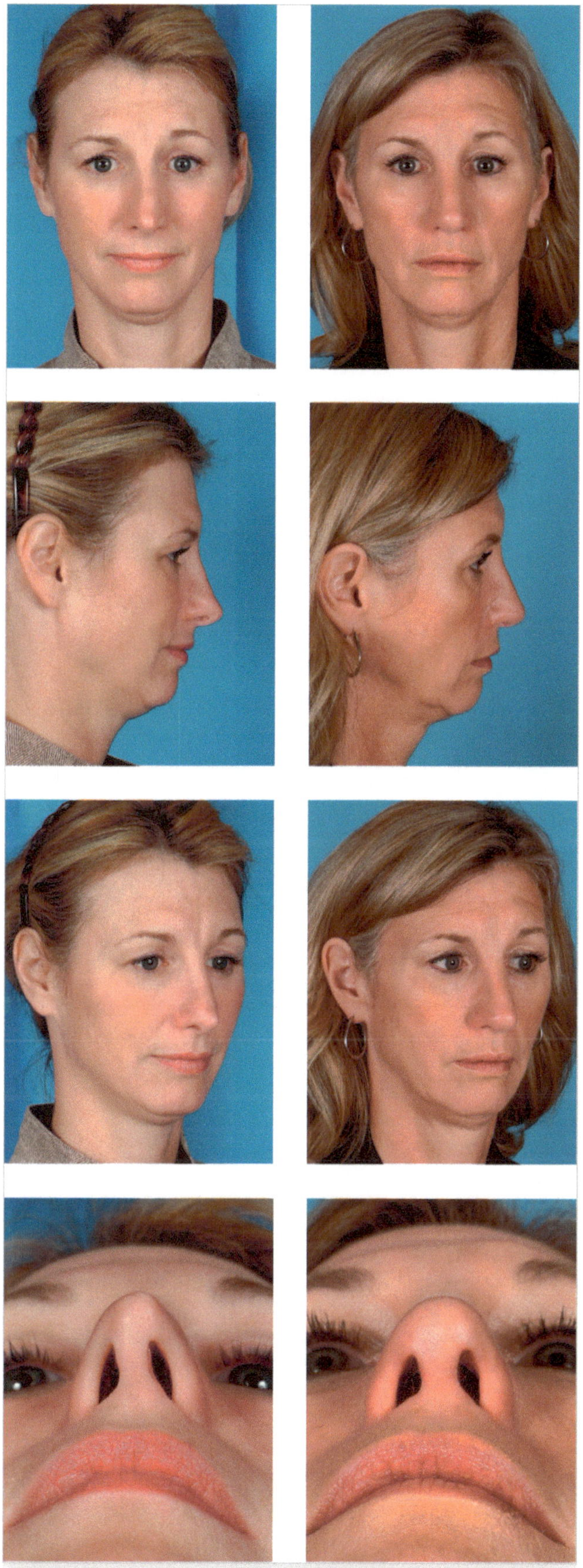

Fig. 19.7 A patient with residual C-shaped cephalocaudal deviation before (left) and after (right) correction of the deformity.

19.4 Case Example

A patient with residual C-shaped cephalocaudal deviation before (left) and after correction of the deformity is shown (▶ Fig. 19.7).

The surgical maneuvers included the following:

- Open technique was used.
- The radix was deepened using a guarded burr.
- The dorsal hump was removed.
- The septoplasty was done through an L-shaped incision.
- Bilateral medial, vertical percutaneous and low-to-low osteotomies were done.
- Right-sided spreader graft was placed.
- A small onlay graft was applied to the dorsum on the right side.
- The medial crura were approximated.
- The fused, distorted domes were lowered beyond what is ideal, proportional to the thickness of the intended tip graft.
- Conchal cartilage was harvested through a posteromedial incision.
- A tip graft was harvested using Guyuron punch from the removed conchal cartilage (Black & Black).
- A thin lobule graft was applied.
- Bilateral alar rim grafts were applied.
- The caudal septum with proportional amount of membranous lining was removed to allow cephalic rotation of the tip.
- Bilateral soft triangle grafts were applied.
- The nose was taped and splinted.

19.5 Conclusion

The septum and nasal bones control the direction of the nose; deviation can result from misalignment of one or the other, or a combination of both. Deviation of the lower nose may involve the caudal septum, anterior nasal spine, and lower lateral cartilages.

There are six classes of septal deviation: septal tilt, C-shaped anteroposterior deviation, C-shaped cephalocaudal deviation, S-shaped anteroposterior deviation, S-shaped cephalocaudal deviation, and localized deviation or spur. These must be identified and properly addressed to obtain a successful outcome.

Residual or persistent deviations are often due to failure to recognize the full extent of the structural deviations. Adjustment in the size of the turbinates plays a cardinal role in the restoration of nasal function following correction of nasal deviation.

Further Readings

Ahmad J, Rohrich RJ. The crooked nose. Clin Plast Surg. 2016; 43(1):99–113

Gunter JP, Rohrich RJ. Management of the deviated nose: the importance of septal reconstruction. Clin Plast Surg. 1988; 15(1):43–55

Guyuron B, Behmand RA. Caudal nasal deviation. Plast Reconstr Surg. 2003; 111(7): 2449–2457, discussion 2458–2459

Guyuron B, Uzzo CD, Scull H. A practical classification of septonasal deviation and an effective guide to septal surgery. Plast Reconstr Surg. 1999; 104(7):2202–2209, discussion 2210–2212

Stepnick D, Guyuron B. Surgical treatment of the crooked nose. Clin Plast Surg. 2010; 37(2):313–325

20 The Ethnic Nose

Shahryar Tork and Ashkan Ghavami

Abstract

Success in ethnic rhinoplasty can be achieved through accurate preoperative analysis, recognition of the common and variable features within each ethnic group, and precise technical maneuvers. The open approach allows for precise intraoperative anatomic diagnosis and the construction of an ethnically congruent nose. Familiarity with a range of cartilage grafting techniques is critical to the surgeon's repertoire. A combination of tip suturing techniques is needed in ethnic rhinoplasty; however, overly exaggerated modification is to be avoided. Skin redraping is done throughout the process of dorsal modification and tip shaping to assess the influence of each maneuver on the external surface. The cartilaginous frame should be fashioned by maneuvers that increase tip support and add refinement. Selective debulking of the nasal skin/soft tissue envelope improves its contractile response to the underlying architecture. Ethnic patients, in particular, are counseled on the prolonged postoperative healing and instructed on self-taping to help with edema.

Although ethnic rhinoplasty is far more complicated than in Caucasian patients, excellent outcomes can be obtained by experienced surgeons who recognize that the ultimate goal is nasofacial harmony.

Keywords: Ethnic rhinoplasty, open rhinoplasty, African nose, Middle Eastern nose, Hispanic nose

Key Points

- Patient selection and management of expectations are prerequisites to achieving good outcomes and patient satisfaction in ethnic rhinoplasty.
- Although a variable spectrum of nasal morphology exists within each ethnic group, certain characteristics are generally present and can overlap with other ethnicities (▶ Table 20.1).
- Patients generally fall into two categories: those whose desire a nose aligned with Caucasian ideals, and those who want to preserve their ancestral traits.
- The surgeon must recognize which presenting traits require which treatments and what combination of techniques will ultimately produce a racially congruent aesthetic result.
- Familiarity with a range of cartilage grafting techniques is critical to the surgeon's repertoire.
- A combination of tip suturing techniques is needed in ethnic rhinoplasty; however, overly exaggerated modification is to be avoided.
- Regardless of ethnic origin, the ultimate goal is to create nasofacial harmony.

20.1 Preoperative Steps

- A thorough approach to nasofacial analysis is critical to achieving harmony and balance in ethnic rhinoplasty.
    - Appreciate the most common goals in rhinoplasty among different ethnic groups (▶ Table 20.2).
    - Evaluate each nose individually, define problematic areas across nasofacial morphologies, and recognize anatomical features that allow for ethnic congruity (Fig. 20.1a–c).

20.2 Operative Steps

The following is our general approach to any ethnic rhinoplasty.

20.2.1 Opening the Nose

- Inverted-"V" transcolumellar incision joined to bilateral infracartilaginous incisions.
- Wide undermining is necessary in patients with a thick, amorphous skin/soft tissue envelope.

20.2.2 Component Dorsum via Anterior-Inferior Approach

- Bilateral mucoperichondrial flaps are raised with a Cottle elevator.
- Upper lateral cartilages are separated from the septum with a #15 blade.
- Septal harvest is performed, preserving at least a 10-mm L-strut.
- *Dorsal reduction (when indicated):*
    - Using a graduated approach, excess cartilaginous septum is excised with angled septal scissors and the bony dorsum is reduced with a rasp.
        - When an open roof is very cephalad, ULC length may be inadequate and true spreader grafts will be required.
    - Reduction of a large dorsal hump, coupled with a low radix, usually requires augmentation with grafting techniques.
    - For augmentation of the radix, we prefer to use diced cartilage facial graft (DCFG) from the concha, rather than an intact onlay graft.
- Dorsal augmentation (when indicated):
    - Generally required in African and Asian noses.
    - The final assessment for dorsal augmentation is made after the osteotomies (when indicated) and tip enhancement.
    - The gold standard is rib cartilage. If the patient does not desire this or requires less than 6 mm of augmentation, then we prefer septal grafting with fascia, AlloDerm (LifeCell Corp., Branchburg, NJ) overlay, or DCFG (▶ Fig. 20.2).
    - *Note: The main concerns of African American patients are usually focused on the nasal tip and nostrils; they may not perceive the extent of their dorsal deficiency.*

20.2.3 Midvault Stabilization

- Achieved with spreader flaps or upper lateral cartilage tension spanning sutures.

Table 20.1 A summary of ethnic variations and common anatomic features in the African, Middle Eastern, and Hispanic nose

	Caucasian	Black	Middle Eastern	Hispanic			
				Castilian	Mexican American	Mestizo	Creole
Frontal view	Equally proportioned vertical fifths and horizontal thirds of face	Wider middle fifth, shorter middle third of face	Equally proportioned vertical fifths and horizontal thirds of face	Equally proportioned vertical fifths and horizontal thirds of face	Equally proportioned vertical fifths and horizontal thirds of face	Variable vertical fifths and horizontal thirds of face	Wider middle fifth, shorter middle third of face
	Nasal length two-thirds of midfacial height	Short nasal length	Short nasal length	Nasal length two-thirds of midfacial height	Nasal length two-thirds of midfacial height	Nasal length two-thirds of midfacial height	Short nasal length
	Symmetric DAL	Symmetric DAL	Asymmetric DAL	Symmetric DAL	Symmetric DAL	Symmetric DAL	Symmetric DAL
	Bony vault 80% of base width	Wide dorsum	Wide dorsum	Bony vault 80% of base width	Bony vault 80% of base width	Wide dorsum	Wide dorsum
	Alar base width equals intercanthal distance	Wide alar base width	Alar base width equal to or less than intercanthal distance	Alar base width equals intercanthal distance	Alar base width equals intercanthal distance	Wide alar base width	Wide alar base width
	Symmetric tip defining points	Bulbous tip; less-defined tip defining points	Bulbous tip; less-defined tip defining points	Symmetric tip defining points	Symmetric tip defining points	Bulbous tip; less-defined tip defining points	Bulbous tip; less-defined tip defining points
Lateral view	Radix between lash line and supratarsal crease	Less projected and caudally located radix	Overprojected and cranially located radix	Radix between lash line and supratarsal crease	Caudally located radix	Radix between lash line and supratarsal crease	Less projected and caudally located radix
	Smooth dorsum	Low dorsum	Dorsal hump	Increased projection	Illusion of dorsal hump	Underprojected tip	Low dorsum
	Projection two-thirds of ideal length	Decreased projection	Increased projection	Projection two-thirds of ideal length	Decreased projection	Projection two-thirds of ideal length	Decreased projection
	Supratip break	No supratip break	No supratip break	Supratip break	No supratip break	Supratip break	Supratip break
	NLA (male, 90–95 degrees; female, 95–100 degrees)	Increased NLA; retracted columella	Decreased NLA; hanging columella; dependent tip	NLA (male, 90–95 degrees; female, 95–100 degrees)	Decreased NLA	NLA (male, 90–95 degrees; female, 95–100 degrees)	Increased NLA
Basal view	Appears as equilateral triangle	Variable shape	Deviated and overprojected tip	Appears as equilateral triangle	Underprojected tip	Underprojected tip	Variable shape
	Tip to columella ratio is 1:2	Short columella	Short columella	Tip to columella ratio is 1:2	Tip to columella ratio is 1:2	Short columella	Short columella
	Symmetric nostrils with teardrop shape	Horizontally oriented nostrils; splayed MFP	Asymmetric nostrils; splayed MFP; deep soft triangles	Symmetric nostrils with teardrop shape	Symmetric nostrils with teardrop shape	Symmetric nostrils	Asymmetric nostrils; splayed MFP

Abbreviations: DAL, dorsal aesthetic lines; MFP, medial crural footplates; NLA, nasolabial angle.
Source: Adapted from Villanueva NL, Afrooz PN, Carboy, JA, Rohrich RJ. Nasal analysis: considerations for ethnic variation. Plast Reconstr Surg 2019;143(6).

Table 20.2 A summary of the most common goals in rhinoplasty for the African, Middle Eastern, and Hispanic nose

Black	Middle Eastern	Hispanic		
		Castilian	Mexican American	Mestizo and Creole
• Correct dorsal/base disproportions • Balance rhinoplasty • Dorsal augmentation with/without osteotomies usually needed • Skin/soft tissue debulking and wide undermining needed; helps with lateral redraping of nasal skin envelope • Enhanced tip projection and definition • Reduce, yet maintain subtle alar flaring • Decrease interalar distance	• Smaller nose • Functional reduction rhinoplasty with a moderate dorsal (avoid over resection) • Narrow the wide and long nasal bones • Debulk fibrofatty tissue (especially in the supratip and paradomal areas) • Define nasal tip through controlled, cartilage preserving techniques • Avoid overcorrection of NLA and over-rotation of nasal tip • Correct tip under-projection with proper rotation and middle/medial crura suturing • Address hyperdynamic tip through treatment of depressor septi nasi muscle • Reposition/reduce alar bases Correct nostril tip imbalance • Use struts and invisible grafting techniques whenever possible	• Smaller nose • Functional reduction rhinoplasty with a significant dorsal reduction • Radix may require reduction/deepening to distinguish nasal root and dorsal profile • Usually tip is adequately projected or evenly overprojected, (address through simple volume reduction and tip refinement) • Spreader graft if significant open roof or deviation present • Need substantial narrowing of the bony vault (use low-to-low and transverse osteotomies for complete mobilization)	• Straighter profile with gentle set-off of the tip • Finesse rhinoplasty • DCFG for radix/dorsal augmentation (avoid partial length grafts); become visible under the thin skin near the rhinion • Usually does not require osteotomies nor caudal septal resection • Open tip suture technique to reposition/shape alar cartilages (minimal resection) • Onlay tip grafts to gain projection and definition if tip suturing alone is inadequate	• Correct dorsal/base disproportions • Balance rhinoplasty • Maximally change the base first, then dorsal augmentation, only if required • Skin/soft tissue debulking and wide undermining needed; helps with lateral redraping of nasal skin envelope • DCFG if radix/dorsal augmentation needed (common for Creole nose) • Usually combined nostril sill/alar wedge resection is needed (reduces both nostril size and alar flaring) • Use alar rim grafts to avoid notching of the alar rim • Usually no need for osteotomies • Tip definition

Abbreviations: DCFG, diced cartilage facial graft; NLA, nasolabial angle.
Source: Adapted from Rohrich RJ, Ghavami A. Rhinoplasty for the Middle Eastern nose. Plast Reconstr Surg 2009;123(4).

- If a large dorsal reduction was performed (>6mm), the upper lateral cartilages are weak, or the nasal bones are short, spreader grafts are used.

20.2.4 Soft Tissue Debulking (▶ Fig. 20.3)

- Generally indicated for tip refinement in African and Middle Eastern noses.
- A thick and inelastic nasal skin envelope blunts changes made to the underlying architecture.
  - The undersurface of the nasal skin, particularly in the supratip, domal, and peridomal region, is trimmed to, but not past, the level of the subdermal plexus.
  - Thickness of the tip skin will determine the dimensions and thickness of any tip grafts.
- Note: Debulking should NOT be a reflexive maneuver by the surgeon. Skin redraping is done throughout the process of dorsal modification and tip shaping to assess the influence of each maneuver on the external surface.

20.2.5 Tip Projection and Shaping

- Construct the cartilaginous frame/shape with maneuvers that will increase tip support and add refinement.
- A septal extension graft or columellar strut is used for tip stabilization.
- Avoid overcorrection of nasolabial angle and over-rotation of the nasal tip.
- *Note: A combination of tip suturing techniques is needed in ethnic rhinoplasty; however, overly exaggerated modification is to be avoided.*
- A cephalic trim (when indicated) is performed with preservation of at least 6 mm of lower lateral cartilage.
- Lateral crural turnover flap is a highly effective technique in ethnic patients because irregularities in the lateral crura are corrected while simultaneously improving rim support (▶ Fig. 20.4).
- Low and high intercrural sutures are placed followed by transdomal and interdomal sutures, as needed.
- Additional crushed graft remnants can be placed after closure of the columella to obliterate residual dead space and add further tip refinement.
- Excess columellar show is corrected with medial crural septal sutures.
  - Footplate excision or a cinching mattress suture across the columellar base, along with intercrural space soft tissue excision, is performed to further enhance the alar base–nostril relationship.
- Note: Overcorrection of the nasolabial angle leads to racial incongruity.

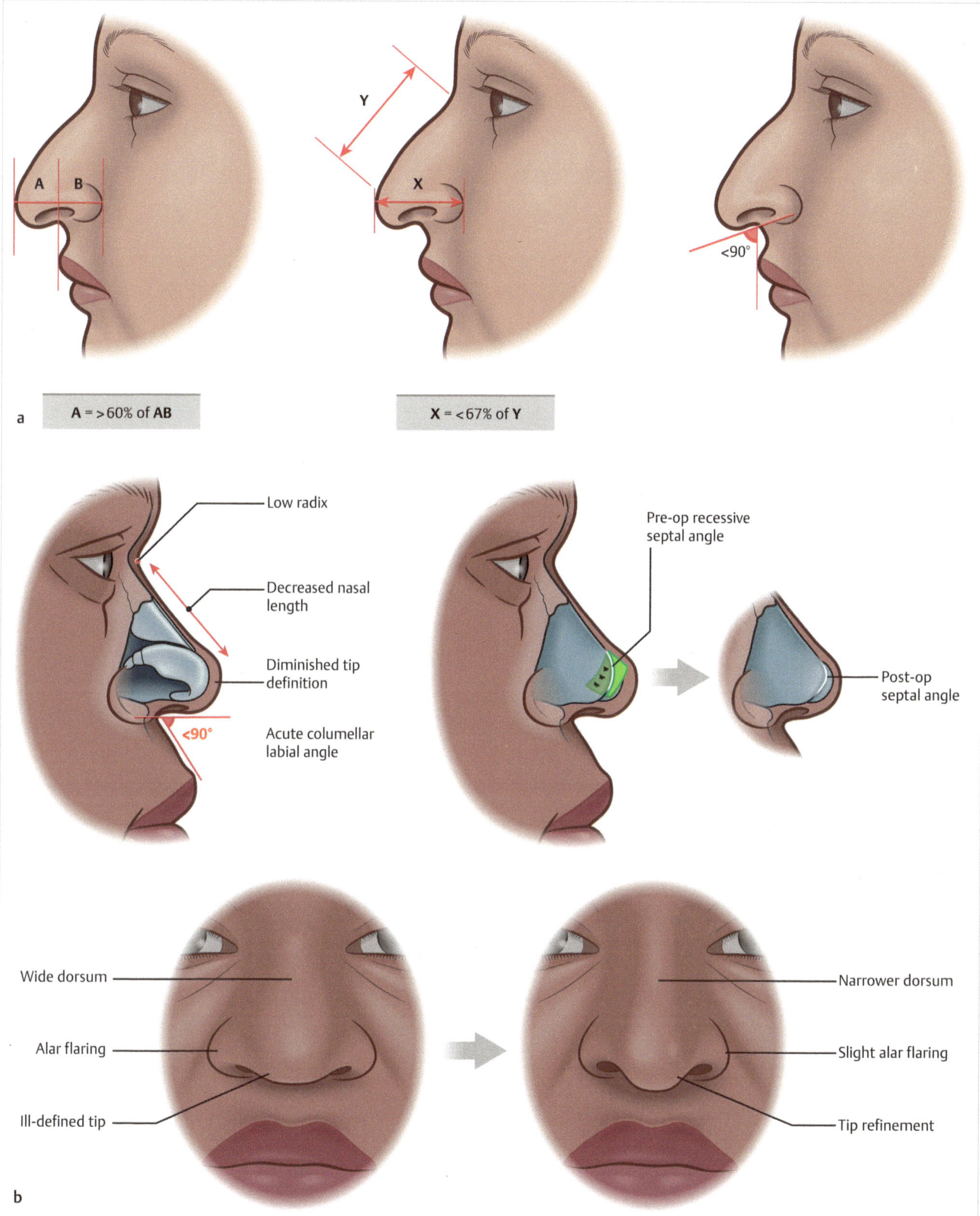

Fig. 20.1 **(a)** Middle Eastern nasofacial morphology. **(b)** African American nasofacial morphology.

(Continued)

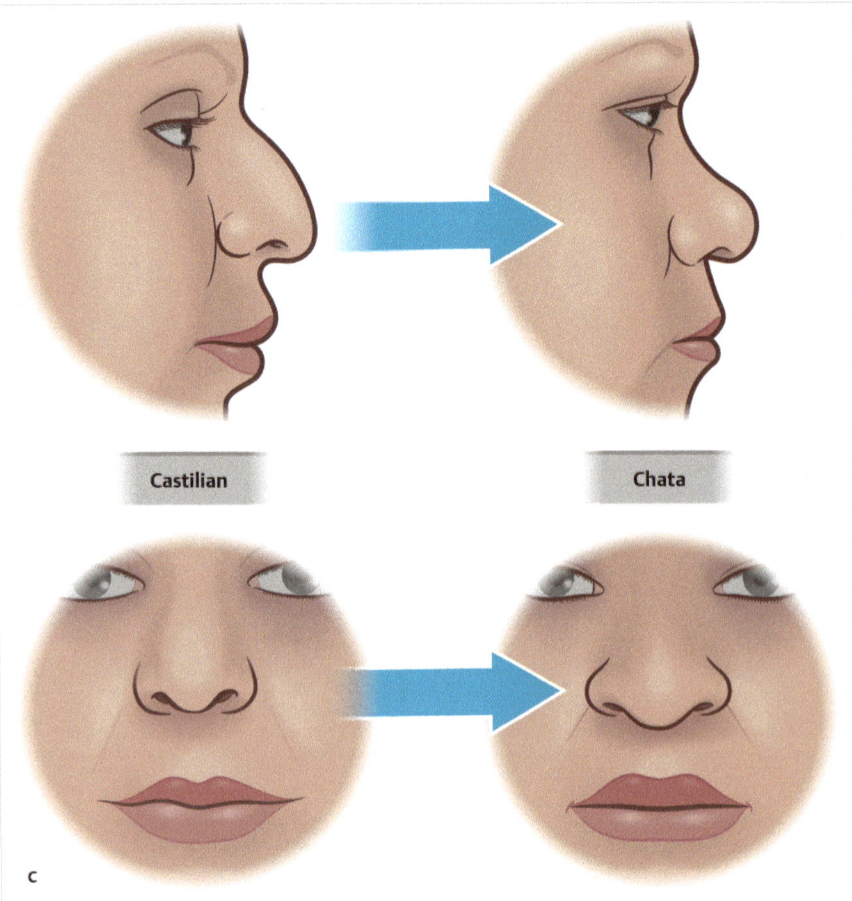

Fig 20.1 *(Continued).* **(c)** Hispanic nasofacial morphology.

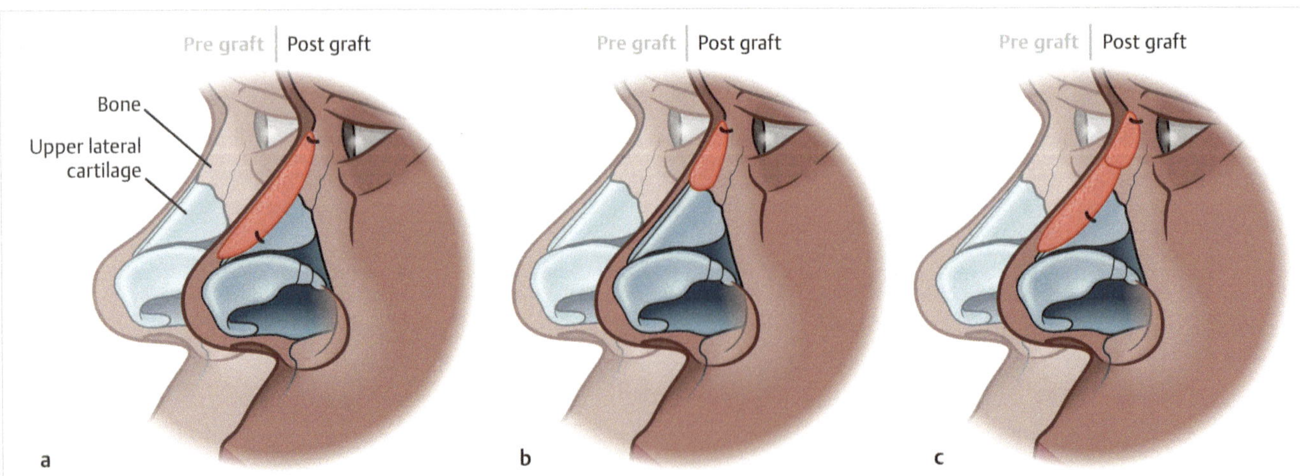

Fig. 20.2 (a) Lateral view of typical diced cartilage facial graft (DCFG) seating and suturing for dorsal augmentation. **(b)** Lateral view showing DCFG for radix-only augmentation. **(c)** Lateral view: variation of using two DCFG constructs.

20.2.6 Osteotomies

- Nasal bones are commonly short in African and Asian patients. Dorsal aesthetic lines can be narrowed with grafting alone.
- Osteotomies (when indicated) are performed in a low-to-low fashion with a super "hinge" greenstick segment, for a natural transition between the maxilla and nasal sidewall (▶ Fig. 20.5).
  - Medial osteotomies are necessary when the cephalad nasal bones are thick.
  - *Note: Aggressive narrowing of a wide bony base can result in the appearance of increased interpupillary distance and disruption to nasofacial harmony.*

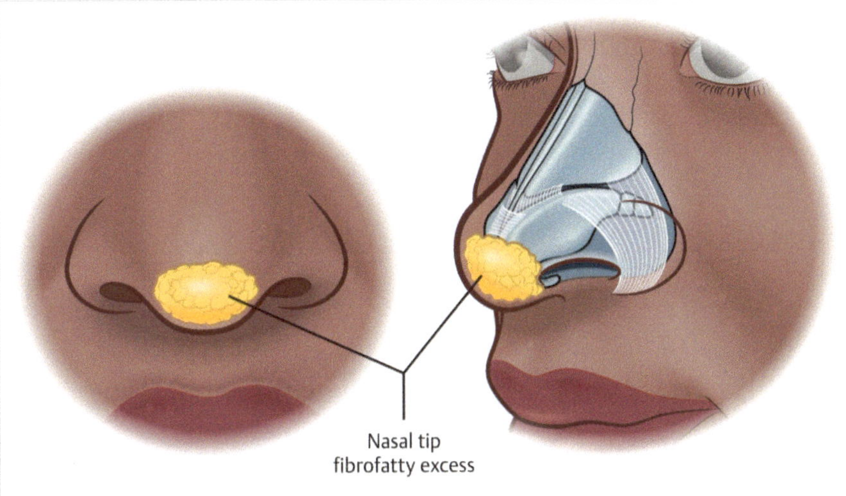

Fig. 20.3 Soft tissue debulking. The undersurface of the nasal skin, particularly in the supratip, domal, and peridomal region, is trimmed to, but not past, the level of the subdermal plexus.

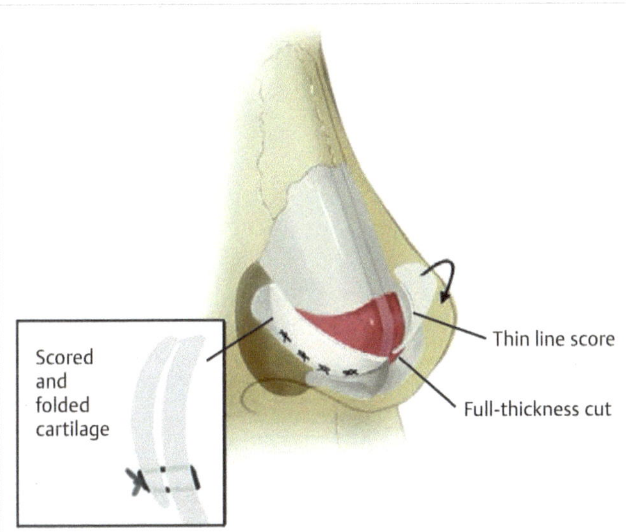

Fig. 20.4 Demonstration of the lower lateral crural turnover flap. The cephalic aspect of the lateral crus is dissected from the underlying vestibular skin inferiorly. A #15 blade is used to score the cartilage, and 2-mm full-thickness cuts are made at the medial and lateral ends of the horizontal line. The flap is turned over while maintaining a minimum of 6 mm width. The caudal edge is secured with multiple horizontal mattress sutures.

20.2.7 Alar Contour Grafts

- Used to prevent notching or retraction of the alar rim and soft triangle, which can readily present in African and Asian patients due to their round nostril shape, and wide interalar distance that is later reduced.
- Addition of a crushed soft triangle graft will offset buckling of the excess alar tissue during tip shaping maneuvers.

20.2.8 Alar Base Reduction (▶ Fig. 20.6)

- Correct alar base discordance through sill and/or alar flare reduction at the end of operation, after columellar closure.
- *Note: Avoid excessive narrowing of the alar base. Additional resection can be performed in office.*
- The techniques for alar base refinement are described in *Chapter 27 Alar Base Surgery.*

20.2.9 Closure

- Transcolumellar incision is closed with 5–0 nylon sutures.
- Only one lateral suture, with 5–0 plain gut, is used to close the infracartilaginous incisions to avoid notching.
- Bacitracin impregnated Surgicel® (Ethicon, Somerville, NJ) is placed in the soft triangles.
- Dead space closure is critical and may include use of lateral sidewall splints.
- Alcohol, skin prep, Steri-Strips, and a Denver splint are placed. Uniform application of the splint is critical, particularly after placement of DCFG.

20.3 Postoperative Care

- Rest and sleep with head elevated. Intermittent cold compresses to eyes and face for the first 72 hours, avoiding direct pressure on the nose.
- Gentle daily cleansing of the columellar and alar base incisions with dilute hydrogen peroxide, followed by antibiotic ointment.
- Nasal splint removed 6 to 7 days postoperatively.
- Sutures removed 6 to 7 days postoperatively.
- Retaping is routinely done to help with edema and the patient is given instructions to tape nightly for 7 to 21 days (depending on amount of swelling observed at the tip).
- DCFG remains malleable for first 3 weeks postoperatively, and if needed, contour irregularities are improved with steady, gentle, yet firm, pressure.
  - "Redness" of the skin overlying the DCFG (when used) has been observed by the authors, which typically subsides without intervention.
- Ethnic patients in particular are counseled on the expected prolonged healing and associated edema after rhinoplasty.

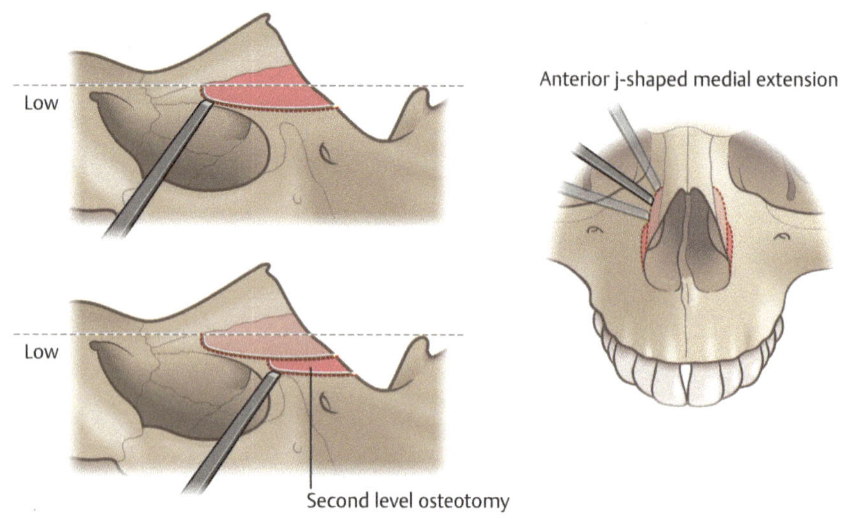

Fig. 20.5 Osteotomies are performed in low–low "J-shaped" fashion to address the dorsal width beginning at the maxillary process and allow for a natural curvilinear line that mimics native bony anatomy. A double level is often needed to further improve the step-off.

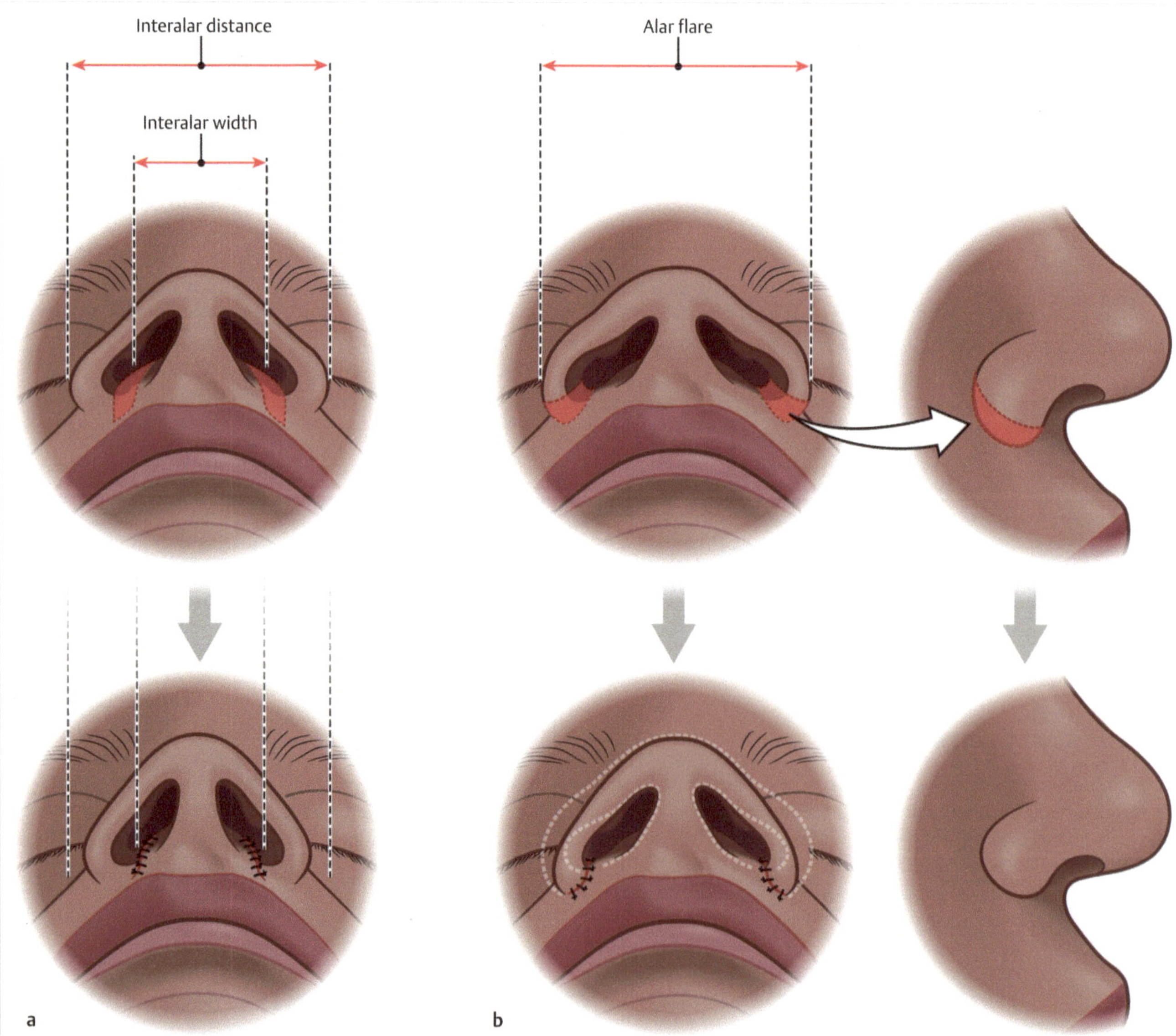

Fig. 20.6 **(a)** Nasal sill and **(b)** alar base resection techniques.

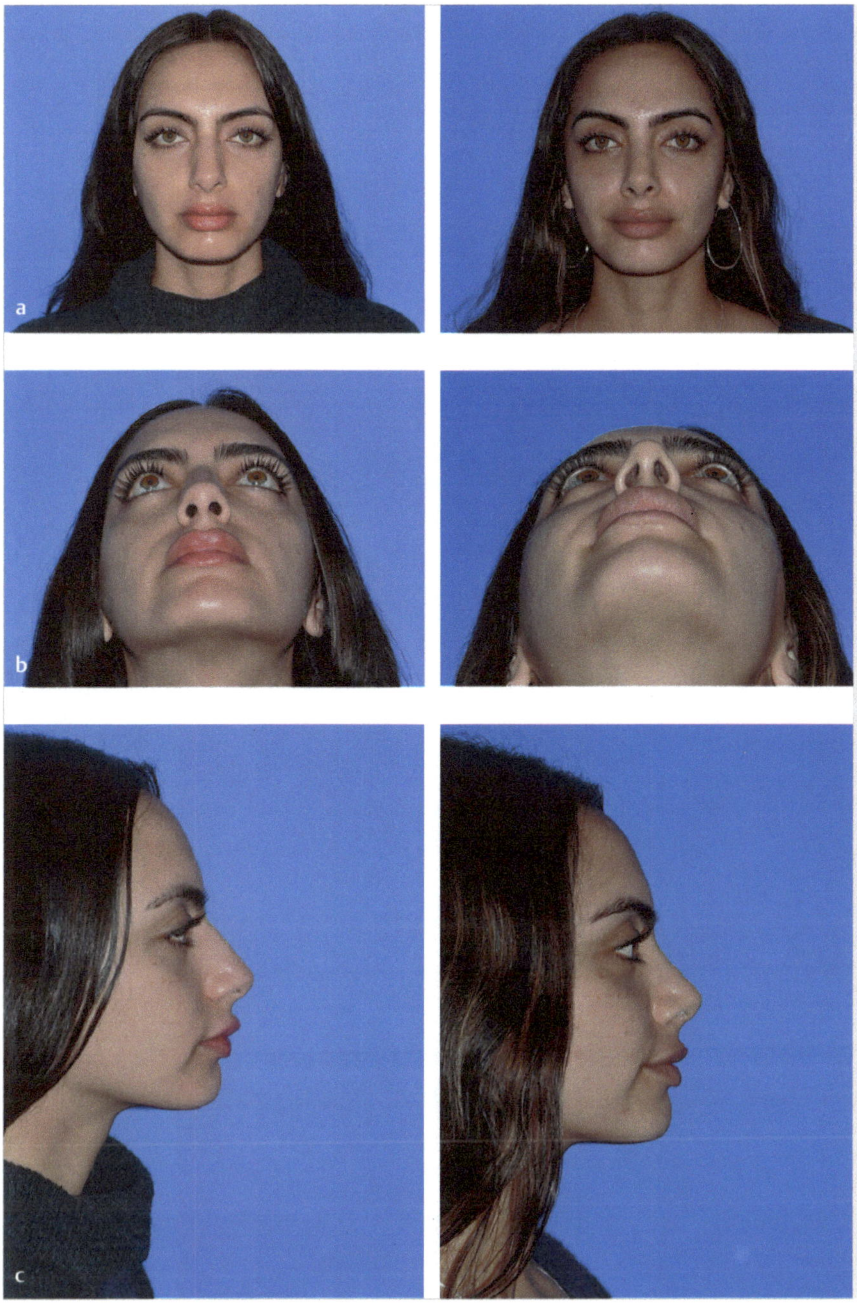

Fig. 20.7 **(a)** Frontal, **(b)** basal, and **(c)** lateral views before and after primary rhinoplasty in a 28-year-old Middle Eastern female to correct wide, asymmetric dorsal aesthetic contour lines, a dorsal hump, and a wide, boxy tip.

20.4 Case Example

Frontal, basal, and lateral views before and after primary rhinoplasty in a 28-year-old Middle Eastern female to correct wide, asymmetric dorsal aesthetic contour lines, a dorsal hump, and a wide, boxy tip (▸ Fig. 20.7a–c).

20.5 Conclusion

Attaining balanced aesthetic results in ethnic rhinoplasty is significantly more complex than in Caucasian patients.

To achieve natural, yet effective, reshaping in the Middle Eastern, Hispanic, and African American nose, the rhinoplasty surgeon must be familiar with the variable nasofacial morphology that exists within an ethnic group and be adept at a number of surgical techniques tailored to each patient's unique anatomy and desired preferences.

No universal parameter can define ideal aesthetics across cultures or ethnic backgrounds; however, the ultimate goal is to achieve nasofacial harmony.

See **Video 20.1**.

Further Readings

Dhir K, Ghavami A. Reshaping of the broad and bulbous nasal tip. Clin Plast Surg. 2016; 43(1):115–126

Ghavami A, Rohrich RJ. The ethnic rhinoplasty. In: Aston SJ, Steinbrech DS, Walden JL, eds. Aesthetic Plastic Surgery. London, UK: Saunders; May 2009

Ghavami A. Tip shaping in primary rhinoplasty. In: Shiffman M, Di Giuseppe A, eds. Advanced Aesthetic Rhinoplasty. Berlin, Heidelberg: Springer; 2013: 853–868

Ghavami A. Secondary rhinoplasty in the Middle Eastern patient. In: Shiffman M, Di Giuseppe A, eds. Advanced Aesthetic Rhinoplasty. Berlin, Heidelberg: Springer; 2013:983–1000

Ghavami A. Indication and technique for diced cartilage and fascia grafting in rhinoplasty. In: Operative Techniques in Plastic Surgery. Vol. 1. 1st ed. Philadelphia: Wolters Kluwer; 2019

21 The Preservation Rhinoplasty

Aaron M. Kosins

Abstract

Preservation rhinoplasty (PR) is a new chapter in rhinoplasty history. The term was first coined by Daniel in 2018, and represents a fundamental change in philosophy. Just as the open approach transformed rhinoplasty surgery, so has PR as surgeons rethink traditional dogma. In certain cases, the standard teaching of reduce and rebuild can be replaced with preserve and reshape. Structural rhinoplasty evolved as surgeons realized that when nasal anatomy is taken apart and/or made smaller, structures must be rebuilt and strengthened to resist the forces of scar contracture. However, if anatomy is preserved less structural rebuilding is necessary. This chapter details the PR, which includes preservation of the soft tissue envelope, alar cartilages, and osseocartilaginous dorsum.

Keywords: Rhinoplasty, preservation, subperichondrial, push down, letdown, polygons

Key Points

- Preservation rhinoplasty involves preservation of the soft tissue envelope, ligaments, alar cartilages, and dorsum.
- Preservation rhinoplasty is a change in rhinoplasty philosophy where resection is replaced with reshaping.
- Preserve as much of the native structures of the nose as possible and the surgeon will have less to rebuild and less chance for scar contracture, warping, and distortion in the future.

21.1 Preoperative Steps

- The patient is evaluated during consultation by asking what three things the patient wants to change about his or her nose.
- Physical examination is done sequentially with a focus on the ability to preserve all aspects of the nose including the soft tissue envelope, the nasal ligaments, the alar cartilages, and the dorsum.
- The author begins with an evaluation of the thickness and quality of the soft tissue envelope to assess the surgical plane of dissection for both the tip and the dorsum—subSMAS, subperichondrial, or subdermal.
- Evaluation of the alar cartilages is then performed with a focus on the volume and the strength of the lower lateral cartilages. The anterior strength and projection of the alar cartilages against the soft tissue envelope of the nose will determine the crispness of the nasal polygons.
- Finally, the dorsum is evaluated first on anterior view, and then on profile view, for suitability of dorsal preservation—a two-step procedure where a septal strip is removed followed by osteotomies to lower the dorsal profile and to maintain the patient's natural dorsal aesthetic lines without opening the cartilaginous vault.

21.2 Operative Steps

See **Video 21.1**.

21.2.1 Soft Tissue Envelope Preservation

- Preservation of the soft tissue envelope can be done in the open or closed approach. Described below will be the open approach for the purposes of this text.
- A unilateral hemitransfixion incision is made and the anterior septal angle is exposed. Using sharp scissors, the subperichondrial plane is found and dissected laterally to the intersection of the vertical and longitudinal scroll ligaments bilaterally. This subperichondrial dissection is continued up to the caudal portion of the nasal bones where a subperiosteal plane is entered up to the nasal radix and down to the cheeks in preparation for piezoelectric surgery. This is the extended open approach of the nasal dorsum.
- Bilateral infracartilaginous incisions are made and at the turning point of the lateral crura, the backside of a #15 blade is used to scrape the perichondrium. Once a subperichondrial plane is developed, it is dissected to the midline and over the domes.
- A transcolumellar incision is made, dividing the superficial Pitanguy's ligament. The deep Pitanguy's ligament is encountered in the midline along with its lateral vertical scroll attachments. The deep Pitanguy's ligament is marked with a pen or two sutures and divided. The vertical scroll attachments are carefully divided, connecting the subperiochondrial dissection of the tip and dorsum. If done correctly, the scroll sesamoid cartilages should move up on the skin flap (▶ Fig. 21.1).
- In this way, a full subperichondrial-subperiosteal dissection of the nose is done and the ligaments are preserved for reattachment at the end of the rhinoplasty surgery.

21.2.2 Dorsal Preservation (High Septal Strip)

- For the purpose of this text, I will be describing the high, subdorsal strip pushdown procedure as popularized by Saban.
- At the point where the caudal upper lateral cartilages attach to the dorsal septum (the W-point, which is often 1 cm cephalic to the anterior septal angle), a subdorsal cut is made directly under the dorsum up to the perpendicular plate of ethmoid (PPE). A second cut is made 2 mm below and a cartilaginous strip is removed. At times, a small amount of PPE is removed with a rongeur directly under the dorsum to allow space for downward impaction of the dorsum. At this point, the osseocartilaginous vault is released from the septum (▶ Fig. 21.2).
- Using straight and curved piezoelectric saws, bilateral low-to-low osteotomies are connected to bilateral transverse osteotomies and a radix osteotomy. At this point, the

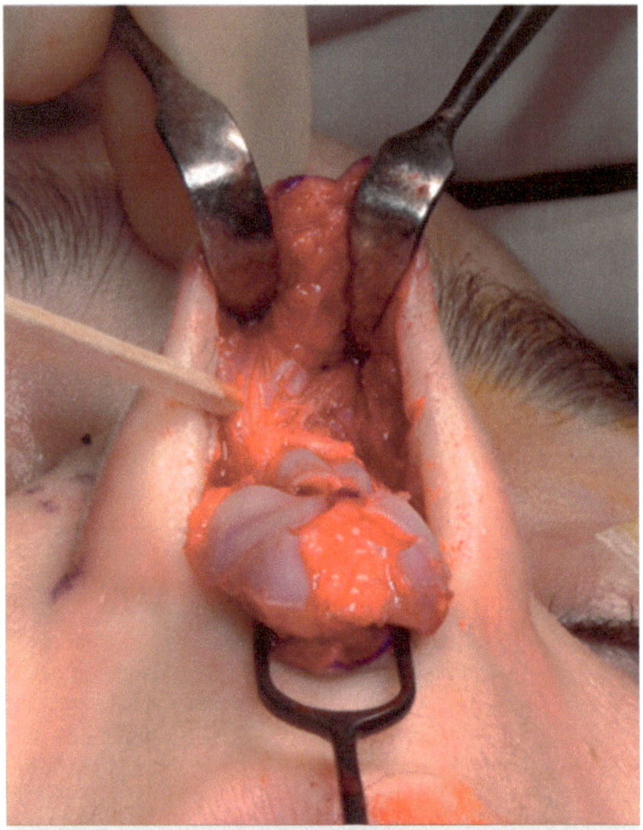

Fig. 21.1 Preservation of the soft tissue envelope involves a full subperichondrial-subperiosteal dissection of the nasal tip and dorsum. Pitanguy's ligament and the scroll ligaments are marked when opening the nose so that they may be reattached during closure. If done properly, the sesamoid cartilages will be lifted with the skin sleeve.

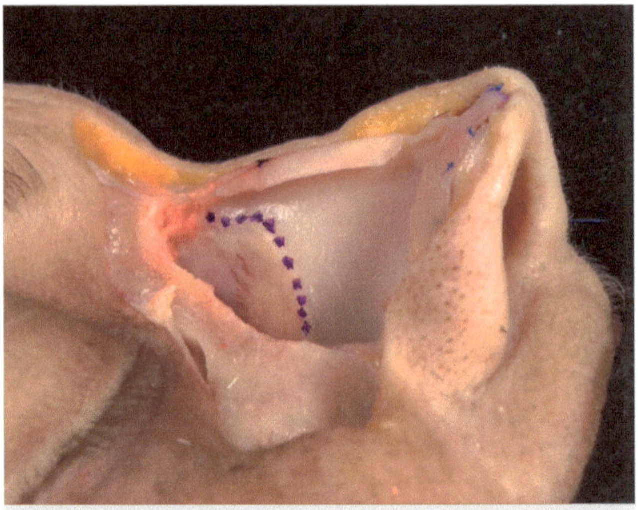

Fig. 21.2 In a high subdorsal strip resection, a strip of septal cartilage is removed from directly underneath the dorsum. If needed, a small amount of perpendicular plate of ethmoid is also removed to allow for impaction of the nose.

osseocartilaginous pyramid has been released not only from the septum, but also from face. A side-to-side movement confirms mobility of the nasal pyramid. Once this is confirmed, the dorsum is squeezed and "pushed down" into the pyriform aperture.
- Incremental strips of cartilage can be removed for further lowering and flexion of the osseocartilaginous joint.
- If the surgeon is having trouble with descent of the dorsum, several blocking points are checked including all osteotomy lines, the separation of the dorsum from the septum, and that space has been created laterally for descent into the pyriform aperture.
- Once the dorsum has been lowered and the surgeon is satisfied, at least one suture is used to reattach the dorsum to the septum at the W-point. More sutures can be added to the keystone area between the dorsum and subdorsal septum as needed, but is not mandatory. Finally, the W-ASA segment (the area between the W-point and anterior septal angle) can be modified to adjust the height at the supratip.

21.2.3 Alar Preservation

- Once the dorsal height and shape are satisfactory, either a columellar strut or septal extension graft is used to support the nasal tip. The type of support is based on the quality of cartilage, volume of cartilage, thickness of the soft tissue envelope, and desired projection. Decisions are made to make sure that enough force is transmitted by the alar cartilages against the soft tissue envelope to create defined nasal polygons.
- Most often, domal creation sutures are combined with a lateral steal procedure to increase the projection and rotation of the nasal tip. These techniques combine to tension the lateral crura and to create central tip support. When combined with a columellar strut or septal extension graft, tension is applied to the soft tissue envelope centrally and laterally.
- In over 50% of patients, nothing is removed from the lateral crura cephalically. If excess bulk lies in the supratip or the cartilages are particularly convex in the transverse axis, a slide under procedure is performed. A cut is made 7 to 8 mm back from the caudal border of the lateral crura, and the cephalic island is slid under the remaining lateral crura and secured with at least two sutures. This technique decreases the volume of cartilage, while straightening/strengthening the lateral crura, and does not sacrifice the longitudinal scroll ligament. In this way, all of the alar cartilage is preserved.

21.2.4 Closure and Ligament Preservation

- For closure, the perichondrium is first reattached to the anterior septal angle. The vertical scroll ligaments are reattached to the intact longitudinal scroll ligaments bilaterally. Finally, the Pitanguy's ligament is reattached in the midline. If an unnatural supratip break point is formed by the reattached deep Pitanguy's ligament, it is excised so as not to form a soft tissue pollybeak.
- Final closure of all incisions is done in the standard fashion. Drains made from angiocatheters are placed in the lateral nasal wall gutters to facilitate hematoma drainage. Doyle splints and a cast are placed for approximately 1 week.

21.3 Postoperative Care

- Patients sleep with their head elevated as well as with an ice pack over their eyes during the first 72 hours.
- The columellar incision is cleaned with hydrogen peroxide and Bactroban is applied around the nostrils for 5 days.
- The nasal splint is removed in 6 to 7 days postoperatively.
- Sutures are removed in 6 to 7 days postoperatively.
- Afrin is used for 3 days after splint removal followed by a steroid spray for 2 to 3 months daily.

21.4 Case Example

Preoperative and 13-month postoperative views of a 22-year-old female patient with a dorsal hump and plunging tip. The patient has ideal dorsal aesthetic lines on front view and therefore, the dorsum was preserved. At 1 year, good dorsal aesthetic lines are seen as well as a nice profile and symmetric basal view. The soft tissue envelope was preserved and all ligaments were reattached. The alar cartilages were likewise preserved. This patient had total PR as nothing was removed from the nose and the structures were simply reshaped (▶ Fig. 21.3a–e).

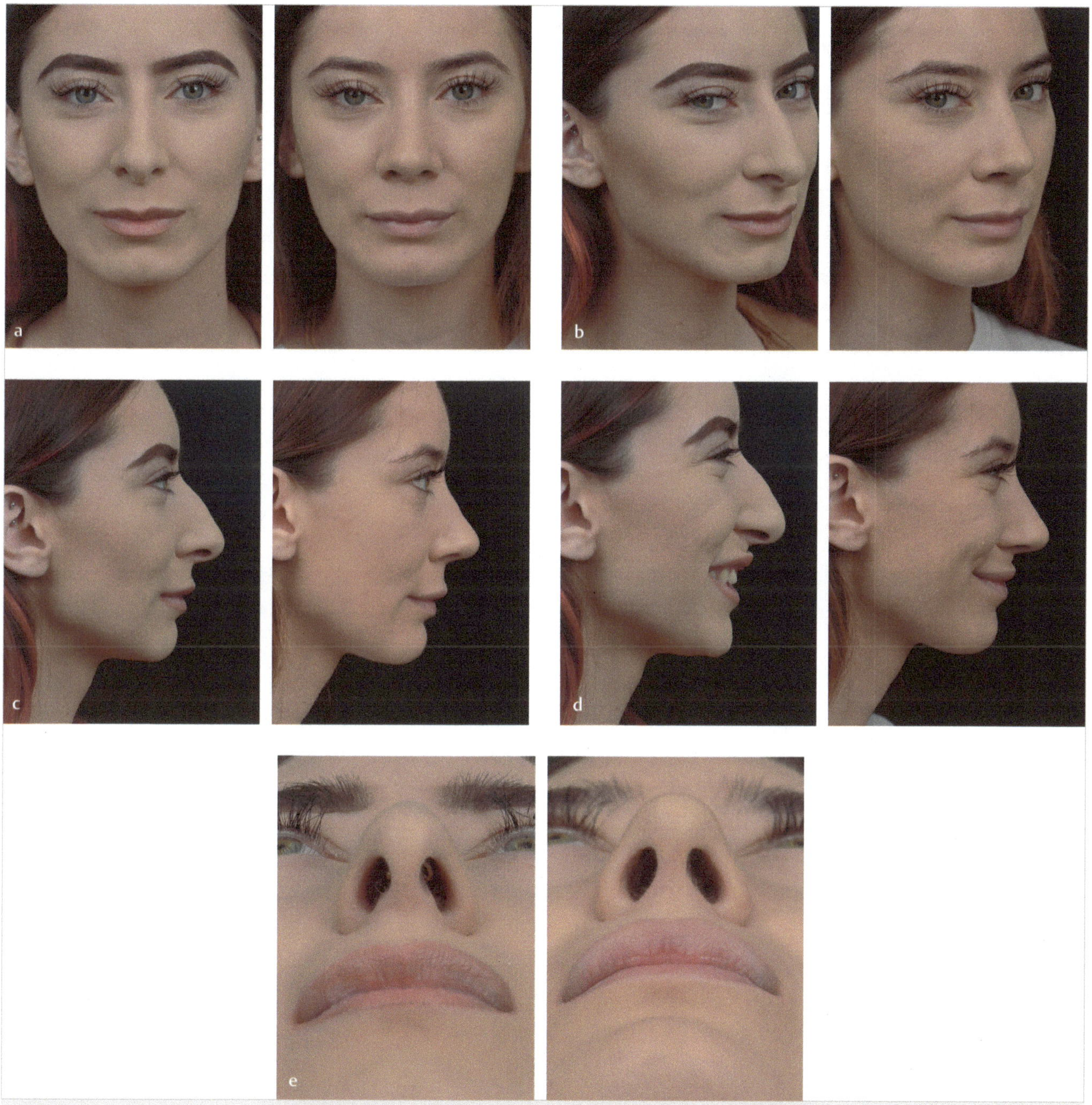

Fig. 21.3 (a–e) Preoperative and 13-month postoperative views of a 22-year-old female patient with a dorsal hump and plunging tip. The patient has ideal dorsal aesthetic lines on front view and therefore, the dorsum was preserved. At 1 year, good dorsal aesthetic lines are seen as well as a nice profile and symmetric basal view. The soft tissue envelope was preserved and all ligaments were reattached. The alar cartilages were likewise preserved. This patient had total preservation rhinoplasty as nothing was removed from the nose and the structures were simply reshaped.

21.5 Conclusion

Preservation rhinoplasty involves preservation of the soft tissue envelope, ligaments, alar cartilages, and dorsum. Preservation rhinoplasty is a change in rhinoplasty philosophy where resection is replaced with reshaping. Preserve as much of the native structures of the nose as possible and the surgeon will have less to rebuild and less chance for scar contracture, warping, and distortion in the future.

Further Readings

Cakir B, Oreroğlu AR, Doğan T, Akan M. A complete subperichondrial dissection technique for rhinoplasty with management of the nasal ligaments. Aesthet Surg J. 2012; 32(5):564–574

Gerbault O, Daniel RK, Kosins AM. The role of piezoelectric instrumentation in rhinoplasty surgery. Aesthet Surg J. 2016; 36(1):21–34

Kosins AM. My first 50 dorsal preservation rhinoplasties. In: Cakir B, Saban Y, Daniel RK, Palhazi P, eds. Preservation Rhinoplasty. Istanbul: Septum Publications; 2018:127–137

Kosins AM, Daniel RK. Decision making in preservation rhinoplasty: a 100 case series with one-year follow-up. Aesthet Surg J. 2020; 40(1):34–48

Saban Y, Daniel RK, Polselli R, Trapasso M, Palhazi P. Dorsal preservation: the push down technique reassessed. Aesthet Surg J. 2018; 38(2):117–131

22 Ancillary Maneuvers in Rhinoplasty: Spreader Grafts

C. Spencer Cochran and Paul N. Afrooz

Abstract

The aesthetic uses of spreader grafts include straightening or strengthening a dorsally deviated septum, preventing or correcting a narrow midvault, and establishing uniform and symmetric dorsal aesthetic lines, and in some cases widening a narrow middle vault. It is this tendency to overly-widen the dorsum which surgeons find objectionable and the reason why many opt not to employ spreader grafts. However, spreader grafts can be recessed slightly below the height of the dorsum to alleviate undesired widening of the nose while still maintaining their usefulness.

Keywords: Rhinoplasty, spreader grafts, internal valve collapse, deviated septum, dorsal aesthetic lines

Key Points

- The aesthetic uses of spreader grafts (▶ Fig. 22.1) include straightening or strengthening a dorsally deviated septum, preventing or correcting narrowing of the midvault, and establishing uniform and symmetric dorsal aesthetic lines, and in some cases widening a narrow middle vault.
- Spreader grafts should be placed bilaterally.
- Recess the spreader grafts 1 to 2 mm to prevent undesired widening of the dorsum (▶ Fig. 22.2).
- The upper lateral cartilages are trimmed to the appropriate height and sutured to the spreader graft–septum complex with simple sutures to recreate an anatomic configuration of the midvault.

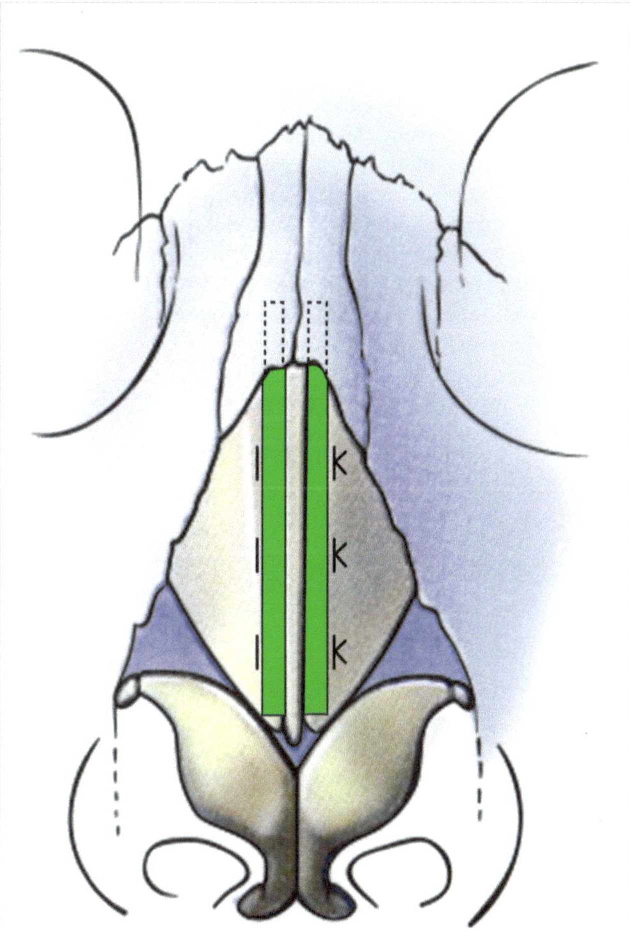

Fig. 22.1 Spreader grafts are usually paired, longitudinal grafts placed between the dorsal septum and the upper lateral cartilages.

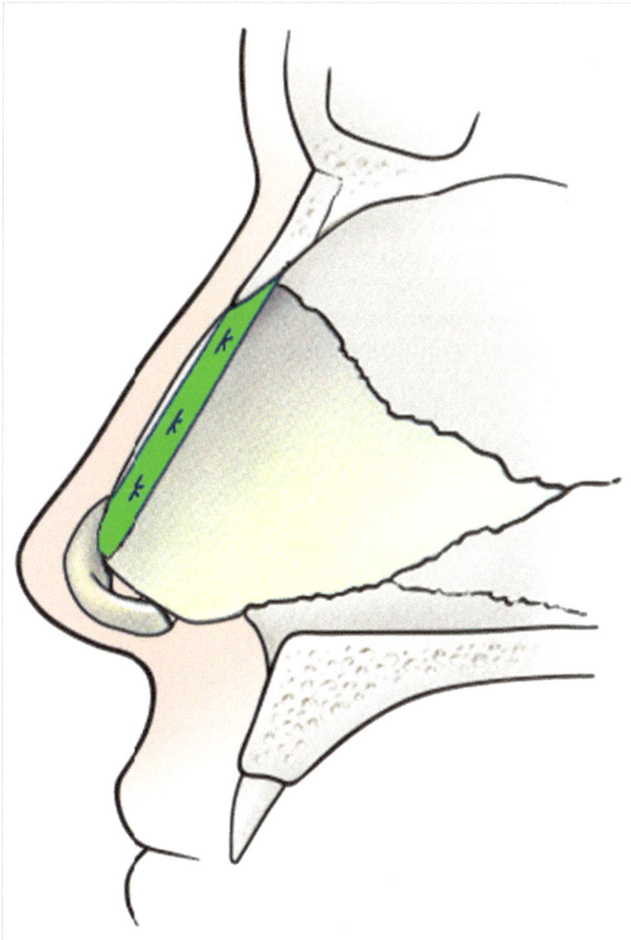

Fig. 22.2 Recessing spreader grafts 1 to 2 mm below the dorsal septum can help to prevent undesired widening of the dorsum.

22.1 Preoperative Steps

- Proper preoperative analysis should be performed and surgical goals established.
- Particular attention should be paid to the dorsal width and the need to maintain dorsal width versus narrowing or widening the midvault.

22.2 Operative Steps

- An open approach is favored to allow adequate visualization of the osseocartilaginous framework.
- Divide the upper lateral cartilages from the dorsal septum and perform a component dorsal reduction if necessary, while leaving the upper lateral cartilages untrimmed until subsequent operative steps (see below).
- Harvest septal cartilage for grafting.
- Fabricate two spreader grafts measuring approximately 4 mm in height. The length should be sufficient to span the entire length of the midvault from the keystone to the septal angle.
- Place the spreader grafts on either side of the septum and secure in two to three locations with horizontal mattress sutures. If no widening of the dorsum is desired, the spreader grafts should be recessed 1 to 2 mm below the height of the dorsal septum (▶ Fig. 22.3).
- The upper lateral cartilages are trimmed to the height of the dorsal septum and sutured to the spreader graft–septum complex with simple sutures tied across the top of the dorsum so that the upper lateral cartilages meet the side of the dorsal septum and cover the top of the spreader grafts (▶ Fig. 22.4).
- If lateral osteotomies are to be performed, these should be done after the midvault has been reconstituted.
- See **Video 22.1**.

22.3 Postoperative Care

- At the conclusion of the case, surgical tape should be applied to the nose from the radix to the supratip to control edema and to eliminate potential dead space beneath the soft tissue envelope.
- External dressings should be removed 1 week after surgery and the skin gently cleansed.
- Patients are instructed not to manipulate their nose for 4 to 6 weeks following surgery.
- For persistent supratip edema and fullness after the perioperative period, selective taping can be performed by applying a compressive tape such as Blenderm™ (3 M Corp) nightly to the dorsum overlying the area.

22.4 Case Example

Preoperative versus postoperative photos of a primary rhinoplasty patient in whom spreader grafts were used to maintain proper dorsal aesthetic lines following a component dorsal reduction are shown (▶ Fig. 22.5a–d).

22.5 Conclusion

The aesthetic uses of spreader grafts include straightening or strengthening a dorsally deviated septum, preventing or correcting narrowing of the midvault, and establishing uniform and symmetric dorsal aesthetic lines, and in some cases widening a narrow middle vault. It is this tendency to overly-widen the dorsum which surgeons find objectionable and the reason why many opt not to employ spreader grafts. However, spreader grafts can be recessed slightly below the height of the dorsum to alleviate undesired widening of the nose while still maintaining their usefulness.

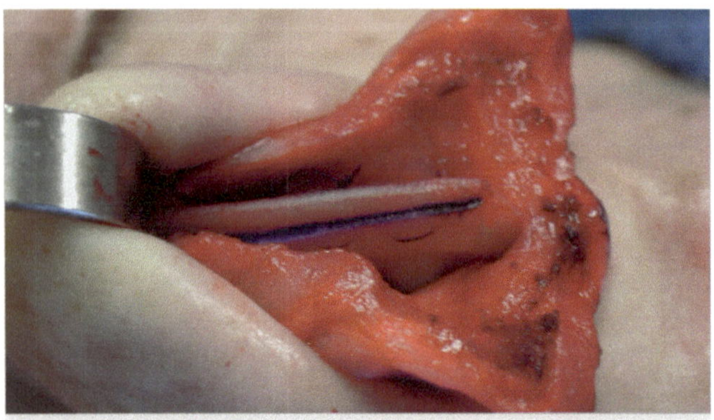

Fig. 22.3 Place the spreader grafts on either side of the septum and secure in two to three locations with horizontal mattress sutures. If no widening of the dorsum is desired, the spreader grafts should be recessed 1 to 2 mm below the height of the dorsal septum.

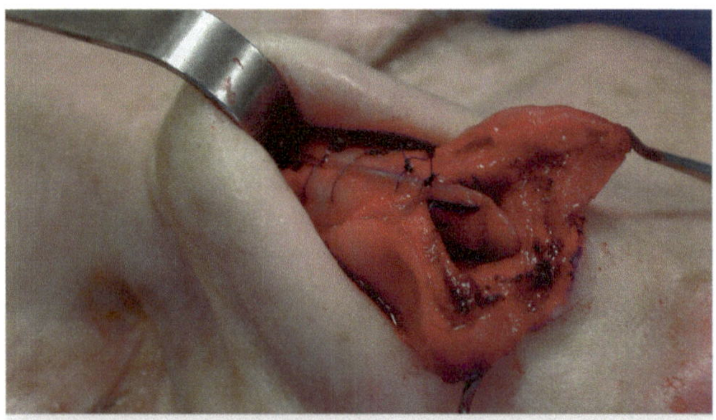

Fig. 22.4 The upper lateral cartilages are sutured to the spreader graft–septum complex with simple sutures tied across the top of the dorsum so that the upper lateral cartilages meet the side of the dorsal septum and cover the top of the spreader grafts.

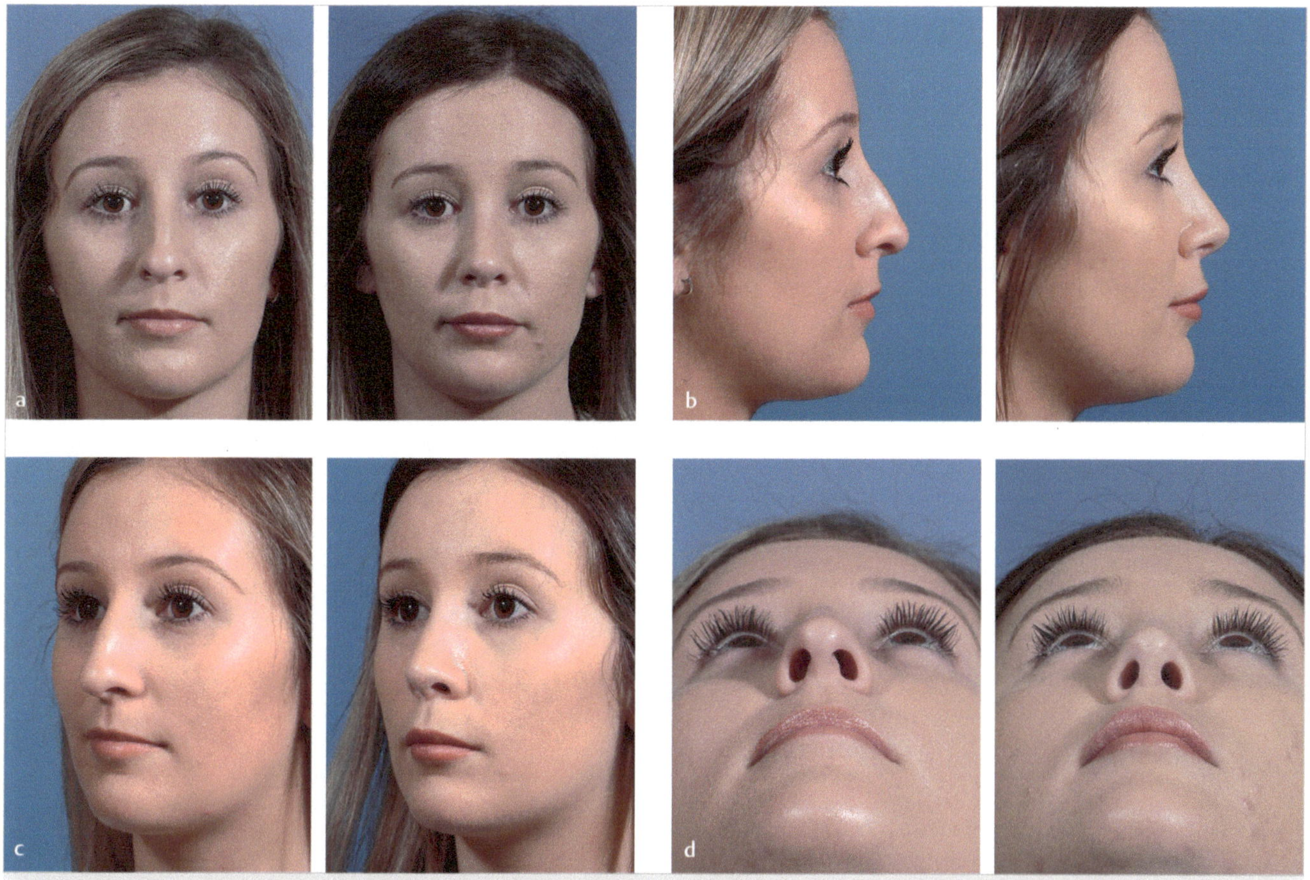

Fig. 22.5 (a–d) Preoperative versus postoperative photos of a primary rhinoplasty patient in whom spreader grafts were used to maintain proper dorsal aesthetic lines following a component dorsal reduction.

Further Readings

Byrd HS, Salomon J, Flood J. Correction of the crooked nose. Plast Reconstr Surg. 1998; 102(6):2148–2157

Gunter JP, Landecker A, Cochran CS. Frequently used grafts in rhinoplasty: nomenclature and analysis. Plast Reconstr Surg. 2006; 118(1):14e–29e

Kim L, Papel ID. Spreader grafts in functional rhinoplasty. Facial Plast Surg. 2016; 32 (1):29–35.– Review

Rohrich RJ, Hollier LH. Use of spreader grafts in the external approach to rhinoplasty. Clin Plast Surg. 1996; 23(2):255–262

Sheen JH. Spreader graft: a method of reconstructing the roof of the middle nasal vault following rhinoplasty. Plast Reconstr Surg. 1984; 73(2):230–239

23 Ancillary Maneuvers in Rhinoplasty: Spreader Flaps

Rod J. Rohrich and Paul D. Durand

Abstract

The spreader (or *autospreader*) flap offers an alternative to the traditional spreader graft in reconstructing the dorsal midvault and preserving internal valve function. This is of particular importance after an aggressive dorsal hump reduction, which has the potential to result in an inverted-V deformity, dorsal narrowing, or saddle-nose deformity. In this chapter, the authors describe a four-step spreader flap technique that offers a simple, reproducible method of shaping the dorsal midvault while preserving internal valve function.

Keywords: Spreader flap, autospreader flap, rhinoplasty

Key Points

- The spreader (or *autospreader*) flap offers an alternative to the traditional spreader graft in reconstructing the dorsal midvault and preserving internal valve function.
- Spreader flaps are of particular importance after an aggressive dorsal hump reduction, which has the potential to result in an inverted-V deformity, dorsal narrowing, or saddle-nose deformity.
- The four-step spreader flap technique described by the authors offers a simple, reproducible method of shaping the dorsal midvault while preserving internal valve function; especially in a primary rhinoplasty with the following: (a) >3 mm of dorsal hump reduction; (b) strong upper lateral cartilages (ULCs); and (c) long nasal bones (▶ Table 23.1).

23.1 Preoperative Steps

- Proper preoperative nasofacial analysis and planning are key to any successful rhinoplasty procedure (refer to Chapter 11 for the 10–7–5 nasal analysis).
- Determine if the following are present or required:
  - More than 3 mm of dorsal hump reduction.
  - Strong ULCs.
  - Long nasal bones.
- Pay particular attention to the dorsal aesthetic lines and if these need modifications due to asymmetry, excessive width, or poor definition.

Table 23.1 Indications for spreader flaps versus spreader grafts

Spreader flaps	Spreader grafts
Primary rhinoplasty	Secondary rhinoplasty
Long nasal bones	Short nasal bones
>3 mm reduction	Deviated nose (esp. high)
Short dorsum	Narrow midvault
Strong ULC	Need for additional width or strength

Abbreviation: ULC, upper lateral cartilage.

23.2 Operative Steps

- Adhering to the principles of component dorsal hump reduction allows for maximal preservation of the ULCs, a crucial element in the successful implementation of the autospreader flap technique.
- ULCs are sharply separated from the cartilaginous septum, in a 30-degree oblique angle so as to preserve the maximum length of ULC.
- Following component dorsal hump reduction, the following four steps are performed in order to reconstitute the nasal dorsum.
- See **Video 23.1**.

23.2.1 Pull-Twist-Turn

- After the ULCs have been freed from the septum and their underlying mucoperichondrium, the caudal edge of these can be trimmed if needed.
- The transverse component of each ULC is then gently pulled and infolded medially. This allows for the folded transverse portion of the ULCs to be effectively "sandwiched" directly abutting the most dorsal aspect of the cartilaginous septum (▶ Fig. 23.1).

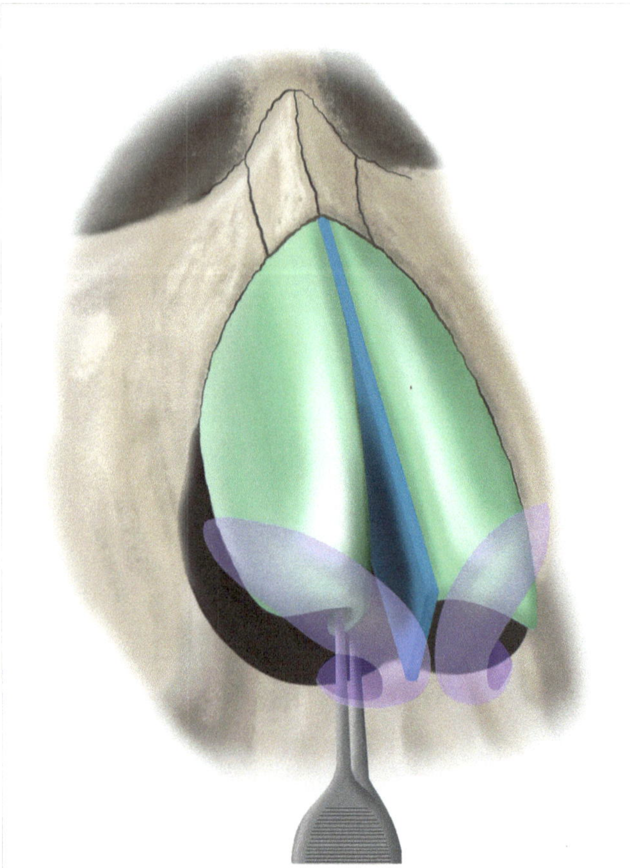

Fig. 23.1 The "*pull-twist-turn*" technique.

23.2.2 Horizontal Mattress Sutures

- A 5–0 polydioxanone suture is placed from the folded portion of the ULC on one side, through the folded ULC in the other side and then back through the distal septum, advancing both the ULCs distally along the septum.
- The suture above helps to stabilize the ULCs to the septum on slight tension, facilitating a straighter septum.
- Another 5–0 polydioxanone suture is performed proximally just distal to the keystone area in a similar fashion providing extra support and stability.
- Adequate dorsal aesthetic lines are then confirmed through direct visualization and palpation of the nasal dorsum. The "three-point palpation test" using the dominant index finger moistened with saline is performed for both the left and right dorsal aesthetic lines, as well as centrally to detect any contour abnormalities (▶ Fig. 23.2).

23.2.3 Low-to-Low Percutaneous Osteotomies

- In noses with wide or asymmetric nasal bones, or in those with an open roof after an aggressive dorsal reduction, an osteotomy is recommended.
- A lateral percutaneous osteotomy is performed as it minimizes the trauma to nasal mucosa, while allowing for maximum control.
- The senior author prefers a low-to-low osteotomy in most cases.
- A 2-mm straight osteotome is introduced through facial skin directly on the midportion of the bony nasal pyramid. This is done in a horizontal plane parallel to the anterior surface of the maxilla and at the level of the inferior orbital rim.
- In a subperiosteal plane and while exerting constant digital pressure, the osteotome is then swept down the lateral nasal wall and laterally along the frontal processes of the maxilla until one reaches the site of the first osteotomy. If performed in the right plane, this maneuver allows for displacement of the angular artery, minimizing the possibility of injury.
- Several perforated 2-mm osteotomies are performed in the maxilla at the pyriform level. Medially, the osteotome is directed just inferior to the medial canthus. Care should be taken to leave 2 mm of untouched bone between osteotomies.
- After this is completed on both sides of the nasal wall, a greenstick fracture is done with the thumb and forefinger. A Boies nasal elevator can then be used to out-fracture and ensure proper final bony alignment (▶ Fig. 23.3).

23.2.4 "The Texas Stitch": Simple Interrupted Suturing

- Using 4–0 polyglactin suture in a simple interrupted fashion, the entire construct consisting of both autospreader flaps and dorsal cartilaginous septum is buttressed and further secured. This is typically performed at least both cephalically, near the keystone area, as well as closer to the caudal edge of the ULCs.
- Visual inspection and gentle palpation are then performed to ensure structural uniformity of the reconstituted dorsum.
- Extra simple interrupted sutures can be placed to reinforce the construct if needed (▶ Fig. 23.4).

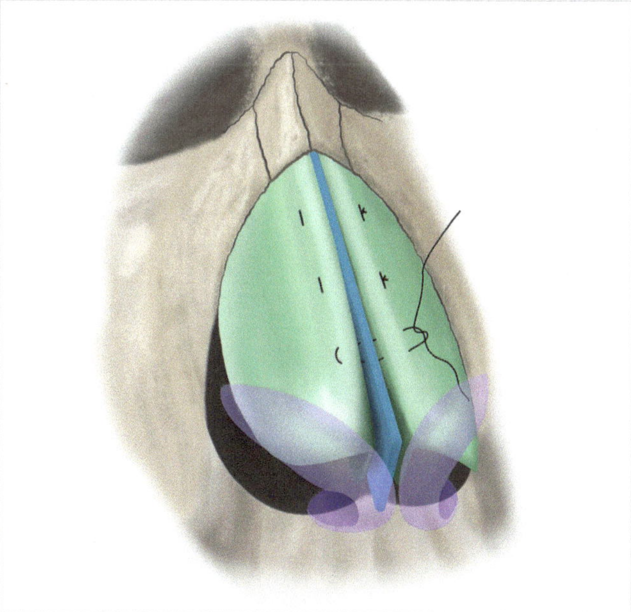

Fig. 23.2 Horizontal mattress sutures through the upper lateral cartilages (ULCs) and septum.

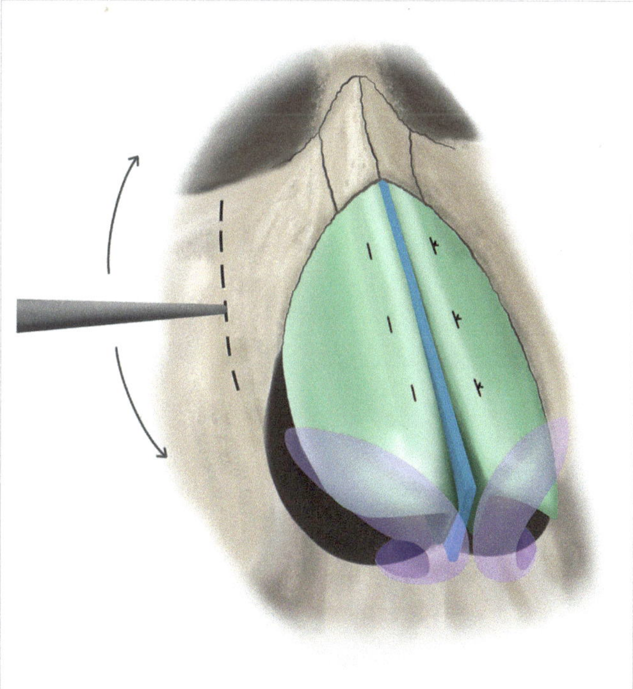

Fig. 23.3 Low-to-low percutaneous osteotomies.

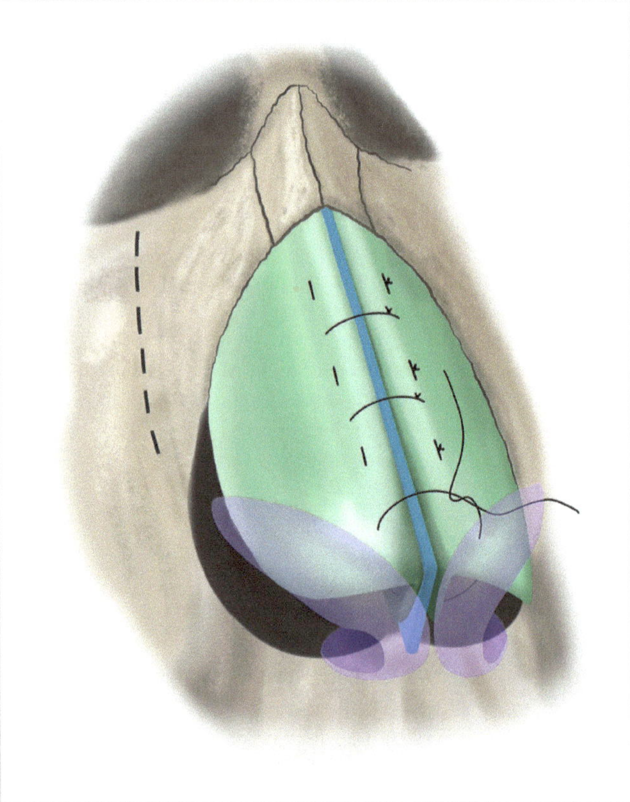

Fig. 23.4 "The Texas Stitch"—vest over pants simple interrupted suture.

23.3 Postoperative Care

- Postoperative care is the same as for open rhinoplasty.
- Patients are instructed to rest and sleep with head elevation.
- Cold compresses are used over the eyes and face intermittently for the first 72 hours postoperatively, taking care to avoid pressure on the nose.
- The columellar and alar base incisions are cleaned with dilute hydrogen peroxide daily, followed by application of antibiotic ointment.
- The nasal splint is removed in 6 to 7 days postoperatively.
- Sutures are removed in 6 to 7 days postoperatively.

23.4 Case Example

A 20-year-old patient who underwent open rhinoplasty with dorsal component reduction and four-step spreader flap technique. Before (left) and after (right) photos in three views are provided (▶ Fig. 23.5a–c).

23.5 Conclusion

The four-step spreader flap technique is a simple and easily reproducible method of shaping the dorsal midvault while preserving internal valve function. In primary rhinoplasty, it obviates the use of spreader grafts in a select patient population who would otherwise be at a high risk of internal valve collapse after aggressive dorsal hump reduction.

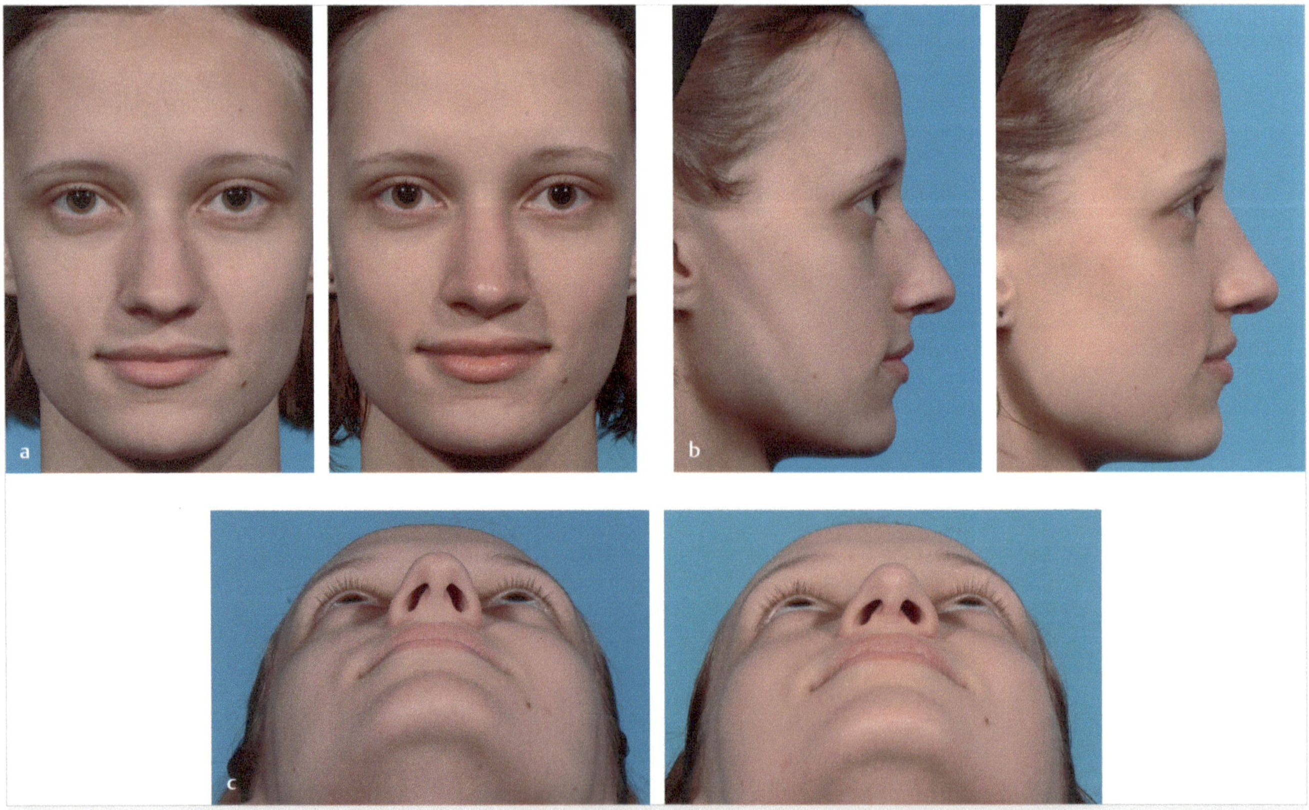

Fig. 23.5 (a–c) A 20-year-old patient who underwent open rhinoplasty with dorsal component reduction and four-step spreader flap technique. Before (left) and after (right) photos in three views are provided.

Further Readings

Byrd HS, Meade RA, Gonyon DL, Jr. Using the autospreader flap in primary rhinoplasty. Plast Reconstr Surg. 2007; 119(6):1897–1902

Courtiss EH, Goldwyn RM. The effects of nasal surgery on airflow. Plast Reconstr Surg. 1983; 72(1):9–21

Moubayed SP, Most SP. The autospreader flap for midvault reconstruction following dorsal hump resection. Facial Plast Surg. 2016; 32(1):36–41

Rohrich RJ, Ahmad J. Rhinoplasty. Plast Reconstr Surg. 2011; 128(2):49e–73e

Rohrich RJ, Krueger JK, Adams WP, Jr, Hollier LH, Jr. Achieving consistency in the lateral nasal osteotomy during rhinoplasty: an external perforated technique. Plast Reconstr Surg. 2001; 108(7):2122–2130, discussion 2131–2132

Rohrich RJ, Muzaffar AR, Janis JE. Component dorsal hump reduction: the importance of maintaining dorsal aesthetic lines in rhinoplasty. Plast Reconstr Surg. 2004; 114(5):1298–1308, discussion 1309–1312

Roostaeian J, Unger JG, Lee MR, Geissler P, Rohrich RJ. Reconstitution of the nasal dorsum following component dorsal reduction in primary rhinoplasty. Plast Reconstr Surg. 2014; 133(3):509–518

Sheen JH. Spreader graft: a method of reconstructing the roof of the middle nasal vault following rhinoplasty. Plast Reconstr Surg. 1984; 73(2):230–239

Villanueva NL, Afrooz PN, Carboy JA, Rohrich RJ. Nasal analysis: considerations for ethnic variation. Plast Reconstr Surg. 2019; 143(6):1179e–1188e

Yoo S, Most SP. Nasal airway preservation using the autospreader technique: analysis of outcomes using a disease-specific quality-of-life instrument. Arch Facial Plast Surg. 2011; 13(4):231–233

24 Ancillary Maneuvers in Rhinoplasty: Columellar Strut

Rod J. Rohrich and Jon Kurkjian

Abstract
The columellar strut is a key rhinoplasty maneuver to unify the nasal tip and maintain tip position. This chapter will give a detailed description of proper indications and technique for use of the columellar strut.

Keywords: Columellar strut graft, nasal tip projection, nasal tip rotation, unification of the nasal tip

Key Points

- Columellar struts are a key maneuver to unify the nasal tip through stabilization and equalization of the medial and intermediate crura of the lower lateral cartilages.
- Technical variations of the columellar strut can be applied to address a wide range of nasal deformities.
- Columellar strut grafts can be placed in a dynamic fashion to help increase tip projection or they can be used in a static fashion to simply maintain tip projection.

24.1 Preoperative Steps

- Perform complete full facial analysis with a focus on nasal tip projection, rotation, and symmetry.
- Confirm adequate cartilage availability for the length and strength of the columellar strut that will be required to address the specific aesthetic and functional goals.

24.2 Operative Steps

- Harvest cartilage that is of the proper size and strength for a columellar strut. Ideally, septal cartilage is preferred for a primary rhinoplasty. Costal cartilage is used for columellar struts in secondary rhinoplasty cases where the septal cartilage is inadequate or in patients with a need for significant tip support. Auricular cartilage can be used, but may require multiple fragments to be sutured together to construct an adequately strong and symmetric columellar strut graft.
- Harvested cartilage is carved into a quadrangular shape that is 2 to 4 mm wide, 15 to 25 mm long, and 2 mm thick.
- Avoid warped or twisted portions of cartilage so as to maximize symmetry in the final construct.
- The cartilage should be shaped to create a slight angle at each end. These angled ends are ideal for placement into the soft tissue pocket proximally and distally while also creating the proper transition from the infratip lobule to the nasal tip.
- Dissect a soft tissue pocket between the medial crura posteriorly toward the maxilla leaving a portion of soft tissue intact to prevent postoperative "clicking" of the columellar strut on the maxillary crest. The pocket dissection depth is critical as it must match the goals for the columellar strut (▶ Fig. 24.1). A limited depth pocket is ideal if the strut graft is to be used dynamically to project the nasal tip and/or if the strut graft cartilage is short. A deeper pocket may be ideal if there is adequate graft material and/or if the graft will be used in a static fashion to only maintain tip projection.
- A double hook is used to retract the lower lateral cartilages anteriorly while advancing the columellar strut graft posteriorly in relation to one another based on the desired effect on tip projection (▶ Fig. 24.2). If more projection is desired, the lower lateral cartilages can be advanced anteriorly while the columellar strut is displaced posteriorly. The graft–lower lateral cartilage interface tension can then be set with a 25-gauge needle placed through the medial crura and graft construct.
- The interrelationship of the structures is then assessed and sutured together using 5–0 PDS sutures in a horizontal mattress fashion. Sutures are placed inferiorly and then again in the infratip area. Careful attention is paid to ensure the medial crura are oriented in a symmetric fashion in all planes.

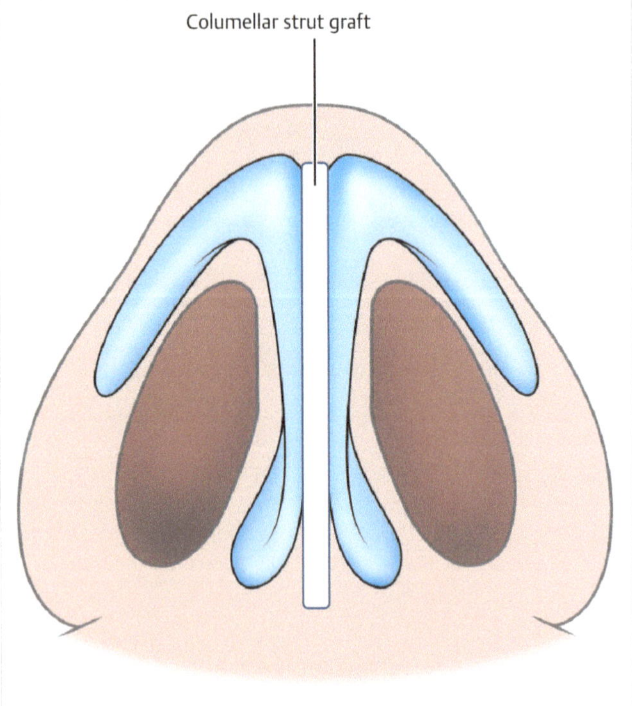

Fig. 24.1 Standard placement of the columellar strut to maintain tip projection and fortify the medial crura.

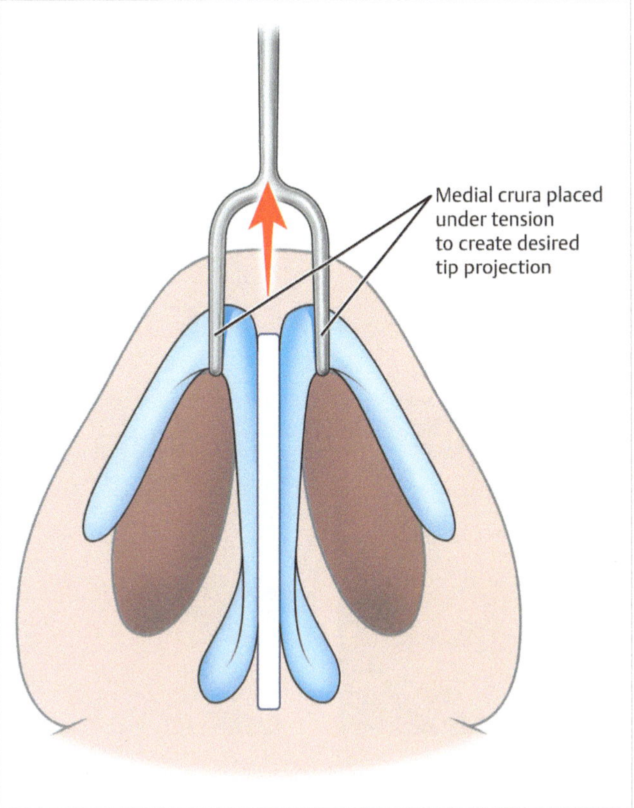

Fig. 24.2 The medial crura are pulled anteriorly (*arrow*) and advanced along the length of the columellar strut in order to increase tip projection.

- If an increase in projection is desired, and a dynamic columellar strut has been placed, the surgeon can expect a 1 to 2 mm decrease in projection over time as the nose heals. This often means that an overcorrection of tip projection is required when using a columellar strut to increase tip projection.
- The columellar strut graft is placed to ensure that it is an invisible graft, which is used to structurally support the lower lateral cartilages and avoid any direct contact with the skin. Particularly in the interdomal area, any visibility of the graft beyond the lower lateral cartilage is to be avoided.
- See **Video 24.1**.

24.3 Postoperative Care

- Taping and nasal splints should be applied to limit the impact of edema on the skin envelope and osseocartilaginous infrastructure.
- After surgery, the head should be elevated to minimize edema.
- Gauze soaked with ice water or ice packs should be applied to the eyes.
- Great care should be taken to avoid any trauma to the nose in the first 4 to 6 weeks after surgery.
- Limit salt intake for the first 3 weeks following surgery.

24.4 Case Example

Photos of a primary rhinoplasty 1 year after surgery are shown. A columellar strut graft was used in a static fashion to maintain tip projection (▶ Fig. 24.3a–l).

24.5 Conclusion

The columellar strut is primarily used to fortify nasal tip projection by giving structural support and shape to the medial and intermediate crura of the lower lateral cartilages. The dimensions and inherent strength of the cartilage graft as well as the pocket dissection can be adjusted to the anatomical needs of the patient.

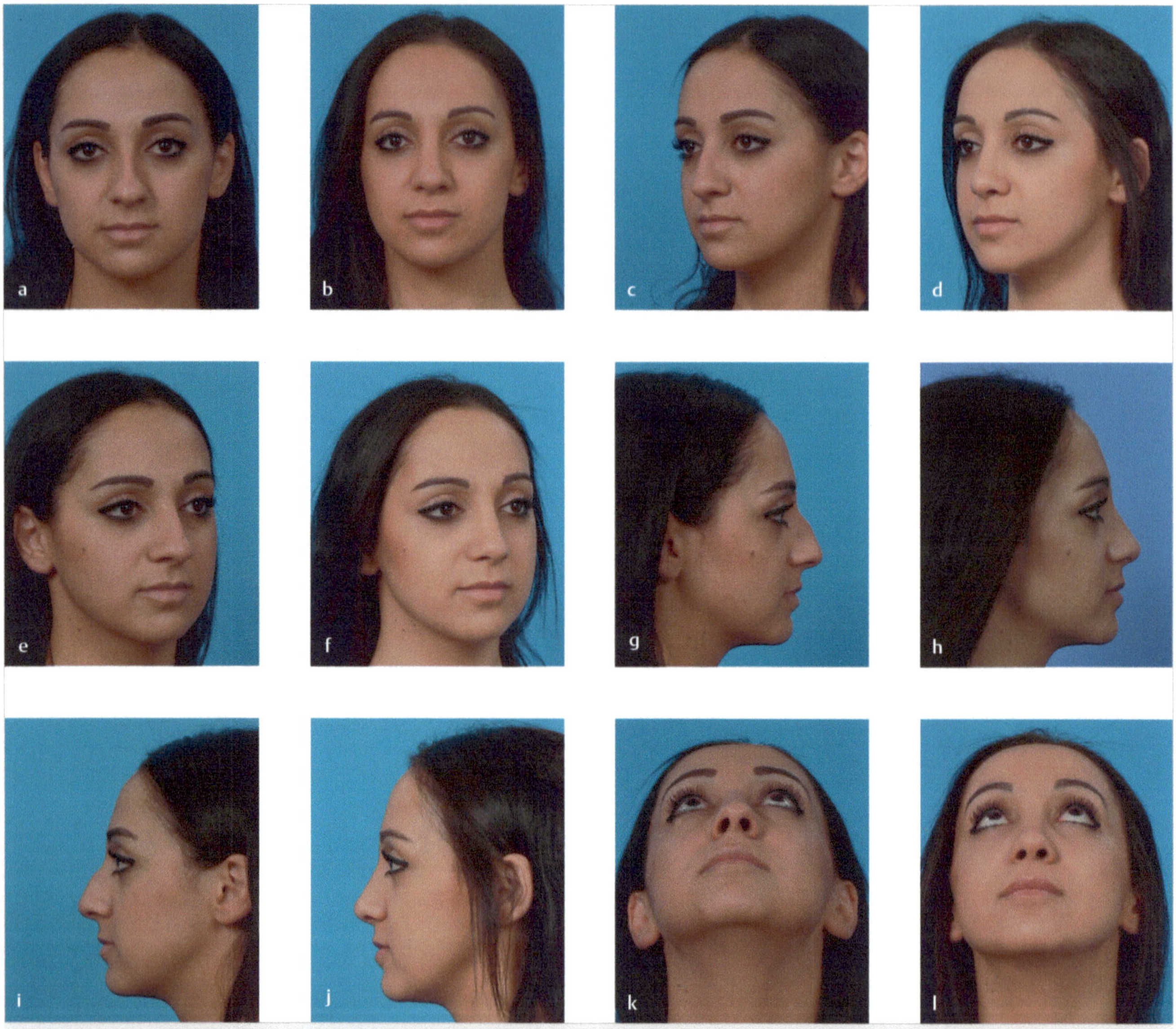

Fig. 24.3 (a–l) Photos of a primary rhinoplasty 1 year after surgery. Columellar strut graft was used in a static fashion to maintain tip projection.

Further Readings

Hackney HL, Gunter JP. Increasing and decreasing tip projection in rhinoplasty. Operat Tech Plast Reconst Surg. 2000; 7(4):168–174

Rohrich RJ, Hoxworth RE, Kurkjian TJ. The role of the columellar strut in rhinoplasty: indications and rationale. Plast Reconstr Surg. 2012; 129(1):118e–125e

Rohrich RJ, Kurkjian TJ, Hoxworth RE, Stephan PJ, Mojallal A. The effect of the columellar strut graft on nasal tip position in primary rhinoplasty. Plast Reconstr Surg. 2012; 130(4):926–932

Rohrich RJ, Liu JH. The dorsal columellar strut: innovative use of dorsal hump removal for a columellar strut. Aesthet Surg J. 2010; 30(1):30–35

25 Ancillary Maneuvers in Rhinoplasty: Alar Rim Grafts

Jason Roostaeian and Sean Saadat

Abstract

Cartilage grafts have long been used in all aspects of both aesthetic and functional rhinoplasty to help correct deformities and provide a sound structural support to the nasal complex. The alar rim is naturally composed of fibrofatty tissue with no cartilaginous support, thus leading to a high incidence of deformities especially after trauma or prior rhinoplasty. Alar notching is a significant deformity that can occur for multiple reasons and cannot be corrected without some form of support to smooth out any irregularities in the nasal skin envelope. Multiple techniques including dermal grafts, fat grafting, and skin redraping techniques have been described to try and correct notches in the alar rim, but none of these options have proven as successful as the alar contour graft. As described in this chapter, alar contour grafts, which are composed of a strip of autologous or cadaveric cartilage, are a key component when correcting alar deformities such as notching or collapse. The cartilage is placed into a bluntly dissected subcutaneous pocket at the alar margin as a last step in the procedure. Alar contour grafts are a key component of rhinoplasty and their routine use has been shown to consistently improve overall nasal function and aesthetic outcomes.

Keywords: Nasal ala, rhinoplasty, alar contour graft, alar rim, cartilage grafting, nasal aesthetics, nasal reconstruction, alar reconstruction

Key Points

- Without the proper structural support, the nasal ala can retract, notch, or collapse, leading to both aesthetic and functional deficits in the nasal complex.
- Alar rim grafts are an effective way of correcting alar notching or asymmetries of the alar rims in both primary and revision rhinoplasty as well as nasal reconstruction.
- The alar rim is ideally located <2 mm from the long axis of the nostril.
- It is important to remember that the basal view of the nasal complex should be an equilateral triangle with an alar to lobular ratio of 2:1 (▶ Fig. 25.1c).
- The aesthetic goal should be to achieve a gentle gull-in-flight appearance on anteroposterior view (▶ Fig. 25.1b).

25.1 Preoperative Steps

25.1.1 Initial Assessment of Need for Alar Rim Grafts

- Indications for alar rim graft placement include weak and asymmetric alar rims; a ptotic, boxy, or bulbous nasal tip; secondary rhinoplasty requiring a correction of alar notching; and nasal reconstruction after the compromise of the nasal–alar complex (▶ Fig. 25.2).

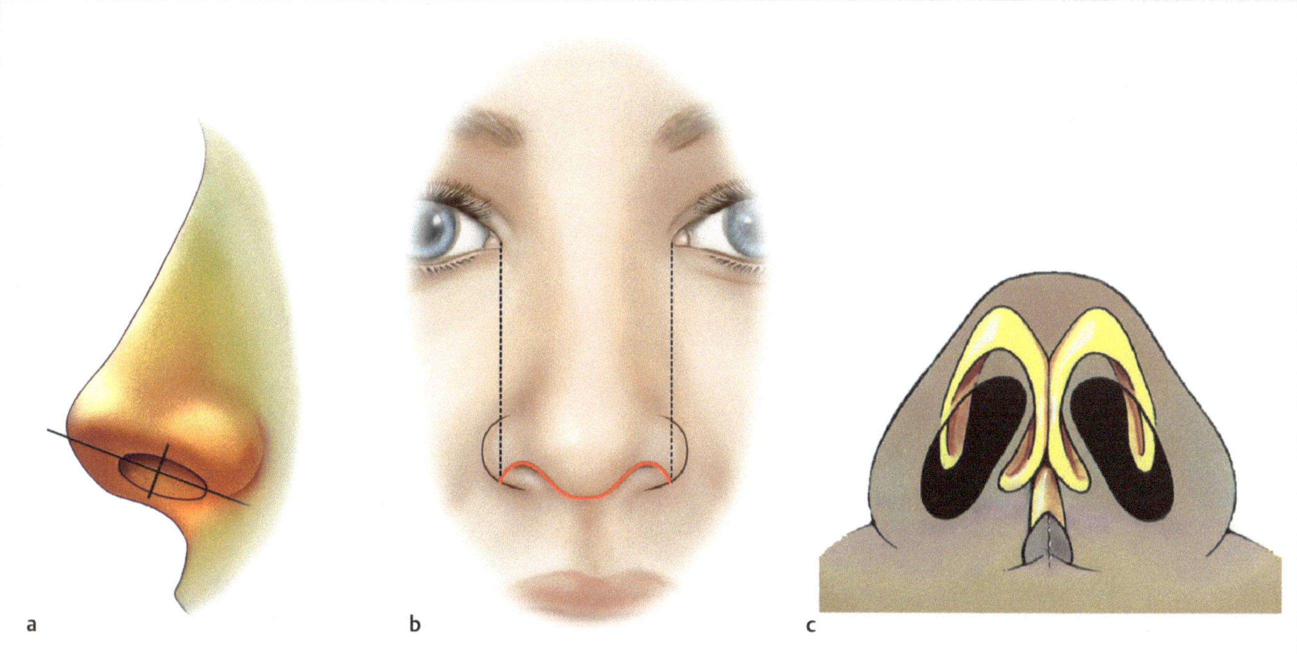

Fig. 25.1 (a–c) Overview of alar aesthetic and functional position. **(a)** The alar position of profile view is key to ensuring the nose does not appear notched or have excessive columellar show. **(b)** A gentle gull-in-flight appearance on anteroposterior view. **(c)** Basal view of the nasal complex should be an equilateral triangle with an alar to lobular ratio of 2:1. (Reproduced with permission from Dallas Rhinoplasty Meeting Alar Contour Grafting Presentation by Dr Jason Roostaeian, originally from Dallas Rhinoplasty.)

- Alar contour grafts are also an important adjunct to other alar grafts such as the alar batten graft or lateral crural strut graft.
- Be sure to determine the strength and position of the lower lateral cartilages, as this may reveal a need for further support in addition to alar contour grafts to correct significant alar deformities.
- On functional examination, have the patient take a deep nasal inhalation, and repeat while manually blocking the left or right nostril sequentially to reveal if there is marked collapse of either nostril indicating a lack of structural support in the ala.

25.2 Operative Steps

See **Video 25.1**.

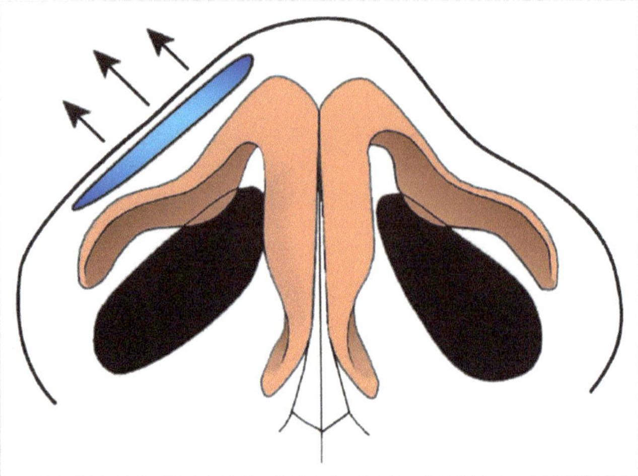

Fig. 25.2 Alar rim grafts act to stent open the nasal ala for both functionally and aesthetically optimal results. (Reproduced with permission from Dallas Rhinoplasty Meeting Alar Contour Grafting Presentation by Dr Jason Roostaeian, originally from Dallas Rhinoplasty.[4])

25.2.1 Open Technique

- To be done as last step prior to closure of the nasal skin envelope.
- Create subcutaneous pocket parallel to alar rim using sharp tenotomy scissors from the dome laterally to the ala (▶ Fig. 25.3a, b).
- Carefully tailor cartilage grafts into segments of equal strength and length in order to prevent asymmetry or unilateral weakness.
- Grafts are ideally 2 to 3 mm wide and roughly 15 mm in length (although this may change depending on nasal projection).
- Once placed, redrape the skin envelope to assess the appearance and palpability of the graft prior to closing the nose.
- If necessary, the alar rim graft can be sutured to the underside of the domal complex of the lower lateral cartilages to help support the dome and prevent visibility or migration of the graft.

25.2.2 Closed Technique

- Similar to the open technique, this is also done as the last step of rhinoplasty surgery prior to closure of intranasal incisions.
- Create a separate incision at the deep surface of the nasal dome and dissect laterally with scissors to carefully create a pocket along the alar rim.
- Use the same dimensions as in the open technique.
- Care should be taken to prevent palpable edges by tapering and shaping the graft.
- In both open and closed rhinoplasty, the cartilage may be harvested from septum, ear, or rib.
- As septal cartilage is often absent or minimal in revision rhinoplasty patients; ear cartilage can sometimes be used for alar rim grafts, and is in some ways ideal due to its natural curvature. However, its softer texture in comparison to rib cartilage offers less support.

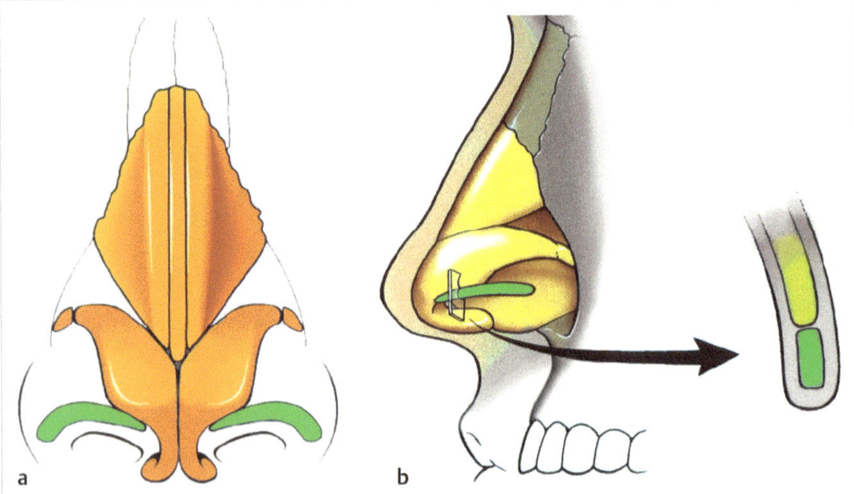

Fig. 25.3 **(a, b)** Alar rim grafts are placed in the subcutaneous pocket dissected along the alar rim and medially abut the intermediate crura of the lower lateral cartilages. (Reproduced with permission from Dallas Rhinoplasty Meeting Alar Contour Grafting Presentation by Dr Jason Roostaeian, originally from Dallas Rhinoplasty.)

25.3 Postoperative Care

- Alar rim grafts do not require specific postoperative care beyond that of a standard rhinoplasty.
- Postoperatively, patients will have internal Doyle splints sutured in place at the septum using a single mattress 3–0 Prolene suture to stent the nasal complex, support the septum, and prevent obstruction of breathing during the immediate recovery.
- Saline nasal rinses are encouraged at least three times daily or as often as the patient feels it would be beneficial in order to keep the nasal splints clean and also prevent any obstruction of the airway with nasal secretions or postoperative drainage.
- In the setting of open rhinoplasty or alar base resection, any external incisions are cleaned daily with dilute peroxide to prevent crusting of blood and drainage, and to make suture removal easier for both the surgeon and patient in the postoperative visit.
- Patients are to avoid any blowing of the nose or undue pressure to the exterior of the nasal complex postoperatively as this could lead to an alteration or violation of the final result both aesthetically and functionally.

25.4 Case Example

The selected case shows a 32-year-old woman who underwent open rhinoplasty to reduce the dorsal hump, improve tip projection and rotation, and address general concerns with the larger unrefined appearance of her nose. Spreader grafts were placed, as well as dorsal hump reduction, lateral osteotomies, septal extension graft, and alar contour grafts were used to address excessive columellar show and alar retraction. The postoperative photos are taken 1 year after her surgery (▶ Fig. 25.4a–c).

25.5 Conclusion

A clear understanding of nasal anatomy is key to performing a proper rhinoplasty that aesthetically refines the nose while maintaining function. There are improved outcomes in primary rhinoplasty with routine use of alar rim grafts. Alar rim grafts provide additional structural support to the external nasal valve. There is increasing use of alar rim grafts among rhinoplasty surgeons due to ease of placement, low complication profile, and minimal cartilage requirement. Precise tailoring of the grafts is essential to avoid graft visibility.

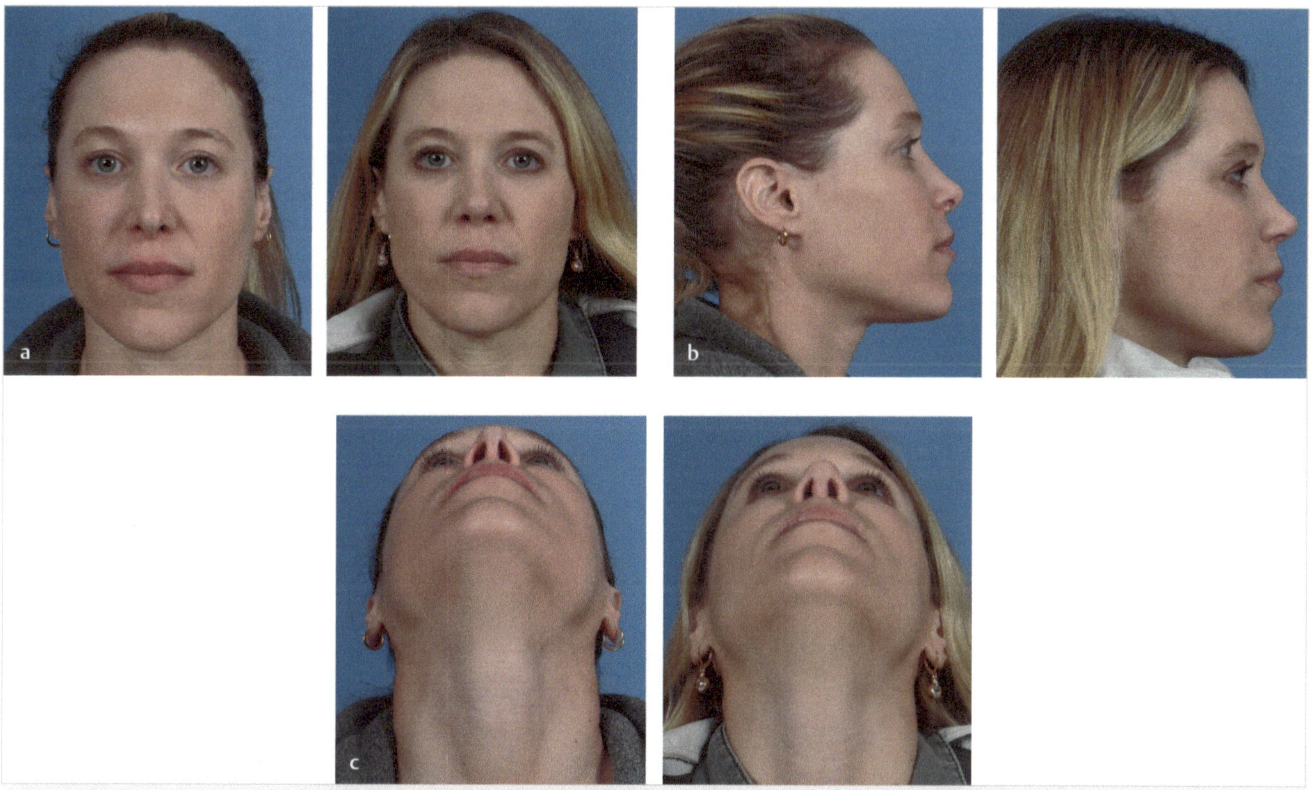

Fig. 25.4 **(a)** Frontal, **(b)** basal, and **(c)** lateral before and after views to correct alar retraction and excessive columellar show.

Further Readings

Gunter JP, Rohrich RJ, Friedman RM. Classification and correction of alar-columellar discrepancies in rhinoplasty. Plast Reconstr Surg. 1996; 97(3): 643–648

Rohrich RJ, Raniere J, Jr, Ha RY. The alar contour graft: correction and prevention of alar rim deformities in rhinoplasty. Plast Reconstr Surg. 2002; 109(7):2495–2505, discussion 2506–2508

Roostaeian J, Jamil K, Rohrich RJ. Correction and prevention of alar rim deformities: alar contour grafts. In: Dallas Rhinoplasty. 3rd ed. St Louis, Missouri: Quality Medical Publishing

Rohrich RJ, Malafa MM, Ahmad J, Basci DS. Managing alar flare in rhinoplasty. Plast Reconstr Surg. 2017; 140(5):910–919

Unger J, Roostaeian J, Small K, Pezeshk R, Lee M, Harris R, Rohrich R. Alar contour grafts in rhinoplasty: a safe and reproducible way to refine alar contour aesthetics. Plast Reconstr Surg. 2016; 137(1):52–61

26 Ancillary Maneuvers in Rhinoplasty: Septal Extension Grafts

David M. Kowalczyk and Dean M. Toriumi

Abstract

Caudal septal extension grafts stabilize the nasal base and set nasal tip position. The airway should be carefully evaluated for signs of severe septal deviation, perforation, nasal valve obstruction, or turbinate hypertrophy. There are seven subtypes of grafts available depending on the patient's nasal deformity. The most commonly used grafts are the superiorly based end-to-end and rectangular-shaped. It is imperative that the surgeon counsel the patient regarding possible outcomes, which include a horizontal, upper lip crease with smiling and stiffness of the nasal tip. Proper, aesthetic nasal proportions and patient's desires should always be kept in mind when using these techniques.

Keywords: Caudal septal extension grafts, tip projection, tip rotation, nasal base, nasal obstruction, septal deviation

Key Points

- Caudal septal extension grafts stabilize the nasal base and set nasal tip position.
- There are seven subtypes of grafts available depending on the patient's existing nasal deformity.
- Regardless of the chosen technique, care should be taken to avoid obstructing the nasal airway.

26.1 Preoperative Steps

- On profile view, the tip projection and rotation, alar–columellar relationship, and premaxilla must be carefully evaluated.
- Whether via anterior rhinoscopy and/or rigid endoscope, the septum should be visualized and examined for severe deviation, septal perforation, nasal valve blockage, or turbinate hypertrophy.
- The caudal septum should be straight and in a midline position; caudal septal deviations must be corrected prior to placing a caudal septal extension graft.
- There must be sufficient vestibular skin available to position the caudal septal extension graft.
- The patient should be advised that graft placement will make the tip stiff and have less recoil; additionally, the upper lip may become rigid or develop a horizontal crease.

26.2 Operative Steps

See **Video 26.1**.

26.2.1 Incisions and Dissection

- After sterile preparation and positioning, the nose is infiltrated with 1% lidocaine with 1:100,000 epinephrine.
- Attention is directed to the posteroinferior septum whereupon a segment of cartilage is removed while preserving at least a 1.5 cm L-strut of native septum; if the caudal septum is deviated, bilateral splinting spreader grafts can be used to straighten the caudal septum.
- An external rhinoplasty approach is then initiated carefully exposing the lower lateral cartilages, caudal septum, and middle vault.

26.2.2 Graft Selection and Placement

- Most grafts are designed as a right-angle triangle with the longer margin oriented superiorly to control tip position and prevent over-rotation of the tip.
- There are seven subtypes of grafts if the standard, right-angle triangle is not suitable for the patient.

Superiorly Based End-to-End Caudal Septal Extension Graft (▶ Fig. 26.1)

- It is the most commonly used type of extension graft.
- This graft will support the nasal base with minimal effect on the upper lip.
- It is less likely to create stiffness in the upper lip.
- This graft does not extend to the nasal spine and should be used in conjunction with a medial crural footplate suture and a nasolabial angle plumping graft.
- Softer cartilage with attached soft tissue should be used for the plumping graft and can be secured transcutaneously if needed.

Rectangular-Shaped Caudal Septal Extension Graft (▶ Fig. 26.2a, b)

- Used for significant increases in tip projection as the graft should extend beyond the anterior septal angle.
- Helps support a weak base.
- Ethnic populations (i.e., Asians), congenital defects, and secondary rhinoplasty patients are ideal candidates.
- Avoid tacking to nasal spine to minimize effect on upper lip.
- Can be used to open the nasolabial angle.
- May create stiffness in the upper lip.

Wide-Base Caudal Septal Extension Graft (▶ Fig. 26.3)

- It is useful in patient with an acute nasolabial angle and/or ptotic tip.
- Graft is narrower anteriorly and wider posteriorly.
- Inferior margin should be sutured to posterior septal angle above nasal spine.

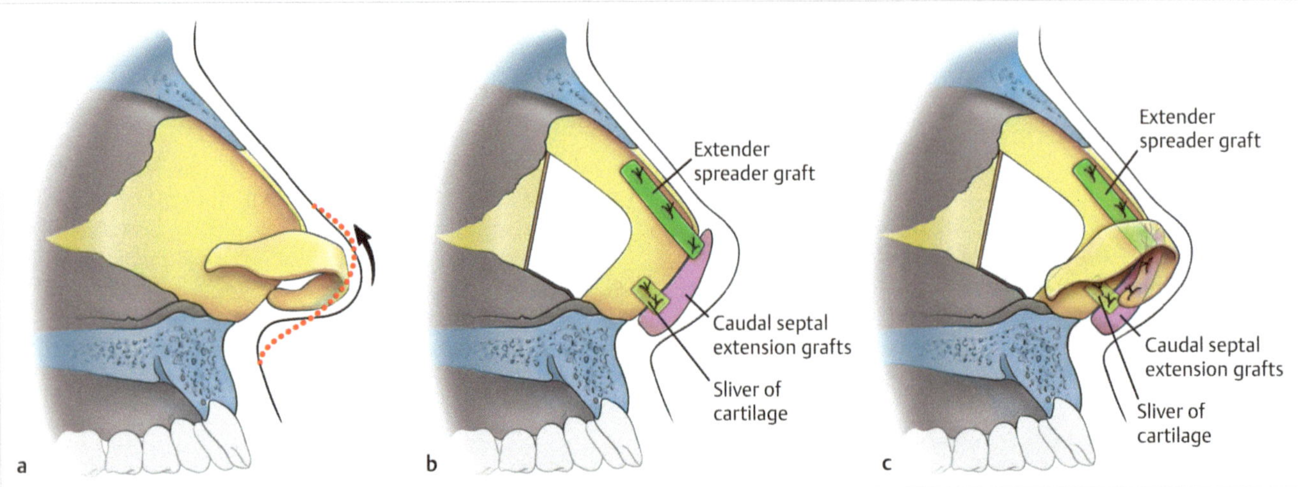

Fig. 26.1 **(a)** Desired goal of counterrotation of the nasal tip. **(b)** Superiorly based caudal septal extension graft. **(c)** Medial crura repositioned. (Reproduced with permission from Rohrich R, Adams W, Ahmad J, et al, eds. Dallas Rhinoplasty. 3rd ed. Thieme; 2014.)

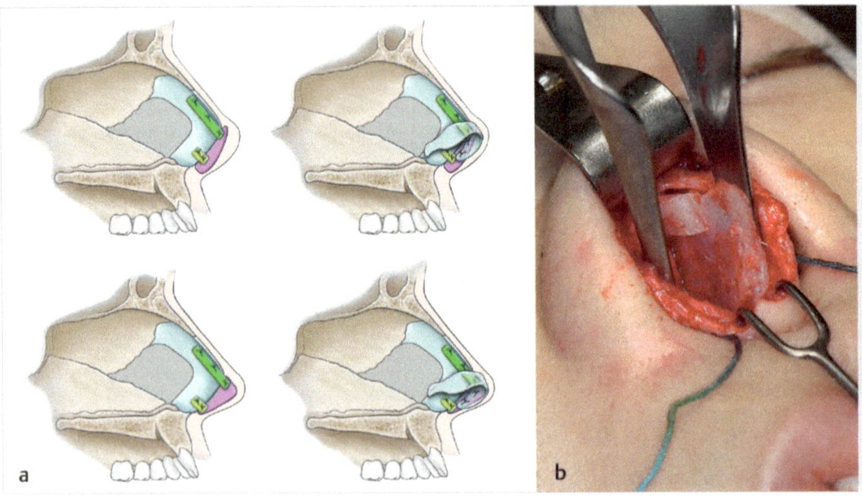

Fig. 26.2 **(a)** Inferiorly based caudal septal extension graft. **(b)** Intraoperative photo with the graft sutured in position.

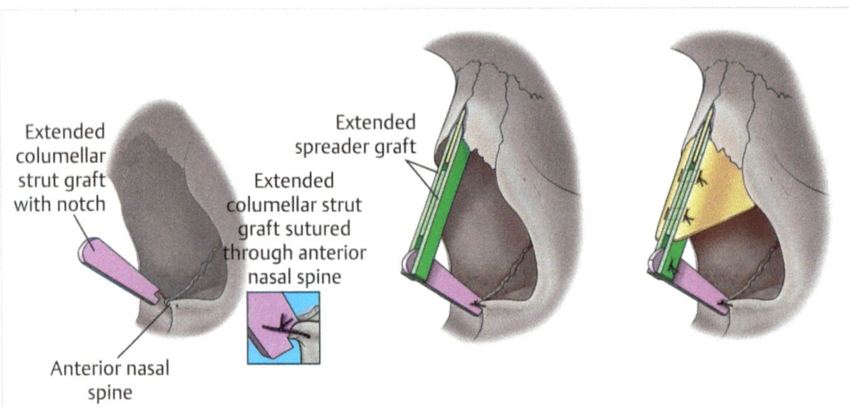

Fig. 26.3 Wide-base caudal septal extension graft. (Reproduced with permission from Rohrich R, Adams W, Ahmad J, et al, eds. Dallas Rhinoplasty. 3rd ed. Thieme; 2014.)

- Thin slivers of cartilage or ethmoid bone should be used to secure the graft inferiorly.
- Avoid using this technique in patients whose oral commissures elevate upon smiling, otherwise a deep crease in the upper lip may ensue.

Caudal Septal Replacement Graft with Advancement of Medial Crura (▶ Fig. 26.4)

- It is used in cases where the caudal septum is severely damaged and cannot be straightened using typical splinting techniques.

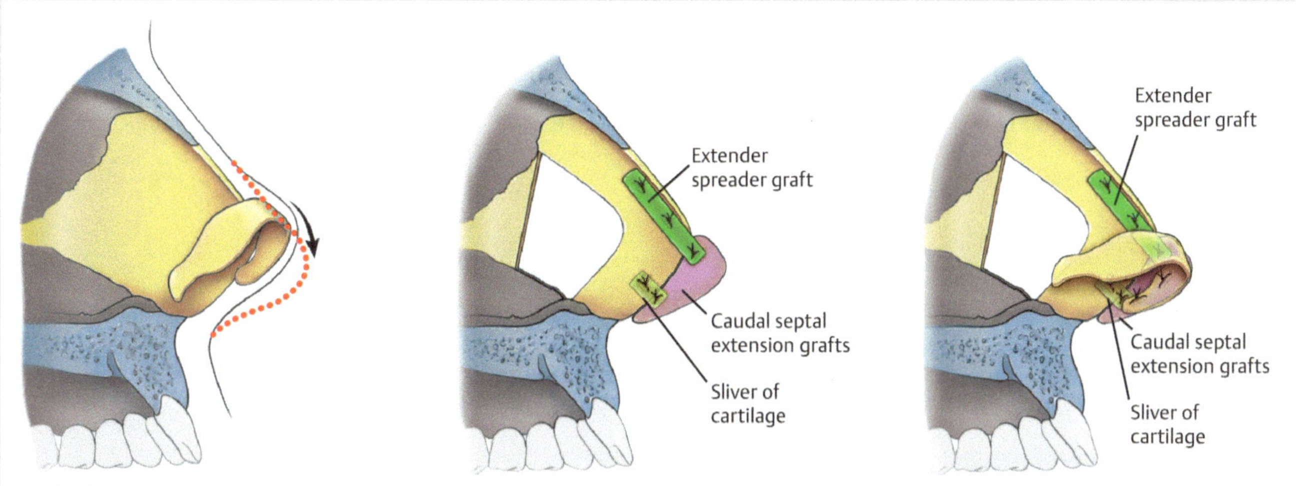

Fig. 26.4 Caudal septal replacement graft with advancement of medial crura. (Reproduced with permission from Rohrich R, Adams W, Ahmad J, et al, eds. Dallas Rhinoplasty. 3rd ed. Thieme; 2014.)

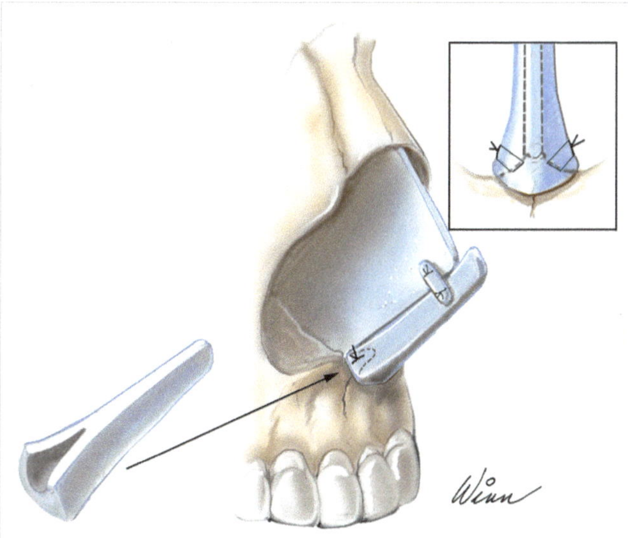

Fig. 26.5 Flared-base caudal septal replacement graft.

- Weak or deformed caudal septum is removed.
- The caudal septal replacement graft is sutured to the nasal spine and stabilized with two extended spreader grafts.
- This graft may limit upper lip excursion creating a risk of a crease in the upper lip when the patient smiles.
- The medial crura are advanced onto the graft and sutured with a 4–0 plain on a straight septal needle and a 5–0 PDS intercrural suture.

Flared-Base Caudal Septal Replacement Graft (▶ Fig. 26.5)

- This graft fits over the nasal spine but is flared at its base to provide augmentation of the premaxilla.
- The ideal patient needs significant augmentation of the nasolabial region and/or has a thin nasal spine which cannot be split without shattering.

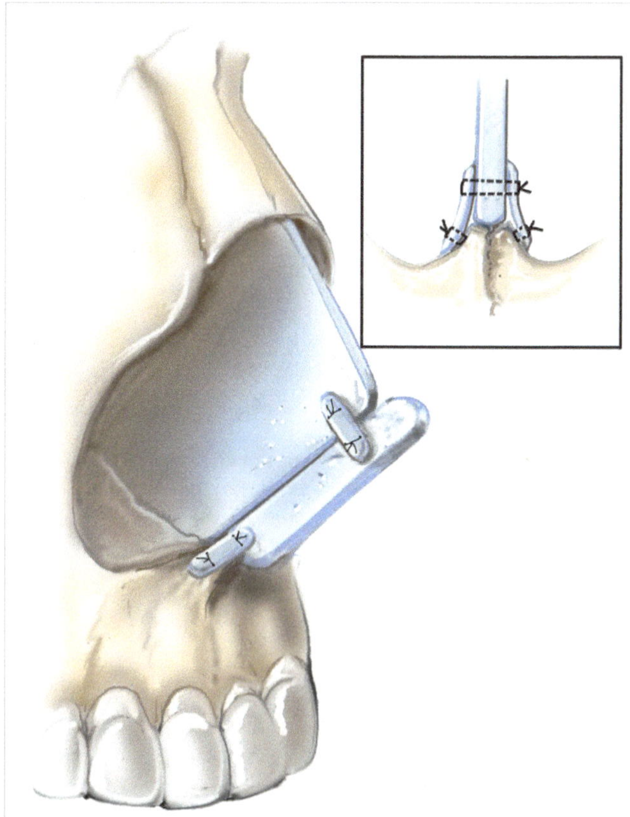

Fig. 26.6 Caudal septal replacement graft with splinting grafts over nasal spine.

Caudal Septal Replacement Graft with Splinting Grafts Over Nasal Spine (▶ Fig. 26.6)

- These are placed around the base of the strut to allow fixation around the nasal spine, which helps prevent displacement.

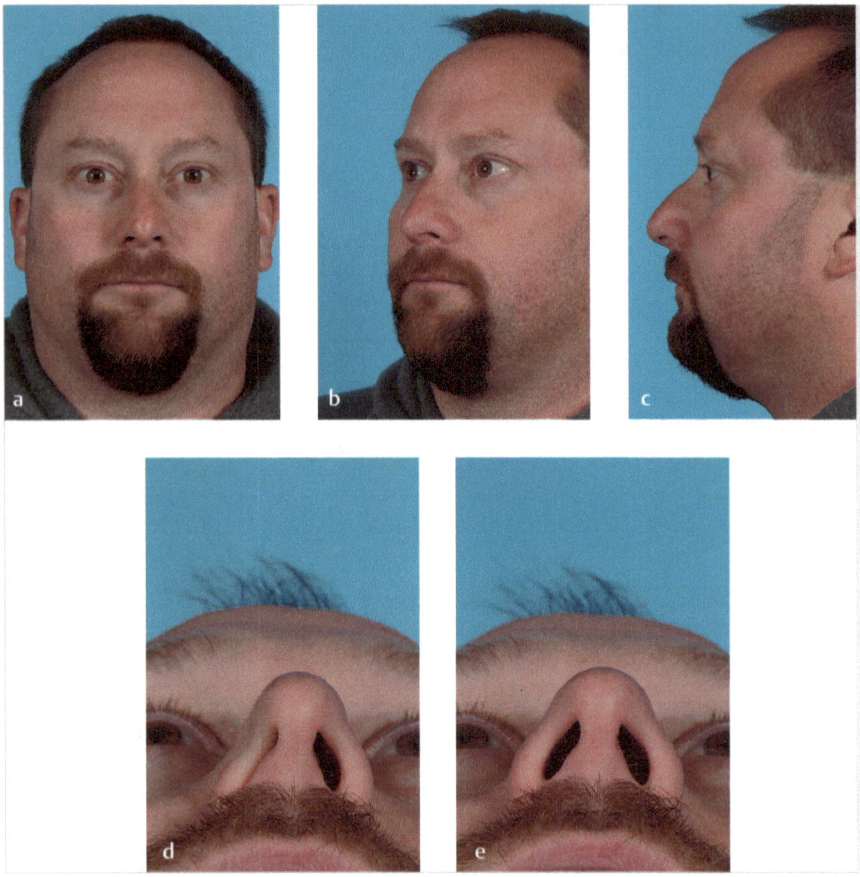

Fig. 26.7 (a–e) A 42-year-old male who presented for a primary functional and cosmetic rhinoplasty. On frontal view, he demonstrates a narrow tip and mild alar retraction. His lateral view highlights a prominent dorsal hump and an obtuse nasolabial angle. On base view, he has a pinched tip with narrow nostrils and flared medial crural footplates.

- This technique is used for those who need premaxillary augmentation in light of an acute nasolabial angle.
- The graft should be sized larger and trimmed once in position and evaluated with the skin-soft tissue envelope redraped for the most accurate assessment.
- The nasal airway should be examined after graft placement to ensure the nasal valve or vestibule is not blocked.
- Great care is taken to ensure proper positioning of the crura to achieve 3 to 4 mm of columella show; the domes should be 5 to 8 mm above the nasal dorsum.

26.2.3 Closure

- Once the graft is fully secured, the septum should be reapproximated with a 5–0 plain gut suture in a quilting fashion.
- The upper lateral cartilages must be resecured to the dorsal septum in order to prevent inferomedial collapse of the upper lateral cartilages with subsequent midvault deformity.
- The nose is taped and dressed with a cast in the standard fashion.

26.3 Postoperative Care

- The patient is prescribed oral antibiotics for a minimum of 7 days, which should include cartilage coverage.
- The tape, nasal cast, external sutures, and internal splints can be removed and the nose gently cleansed after 7 days.
- The patient should be encouraged to ambulate multiple times per day, follow a low salt diet, and avoid any manipulation of the nose.

26.4 Case Example

A 42-year-old male presented for a primary functional and cosmetic rhinoplasty. On frontal view, he demonstrates a narrow tip and mild alar retraction. His lateral view highlights a prominent dorsal hump and an obtuse nasolabial angle. On base view, he has a pinched tip with narrow nostrils and flared medial crural footplates. His 4-month, postoperative photos show symmetric brow-tip aesthetic lines, straight dorsum, and counterrotation of the nasal tip with natural definition, favorable alar–columellar relationship, and improved patency of both nostrils (▸ Fig. 26.7a–e and ▸ Fig. 26.8a–e).

26.5 Conclusion

Caudal septal extension grafts are best used for deficiencies of the caudal septum and a weak base. Dramatic changes in tip position and rotation, as well as upper lip excursion, can occur as a result of placement of these types of grafts. Proper, aesthetic nasal proportions and patient's desires should be kept in mind when using these techniques.

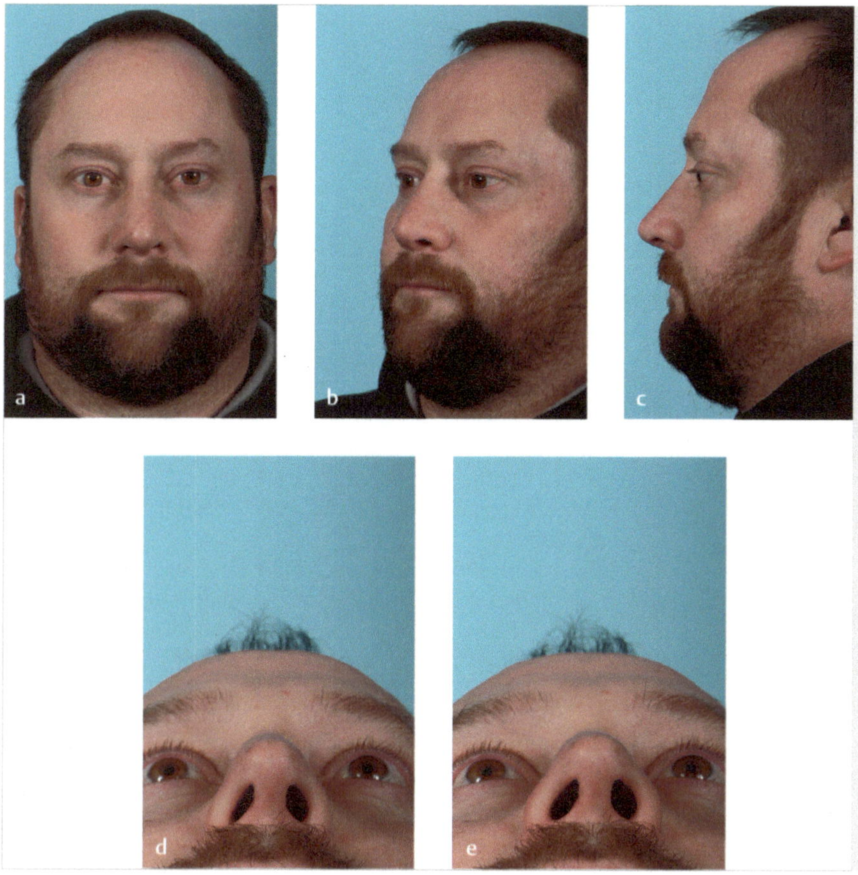

Fig. 26.8 (a–e) The same patient as in ▶ Fig. 26.7, 4-month, postoperative photos show symmetric brow-tip aesthetic lines, straight dorsum, and counterrotation of the nasal tip with natural definition, favorable alar–columellar relationship, and improved patency of both nostrils.

Further Readings

Toriumi DM. Caudal septal extension graft for correction of the retracted columella. Oper Tech Otolaryngol–Head Neck Surg. 1995; 6(4):311–318

Toriumi DM. Stabilizing the nasal base and caudal septal extension grafts. In: Structure Rhinoplasty: Lessons Learned in 30 Years. Chicago: DMT Solutions; 2019;1:279–416

Toriumi DM, Asher SA. Lateral crural repositioning for treatment of cephalic malposition. Facial Plast Surg Clin North Am. 2015; 23(1):55–71

Toriumi DM, Bared A. Revision of the surgically overshortened nose. Facial Plast Surg. 2012; 28(4):407–416

Toriumi DM, Becker DG. Other maneuvers: caudal extension grafts. In: Rhinoplasty Dissection Manual. Philadelphia: Lippincott; 1999:118–121

27 Alar Base Surgery

Rod J. Rohrich, Jamil Ahmad, Yash J. Avashia, and Ira L. Savetsky

Abstract

Alar base surgery is a powerful aspect of rhinoplasty. Due to the changes imparted by maneuvers that adjust tip projection, this portion is performed as the last step of the open rhinoplasty. Alar base width and alar flare are two separate entities. Management for them can be separate or combined depending on each case. The three-dimensional nature of the alar base requires detailed analysis and consistent points of reference for marking base width and flare reductions. A systematic approach to managing increased alar base width and/or alar fare will aid in achieving consistent results.

Keywords: Alar base, alar flare, tip projection, alar base reduction, alar base surgery

Key Points

- The alar base is the caudal-most point of the nasal ala at the alar–facial junction.
- Alar base width should approximate the intercanthal distance (31–33 mm).
- Interalar distance is the distance between the lateral-most points of the ala.
- Alar flare is present when the interalar distance is greater than the alar base width (▶ Fig. 27.1).
- A larger degree of alar flaring is accepted in non-Caucasian patients.
- Alar flare and alar base reduction are not mutually exclusive but represent separate anatomic entities.

27.1 Preoperative Steps

- Preoperative assessment of the alar base is performed from the basal view.
- Both alar base width and interalar distances are measured.
- A difference greater than 2 mm between these values on each side defines alar flare.
- Rohrich et al describe four morphologies of alar flare depending on the location of the lateral-most point along the ala in comparison to the nasal base.
  - Type 1: Lateral point is close to the alar–facial groove and is inferior to the level of the sill–base junction.
  - Type 2: Lateral point is at the same level of the sill–base junction.
  - Type 3: Lateral point is superior to the level of the sill–base junction.
  - Type 4: This is a combination of Type 3 flare with a widened nasal base.

27.2 Operative Steps

See **Video 27.1**.

- Changes in nasal tip projection and rotation directly influence alar base width and flare.
  - The decision to perform alar base and/or alar flare reduction should be made at the completion of the rhinoplasty after the transcolumellar incision has been closed.
  - If the indication is not clear, reduction is postponed until postsurgical swelling has subsided in 6 to 12 months.
- Alar flare reduction is a powerful technique to reduce interalar distance without the scar burden associated with more aggressive techniques for alar base medialization.

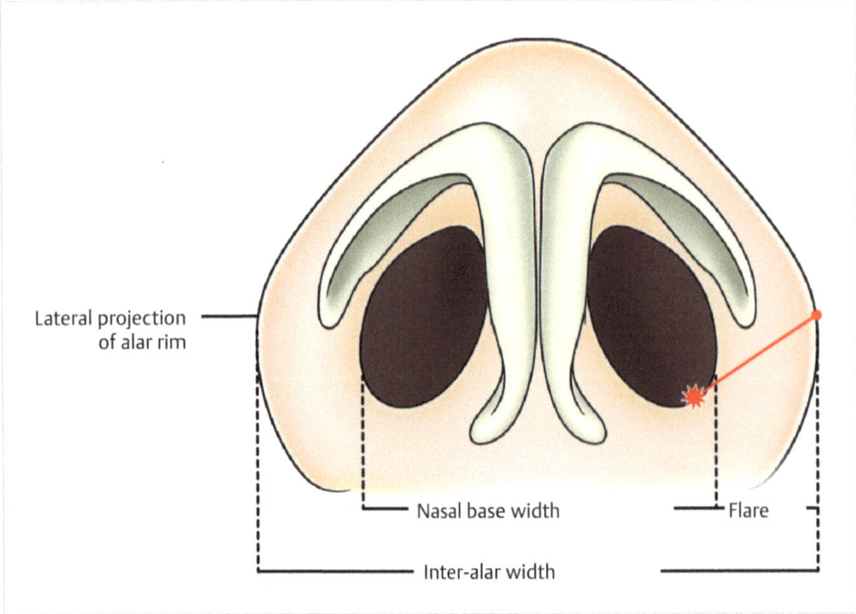

Fig. 27.1 Basal view of the nose. The *double-headed red arrow* is drawn from the lateral-most point along the alar rim to the point where the alar base meets the nasal sill along the nostril, the "sill-base junction." The relative vertical relationship between these two points on the basal view analysis characterizes the flare morphology and guides excision pattern design.

- The goal of flare reduction is to reduce nostril flare and improve nasal harmony.
- Understanding the alar flare type aids in excision design.
- The excised amount progressively increases with each type (1 through 3).
- Alar flare reduction marking (▶ Fig. 27.2):
  - Point 1: The lateral-most point is marked at the alar–facial groove.
  - Point 2: The sill–base junction is marked.
  - Point 3: A point 2 mm inferior to the sill–base junction is marked.
  - Line 1: A curved line in the alar–facial groove is made from Point 1 to Point 3.
  - Line 2: A curved line along the ala is made from Point 1 to Point 3 creating a final ellipse. The width of the ellipse increases with the degree of alar flare (Types 1 through 3).
  - If the inferior incision is made more than 1 mm above the groove, one risks having a visible scar.
  - The medial corner of the elliptical excision should not go beyond the sill–base junction, into the nasal sill. Incisions in this region will narrow the nasal sill and further distort the nostril size.
  - It is always safer to take less tissue, allowing a milder degree of alar flare, than to overresect and distort the nasal harmony.
- Alar base reduction marking (▶ Fig. 27.2):
  - Alar base reduction can be performed either with or without alar flare reduction.
  - When performed with alar flare reduction, a nostril sill excision is performed to narrow the base width.
  - Starting from Point 2, an elliptical excision of the nasal sill is performed in the sagittal plane to narrow the base width.
    - The sill–base junction should be preserved.
  - The sill–base junction to columellar–sill junction should be equivalent on both sides.
- Surgical technique:
  - Infiltrate 0.25% Marcaine with 1:100,000 epinephrine at the proposed flare reduction site.
  - Using a #15 blade, the marked wedge is excised including the skin and subcutaneous tissue. It is important not to excise the deeper layers including the muscle.
  - Hemostasis is achieved with a fine tip electrocautery.
  - Closure is performed in one layer using simple interrupted 6-0 nylon sutures.
  - Deep sutures are not advised as they run a high risk of extrusion and inflammatory scarring in this area.
  - During closure, the first stitch should be placed where the curvature of the alar rim meets with the upper lip.
  - Every stitch should be meticulously placed including full-thickness bites of skin and subcutaneous tissue.

27.3 Postoperative Care

- Half of the sutures are removed on postoperative day 7.
- The remaining sutures are removed on postoperative day 10.

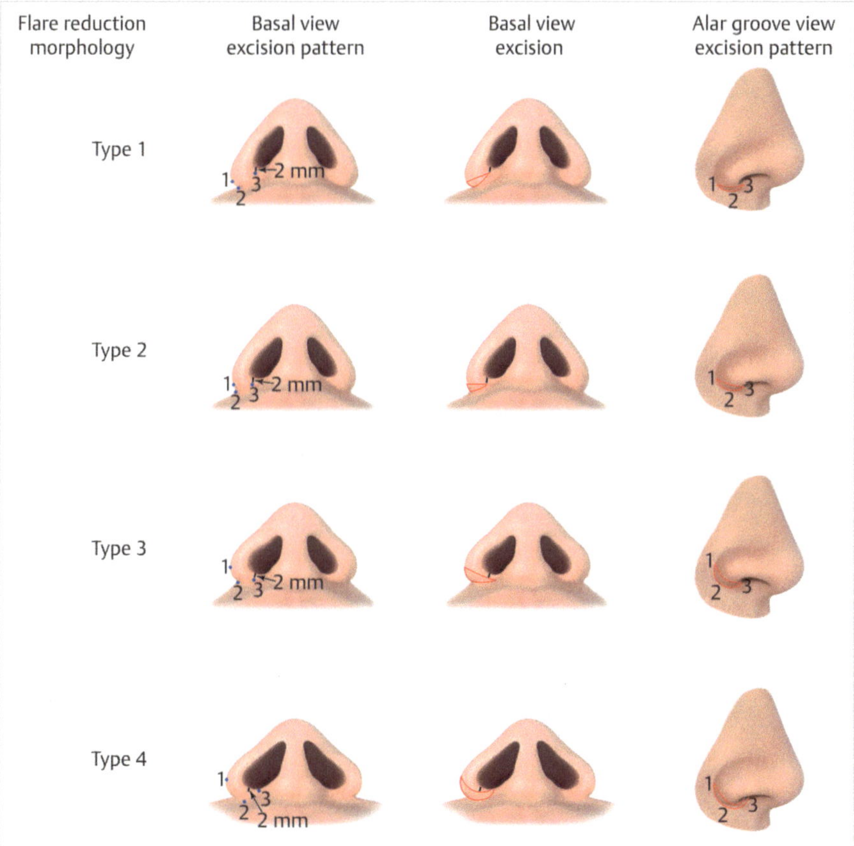

Fig. 27.2 Alar flare types and excision patterns. Flare is classified according to where the most lateral point along the alar rim occurs relative to the level of the sill–base junction on basal view. In Type 1 flare, the lateral-most point (Point 1) on the rim is below the sill–base junction such that a straight line from sill–base junction to the lateral-most point on the ala will slant inferiorly. In Type 2 flare, this line is horizontal. In Type 3 flare, the line slants superiorly from sill–base junction to lateral-most point (Point 1) along the alar rim. In Type 4, it is a combination of Type 3 flare with a widened nasal base. Alar flare reduction marking is performed by marking the lateral-most point at the alar–facial groove (Point 1) followed by marking the sill–base junction (Point 2). A point 2 mm inferior to the sill–base junction is then marked (Point 3). A curved line in the alar–facial groove is then drawn from Point 1 to Point 3 (Line 1). Finally, an additional curved line is drawn along the ala from Point 1 to Point 3 creating a final ellipse. The width of the ellipse increases with the degree of alar flare (1 through 3). It is essential to preserve 2 mm of the vertical cutaneous portion of the sill to avoid notching and maximize the aesthetic outcome. For Type 4, alar flare reduction with a nostril sill excision is performed. Starting from Point 2, an elliptical excision of the nasal sill is performed in the sagittal plane to narrow the base width. Once again, 2 mm of the vertical cutaneous portion of the sill is preserved to avoid notching and maximize the aesthetic outcome.

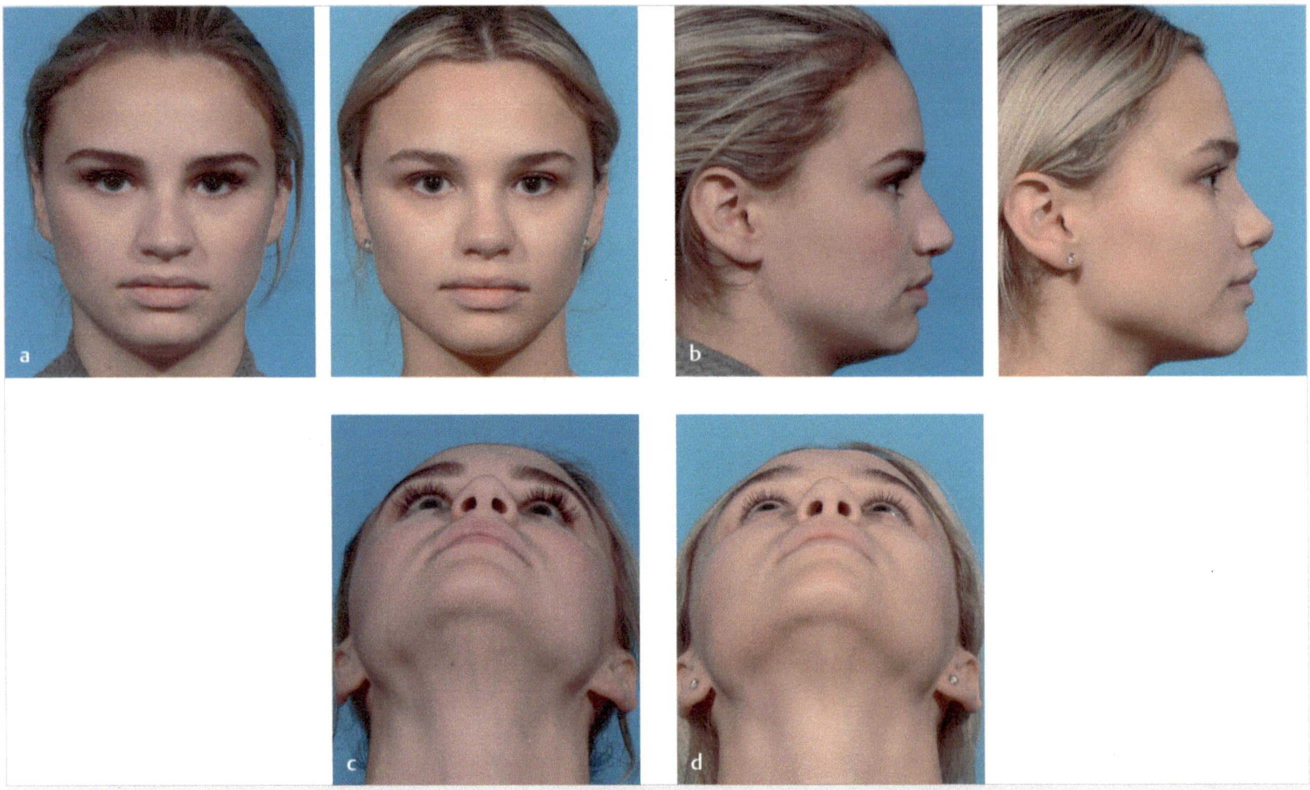

Fig. 27.3 (a–d) Example of preoperative alar flaring (R – Type 2, L – Type 3) treated with alar flare reduction. Preoperative photos on the left, and 1-year postoperative photos on the right.

27.4 Case Example

Example of preoperative alar flaring (R – Type 2, L – Type 3) treated with alar flare reduction. Preoperative photos on the left, and 1-year postoperative photos on the right (▶ Fig. 27.3a–d).

27.5 Conclusion

Alar base surgery is a powerful technique in rhinoplasty. Preoperative and intraoperative evaluations are critical to making the appropriate decision for alar flare reduction. A systematic approach to marking alar flare and alar base reductions allows for consistent results.

Further Readings

Kridel RW, Castellano RD. A simplified approach to alar base reduction: a review of 124 patients over 20 years. Arch Facial Plast Surg. 2005; 7(2):81–93

Rohrich RJ, Ahmad J. A practical approach to rhinoplasty. Plast Reconstr Surg. 2016; 137(4):725e–746e

Rohrich RJ, Afrooz PN. Primary open rhinoplasty. Plast Reconstr Surg. 2019; 144(1): 102e–117e

Rohrich RJ, Malafa MM, Ahmad J, Basci DS. Managing alar flare in rhinoplasty. Plast Reconstr Surg. 2017; 140(5):910–919

28 Revision Rhinoplasty

Rod J. Rohrich, Jamil Ahmad, and Ira L. Savetsky

Abstract
Rhinoplasty remains one of the most challenging operations performed by plastic surgeons. The complexity lies in the ability to have a consistent and predictable aesthetic result. The unpredictability is mainly due to the interplay of manipulated internal structures and wound healing dynamics. In addition, setting realistic expectations with the patient is essential in achieving high postoperative patient satisfaction. An open rhinoplasty approach enables an accurate and in-depth evaluation and intervention. We provide a detailed analysis and discussion on why primary rhinoplasty fails and the surgical approach to prevent these failures.

Keywords: Rhinoplasty, revision rhinoplasty, open rhinoplasty, secondary rhinoplasty, spreader flaps, spreader grafts, alar contour grafts, septal extension graft, columellar strut graft

Key Points

- A comprehensive and systematic nasofacial analysis is critical in establishing goals and formulating a precise surgical plan for aesthetic nasal surgery.
- Setting realistic expectations with the patient is essential for achieving high postoperative patient satisfaction.
- Using structural support and closing dead space will result in a more consistent, predictable result while minimizing primary rhinoplasty failures.
- An open rhinoplasty approach enables an accurate and in-depth evaluation and intervention.

28.1 Preoperative Planning

28.1.1 Nasal History and Physical Examination

- Have the patients list their top three nasal aesthetic and/or function concerns and record them precisely.
- Note any prior nasal trauma and operations including rhinoplasty, septal reconstruction/septoplasty, and sinus surgery and, when possible, prior operative reports should be reviewed.
- An internal nasal examination should include assessment of the septum, turbinates, and internal and external valves.
- Palpate the nose to assess the length of the nasal bones and strength of the lower lateral cartilages.

28.1.2 Nasofacial Proportions and Systematic Nasal Analysis: "10–7–5" Nasal Analysis (▶ Table 28.1)

- The front view evaluation should include 10 key areas: Facial proportions, skin type/skin thickness, symmetry/nasal deviation, bony vault width, midvault asymmetry, dorsal aesthetic lines, tip shape/tip-defining points, alar rims/base, infratip lobular projection, and periapical hypoplasia/upper lip length.
- The profile view includes 7 areas: Radix height and position, dorsal convexity, nasal length, tip projection, tip rotation, alar–columellar relationship, and chin projection.
- Use the base view to assess 5 areas: Nasal projection, nostril shape/symmetry, columella symmetry/width, alar base width, and alar rim flaring.

28.2 Operative Steps

- We have shown the safety of ignoring prior incisions in the columella and basing the new scar location based on where the surgeon feels is ideal (Unger et al. 2013.).
- The nose should be approached using an open technique as described in *Chapter 15 Open Rhinoplasty Finesse*. It is critical that dissection remains deep to the scar tissue.
- See **Video 28.1.**

28.2.1 Nasal Dorsum and Midvault

- Deformities of the nasal dorsum are commonly found in revision rhinoplasty and can not only lead to irregularities and disruption of the dorsal aesthetic lines but also lead to compromise of the internal nasal valve.
- Inadequate support can lead to midvault collapse resulting in an aesthetically displeasing inverted-V deformity. Maximal control with a graduated approach of the dorsum is critical.
- Use of the senior author's "4Rs" component dorsal hump reduction is recommended when addressing this area: (1) **R**elease the upper lateral cartilages from the septum, (2) incrementally **R**esect the septum proper, (3) **R**asp the bony dorsum, and (4) **R**estore the dorsal aesthetic lines. Deformities of the nasal dorsum are commonly found and can lead to irregularities and disruption of the dorsal aesthetic lines (▶ Fig. 28.1).
- When sufficient upper lateral cartilage volume is present, restoration of the dorsal aesthetic lines is predictably achieved by using the senior author's four-step approach for autospreader grafts: (1) pull-twist-turn, (2) horizontal mattress sutures, (3) percutaneous osteotomies, and (4) simple interrupted sutures.
- Spreader grafts should be used selectively when additional midvault infrastructure is needed (▶ Fig. 28.2a–c).
- External nasal valve compromise is also commonly encountered in revision rhinoplasty. This area is particularly prone to late changes due to wound contraction and scarring of the soft triangles and the lack of structural support in this region.
- Alar collapse due to misplaced alar grafts causing obstruction is commonly encountered.
- Removal of obstructing alar grafts and replacement with appropriate structural support will open the external nasal valve and restore air flow.

Table 28.1 Evidence-based nasal analysis: The 10–7-5 method

Nasal view	Analysis
Frontal	
1. Facial proportions	Height (thirds), width (fifths), symmetry
2. Skin type/quality	Fitzpatrick type, thin or thick, sebaceous
3. Symmetry/nasal deviation	Midline, dorsal deviation, C-, reverse C-, or S-shaped deviation
4. Dorsal aesthetic lines	Straight, symmetric or asymmetric, well- or ill-defined, narrow or wide
5. Bony vault	Narrow or wide, asymmetric, short or long nasal bones
6. Midvault	Narrow or wide, collapse, inverted-V, saddle deformity
7. Nasal tip	Ideal/bulbous/boxy/pinched, supratip, tip-defining points, infratip lobule
8. Alar rims	Gull-shaped, facets, notching, retraction
9. Alar base	Width
10. Upper lip	Long or short, dynamic depressor septi, upper lip crease
Lateral	
1. Nasofrontal angle and radix	Acute or obtuse, high or low radix, prominent or low nasion
2. Nasal length, dorsum and supratip	Length: long or short Dorsum: smooth, hump, scooped out Supratip: break, fullness, pollybeak, overprojected or underprojected
3. Tip projection	Overprojected or underprojected
4. Tip rotation	Overrotated or underrotated
5. Alar–columellar relationship	Hanging or retracted ala, hanging or retracted columella Maxillary or soft tissue deficiency
6. Periapical hypoplasia	Maxillary or soft tissue deficiency
7. Lip–chin relationship	Normal, overprojected or underprojected chin
Basal	
1. Nasal projection	Overprojected or underprojected, well- or ill-defined tip-defining points, columellar-to-lobule ratio
2. Nostril	Symmetry, long/narrow or short/wide nostril, nostril–tip ratio, concave or convex ala
3. Columella	Caudal septal deviation, flaring of medial crura
4. Alar base	Width
5. Alar flaring	

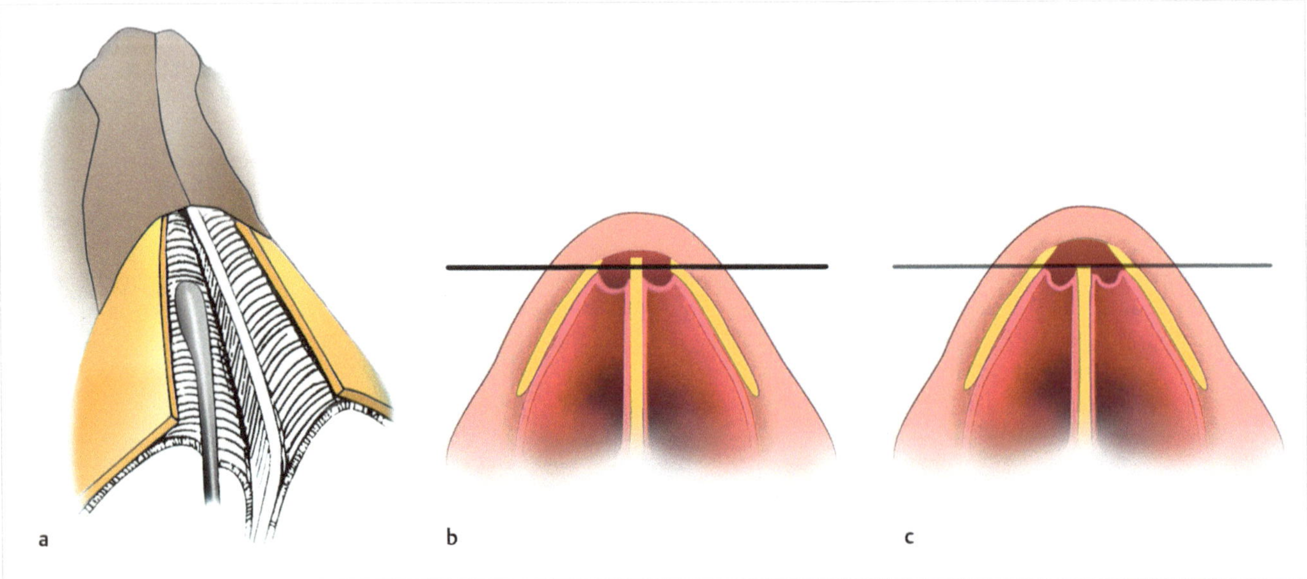

Fig. 28.1 (a–c) Component dorsum. Surgical approach to the dorsum: separation of the upper lateral cartilages from the septum. The mucoperichondrium of the dorsal septum is elevated, from caudal to cephalad, until the elevator reaches the nasal bones. (Reproduced with permission from Rohrich R, Ahmad J, eds. The Dallas Rhinoplasty and Dallas Cosmetic Surgery Dissection Guide. 1st ed. Thieme; 2018.)

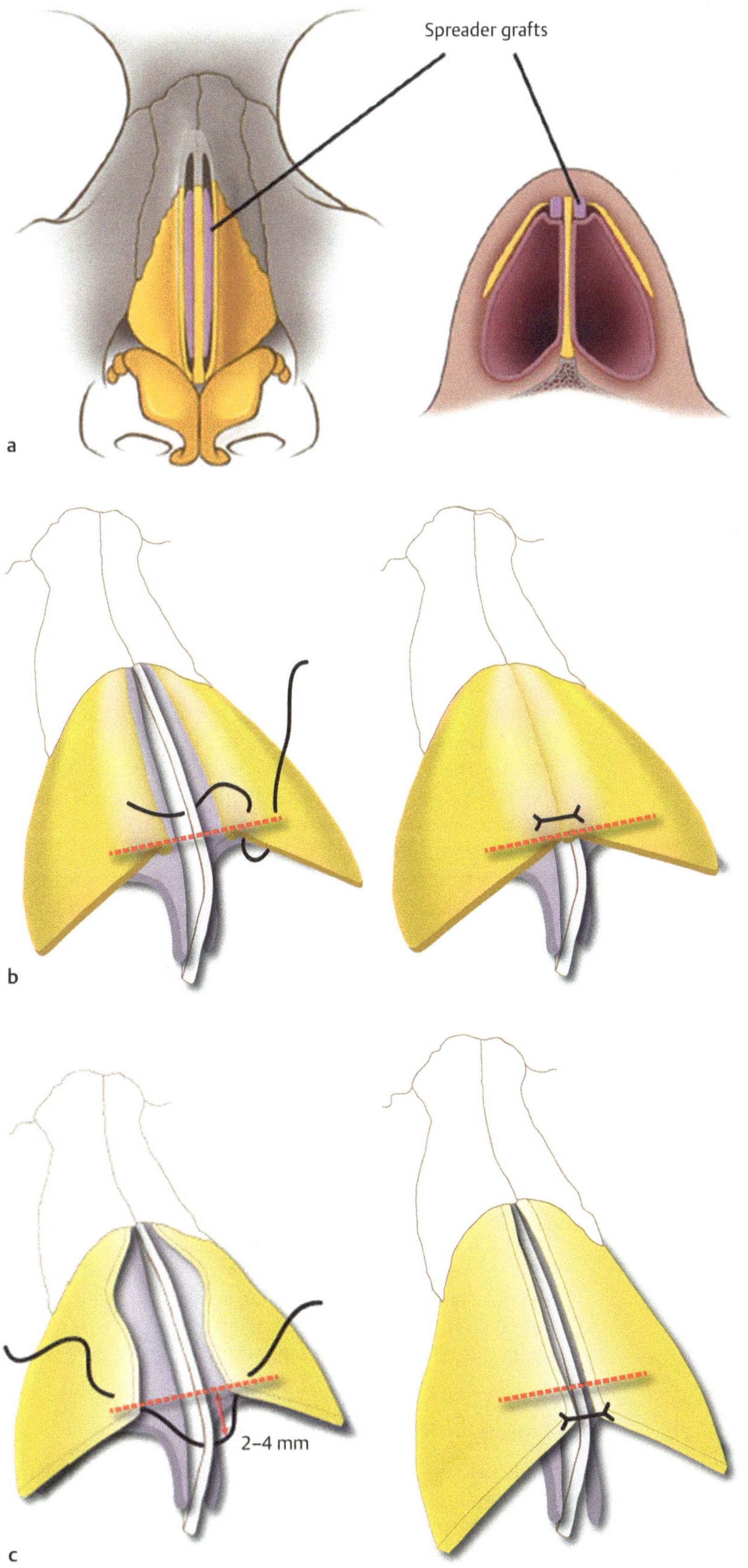

Fig. 28.2 **(a)** Spreader grafts. Reconstitution of the dorsum: spreader grafts. Spreader grafts may be positioned at or above the plane of the dorsal septum to be visible for aesthetic indications or below it as invisible grafts for purely functional indications. (Reproduced with permission from Rohrich R, Ahmad J, eds. Secondary Rhinoplasty by the Global Masters. 1st ed. Thieme; 2016.)
(b) Spreader flaps. Reconstitution of the dorsum: Type 3: midvault restoration with spreader flap modification. The 5–0 PDS sutures are placed caudal to the upper edge of the upper lateral cartilages, thereby infolding the superior edge of the upper lateral cartilages. This serves a spreader-type function. This technique should be employed when attempting to widen the midvault. **(c)** Upper lateral cartilage tension spanning sutures. (Reproduced with permission from Rohrich R, Adams W, Ahmad J, et al, eds. Dallas Rhinoplasty: Nasal Surgery by the Masters. 3rd ed. Thieme; 2014.)

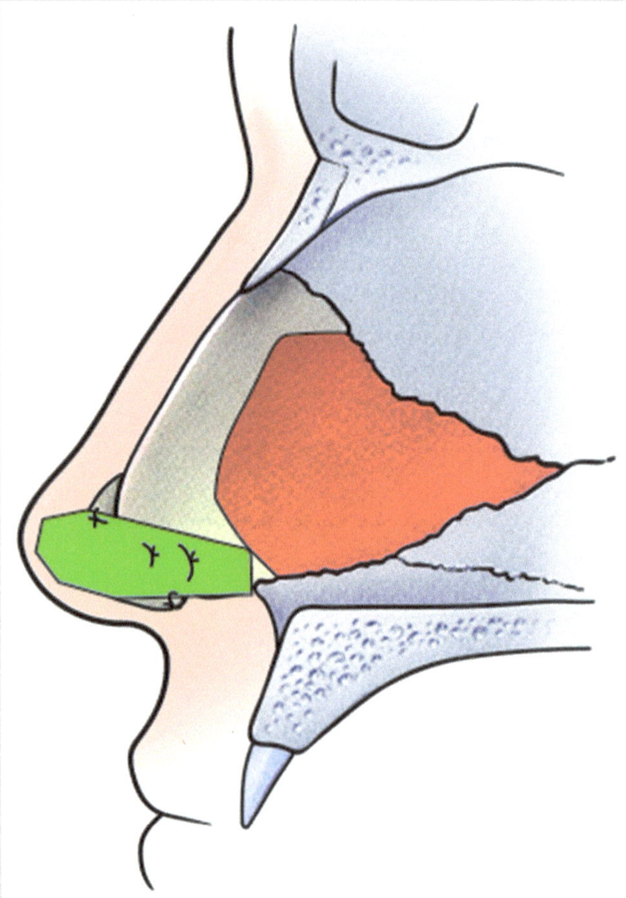

Fig. 28.3 Septal extension graft four-step suture technique.

- Proper and routine placement of extended alar contour grafts in primary rhinoplasty is advocated as it helps to prevent external nasal valve collapse secondarily.

28.2.2 Wound Healing

- The unpredictability of wound healing in rhinoplasty is often the key determinant of a good versus a bad result.
- The creation of dead space in rhinoplasty creates an environment for erratic soft tissue contraction.
- To minimize the effect of scar tissue formation, surgical technique with precise and minimal dissection while maintaining the correct plane of dissection is critical.
- The minimal amount of internal structure resection should be performed to obtain the desired result.
- Meticulous hemostasis and the use of tranexamic acid have been transformational in the senior author's practice.

28.2.3 Structural Support

- Soft tissue contraction is exacerbated by the lack of structural support, which is often seen in revision rhinoplasty.
- The loss of tip projection after a primary rhinoplasty is not uncommon and is only worsened with zero-to-minimal structural support.

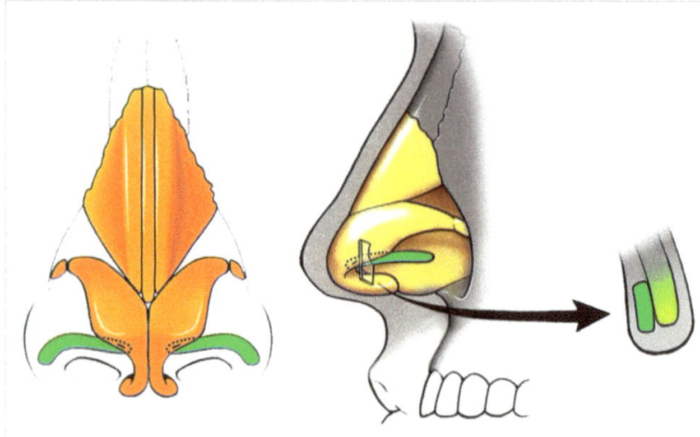

Fig. 28.4 The extended alar contour graft has been used to prevent notching of the anterior alar rim where the lateral crus begins to diverge from the alar rim as it courses to the pyriform aperture. (Reproduced with permission from Rohrich R, Adams W, Ahmad J, et al, eds. Dallas Rhinoplasty: Nasal Surgery by the Masters. 3rd ed. Thieme; 2014.)

- It is the senior author's preference to use a septal extension graft to control both tip rotation and projection.
- The septal extension graft is keel-shaped to mimic the inferior margin of the middle crura.
- It is placed onto the anterior septal angle as a "fixed-floating" graft with extension beyond the anterior septal angle into the interdomal space with the most caudal and inferior portion of the graft placed on the cephalic border of the medial crus at the columellar–lobular angle.
- A four-step suture technique is performed (▶ Fig. 28.3): (1) Body fixation horizontal mattress suture, (2) superior stabilization suture, (3) inferior stabilization suture, and (4) body stabilization horizontal mattress suture.
- Alar rim deformities are one of the more common problems encountered in revision rhinoplasty. They range from alar notching to retraction, collapse, and asymmetry. These deformities have been well characterized by the alar–columellar relationship.
- This area is particularly prone to late changes due to wound contraction and scarring of the soft triangles and the lack of structural support in this region.
- It is the senior author's preference to use an extended alar contour graft routinely in primary rhinoplasty given its clear improvement on alar aesthetics (▶ Fig. 28.4).
- If there is any residual notching or asymmetry after placement of the extended alar contour graft, a retrograde or dual alar contour graft is placed through a separate stab incision below the extended alar contour graft (▶ Fig. 28.5).

28.2.4 Dead Space Closure

- Obliteration of dead space is a key component in rhinoplasty as it minimizes soft tissue contraction resulting in a more predictable outcome.
- Dead space closure is performed in a systematic five-step manner: (1) Infratip lobule butterfly graft, (2) membranous septum closure, (3) septal splints, (4) external splint, and

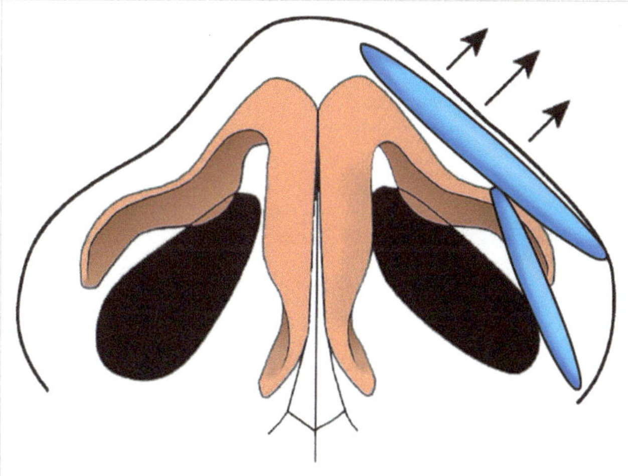

Fig. 28.5 Retrograde or dual alar contour graft.

(5) soft tissue triangle Surgicel® impregnated with mupirocin application.

- The infratip lobule butterfly graft is used to obliterate the dead space above the lower lateral cartilage after the cephalic margin of the lower lateral cartilage is removed. This minimizes scarring and retraction of the alar rim. It is a soft graft, typically obtained from the cephalic trim cartilage. This graft also provides support and continuity between the tip and alar lobule, which is otherwise prone to collapse and contour irregularities (▸ Fig. 28.6).
- Closure of the membranous septum after septal reconstruction and closure around the septal extension graft are important in minimizing fluid around the septum and septal extension graft.
- Closure also eliminates the soft tissue memory caused by the deviated septum and further stabilizes the septal extension graft. This is performed using horizontal absorbable mattress sutures. It is also the senior author's preference to leave a posterior unilateral drainage port to allow any fluid to egress easily.
- To further close the membranous septum dead space, mupirocin-coated intranasal Doyle open lumen splints are then placed and sutured in place.
- When needed, external splints, which are used as a soft silicone bolster, provide external soft tissue support and control soft tissue memory of the ala and nasal sidewalls.
- The soft tissue triangle is never sutured closed given the high risk of poor wound healing and subsequent alar notching and retraction. Therefore, Surgicel® impregnated with mupirocin is placed inside the soft tissue triangle to eliminate dead space and support this region. This will autocoagulate in 3 to 5 days.

28.3 Postoperative Care

- When sleeping, keep your head elevated on two pillows for the first 7 days after surgery.
- During the day for the first 72 hours after surgery, apply crushed ice in an ice bag or Swiss eye pads to minimize swelling and bruising. Do not put pressure on the nasal splint.
- It is normal to continue to swell after the first 48 hours. Swelling reaches its peak at 48 to 72 hours.

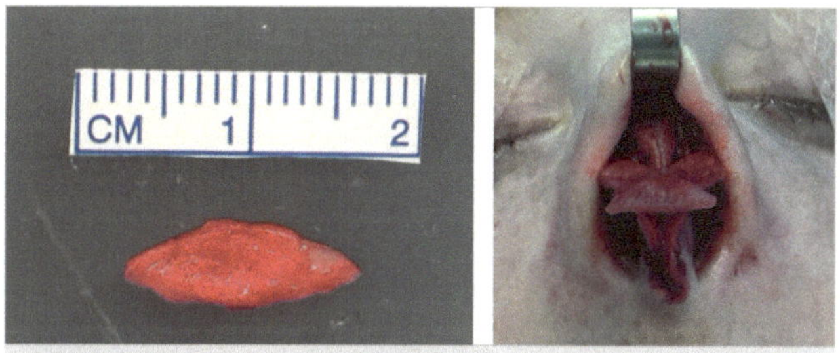

Fig. 28.6 Infratip lobule butterfly graft.

- If you have pain, take the pain medication every 4 to 6 hours.
- If you feel anxious, take the anti-anxiety medication (Xanax) every 8 hours for the first 24 to 48 hours.
- Following surgery begin with a light diet, liquids only. The next day you can begin a soft, regular diet, but for 2 weeks avoid foods that require excessive lip movement.
- You will probably have a bloody nasal discharge for 3 to 4 days and may change the drip pad under your nose as often as needed. Do not rub or blot your nose, as this will tend to irritate it.
- To prevent bleeding, do not sniff or blow your nose for the first 4 weeks after surgery. Try not to sneeze, but if you do, sneeze through your mouth.
- While the nasal splint is on, you may have your hair washed in beauty salon fashion. Take care to prevent the nasal splint from getting wet.
- Keep the inside edges of your nostrils and any stitches clean by using a Q-tip saturated with hydrogen peroxide followed by a thin coating of Polysporin, which is an over-the-counter antibiotic ointment. This is done in a circular manner. Please do this at least four to five times per day.
- Avoid hitting or getting bumped in your nose for 4 weeks after surgery.
- After the splint is removed, do not wear glasses or allow anything else to rest on your nose for 4 weeks.
- Protect the incision line from sun exposure for 12 months.
- The nasal splint will be removed in 6 to 7 days after surgery.
- After your sutures are removed and the internal/external splints are removed, it is recommended that you use two squirts of a saline solution (salt water), in each nostril, six to eight times daily, to gently remove crusty formation from inside your nose.
- You can use nasal spray (Afrin) intermittently *only* after the first week postoperatively for improved nasal breathing, and then stop it after 5 to 7 days.
- If you experience increased nasal bleeding with bright red blood (with a need to change nasal pad every 30–40 minutes), notify you doctor immediately. You should sit up and apply pressure to the end of your nose for 15 minutes and you can use Afrin spray to stop the oozing in the interim. Bleeding usually stops with these maneuvers.

28.4 Case Example

A 41-year-old woman presented to the senior author (Rod J. Rohrich) for secondary rhinoplasty. (Left) The patient had persistent nasal deviation with concavity of the left middle third

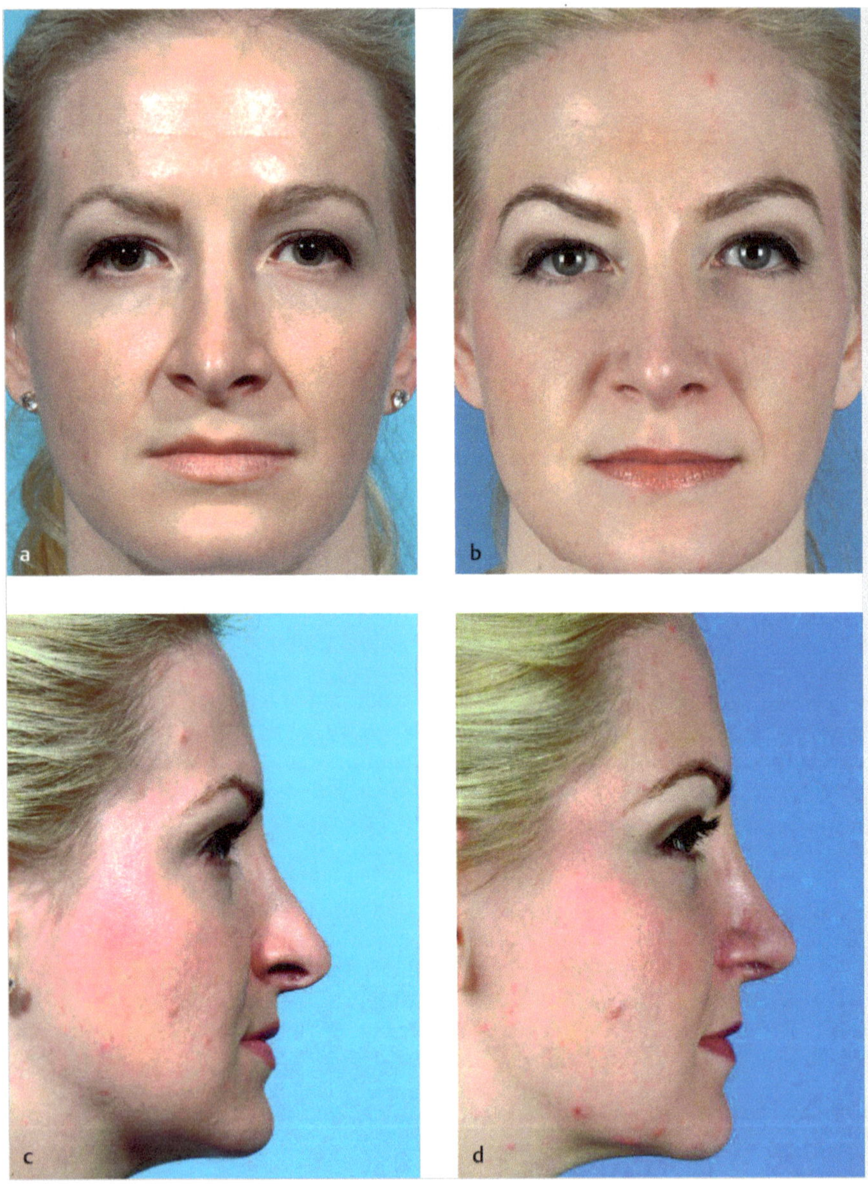

Fig. 28.7 (a–d) A 41-year-old woman presented to the senior author (Rod J. Rohrich) for secondary rhinoplasty. (Left) The patient had persistent nasal deviation with concavity of the left middle third and distorted dorsal aesthetic lines. In addition, she suffered from residual dorsal hump, a narrow tip, a wide nasal base, an excessive infratip lobule, and alar flaring. (Right) The patient is shown at her 12-month follow-up. Note correction of the bony deviation and re-establishment of the dorsal aesthetic lines. Hump removal allows for a slightly concave dorsum, although it does lack a supratip break. The concavity of the left middle third has been corrected and the alar base reduced to approximate the intercanthal distance. Also, note the infratip lobule, as this region is much improved, and her alar flaring is corrected.

and distorted dorsal aesthetic lines. In addition, she suffered from residual dorsal hump, a narrow tip, a wide nasal base, an excessive infratip lobule, and alar flaring. (Right) The patient is shown at her 12-month follow-up. Note correction of the bony deviation and re-establishment of the dorsal aesthetic lines. Hump removal allows for a slightly concave dorsum, although it does lack a supratip break. The concavity of the left middle third has been corrected and the alar base reduced to approximate the intercanthal distance. Also, note the infratip lobule, as this region is much improved, and her alar flaring is corrected (▶ Fig. 28.7a–d). Preoperative oblique and basal views (Left), and (Right) postoperative views at 12-month follow-up are shown (▶ Fig. 28.8a–d).

28.5 Conclusion

The complex interplay between the dead space, lack of structural support, soft tissue memory, and wound healing can make rhinoplasty outcomes unpredictable.

By carefully selecting our patients, performing precise preoperative nasofacial analysis, using structural support, and

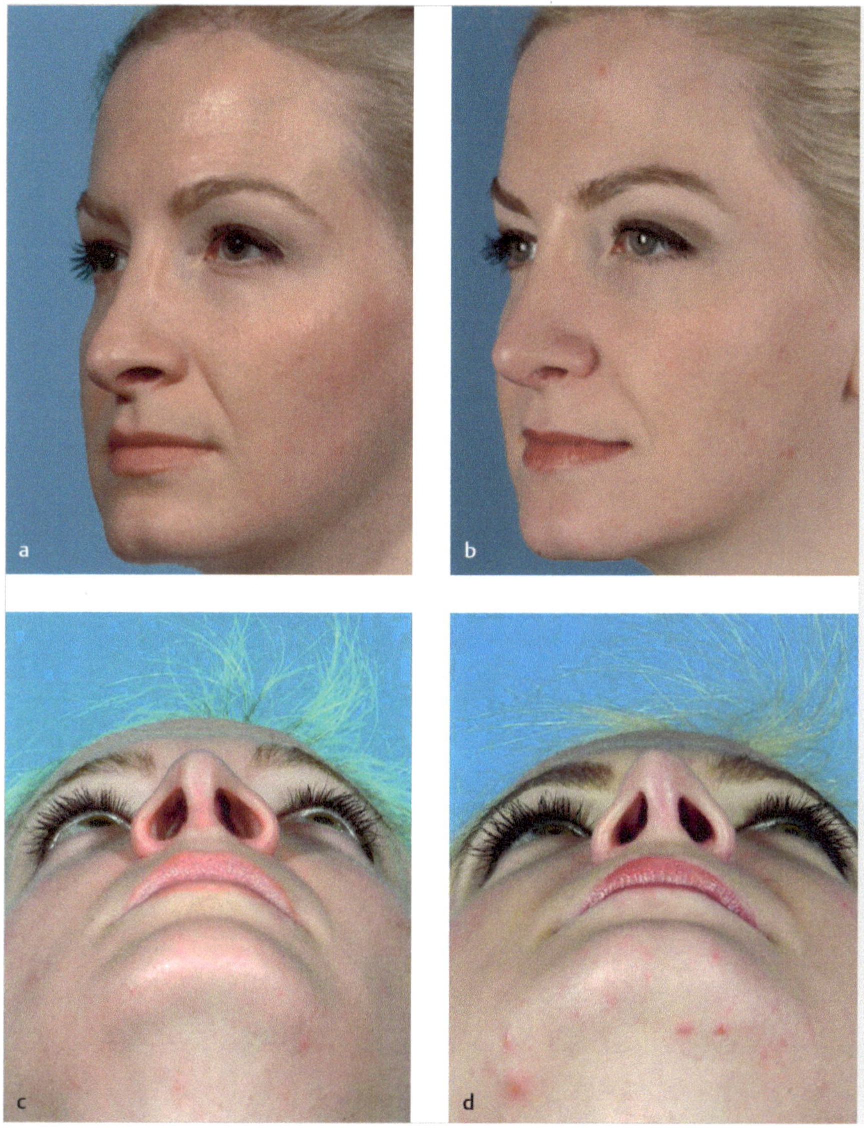

Fig. 28.8 (a–d) Oblique and basal views of the patient shown in ▶ Fig. 28.7. (Left) Preoperative views. (Right) Postoperative views at 12-month follow-up.

closing dead space, the results will be more consistent, predictable, functional, and aesthetic, while minimizing rhinoplasty failures.

Further Readings

Lehrman CR, Lee MR, Ramanadham S, Rohrich RJ. Digital imaging in secondary rhinoplasty. Plast Reconstr Surg. 2016; 137(6):950e–953e

Mohan R, Shanmuga Krishnan RR, Rohrich RJ. Role of fresh frozen cartilage in revision rhinoplasty. Plast Reconstr Surg. 2019; 144(3):614–622

Rohrich RJ, Dauwe PB, Pulikkottil BJ, Pezeshk RA. The importance of the anterior septal angle in the open dorsal approach to rhinoplasty. Plast Reconstr Surg. 2017; 139(3): 604–612

Rohrich RJ, Lee MR. External approach for secondary rhinoplasty: advances over the past 25 years. Plast Reconstr Surg. 2013; 131(2):404–416

Unger JG, Roostaeian J, Cheng DH, et al. The open approach in secondary rhinoplasty: choosing an incision regardless of prior placement. Plast Reconstr Surg. 2013; 132(4):780–786

Part III

Periorbital Rejuvenation

III

29 Periorbital Rejuvenation Consultation

Rod J. Rohrich and Yash J. Avashia

Abstract
Periorbital rejuvenation consultation requires a detailed preoperative analysis to identify all aspects that may be contributing to periorbital aging. The surgeon should have a thorough understanding of periorbital anatomy in order to properly assess the patient. The periorbital examination should be approached in a top-down systematic method. Basic preoperative medical history and a focused ophthalmologic history should be obtained.

Keywords: Periorbital, eye examination, blepharoplasty, brow ptosis, facial rejuvenation

Key Points

- The periorbital region is a critical component of facial rejuvenation.
- A detailed preoperative analysis is critical to identifying all aspects contributing to periorbital aging.
- Thorough preoperative analysis will also help identify patients with anatomic predisposition to lower eyelid malposition or dry eyes.

29.1 Preoperative Steps

- The first step in the consultation is to obtained a through medical history that includes the following:
  - History of hypertension, cardiac disease, bleeding or clotting disorders, diabetes, thyroid dysfunction, and autoimmune disease.
- Once the medical history has been obtained, the surgeon should obtain a focused ophthalmologic history including the following:
  - When was the last time the patient had his or her visual acuity checked?
  - Does he or she use any corrective lenses or glasses?
  - Any prior history of facial or periorbital trauma, glaucoma, excess tearing and/or dry eyes, prior ophthalmologic/periorbital surgery, or LASIK or refractive surgery?
- A systematic approach should be used for the periorbital physical examination:
  - The presence of the protective Bell's phenomenon is documented, which is the upward movement of the globe with eye closure.
  - Forehead and brow examination:
    - Brow and forehead should be part of a comprehensive periorbital examination.
    - Presence of hyperactive frontalis and brow elevation should be noted at baseline. The patient should be asked to relax the forehead in order to determine the resting brow level.
    - In females, the eyebrow should be 1 cm above the supraorbital rim, and slightly peaked at the lateral third. The eyebrow may be at the level of the supraorbital rim in males without peaking laterally.
    - Forehead length should be documented. The normal length is 6 cm.
    - Fat atrophy in the supraorbital region particularly in the central, middle, and lateral temporal fat compartments should be documented.
  - Skeletal support:
    - The underlying skeletal support of the periorbita should be examined. This includes the orbital rim, zygomatic prominence at the malar eminence, and temporal bone of the forehead.
    - Facial aging includes a component of bone resorption, which may also contribute to some of the findings in periorbital aging.
  - Upper eyelid skin quality and quantity (▶ Fig. 29.1):
    - The upper eyelid is examined with the eyebrows at resting neutral position.
    - Dermatochalasis is the extent of excess upper eyelid skin.
    - Supratarsal fold location should be about 6 to 7 mm above the lash line. An elevation in this with eyelid ptosis is indicative of levator dehiscence.
  - Upper eyelid position:
    - The upper eyelid position is determined relative to the superior limbus.
    - Marginal to reflex distance 1 is the measured distance from the upper eyelid to the corneal light reflex. The normal value is 4 mm. Values less than this indicate the degree of blepharoptosis.
  - Levator excursion:
    - This is the value given to the distance the upper eyelid moves from inferior to superior gaze.

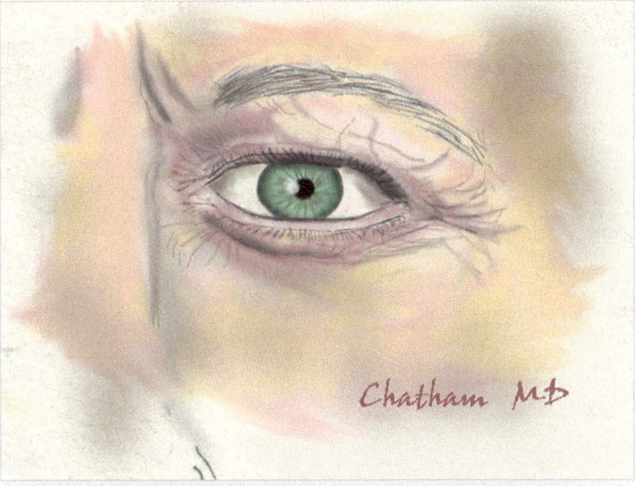

Fig. 29.1 Upper eyelid demonstrating dermatochalasis of the skin with lateral fullness. (Reproduced with permission from Fedok F, Carniol P, eds. Minimally Invasive and Office-Based Procedures in Facial Plastic Surgery. 1st ed. Thieme; 2013.)

- Values for normal function are between 10 and 15 mm, moderate function is 5 to 10 mm, and poor function is 0 to 5 mm.
- ○ Lower eyelid position (▶ Fig. 29.2):
  - The lower eyelid should sit at the inferior corneo-scleral junction. Any scleral show between these points indicates lower eyelid ptosis secondary to one of two common causes: lateral canthal laxity or lower eyelid horizontal excess.

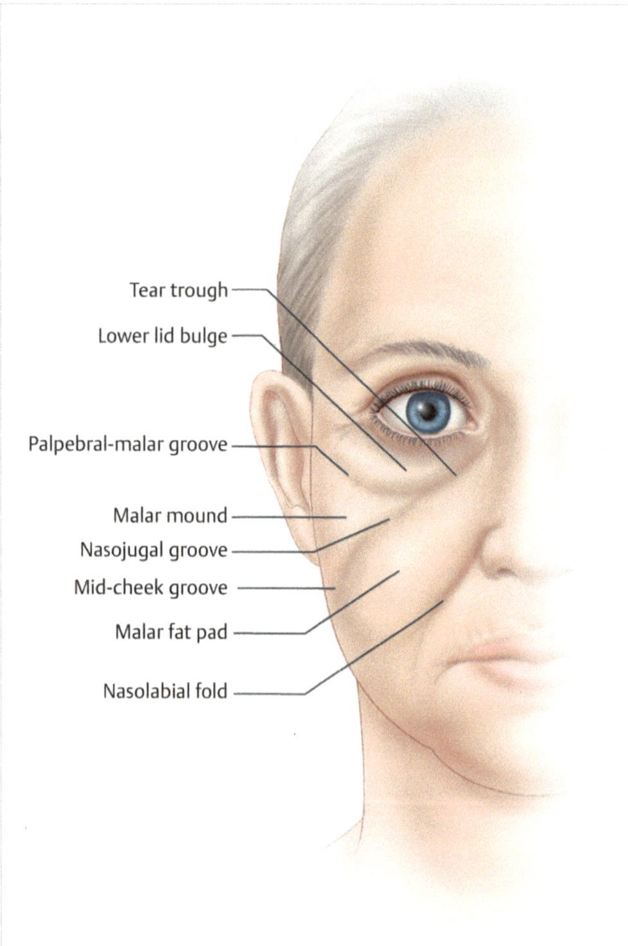

Fig. 29.2 Periorbital aging demonstrating lower eyelid fat compartment herniation, tear trough deformity, and nasojugal folds. (Reproduced with permission from Codner M, McCord C, eds. Eyelid & Periorbital Surgery. 2nd ed. Thieme; 2016.)

  - The lower eyelids should be examined for protuberant fat from the three compartments along with the presence of a tear trough deformity.
- ○ Lateral canthal position (▶ Fig. 29.3a–c):
  - The lateral canthus should be 2 mm superior to the medial canthus with a positive tilt. Lack of a positive tilt indicates lateral canthal laxity.
  - The lateral canthal angle should be sharp. A blunted angle indicates lateral canthal laxity or a history of prior surgery.
- ○ Anterior distraction:
  - The lower eyelid is distracted anteriorly to the globe. A distraction of >6 mm indicates horizontal excess, best managed with a lateral tarsal strip canthoplasty.
- ○ Snapback test:
  - This test evaluates the lower eyelid tone. The lower eyelid is pulled inferiorly and then allowed to return to normal position without the blinking mechanism. A sluggish return to normal indicates poor tone.
- ○ Malar eminence vector (▶ Fig. 29.4):
  - A critical part of the examination is determining whether the patient has a positive or negative vector.
  - A positive vector is demonstrated when the malar eminence is anterior to the corneal surface of the globe on lateral view.
  - A negative vector is demonstrated when the malar eminence is posterior to the corneal surface of the globe.
  - Patients with a negative vector are at an increased risk for lower eyelid malposition after lower eyelid blepharoplasty.
- ○ Dry eye:
  - In patients with a history of dry eye, a Schirmer's test is performed.
  - Patients who demonstrate an abnormal Schirmer's test are referred for ophthalmologic evaluation.

29.2 Case Example

A 65-year-old female with the following findings on periorbital and facial assessment:

- Forehead: Forehead length is an appropriate 6 cm with the eyebrows at the level of supraorbital rim with central and supraorbital fat atrophy of the forehead region. Temporal hollowing is also present.
- Upper eyelid: Generalized atrophy of fat in the upper eyelids. Dermatochalasis is observed on examination.
- Lower eyelid: No inferior scleral show or dermatochalasis. She has a mild tear trough deformity medially.

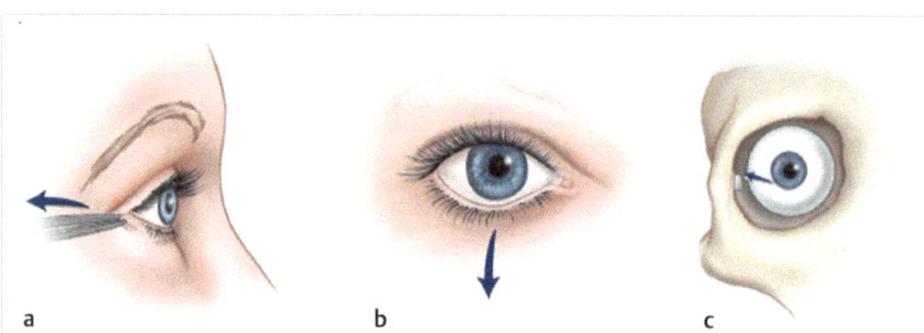

Fig. 29.3 (a–c) Periorbital examination demonstrating lower eyelid scleral show from horizontal eyelid excess, decreased muscle tone, or lateral canthal laxity. (Reproduced with permission from Codner M, McCord C, eds. Eyelid & Periorbital Surgery. 2nd ed. Thieme; 2016.)

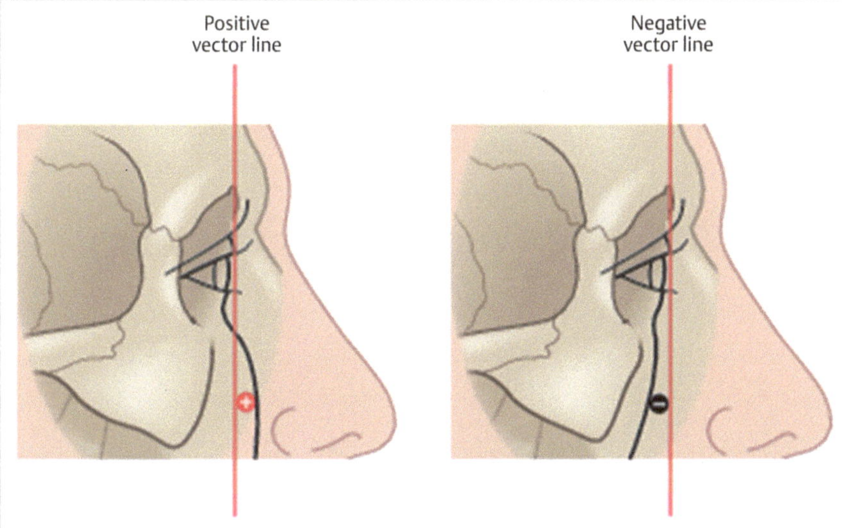

Fig. 29.4 When comparing the anterior surface of the globe to the anterior surface of the malar eminence, a "positive vector" is used to describe patients whose malar eminence is anterior to the globe surface. A "negative vector" is used to describe patients with the opposite. Vector analysis is important in determining lower eyelid support. Patients with negative vectors have inherently unsupported lower eyelids. These patients in particular require malar fat augmentation along with lateral canthopexy to support the lower eyelid and improve the eyelid position after lower eyelid blepharoplasty. (Reproduced with permission from Cohen M, Thaller S, eds. The Unfavorable Result in Plastic Surgery: Avoidance and Treatment. 4th ed. Thieme; 2018.)

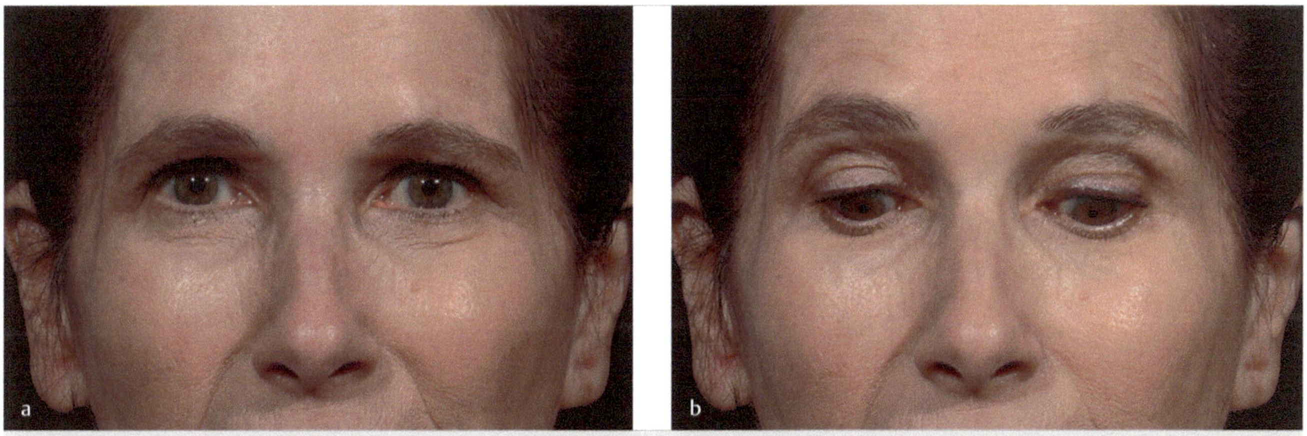

Fig. 29.5 (a, b) A 65-year-old female with the following findings on periorbital and facial assessment: Forehead: Forehead length is an appropriate 6 cm with the eyebrows at the level of supraorbital rim with central and supraorbital fat atrophy of the forehead region. Temporal hollowing is also present. Upper eyelid: Generalized atrophy of fat in the upper eyelids. Dermatochalasis is observed on examination. Lower eyelid: No inferior scleral show or dermatochalasis. She has a mild tear trough deformity medially. The periorbital surgical plan for this patient includes bilateral upper and lower eyelid blepharoplasty. During the upper blepharoplasty, a lateral orbicularis window will allow placement of a lateral retinacular canthopexy. Minimal nasal fat will be removed to avoid secondary excessive hollowing of the upper eyelid and creation of an A-frame deformity. During the lower blepharoplasty, a skin pinch will be performed for removal of the excess skin. Lateral retinacular canthopexy will be used to resuspend the lateral canthus and provide lower eyelid support to avoid eyelid malposition. Additionally, fat augmentation of the deep and superficial malar fat pads will provide additional support to the lower eyelid. Fractionated fat will be placed at the superior and inferior orbital rim. The orbital-malar retaining ligament will be bluntly released while placing fractionated fat at the inferior orbital rim to blend the eyelid–cheek junction. Fat augmentation of the central and supraorbital regions will provide improved aesthetic fullness to this region, and also support the brow placement slightly above the orbital rim.

The periorbital surgical plan for this patient includes bilateral upper and lower eyelid blepharoplasty. During the upper blepharoplasty, a lateral orbicularis window will allow placement of a lateral retinacular canthopexy. Minimal nasal fat will be removed to avoid secondary excessive hollowing of the upper eyelid and creation of an A-frame deformity. During the lower blepharoplasty, a skin pinch will be performed for removal of the excess skin. Lateral retinacular canthopexy will be used to resuspend the lateral canthus and provide lower eyelid support to avoid eyelid malposition. Additionally, fat augmentation of the deep and superficial malar fat pads will provide additional support to the lower eyelid. Fractionated fat will be placed at the superior and inferior orbital rim. The orbital-malar retaining ligament will be bluntly released while placing fractionated fat at the inferior orbital rim to blend the eyelid–cheek junction. Fat augmentation of the central and supraorbital regions will provide improved aesthetic fullness to this region, and also support the brow placement slightly above the orbital rim (▶ Fig. 29.5a, b).

29.3 Conclusion

A detailed understanding of the periorbital anatomy is a prerequisite to periorbital rejuvenation. The preoperative assessment will guide the options available for periorbital rejuvenation. Identifying the high-risk patient for dry eyes or lower eyelid malposition is a critical aspect of the preoperative assessment. These include negative vector, inferior scleral show from horizontal lower eyelid excess, and lateral canthal laxity.

See **Video 29.1**.

Further Readings

Codner MA, Kikkawa DO, Korn BS, Pacella SJ. Blepharoplasty and brow lift. Plast Reconstr Surg. 2010; 126(1):1e–17e

Friedland JA, Lalonde DH, Rohrich RJ. An evidence-based approach to blepharoplasty. Plast Reconstr Surg. 2010; 126(6):2222–2229

Trussler AP, Rohrich RJ. MOC-PSSM CME article: blepharoplasty. Plast Reconstr Surg. 2008; 121(1) Suppl:1–10

30 Eyelids: Upper Blepharoplasty

Rod J. Rohrich and Yash J. Avashia

Abstract

The upper eyelid blepharoplasty focuses on eyelid reshaping with skin reduction, lateral retinacular canthopexy, and fat compartment restoration. Detailed preoperative analysis coupled with well-executed operative technique help to achieve consistent results. The five steps presented by the senior author in upper eyelid blepharoplasty include skin excision, lateral orbicularis window, lateral retinacular canthopexy, fat restoration with fractionated fat, and differential skin closure.

Keywords: Blepharoplasty, dermatochalasis, canthopexy, fat augmentation, ptosis

Key Points

- Upper eyelid blepharoplasty should focus on upper eyelid shaping with skin reduction, lateral retinacular canthopexy, and fat compartment restoration.
- Fat grafting is an important aspect of restoring a youthful upper eyelid and eyebrow.

30.1 Preoperative Steps

- Patient evaluation:
  - Chapter 29 discusses at length the steps involved in a thorough patient evaluation and physical examination for periorbital rejuvenation.
- Upper eyelid blepharoplasty markings (▶ Fig. 30.1):
  - The patient is marked in the upright position with a neutral gaze.
  - The brow is relaxed and positioned appropriately at the level of the supraorbital rim prior to marking.
  - At the midpupillary line, an inferior mark is placed just inferior to the supratarsal fold. This is located 8 to 9 mm above the ciliary margin in women and 7 to 8 mm in men.
  - The superior mark is placed at least 10 mm from the lower edge of the eyebrow. A skin pinch test may also be performed to determine the superior point.
  - The medial mark should not extend beyond the medial canthus as this may cause webbing.
  - Two points are noted laterally: The lateral orbital skin crease and the lateral canthus.

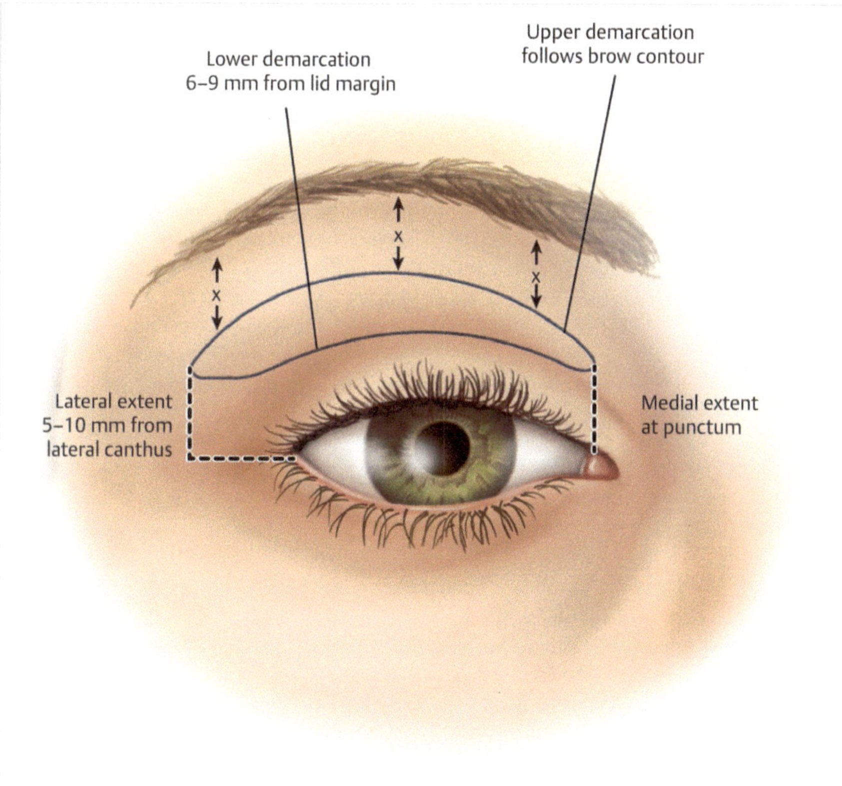

Fig. 30.1 Upper eyelid blepharoplasty marking. The lower incision is made roughly 1 mm below the supratarsal crease or at 6 to 7 mm from the eyelid margin. The superior incision follows the curve of the eyebrow, preserving a minimum of 10 mm of upper eyelid skin (X). The medial extent should not cross the punctum, nor should the lateral extent reach 5 to 10 mm beyond the lateral canthus.

 - The skin excision shape should include the four borders defined above and may be shaped in a lenticular or trapezoidal shape.
 - Laterally the inferior incision line should be 6 mm superior to the ciliary margin at the level of the lateral canthus before curving inferiorly to join the lateral orbital skin crease.

30.2 Operative Steps

See **Video 30.1.**

30.2.1 Incision

- Subcutaneous injection of 3 to 5 mL of 1% lidocaine with 1:100,000 epinephrine with a 27-guage, 1.5 inch needle is performed 7 minutes prior to incision.
- Using a #15 blade scalpel, the presurgical marking is incised beginning with the inferior incision.

30.2.2 Excision

- Using a fine pair of scissors, the skin is excised while preserving the underlying orbicularis muscle.
- A minimal portion of the lateral orbicularis muscle may be excised if there is lateral redundancy or laxity.

30.2.3 Lateral Retinacular Canthopexy (▶ Fig. 30.2)

- In combined upper and lower eyelid blepharoplasty, a lateral canthopexy is advised to provide lower eyelid support and prevent eyelid malposition. The lateral canthopexy is performed through the upper eyelid approach.
- Through an orbicularis window, a 5–0 Vicryl (Ethicon, Inc., Somerville, NJ) suture is used to grasp the lower lateral retinaculum and secure it to the periosteum of the inner upper orbital rim lateral to the lateral limbus. The suture is tensioned depending on the degree of lower eyelid laxity.

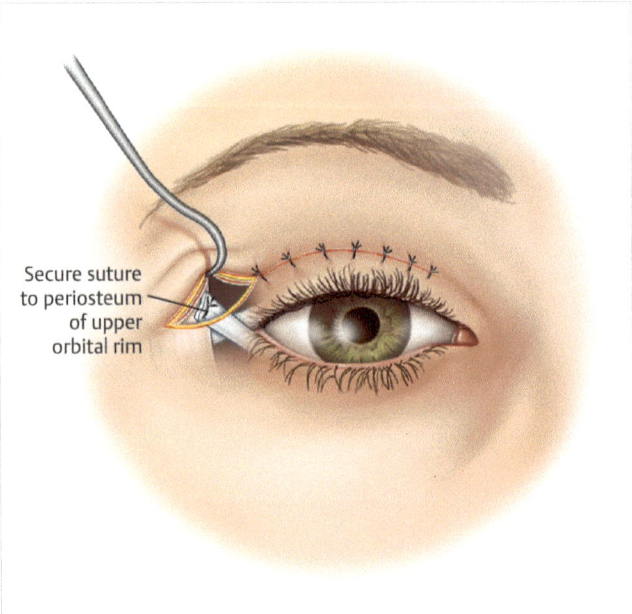

Fig. 30.2 Lower lateral retinacular canthopexy is a lower eyelid tightening technique performed from the upper eyelid blepharoplasty approach. A lateral orbicularis window allows a suborbicularis dissection down to the lateral canthus. Using a 5–0 Vicryl, the lower lateral retinaculum is secured to the superior orbital rim's inner border.

30.2.4 Closure

- Hemostasis is obtained with a pinpoint insulated cautery.
- To correct for the inherent difference in skin thickness between the infra-brow skin and lower eyelid skin, differential skin bite thickness is carried out during closure.
- A running subcuticular 6–0 Prolene (Ethicon) suture is placed, taking a deep path on the eyelid skin and a superficial path on the brow skin to compensate for the difference in skin thickness.
- This is followed by interrupted simple 6–0 nylon sutures placed in a similar differential manner, with superficial passes of the needle in the thicker brow skin and deeper bites in the thinner eyelid skin.

30.2.5 Volume Restoration

- Volume restoration of the upper orbit is performed using fractionated fat.
- The fat is harvested at the beginning of the case from the medial thighs and centrifuged at 2,250 rpm for 3 minutes as described previously.
- The fat is then passed between two syringes through a small Tulip Emulsifier (Tulip Medical Products, San Diego, California) 50 times.
- Then, using a 14-gauge needle, a small stab incision is made in the upper lateral brow and the fractionated fat is injected into a submuscular plane in the upper eyelid and just above the periosteum near the orbital rim using an 18-gauge, 1.5-inch blunt cannula (Micrins; Eriem Surgical, Lake Forest, IL).
- This step improves the volume of the upper eyelid, and the stem cells in the fractionated fat may enhance the skin quality, which has been noted by the senior author in clinical follow-up.

30.3 Postoperative Care

- Suture removal:
  - Suture removal is performed between postoperative day 5 and 7.
- Medications:
  - Daily eye lubrication with artificial tears is applied three times daily and at bedtime.
- Chemosis:
  - Combined ophthalmic antibiotic and steroid drops (Tobramycin and Dexamethasone—Tobradex®) should be used for 1 week.
    - One to two drops applied every 4 to 6 hours.
  - Continue aggressive eye lubrication with artificial tears.
    - Gel lubricants may be used at night for longer application.
    - In severe cases of chemosis, temporary tarsorrhaphy can be performed.

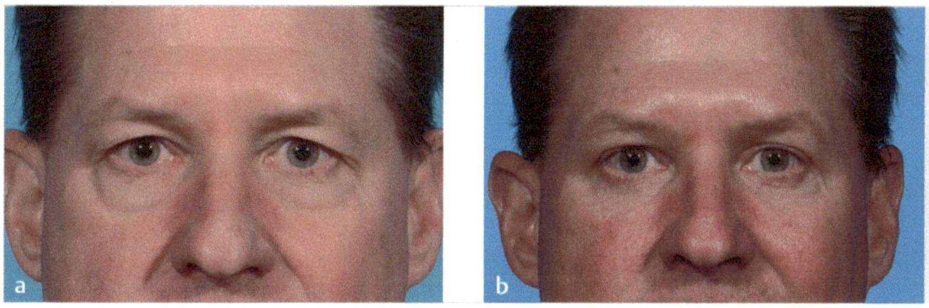

Fig. 30.3 (a, b) A 52-year-old male presenting for periorbital rejuvenation. Focused upper eyelid examination is notable for eyebrow asymmetry, upper eyelid dermatochalasis, minimal upper eyelid nasal fat pad, and lateral canthal laxity. Preoperative and 6-month postoperative examination images shown after four-lid blepharoplasty and facial fat grafting.

30.4 Case Example

A 52-year-old male presenting for periorbital rejuvenation. Focused upper eyelid examination is notable for eyebrow asymmetry, upper eyelid dermatochalasis, minimal upper eyelid nasal fat pad, and lateral canthal laxity. Preoperative and 6-month postoperative examination images shown after upper and lower blepharoplasty with facial fat grafting (▶ Fig. 30.3a, b).

30.5 Conclusion

The upper eyelid blepharoplasty seeks to correct upper eyelid skin excess, medial fat prominence, lateral orbicularis redundancy, and serves as an approach to tightening the lower eyelid via the lateral retinacular canthopexy. Preoperative assessment helps to tailor surgical technique. Postoperative chemosis should be proactively managed to avoid secondary ophthalmologic sequelae.

Further Readings

Rohrich RJ, Mahedia M, Shah N, Afrooz P, Vishvanath L, Gupta RK. Role of fractionated fat in blending the lid-cheek junction. Plast Reconstr Surg. 2018; 142(1): 56–65

Rohrich RJ, Villanueva NL, Afrooz PN. Refinements in upper blepharoplasty: the five-step technique. Plast Reconstr Surg. 2018; 141(5):1144–1146

Trussler AP, Rohrich RJ. MOC-PSSM CME article: blepharoplasty. Plast Reconstr Surg. 2008; 121(1) Suppl:1–10

31 Eyelids: Lower Blepharoplasty

Rod J. Rohrich and Ira L. Savetsky

Abstract
Lower eyelid blepharoplasty is one of the most complex procedures performed by plastic surgeons, and if done improperly may cause significant long-term sequelae. Here we provide a comprehensive and systematic approach to the lower eyelid, which is critical for lower eyelid blepharoplasty success.

Keywords: Blepharoplasty, fat augmentation, canthopexy, tear trough, fractionated fat, orbicularis retaining ligament

Key Points

- A comprehensive and systematic ophthalmic history and examination are critical in establishing goals and formulating a precise surgical plan for lower blepharoplasty.
- Lower eyelid malposition, scleral show, dry eyes, ectropion, and other complications can be prevented with a thorough understanding of periorbital anatomy and precise surgical planning and execution.

31.1 Preoperative Planning

31.1.1 Focused Ophthalmic History

- A thorough medical history and focused ophthalmologic history must be obtained. Please refer to Chapter 29.

31.1.2 Focused Ophthalmic Examination

- Evaluation should include facial proportions, skin type, skin thickness, skin excess, snapback, palpebral fissure size/shape, fat herniation, tear trough, canthal position, extraocular muscle function, Bell's phenomenon, levator function, margin reflex distance, brow and eyelid ptosis, and globe position relative to malar prominence.
- Greater than 6 mm anterior distraction indicates significant skin laxity.
- Lateral canthal tilt is typically 2 mm superior to the medial canthal position (positive canthal tilt).
- Posterior displacement of the orbital rim in relation to the anterior portion of the globe is a negative vector and must be identified in the preoperative consultation.
- Malar anatomy should be evaluated for tear trough deformities or prominent nasojugal folds, which may guide lower eyelid operative plans.

31.1.3 Standardized Photography and Digital Imaging

- Standardized photographs including frontal, lateral, and oblique should be obtained for every patient.
- Additional dynamic views are recommended.

31.1.4 Preoperative Markings

- Markings are performed in the upright position in neutral gaze.
- Areas of volume deflation, fat excess, and the tear trough should be marked.
- Periorbital fine lines should be marked as these may guide incision placement.

31.2 Operative Approach

See **Video 31.1.**

31.2.1 Five-Step Lower Blepharoplasty Technique

- *Step 1: Deep malar fat compartment augmentation:* Fat is injected into the deep malar space from the alar base as an entry point using a 2-mm blunt single side-hole cannula approximately one fingerbreadth below the orbital rim correcting malar deflation (▶ Fig. 31.1).
- *Step 2: Transconjunctival removal of lower eyelid fat (if indicated):* Only a small amount of fat is removed, proceeding from medial to lateral in most cases. In general, the amount of

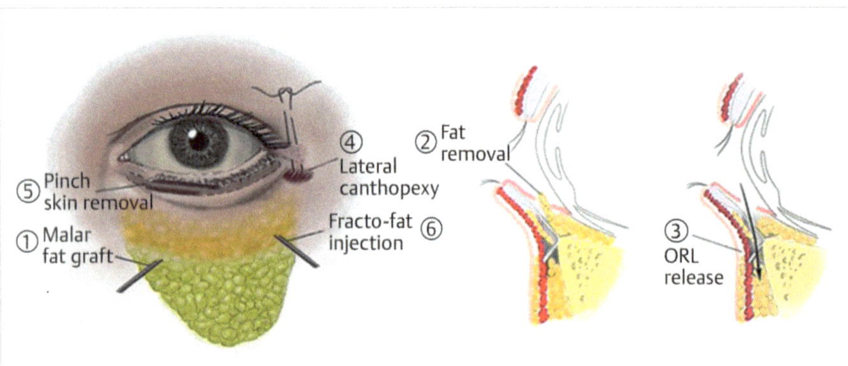

Fig. 31.1 The five-step lower blepharoplasty technique.

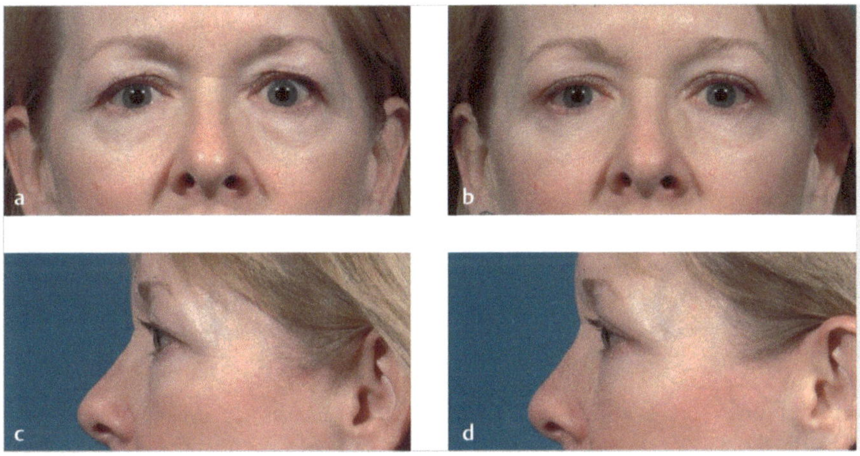

Fig. 31.2 Anteroposterior views of a 56-year-old woman before **(a)** and 1 year after **(b)** five-step lower eyelid blepharoplasty. Preoperative lateral view **(c)** and 1-year postoperative view **(d)**.

fat removed decreases as you proceed from lateral to medial. The lateral deep lower eyelid fat tends to be fuller, more robust, and more vascular. The lateral fat pad is also the most likely to be missed, causing persistent lateral fullness postoperatively (▶ Fig. 31.1).

- *Step 3: Lateral retinacular canthopexy:* An absorbable 5–0 Vicryl (Ethicon, Inc., Somerville, NJ) suture should be used for the lateral canthopexy, to prevent scleral show and lower eyelid malposition without affecting long-term lateral canthal shape. A 5–0 Mersilene (Ethicon, Inc., Somerville, NJ) suture may be necessary in men, secondary lax eyelids, cases of dry eyes, and in negative vector patients (▶ Fig. 31.1).
- *Step 4: Skin pinch removal:* After appropriate markings are made, fine-tooth forceps are used to pinch the excess skin, creating a linear partition to be excised. Curved scissors are then used to carefully excise the skin, maintaining the underlying orbicularis muscle intact (▶ Fig. 31.1).
- *Step 5: Fractionated fat injection and release of the orbicularis retaining ligament:* A stab incision is made laterally, right at the orbital rim, followed by fractionated fat (fracto-fat) injected both above the periosteum and also below the muscle with 50% overcorrection. This is performed using a fine 1-mm cannula with a single side hole. Fat is generally harvested from the inner thigh with a small multiport cannula. The harvested fat is centrifuged with the supranatant and infranatant wasted. The remaining fractionated fat is then run through a tulip connector at least 50 times to allow for true fat fractionation. This excludes viable fat cells and therefore prevents uneven fat take in this area. The medial portion of the orbicularis retaining ligament needs to be released from its maxillary attachments to blend this transition zone. Release is performed laterally using the same fine 1-mm cannula and is gently performed in a blunt manner through the supraperiosteal plane (▶ Fig. 31.1).

31.3 Postoperative Care

- Suture removal:
  - Suture removal is performed between postoperative day 5 and 7.
- Medications:
  - Daily eye lubrication with artificial tears is applied three times daily and at bedtime.
- Chemosis:
  - Combined ophthalmic antibiotic and steroid drops (Tobramycin and Dexamethasone—Tobradex®) should be used for 1 week.
    - One to two drops applied every 4 to 6 hours.
  - Continue aggressive eye lubrication with artificial tears.
    - Gel lubricants may be used at night for longer application.

In severe cases of chemosis, temporary tarsorrhaphy can be performed.

31.4 Case Example

Anteroposterior views of a 56-year-old woman before (above, left) and 1 year after (above, right) five-step lower eyelid blepharoplasty. Preoperative lateral view (below, left) and 1-year postoperative view (below, right) (▶ Fig. 31.2).

31.5 Conclusion

A comprehensive ophthalmic history and examination are crucial for surgical success. The surgeon's goals and patient's expectations must be aligned. The five-step lower blepharoplasty includes malar fat compartment augmentation, transconjunctival removal of lower eyelid fat if indicated, lateral retinacular canthopexy, skin pinch removal, and fractionated fat injection and release of the orbicularis retaining ligament.

Further Readings

Friedland JA, Lalonde DH, Rohrich RJ. An evidence-based approach to blepharoplasty. Plast Reconstr Surg. 2010; 126(6):2222–2229

Pezeshk RA, Sieber DA, Rohrich RJ. The six-step lower blepharoplasty: using fractionated fat to enhance blending of the lid-cheek junction. Plast Reconstr Surg. 2017; 139(6):1381–1383

Rohrich RJ, Mahedia M, Shah N, Afrooz P, Vishvanath L, Gupta RK. Role of fractionated fat in blending the lid-cheek junction. Plast Reconstr Surg. 2018; 142(1): 56–65

Rohrich RJ, Mahedia M, Hidalgo D, Shah N. The evolving role of blending of the lid-cheek junction in lower blepharoplasty. Plast Reconstr Surg. 2018; 142(2): 377–382

Rohrich RJ, Ghavami A, Mojallal A. The five-step lower blepharoplasty: blending the eyelid-cheek junction. Plast Reconstr Surg. 2011; 128(3):775–783

32 Periorbital Fat Grafting

Dino Elyassnia and Timothy Marten

Abstract

The hallmark of a youthful, attractive orbit is fullness. It has become clear that fat atrophy is a significant component of periorbital aging, which results in volume loss and a hollow appearance around the eyes. Traditional blepharoplasty procedures have focused on treating skin laxity, fat herniation, canthal laxity, and levator dehiscence but have largely ignored fat atrophy. This chapter will present a detailed approach to periorbital fat grafting, which represents a new paradigm in eyelid aesthetics. This approach produces a full, healthy appearance to the eyes that has not been possible with traditional blepharoplasty techniques.

Keywords: Augmentation blepharoplasty, periorbital fat grafting, lower eyelid fat grafting, upper eyelid fat grafting, blepharoplasty, periorbital fat atrophy, periorbital rejuvenation

Key Points

- The hallmark of a youthful, attractive orbit is fullness.
- It has become clear that fat atrophy is a significant component of periorbital aging, which results in a hollow appearance around the eyes.
- Traditional blepharoplasty techniques have generally not addressed volume loss.
- Periorbital fat grafting represents a new paradigm in eyelid aesthetics, which focuses on volumetric rejuvenation of the upper and lower eyelids (▸ Fig. 32.1a, b).

32.1 Preoperative Steps

32.1.1 Analysis

- A focused history should include any ophthalmologic conditions, previous blepharoplasties, or filler use.
- As hyaluronic acid filler tends to last especially long in the upper and lower eyelids, knowledge of its use must be obtained so that a decision can be made whether to dissolve the material prior to fat grafting.
- Physical examination of the eyelids should include looking for the presence of ptosis, dermatochalasis, lower eyelid fat herniation, canthal laxity, orbital vector, and degree of fat atrophy of the eyelids, midface, and cheek.
- If problems other than fat atrophy are present such as significant lower eyelid fat herniation or excess skin, traditional blepharoplasty techniques may need to be combined with fat grafting.

32.2 Operative Steps

See **Video 32.1.**

32.2.1 Fat Harvest

- Our preferred areas for fat harvest include the waist, hip, and outer thigh, performed with a limited prep in the semilateral decubitus position (▸ Fig. 32.2).
- Areas from which fat is to be harvested are infiltrated with a dilute 0.1% lidocaine with 1:1,000,000 epinephrine solution using a multiholed infiltration cannula.
- Approximately 1 cc of this solution is injected for every 3 cc of anticipated fat removal. Over-wetting the tissue will result in an over-dilute harvest and more time spent in the harvesting process.
- Fat is harvested with a special harvesting cannula ranging in size from 2.1 to 2.4 mm and 15 to 25 cm long attached to a 10-cc syringe using gently applied syringe suction.
- Sharp hypodermic needles should not be used to harvest fat.
- At least twice as much fat is harvested as is anticipated to be used to insure an adequate amount of processed fat will be available.

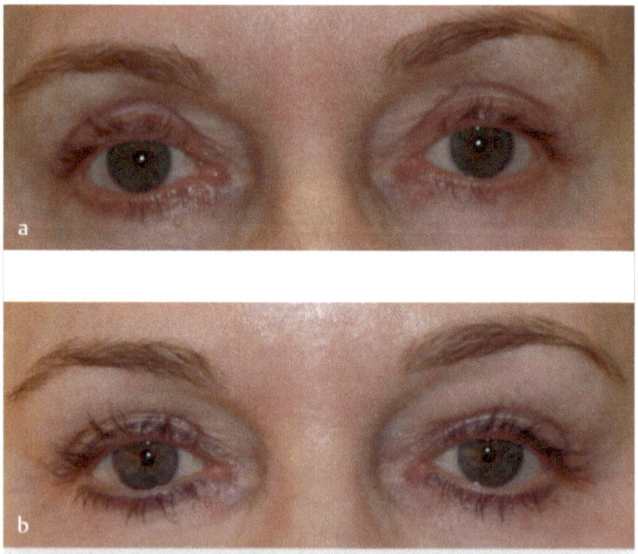

Fig. 32.1 (a, b) Patient with hollow upper and lower orbits before and after fat grafting to the upper and lower orbits (note: the patient also had fat grafting to the midface, cheek, and temple, along with a temple lift and facelift). (Procedure performed by Dino Elyassnia, MD, FACS.)

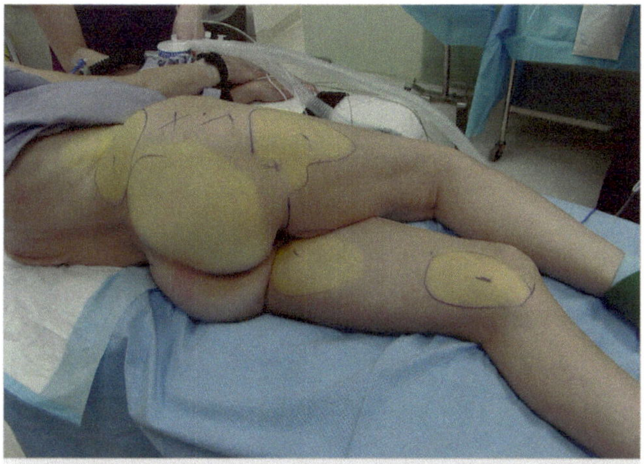

Fig. 32.2 Positioning patient for fat harvest in a semilateral decubitus position.

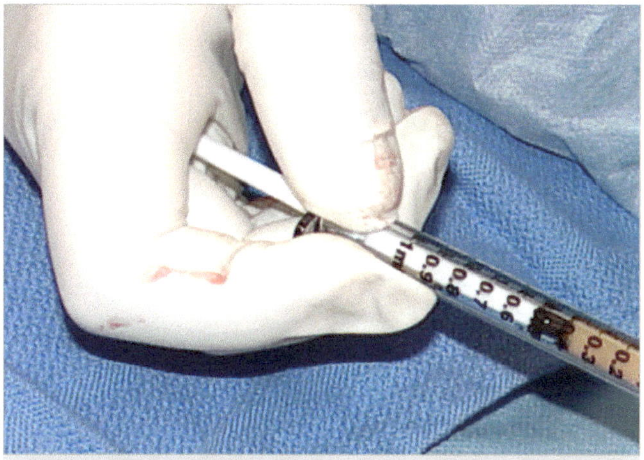

Fig. 32.3 Method of holding syringe to control volume ejected during injection. Held in this manner, a slight closing of the hand results in only a small amount of fat being ejected.

32.2.2 Processing Harvested Fat

- Our preferred method of processing fat is centrifugation.
- First, a sterile disposable plastic cap is placed on the end of the syringe and the syringe plunger removed from the syringe barrel.
- Capped syringe barrels containing unprocessed fat are then spun for 1 to 3 minutes at 1,000 rpm.
- Many centrifuges available for this purpose have rotors that can be sterilized or sterilizable tubes that fit into the rotor so that the syringes containing the fat remain sterile and can be handled by the scrubbed surgical team.
- Once centrifuged, spun fat will be seen to contain an upper oil (ruptured fat cells), central fat, and lower "water" (blood, lidocaine) components.
- The blood-tinged "water" (local anesthetic) component is allowed to run out after removing the cap while the oil fraction is then poured out of the top of the syringe. Telfa sponges can be used to wick up the small amount of residual oil present.
- A laboratory "test tube" type rack to hold and organize the syringes containing fat greatly facilitates fat-processing activities.
- The resultant fat is transferred into 1 cc Luer lock syringes using a transfer coupler.
- The bottom 2 cc's of fat in the syringe containing the highest concentrations of high-density adipocytes are segregated and are used preferentially in the procedure.

32.2.3 Upper Orbit Fat Grafting

- First, nerve blocks are performed with 0.25% bupivacaine with 1:200,000 epinephrine local anesthetic solution.
- Then small stab incisions are made in the medial and lateral extent of the eyebrow with a 20-gauge needle.
- Infiltration is made in multiple passes injecting on both the in and out strokes. Approximately 0.05 cc or less should be injected per pass. This corresponds to 20 to 40 back and forth passes or more for each 1-cc syringe of processed fat.
- Faster movements of the cannula are desirable in that if the injection cannula is constantly in motion intravascular injection or bolus injections are less likely.
- The syringe should be held with the end of the plunger in the palm of the hand as this will help in controlling the volume injected with each pass (▸ Fig. 32.3).
- The goal is to inject the fat in a way that optimizes its chance of developing a blood supply and surviving, and the mental model should be one of scattering tiny particles of fat into the recipient site in multiple crisscrossing fine trails.
- To allow for the deposition of tiny aliquots of fat per each pass, very fine cannulas must be used when fat grafting around the eyes. Currently a 4 cm long, 0.7 mm (22 gauge) cannula is preferred.
- The hollow upper eyelid is restored by placing fat in a deep submuscular/preperiosteal position along the inferior margins of the supraorbital rim. The process is best conceptualized as one of *lowering the supraorbital rim* and filling the upper orbital area to push skin that has retracted up into the orbit down onto the preseptal eyelid to create a full and appropriately creased upper eyelid (▸ Fig. 32.4).
- In general 1.5 to 3 cc of fat must be placed in each upper orbit.
- When grafting the upper orbit one must always be aware of the location of the tip of the cannula in relationship to the ocular globe to prevent any trauma.
- Fat grafting of the upper orbit and "eyelid" is advanced in difficulty, and treatment of this area should be made only after experience has been gained in treating noncritical areas.
- Once that experience is obtained, fat grafting of the upper orbit can be one of the most artistically rewarding uses of autologous fat.

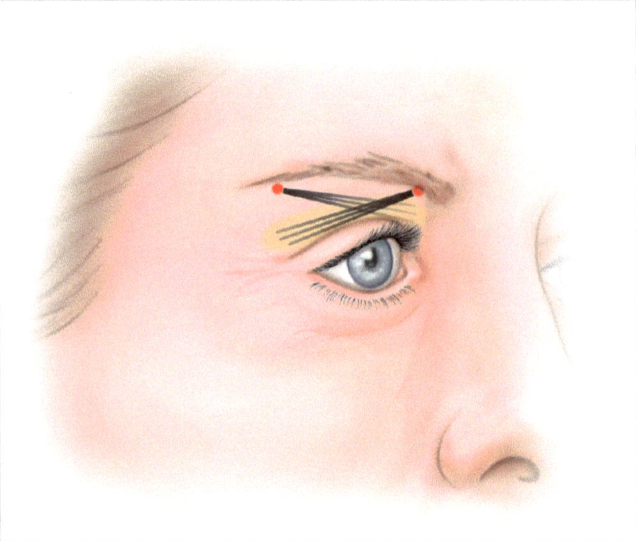

Fig. 32.4 Incision sites and plan for injecting fat into the upper orbital ("upper eyelid") area.

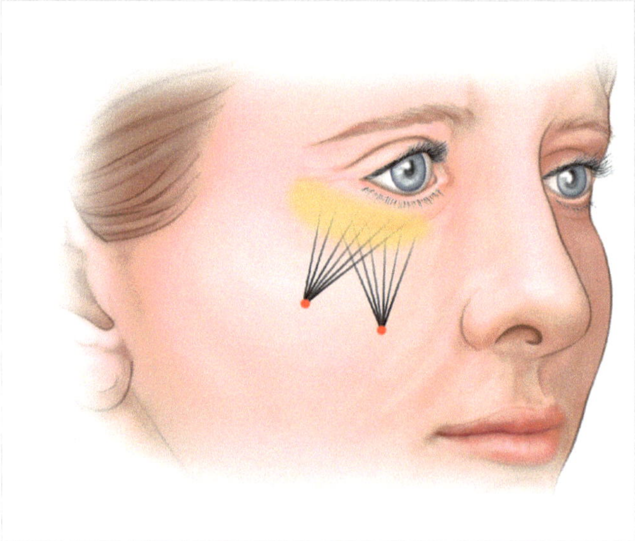

Fig. 32.5 Incision sites and plan for injecting fat into the infraorbital ("lower eyelid") area.

32.2.4 Lower Orbit Fat Grafting

- First, nerve blocks are performed as is done in the upper orbit.
- Unlike the upper orbit, for the lower orbit fat is best and most easily injected *perpendicular* to the infraorbital rim through stab incisions placed in the midcheek or perioral area (▸ Fig. 32.5).
- Like the upper orbit, fat grafting of the infraorbital area is performed with a 4 cm long, 0.7 mm (22 gauge) injection cannula with a focus on placing very small aliquots of fat per each pass using the same basic injection technique described above.
- Also like the upper orbit, fat should be injected deep in a submuscular/preperiosteal plane.
- The technical goal of the procedure should be thought of as raising up and anteriorly projecting the infraorbital rim rather that filling the eyelid itself.
- It is wise to avoid any subcutaneous injection in the infraorbital area due to the extremely thin skin present and the likelihood of creating visible lumps and irregularities. The purported benefit of superficial injections—improving skin texture and color—is too small an improvement in most cases for all but the expert injector.
- When injecting the lower orbit, the surgeon should place her or his index finger of the nondominant (noninjecting) hand firmly on the infraorbital rim to protect the ocular globe.
- Volumes required to obtain corrections in the lower orbit are 2 to 4 cc per side in most cases.

32.3 Postoperative Care

- Regional fat grafting to the periorbita is performed on an outpatient basis. Patients having a combined facelift with fat grafting are typically discharged to an aftercare specialist for the first night.
- Patients are asked to rest quietly and apply cool compresses to their face for 15 to 20 minutes every hour they are awake for the first 3 days after surgery.
- Patients are advised to take a soft diet that is easy to chew and digest for 2 weeks after surgery and are encouraged to avoid salty foods.
- In general, patients are asked to set aside 2 to 3 weeks for recovery and 2 to 3 months prior to any major business presentation or important social function.
- The change in facial contour seen at 4 to 6 months is likely to consist of living fat as most swelling has completely resolved.

32.4 Case Example

Periorbital fat grafting case example. Patient with no previous surgery and hollow appearance around the eyes (▸ Fig. 32.6a). The same patient seen after facial fat injections including to the upper and lower orbits. A healthier, more youthful appearance can be seen (▸ Fig. 32.6b).

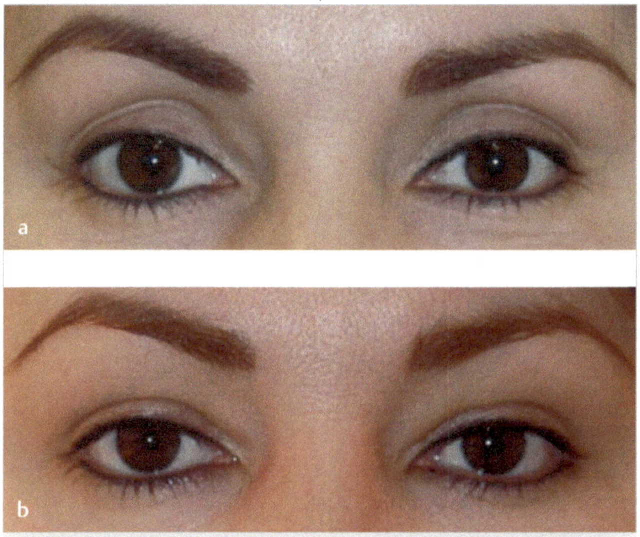

Fig. 32.6 Periorbital fat grafting case example. **(a)** Patient with no previous surgery and hollow appearance around the eyes. **(b)** The same patient seen after facial fat injections including to the upper and lower orbits. A healthier, more youthful appearance can be seen. (Procedure performed by Timothy Marten, MD, FACS—Courtesy of Marten Clinic of Plastic Surgery.)

32.5 Conclusion

Periorbital fat grafting is a powerful tool for eyelid aesthetics that can significantly enhance and sometimes replace traditional blepharoplasty techniques. Fat grafting to the upper and lower orbits should be performed using fine cannulas with fat being placed in a deep plane in very tiny aliquots to avoid irregularity. The role of the nondominant hand is critical to maintaining awareness of the position of the cannula at all times to ensure safety of the ocular globe.

Further Readings

Marten TJ. Simultaneous facelift and fat grafting: combined lifting and filling of the face. In: Nahai F, ed. The Art of Aesthetic Surgery. 2nd ed. Saint Louis: Quality Medical Publishing; 2011

Marten TJ, Elyassnia D. Fat grafting in facial rejuvenation. Clin Plast Surg. 2015; 42 (2):219–252

Marten TJ, Elyassnia D. Simultaneous facelift and fat grafting. In: Connell BF, Sundine MJ, eds. Aesthetic Rejuvenation of the Face and Neck. New York: Thieme; 2016

Marten TJ, Elyassnia D. Simultaneous facelift and fat grafting: combined lifting and filling of the aging face. In: Coleman S, Mazzola R, Pu L, eds. Fat Injection: From Filling to Regeneration. 2nd ed. New York: Thieme; 2018

Rohrich RJ, Pessa JE. The fat compartments of the face: anatomy and clinical implications for cosmetic surgery. Plast Reconstr Surg. 2007; 119(7):2219–2227, discussion 2228–2231

33 Brow and Forehead: Forehead Lift

Christina R. Vargas and Bahman Guyuron

Abstract
Successful forehead lift depends on careful preoperative facial analysis and proper selection of the ideal procedure. Particular attention should be given to the assessment of blepharoptosis, horizontal rhytides indicative of frontalis compensation, corrugator function, hairline, and brow and globe position. Endoscopic and transpalpebral approaches to the forehead provide access for forehead suspension and corrugator resection and isolated corrugator resection, respectively.

Keywords: Forehead, rejuvenation, endoscopic, transpalpebral, suspension, lift, corrugator

Key Points

- Forehead rejuvenation has a significant role in comprehensive facial rejuvenation.
- Circumspect facial analysis provides a crucial foundation in selecting the appropriate surgical technique and in optimizing the final aesthetic outcome.
- The horizontal lines in the forehead denote frontalis compensation of upper eyelid ptosis or dermatochalasia.
- For patients who need a brow lift as well as corrugator muscle resection, an endoscopic procedure would be ideal.
- For patients with close to optimal eyebrow position who have deep frown lines, those with a long or very round forehead, and patients with exophthalmos or proptosis, the transpalpebral approach is more appropriate.
- On patients who have eyelid ptosis or proptosis, elevation of the eyebrows may divulge a condition that otherwise may not be so discernable.

33.1 Preoperative Steps

33.1.1 Analysis

- The facial rejuvenation procedure begins with a thorough preoperative analysis including rhytides, forehead length and contour, brow position, shape, and hairline.
- Special attention should be given to concomitant eyelid ptosis and overactive frontalis, corrugator supercilii, and/or depressor supercilii muscles with dynamic evaluation.

33.2 Operative Steps

See **Video 33.1.**

33.2.1 Endoscopic Forehead Lift

Approach to Endoscopic Access

- Access is gained using five 1.5-cm incisions hidden in the hairline.
- A midline incision is marked vertically at the widow's peak.
- The next two incisions are marked in the temple area, approximately 0.5 to 1 cm behind the hairline; the first about 7 cm from the midline incision and the second about 10 cm from the midline incision (▶ Fig. 33.1).
- The entire forehead and scalp area extending about 8 to 10 cm behind the hairline is infiltrated with 1% lidocaine with 1:100,000 units of epinephrine for non-hair-bearing areas and 1:200,000 units in hair-bearing areas.
- The patient's hair may be braided between the marked incisions or put into rubber bands to avoid interference with the procedure.
- An endoscopic access device (EAD) may be utilized to ease the introduction of instruments during the procedure (▶ Fig. 33.2).
- The most lateral incision on one side is carried through the superficial temporalis fascia down to, but not through, the deep temporal fascia.
- An elevator, such as an Obwegeser periosteal elevator, is used to dissect the tissue at a plane superficial to the deep temporalis fascia to a minimal extent.
- This plane is extended cephalad to a subperiosteal plane, which is located medial to the temporal ridge and therefore overlies only the periosteum, and where the second incision is marked.
- Once the second incision is carried down through the periosteum, the dissection is performed medially under the midline incision.
- The medial incision is made down through the periosteum and into the target plane.

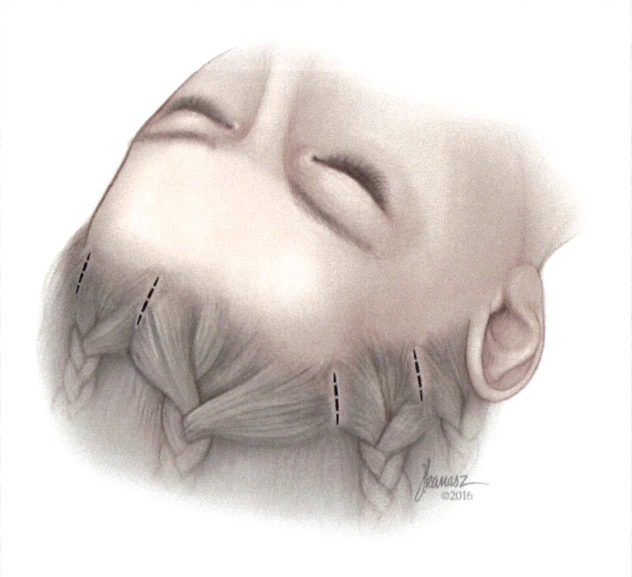

Fig. 33.1 Endoscopic forehead lift. Approach to endoscopic access. Two incisions are marked in the temple area, approximately 0.5 to 1 cm behind the hairline; the first about 7 cm from the midline incision and the second about 10 cm from the midline incision. (Reproduced with permission from Guyuron B. Migraine Surgery. Thieme; 2018.)

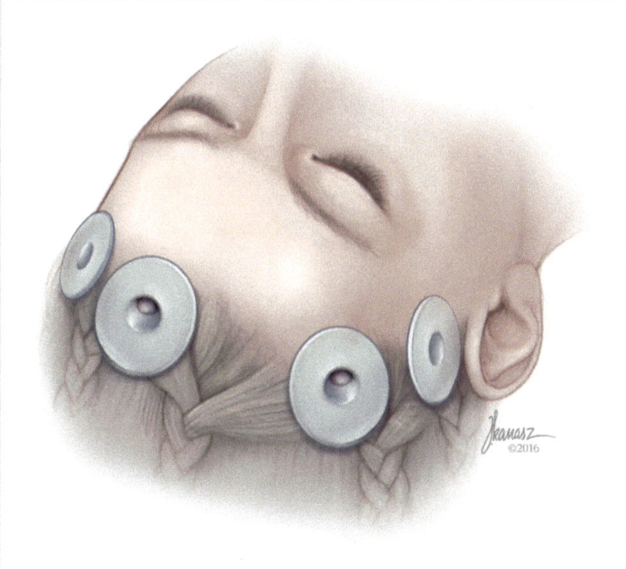

Fig. 33.2 Endoscopic forehead lift. Approach to endoscopic access. An endoscopic access device (EAD) may be utilized to ease the introduction of instruments during the procedure. (Reproduced with permission from Guyuron B. Migraine Surgery. Thieme; 2018.)

- The procedure is repeated on the contralateral side, developing the plane from lateral to medial.
- The two planes are connected using a periosteal elevator and extended cephalad to allow enough tissue laxity for the introduction of the endoscope and related instruments.
- The Obwegeser elevator is used laterally to further skeletonize the deep temporal fascia posteriorly to approach ear level. This plane should remain deep to the superficial temporal fascia, but superficial to the deep temporal fascia.
- The Obwegeser elevator is then introduced through the midline incision and the area 8 to 10 cm behind the middle incision is released in a subperiosteal plane, providing laxity for the procedure.

Endoscopic Dissection

- The endoscope is introduced and dissection of the forehead area is performed under direct visualization in a subperiosteal plane to the supraorbital rim. It is crucial to conduct the dissection immediately superficial to the deep temporal fascia and deep to any piece of fat attached to the superficial temporal fascia to protect the frontal branch of the facial nerve.
- The arcus marginalis and periorbita are released from the superior orbital rim and along the lateral orbital wall and dissection carried medially to the glabellar area.
- The supraorbital and supratrochlear nerves and vessels are identified immediately above and along the medial third of each orbital rim.
- The corrugator muscle lies both deep and superficial to the nerves.
- A Daniel endoscopic grasper is utilized to remove the corrugator muscle as radically as possible.
- The nerves are preserved and may be retracted utilizing a nerve hook.
- Most medially, in the glabellar area, the periosteum is elevated but not transected. Transection is only necessary if there is significant and unusual hyperactivity of the procerus muscle.
- A longer periosteal elevator is utilized to reach the midline areas; this subperiosteal plane is also developed laterally along the orbital rim and down to the zygomatic arch.
- Dissection is carried laterally and efforts made to avoid and preserve the sentinel vein.
- A similar dissection is conducted on the opposite side and the corrugator supercilii muscle is removed.
- Hemostasis is maintained utilizing suction electrocautery.
- The corrugator muscle is replaced with fat graft harvested through a small rent immediately above the zygomatic arch medially deep to the deep temporal fascia, which is facilitated by pressing on the buccal fat pad, or from another site if other procedures are being performed concurrently.

Forehead Suspension

- Suspension is undertaken at one point laterally on each side.
- Skin hooks are placed in a more anterior position at the lateral-most incision and the wound edges are retracted.
- The nondominant index finger is utilized to evert the anterior portion of the wound, exposing the superficial layer of the temporal fascia.
- A 3–0 PDS suture is placed through a substantial amount of this tissue by first going from the outside in and then from the inside out.
- Skin hooks are moved to a more posterior position on the wound and firmly retracted in the direction of the desired vector of pull and lift of the lateral eyebrow, which is commonly 45 degrees in relation to the body axis.
- The suture is passed through the deep temporalis fascia and incrementally tightened until the brow is lifted to the aesthetically desired level; it is then tied and cut. This is done bilaterally.
- When the eyebrows are asymmetric a similar suture is placed through the anterior portion of the second wound. However, because this area is beyond the reach of the temporalis fascia for obtaining the correct vector of lift, the suture is fastened through a bone tunnel rather than the fascia.
- Skin hooks are moved to the posterior portion of the incision and a thin malleable retractor is used to protect the scalp posteriorly.
- A 1.1 mm diameter, 5 mm long drill tip is used to create two drill holes positioned opposite one another at a 45 degrees angle, approximately 4 mm apart.
- The bone is irrigated to avoid thermal damage during drilling.
- The free end of the suture is then passed through the tunnel and is incrementally tightened until the desired lift has been achieved. The procedure is repeated on the opposite side.
- Incisions are repaired with 5–0 Monocryl for the periosteum or the superficial fascia and 5–0 plain catgut for the skin.

33.2.2 Transpalpebral Corrugator Resection

This approach is useful for patients with a high forehead as well as those with hyperactive corrugator muscles causing vertical

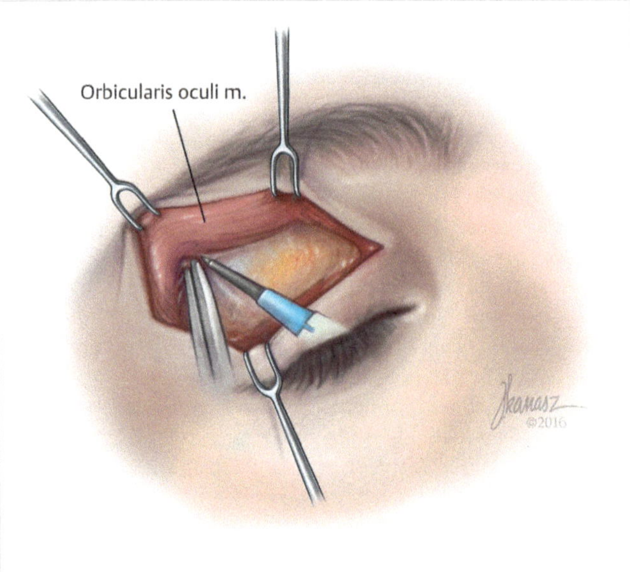

Fig. 33.3 Transpalpebral corrugator resection. The orbital septum is retracted inferiorly and the orbicularis muscle retracted superiorly. (Reproduced with permission from Guyuron B. Migraine Surgery. Thieme; 2018.)

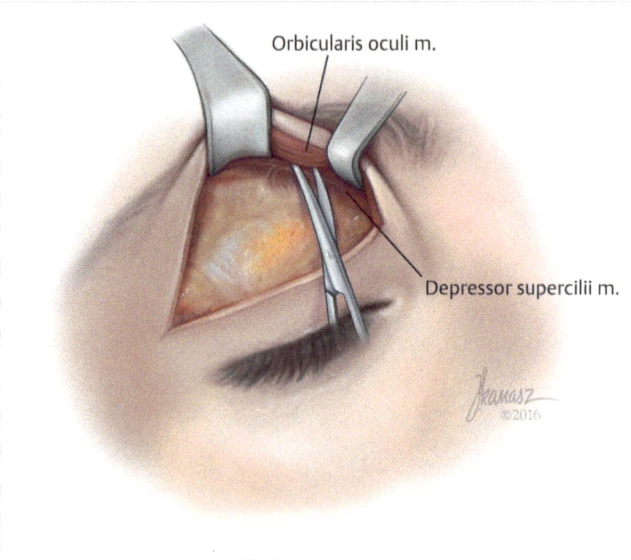

Fig. 33.4 Transpalpebral corrugator resection. A thin layer of depressor supercilii muscle overlying the darker, more friable corrugator supercilii muscle is dissected and excised. (Reproduced with permission from Guyuron B. Migraine Surgery. Thieme; 2018.)

glabellar lines but with otherwise well-positioned eyebrows. It is also indicated for those patients with proptosis, exophthalmos, and eyelid ptosis who would not undergo ptosis correction to prevent elevation of the eyebrows, exaggerating the proptosis or ptosis. This technique is also used by the senior author in patients with frontal migraine headaches without the temporal headaches.

- The supratarsal crease is marked, then infiltrated with 1% lidocaine with 1:100,000 units of epinephrine. The glabellar area is infiltrated with a mixture of 1% xylocaine and 0.5% Naropin with 1:100,000 epinephrine.
- If the patient will also undergo upper blepharoplasty, a standard upper blepharoplasty incision is made. If upper blepharoplasty is not planned, the incision should be limited to the medial half of the upper eyelid.
- The eyelid incision is made and extended through the orbicularis muscle. Excess skin is resected if necessary.
- The orbital septum is retracted inferiorly and the orbicularis muscle retracted superiorly (▸ Fig. 33.3).
- The plane between these two structures is dissected cephalad to the superior orbital rim for 5 to 8 mm until the corrugator muscles are encountered.
- The dissection is continued using baby Metzenbaum scissors and a spreading technique.
- A thin layer of depressor supercilii muscle overlying the darker, more friable corrugator supercilii muscle is dissected and excised (▸ Fig. 33.4).
- A branch of the supraorbital nerve, which pierces the corrugator muscle medially, is identified on the surface and followed into the muscle using a mosquito hemostat. The muscle is lifted and the branch identified above the periosteum and protected (▸ Fig. 33.5).
- The segment of muscle caudal to the nerve is isolated and removed using electrocautery, first medially then laterally. The segment cephalad to the nerve is isolated and removed. The remaining muscle is removed in piecemeal fashion as thoroughly as possible to include lateral fibers of procerus muscle until subcutaneous fat is encountered.
- A fat graft equal in size to the excised corrugator muscle is used, harvested either from the medial compartment of the

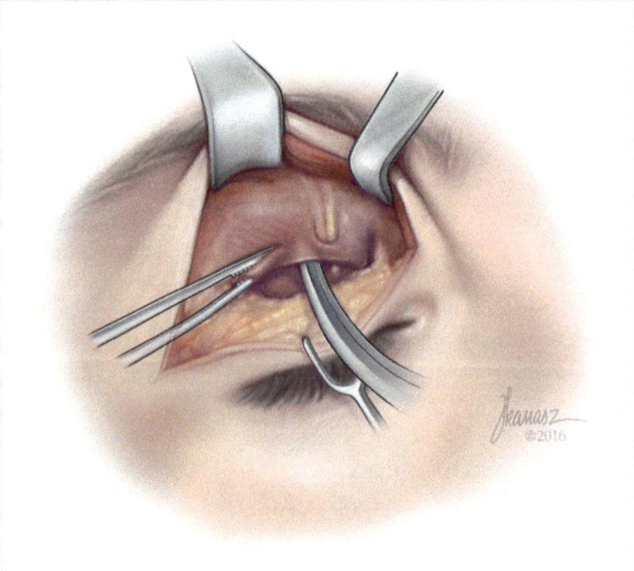

Fig. 33.5 Transpalpebral corrugator resection. A branch of the supraorbital nerve, which pierces the corrugator muscle medially, is identified on the surface and followed into the muscle using a mosquito hemostat. The muscle is lifted and the branch identified above the periosteum and protected. (Reproduced with permission from Guyuron B. Migraine Surgery. Thieme; 2018.)

upper eyelid during upper blepharoplasty or elsewhere in patients who do not have excess upper eyelid fat.

- The fat graft is placed above the periosteum and fixed in place using 6–0 Monocryl, taking care to avoid significant volume overcorrection as take is generally very good.
- Meticulous hemostasis is maintained with electrocautery.
- Skin is reapproximated using 6–0 fast-absorbing plain catgut suture and antibiotic ointment is applied.

33.3 Postoperative Care

- The incisions are cared for with application of Bacitracin ointment for approximately 7 days postoperatively. Sutures are allowed to dissolve.
- The patient may shower after 2 days but should refrain from use of hair dryer and curling irons for at least 2 weeks and with extreme care thereafter to avoid thermal injury.

33.4 Case Examples

33.4.1 Case Example 1

A patient with hyperactive corrugator muscle before (left) and after transpalpebral corrugator resection (right) in repose (above) and on trying to frown (below) (▸ Fig. 33.6).

33.4.2 Case Example 2

A patient with hyperactive corrugator muscle before (left) and following endoscopic forehead rejuvenation (right) in repose (above) and on trying to frown (below) (▸ Fig. 33.7).

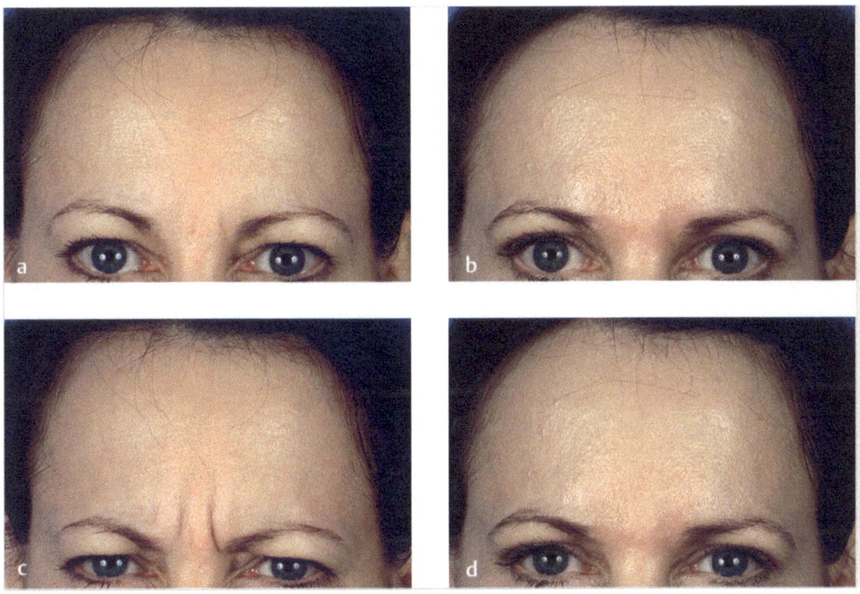

Fig. 33.6 Case 1. A patient with hyperactive corrugator muscle before **(a, c)** and after transpalpebral corrugator resection **(b, d)** in repose **(a, b)** and on trying to frown **(c, d)**.

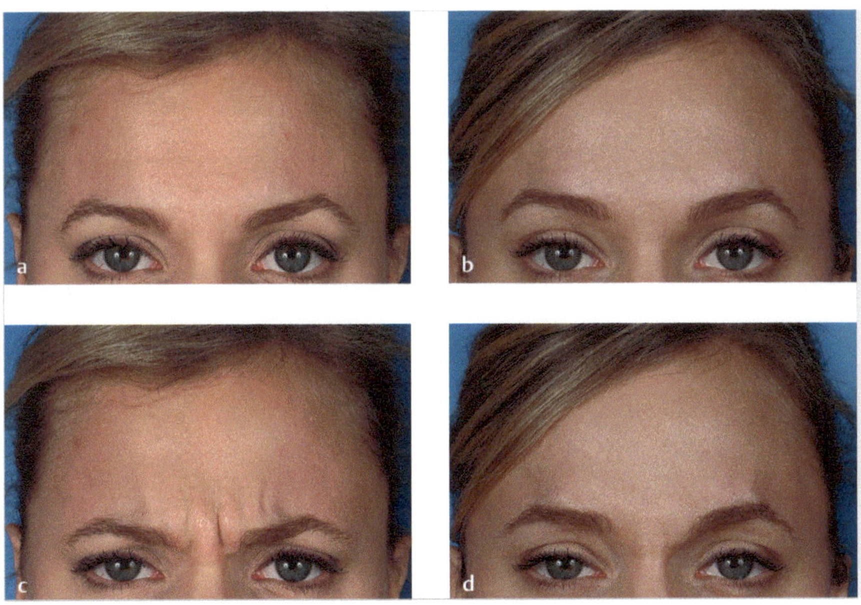

Fig. 33.7 Case 2. A patient with hyperactive corrugator muscle before **(a, c)** and following endoscopic forehead rejuvenation **(b, d)** in repose **(a, b)** and on trying to frown **(c, d)**.

33.5 Conclusion

Forehead rejuvenation can be achieved through the combination of volume restoration and face and neck contouring. Volumization is achieved with autologous fat grafting of the facial fat compartments. Neck contouring is achieved through medial platysma plication and the lateral platysma window. Lateral midface rejuvenation is achieved through superficial musculoaponeurotic system (SMAS) stacking or SMASectomy techniques. Transpalpebral corrugator resection is useful for patients with a long or very round forehead, as well as those with hyperactive corrugator muscles causing vertical glabellar lines but with otherwise well-positioned eyebrows. It is also indicated for those patients with proptosis, exophthalmos, and eyelid ptosis, as well as those with frontal migraine headaches.

Further Readings

Guyuron B, Behmand RA, Green R. Shortening of the long forehead. Plast Reconstr Surg. 1999; 103(1):218–223

Guyuron B, Davies B. Subcutaneous anterior hairline forehead rhytidectomy. Aesthetic Plast Surg. 1988; 12(2):77–83

Guyuron B, Michelow BJ, Thomas T. Corrugator supercilii muscle resection through blepharoplasty incision. Plast Reconstr Surg. 1995; 95(4):691–696

Guyuron B, Michelow BJ. Refinements in endoscopic forehead rejuvenation. Plast Reconstr Surg. 1997; 100(1):154–160

Guyuron B, Son JH. Transpalpebral corrugator resection: 25-year experience, refinements and additional indications. Aesthetic Plast Surg. 2017; 41(2):339–345

34 Brow and Forehead: Endotemporal Brow Lift

Rod J. Rohrich and Min-Jeong Cho

Abstract

The goal of brow rejuvenation is to restore a youthful appearance of the brow and forehead. Plastic surgeons have several options to perform brow lift: direct, endoscopic, hairline, lateral, temporal, and transblepharoplasty brow lift. In this chapter, we discuss the endotemporal brow lift, which combines the strength of endoscopic and temporal brow lift techniques. This technique allows plastic surgeons to treat both medial and lateral brow ptosis in patients with mild to moderate brow ptosis.

Keywords: Brow rejuvenation, brow lift, endotemporal brow lift, endoscopic brow lift, temporal brow lift

Key Points

- Endotemporal brow lift combines the advantages of the endoscopic and temporal brow lift approach.
- It offers treatment for both medial and lateral brow ptosis.

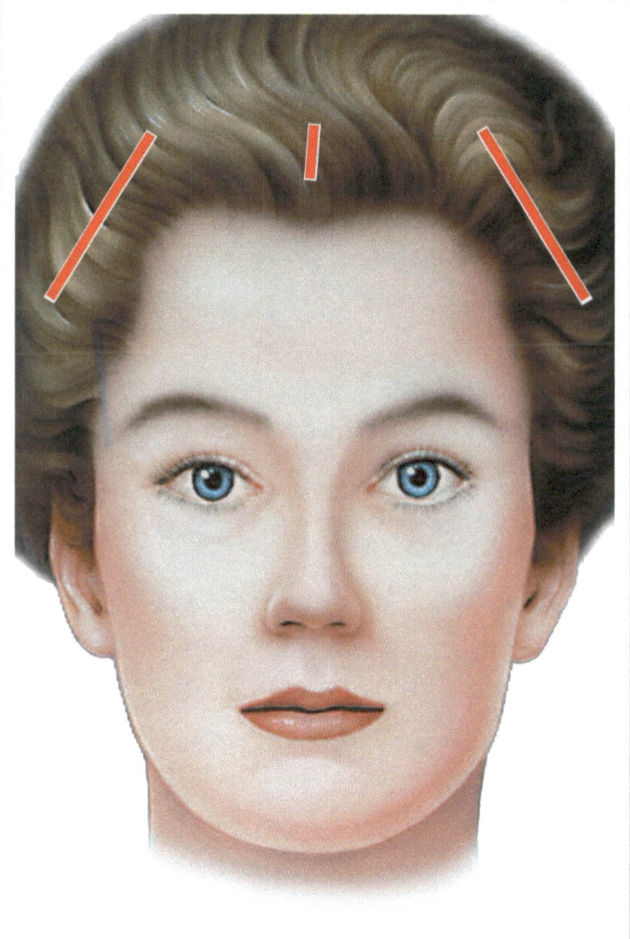

Fig. 34.1 Incisions for anterior and temporal port.

34.1 Preoperative Steps

- Analysis:
  - The brow rejuvenation procedure begins with a comprehensive preoperative facial analysis including horizontal thirds and vertical fifths.
  - Patients with the following are candidates for the endotemporal brow lift:
    - Female: Mild/moderate rhytides with a short forehead.
    - Male: A long forehead with sparse hair.

34.2 Operative Steps

Prior to draping, proposed operative sites are injected with 30 mL of 0.25% of xylocaine with 1:400,000 epinephrine.

34.2.1 Incision Placement

- First, a 6 cm horizontal incision is drawn 5 cm posterior to the temporal hairline (▶ Fig. 34.1). This incision will serve as a temporal port.
- Then, a 2 cm vertical incision is drawn at the midline (▶ Fig. 34.1). This incision will serve as an anterior port.

34.2.2 Temporal Brow Elevation

- The scalp is incised while beveling to prevent damage to the deep hair follicles.
- The scalp is elevated in a subgaleal plane using a periosteal elevator.
- Dissection is continued caudally in the subgaleal plane superficial to the deep temporal fascia (▶ Fig. 34.2).
- At the supraorbital rim, the orbital retaining ligament is released. Then, the zone of adhesion at the temporal fusion line and the temporal ligamentous adhesions are released.

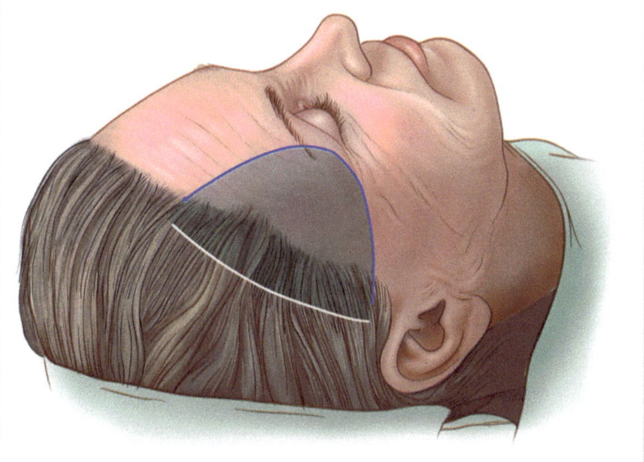

Fig. 34.2 Area of dissection for temporal brow lift. (Reproduced with permission from Codner M, McCord C. Eyelid and Periorbital Surgery. 2nd ed. Thieme; 2016.)

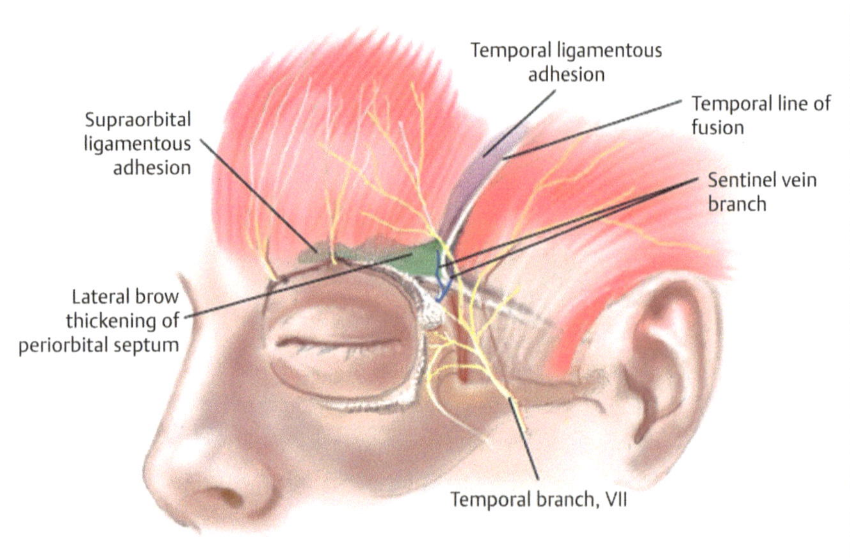

Fig. 34.3 Ligaments that are released during the temporal brow lift. (Reproduced with permission from Codner M, McCord C. Eyelid and Periorbital Surgery. 2nd ed. Thieme; 2016.)

The medial extent of the dissection stops at the lateral two-thirds of the brow (▶ Fig. 34.3).

34.2.3 Medial Brow Elevation

- Using the midline incision, the scalp is elevated in a subgaleal plane using a periosteal elevator until the dissection is carried down to the supraorbital rim (▶ Fig. 34.4).
- Then, the endoscope is inserted into the anterior port, and Takahashi forceps are inserted into the temporal port.
- Under direct visualization using an endoscope, 80 to 95% of the medial corrugators are removed with Takahashi forceps while preserving supraorbital and supratrochlear nerves (▶ Fig. 34.5a, b).
- Then, further presence of rhytides and position of the medial brows are inspected intraoperatively.
- Upon satisfactory removal of the corrugators, and adequate mobilization of the brow, the anterior port can be closed with staples.

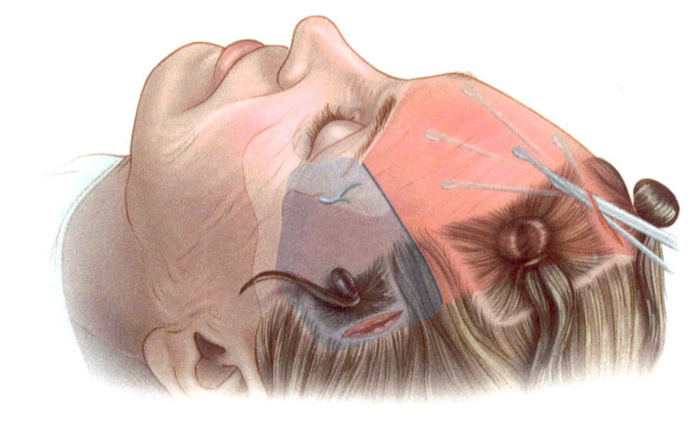

Fig. 34.4 Area of dissection for endoscopic brow lift. (Reproduced with permission from Cohen M, Thaller S. The Unfavorable Result in Plastic Surgery: Avoidance and Treatment. 4th ed. Thieme; 2018.)

34.2.4 Closure

- Once the anterior port is closed, the position of lateral brows is assessed.
- The lateral brows are elevated to the desired height and the excess scalp skin is excised. Then, the galea is approximated using 4–0 Vicryl and tension-free closure of the scalp is performed using staples. Typically, an excision of 1 to 1.5 cm of scalp results in 2 to 3 mm of elevation of the lateral brow.
- A head dressing is applied at the end of the case.

34.3 Postoperative Care

- Patients may take off their head dressing 24 hours after the surgery.
- Patients can begin a light, liquid diet on the day of surgery, and advance to a soft, regular diet the next day.
- Patients are encouraged to apply cold compresses close to the surgery site and eyelids as much as possible, and avoid any type of straining during the first 72 hours after surgery.
- Patients may begin washing their hair 48 hours after surgery.
- Patients can apply eye drops as needed to keep their eyes moist and comfortable.
- Staples are removed in 7 to 10 days.

34.4 Case Example

Preoperative and postoperative photographs of a patient at 20 months following a facelift and endotemporal brow lift in anteroposterior (AP) view (▶ Fig. 34.6a, b).

34.5 Conclusion

Medial and lateral brow rejuvenation can be treated with the endotemporal brow lift technique. This technique combines the advantages of the endoscopic and temporal brow lift.

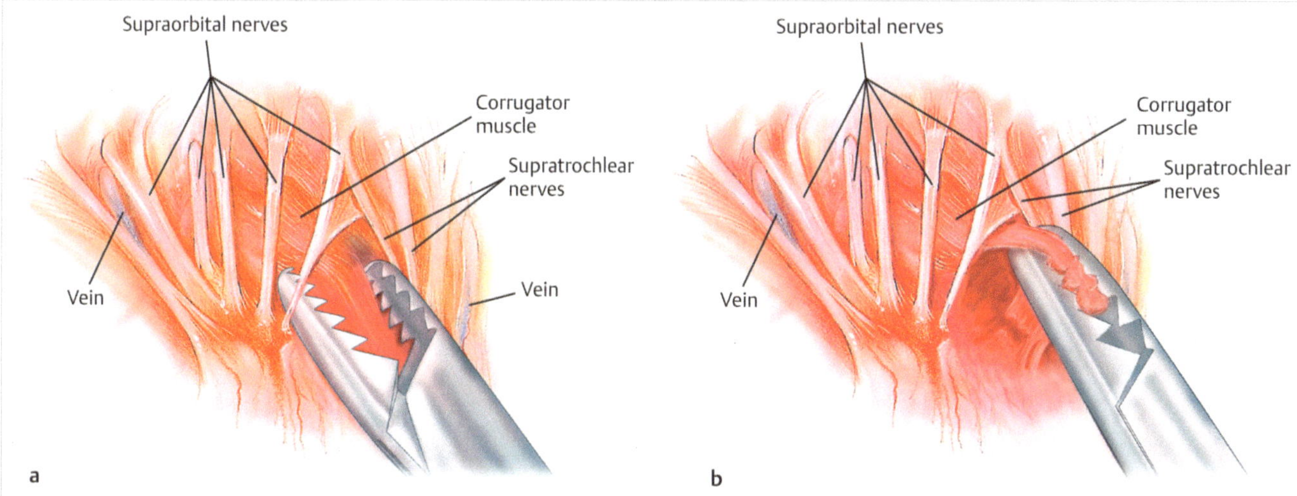

Fig. 34.5 (a, b) Medial corrugator resection. (Reproduced with permission from Cohen M, Thaller S. The Unfavorable Result in Plastic Surgery: Avoidance and Treatment. 4th ed. Thieme; 2018.)

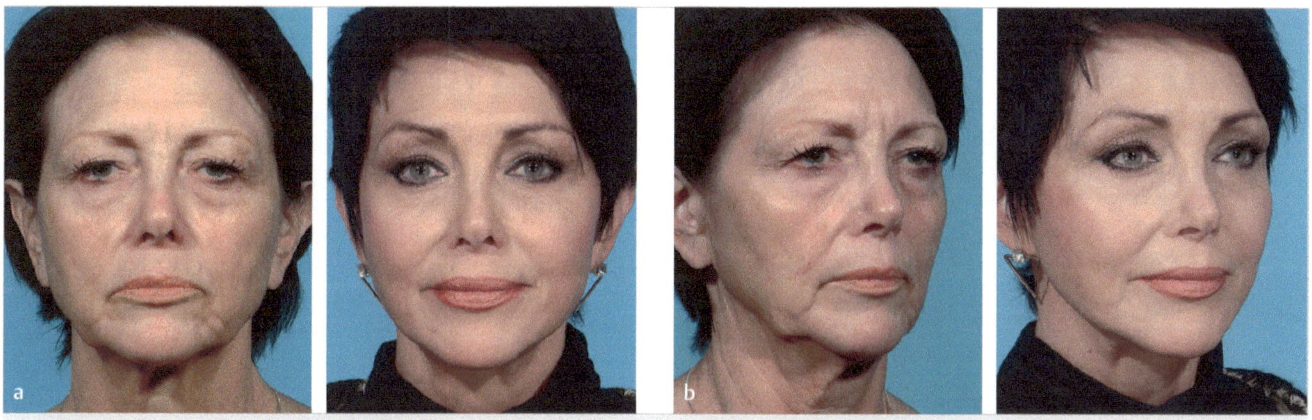

Fig. 34.6 (a) Preoperative and postoperative photographs of a patient at 20 months following a facelift and endotemporal brow lift in anteroposterior (AP) view. **(b)** Preoperative and postoperative photographs of a patient at 20 months following the facelift and endotemporal brow lift in oblique view.

Ideal candidates for this technique are patients with mild to moderate brow ptosis.

See **Video 34.1.**

Further Reading

Cho MJ, Carboy JA, Rohrich RJ. Complications in brow lifts: a systemic review of surgical and nonsurgical brow rejuvenations. Plast Reconstr Surg Glob Open. 2018; 6(10):e1943

Graham DW, Heller J, Kurkjian TJ, Schaub TS, Rohrich RJ. Brow lift in facial rejuvenation: a systematic literature review of open versus endoscopic techniques. Plast Reconstr Surg. 2011; 128(4):335e–341e

Guyuron B. Endoscopic forehead rejuvenation: I. Limitations, flaws, and rewards. Plast Reconstr Surg. 2006; 117(4):1121–1133, discussion 1134–1136

Rohrich RJ, Beran SJ. Evolving fixation methods in endoscopically assisted forehead rejuvenation: controversies and rationale. Plast Reconstr Surg. 1997; 100(6): 1575–1582, discussion 1583–1584

Rohrich RJ, Cho MJ. Endoscopic temporal brow lift: surgical indications, technique, and 10-year outcome analysis. Plast Reconstr Surg. 2019; 144(6):1305–1310

35 Brow and Forehead: Fat Grafting to the Brow, Temples, and Forehead

Rod J. Rohrich and Erez Dayan

Abstract

A modern paradigm shift in facial rejuvenation focuses on volume restoration in addition to facial recontouring. The concept of facial volume restoration has long been advocated, and ultimately accepted into common practice with our improved understanding of facial aging. Forehead and eyebrow revolumization is often neglected during facial fat grafting. The purpose of this chapter is to describe the technique for volume restoration of these areas.

Keywords: Fat grafting, forehead, eyebrow, temporal hollowing, facial revolumization

Key Points

- Fat grafting to the forehead, temples, and brows is a key component of pan facial revolumization (▶ Fig. 35.1 and ▶ Fig. 35.2).
- Injections are performed in the subcutaneous plane.
- Injection of the superior brow regions not only corrects age-related changes, but also creates the illusion of more lifted brows.
- Correction of temporal hollowing requires disruption of the temporal fusion line.

35.1 Preoperative Steps

- Fat harvest is accomplished using manual low-pressure lipoaspiration using a blunt 3-mm cannula.
- Inner thighs and abdomen are the ideal donor sites, which contain the highest concentration of stromal vascular cells with the least amount of pain, as shown in previous studies and clinical experience.
- The lipoaspirate is then processed using centrifugation at 2,250 rpm for 1 minute. The supranatant and infranatant are discarded before transferring the fat graft into 1-cc syringes.
- Fractionated fat is used for periorbital injections. Fat is processed via mechanical emulsification by pushing centrifuged fat between two 10-cc syringes through a 2-mm filter 60 to 80 times. This results in fragmentation of adipose tissue structure.

35.2 Operative Steps

- Temporal and forehead fat grafting addresses age-related hollowing and has the added benefit of mildly lifting the brows.
- Temporal injection is performed using a single port access within the temporal hairline. The key principle is disrupting the temporal fusion line to allow uniform fill. This typically requires 1 cc of fat graft. Another 1 cc injection is then needed to correct the hollowing in a radial fashion just lateral to the lateral brow.

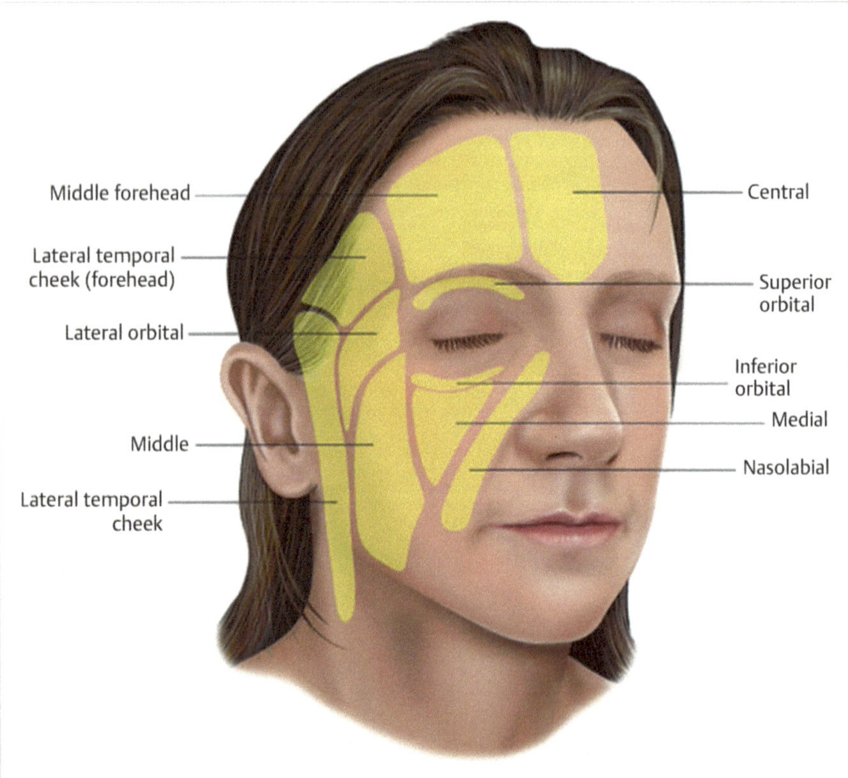

Fig. 35.1 Superficial fat compartments of the face. (Reproduced with permission from Leatherbarrow B, ed. Oculoplastic Surgery. 3rd ed. Thieme; 2019.)

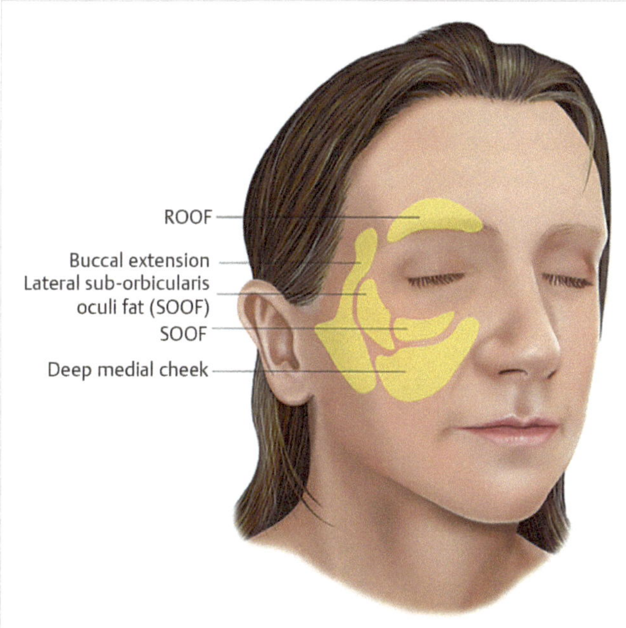

Fig. 35.2 The deep fat compartments of the face. ROOF, retro-orbicularis oculi (muscle) fat; SOOF, lateral sub-orbicularis oculi fat. (Reproduced with permission from Leatherbarrow B, ed. Oculoplastic Surgery. 3rd ed. Thieme; 2019.)

- The central forehead injections must correct three distinct compartments—the glabella and the two superior brow regions. Injection is performed in the subcutaneous plane using a port either in a crease in the mid-forehead for those with a tall forehead, or in the hairline for those with a shorter forehead.
- Injection of the superior brow regions not only corrects age-related changes, but also creates the illusion of more lifted brows. A second stab incision along the medial brow line allows additional access to the superior brow, and disruption of the temporal fusion line from the medial aspect and full correction of temporal hollowing.

35.3 Postoperative Care

Postprocedure care is typically minimal. Patients may return to daily activities while avoiding pressure (i.e., eyeglasses) over grafted regions.

35.4 Case Example

This is a 50-year-old female who is 6 months post-op lift and fill facelift with 35 cc of facial fat augmentation—in the temple 2 cc per side, 4 cc in the brow, and a total of 30 cc in her face, i.e., 4 cc in the deep malar compartments and 4 cc in the superficial fat compartments per side (16), 1 cc in each earlobe (2), 2 cc in chin area (4), and 4 cc in peroral area (8 cc) (▶ Fig. 35.3a–e).

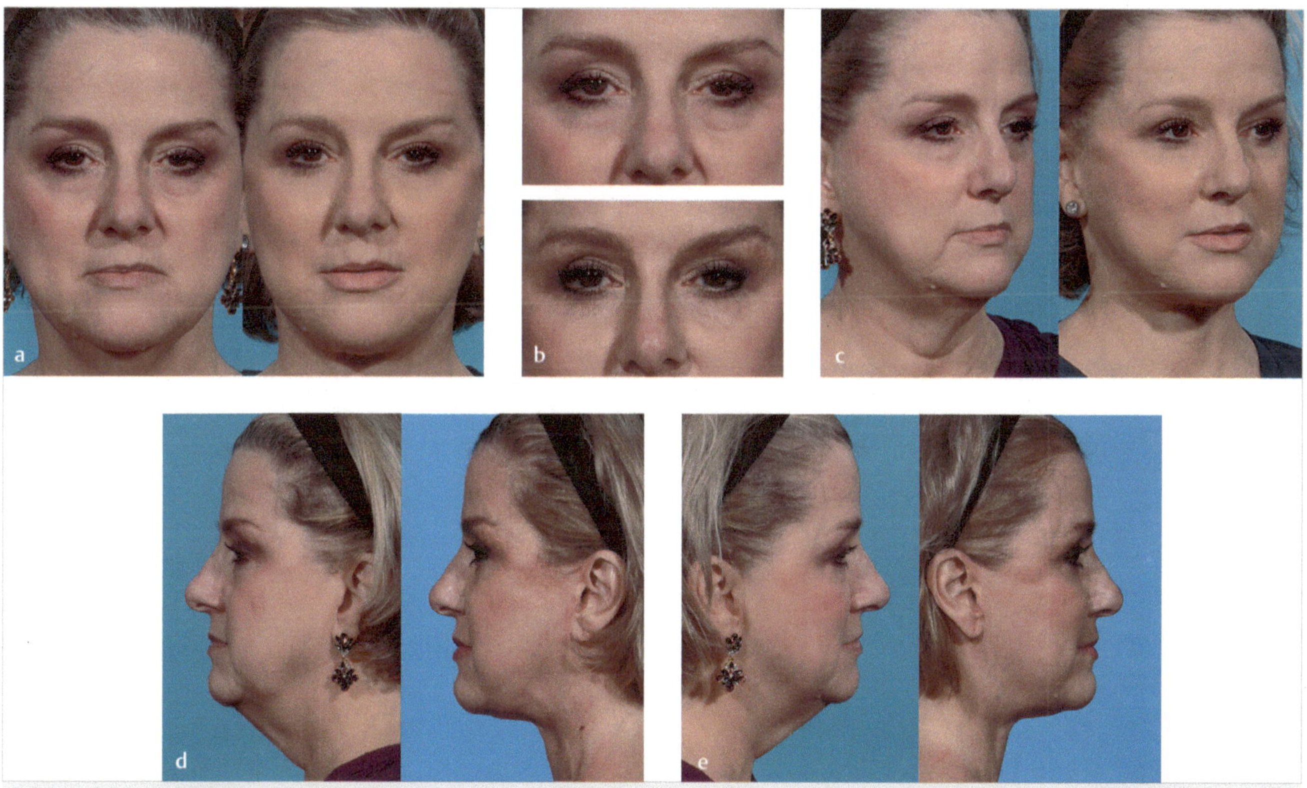

Fig. 35.3 (a–e) This is a 50-year-old female who is 6 months post-op lift and fill facelift with 35 cc of facial fat augmentation—in the temple 2 cc per side, 4 cc in the brow, and a total of 30 cc in her face, i.e., 4 cc in the deep malar compartments and 4 cc in the superficial fat compartments per side (16), 1 cc in each earlobe (2), 2 cc in chin area (4), and 4 cc in peroral area (8 cc).

35.5 Conclusion

Volume restoration with autologous fat of the facial fat compartments is essential to facial rejuvenation. It can be used independently or as an adjunct to rhytidectomy and blepharoplasty. Accurate preoperative facial analysis, knowledge of fat compartment anatomy, and precise intra-operative techniques are needed for successful outcomes. Preoperative bony contour and distribution of fullness dictate the contour and volume of grafting, particularly in the eyebrow, temples, and forehead regions. When used properly, fat augmentation is a powerful tool to ensure optimal restoration to youth.

See **Video 35.1.**

Further Readings

Coleman SR. Facial augmentation with structural fat grafting. Clin Plast Surg. 2006; 33 (4):567–577

Lambros V. Observations on periorbital and midface aging. Plast Reconstr Surg. 2007; 120(5):1367–1376, discussion 1377

Owsley JQ. Lifting the malar fat pad for correction of prominent nasolabial folds. Plast Reconstr Surg. 1993; 91(3):463–474, discussion 475–476

Rohrich RJ, Pessa JE. The fat compartments of the face: anatomy and clinical implications for cosmetic surgery. Plast Reconstr Surg. 2007; 119(7):2219–2227, discussion 2228–2231

Rohrich RJ, Ghavami A, Constantine FC, Unger J, Mojallal A. Lift-and-fill face lift: integrating the fat compartments. Plast Reconstr Surg. 2014; 133(6): 756e–767e

Stuzin JM. Restoring facial shape in face lifting: the role of skeletal support in facial analysis and midface soft-tissue repositioning. Plast Reconstr Surg. 2007; 119(1): 362–376, discussion 377–378

36 Brow and Forehead: Lateral Brow Lift

Thomas A. Mustoe and Sammy Sinno

Abstract

Treatment of the brow is necessary to correct lateral hooding. By lifting the brow in a superior and lateral direction, a tired and aged brow can be rejuvenated. When combined with an upper blepharoplasty, the following technique is very effective and can be performed under local anesthesia.

Keywords: Brow lift, lateral hooding, blepharoplasty, lateral temporal incision, orbital retaining ligament, temporal septum

Key Points

- The width of the area of lateral temporal tissue excision is based on the degree of brow ptosis, approximately a 4:1 ratio (width of tissue excision to expected lateral brow lift) is used.
- Medially, the dissection is in the subperiosteal plane, protecting the supraorbital nerve.
- Laterally, the dissection is deep to the superficial layer of deep temporal fascia (exposing the temporal fat pad), protecting the facial nerve.

36.1 Preoperative Steps

- The procedure is performed via a 4 to 5 cm temporal incision parallel to the brow and 2 to 3 cm posterior to the temporal hairline.
- The width of the scalp excision is planned to effect brow elevation in a 4:1 ratio. Based on this, standard upper blepharoplasty markings are made (▶ Fig. 36.1).
- Scalp incisions allow access to the zones of adhesion.

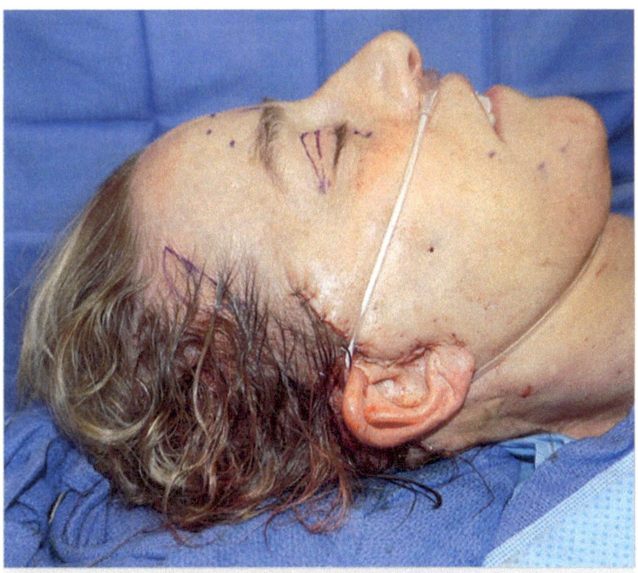

Fig. 36.1 Simplified lateral brow lift markings.

- The upper eyelid approach allows access to the medial brow depressors, lateral temporal area, orbital retaining ligament, and periosteal/galeal attachments.
- Medially, the dissection is in the subperiosteal plane, which protects the supraorbital nerve.
- Laterally, the dissection is deep to the superficial layer of deep temporal fascia (exposing the temporal fat pad) which protects the frontal branch of the facial nerve (▶ Fig. 36.2 and ▶ Fig. 36.3).

36.2 Operative Steps

See **Video 36.1**.

36.2.1 Upper Blepharoplasty Access

- Local anesthesia is infiltrated in all areas of planned dissection.
- The upper blepharoplasty incision is made.
- Medially, the corrugator and procerus are exposed. The corrugator is found deep to the orbicularis oculi.
- A Ragnell retractor can be used to protect the supraorbital artery and nerve.
- The corrugator muscle is divided with fine bipolar cautery.

36.2.2 Lateral Temporal Incision

- A lateral temporal incision is made down to the temporalis fascia.

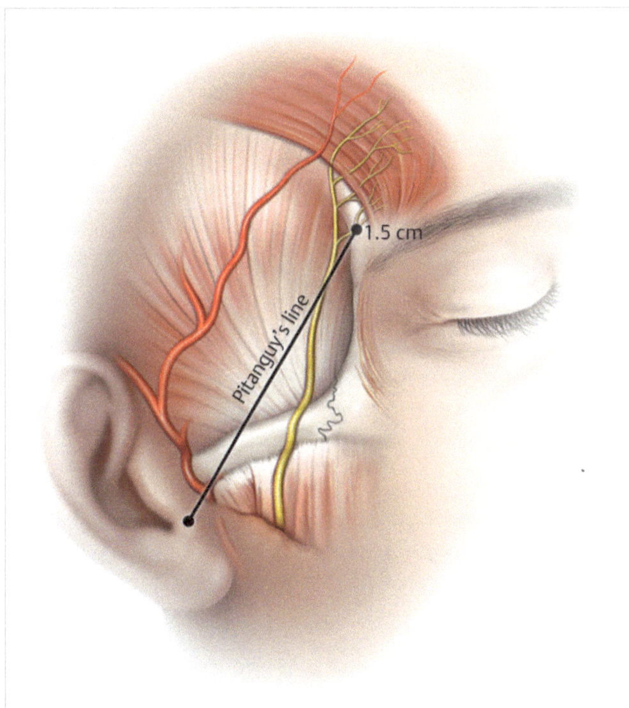

Fig. 36.2 Pitanguy's line is the classic reference line for the general path of the frontal branch within the temporal regions. This landmark is a line from the base of the tragus to 1.5 cm above the eyebrow.

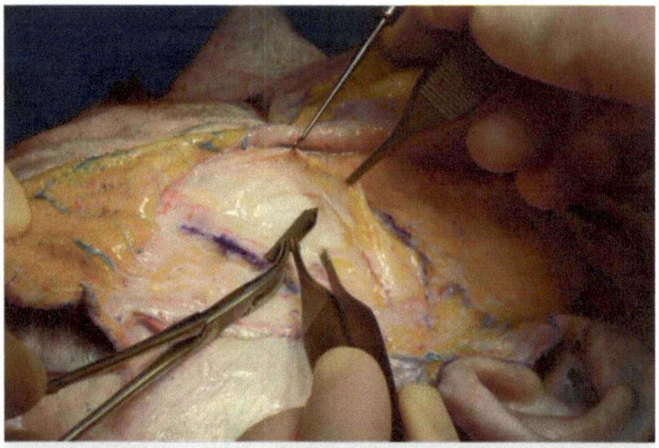

Fig. 36.3 A cadaver dissection demonstrating the frontal branch within the temporal region (*arrow*). The superficial fascia (superficial musculoaponeurotic system [SMAS]) invests the superficial temporal artery, while deep to the SMAS (in the plane between superficial and deep fascia) is the loose areolar layer, termed subaponeurotic fascia, which contains sub-SMAS fat. The frontal nerve branches are situated in the subaponeurotic plane invested in the sub-SMAS fat.

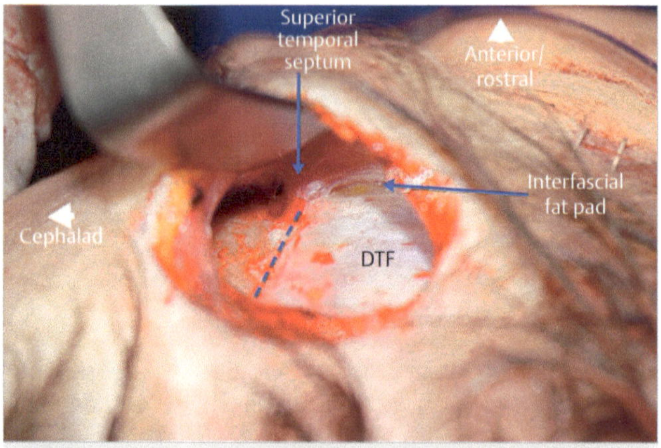

Fig. 36.4 Temporal dissection. Continuity of the cephalad subperiosteal dissection plane and caudal dissection on top of the deep temporal fascia (DTF) is attained by dividing superior temporal septum. Dashed blue line indicates the superior temporal line.

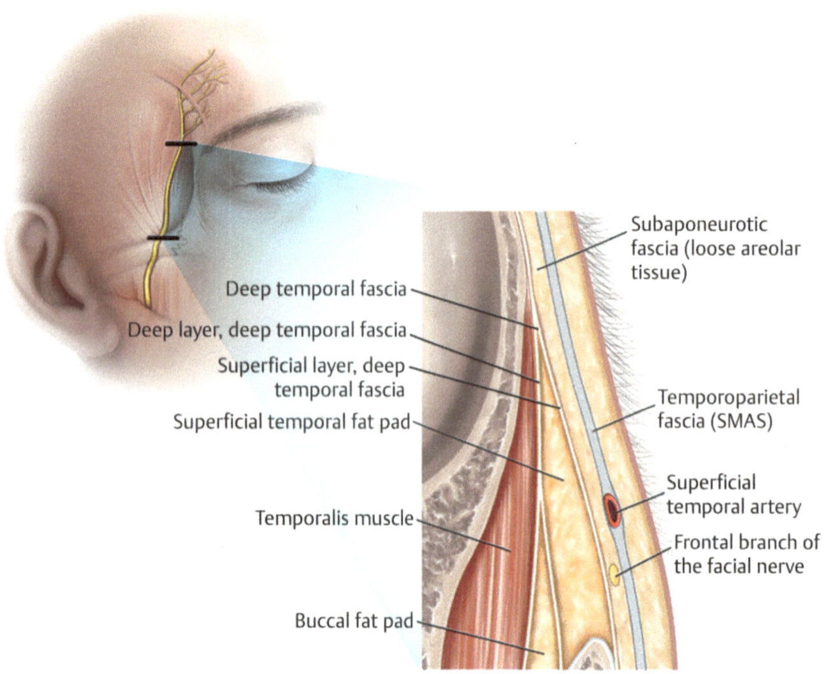

Fig. 36.5 A cross section of the temporal region illustrated in the region between the superior orbital rim and the zygomatic arch. The key to safety when operating in the temporal region is to dissect either superficial or deep to the plane of the frontal branch.

- Dissection is carried out above the deep temporal fascia caudal to the superior temporal septum (▶ Fig. 36.4).
- Cephalad to the septum, dissection is performed inferomedially in a subperiosteal plane toward the superior lateral orbital rim.
- The temporal septum is released joining the two dissection planes.
- Next, the deep layer of deep temporal fascia is incised, thereby exposing the temporal fat pad (▶ Fig. 36.5).
- The entire forehead is undermined in the subperiosteal plane to allow for optimal redraping.

36.2.3 Ligamentous Release

- Attention is turned back to the blepharoplasty incision, where the lateral superior orbital rim periosteum is incised.
- Subperiosteal dissection in the cephalic direction to the level of the lateral canthal tendon releases the lateral orbital thickening (▶ Fig. 36.6).

- The fat pad may be visualized in this area.
- Superomedially, the dissection in this plane releases the orbital retaining ligament and supraorbital ligamentous adhesions.
- Continuity between the temporal and upper blepharoplasty subperiosteal dissection planes is achieved (▶ Fig. 36.7).

36.2.4 Fixation

- Two 3-0 PDS sutures are placed to secure the galea to the mobilized periosteum/superficial temporal fascia layer.

36.2.5 Skin Removal

- The excess skin is excised, approximately 1 to 1.5 cm.
- Staples are used for skin closure.

36.3 Postoperative Care

- The senior author does not use any drains and no compression wrap is needed.
- Patients can shower in 2 days.
- Ice can be applied to the incisions for 3 to 5 days.
- Staples are removed in 7 days.
- Aquaphor is applied to the incisions twice daily for 2 weeks.

36.4 Case Example

Preoperative and postoperative photos of a 51-year-old woman at 1-year follow-up after upper and lower blepharoplasty and lateral brow lift bilaterally (▶ Fig. 36.8).

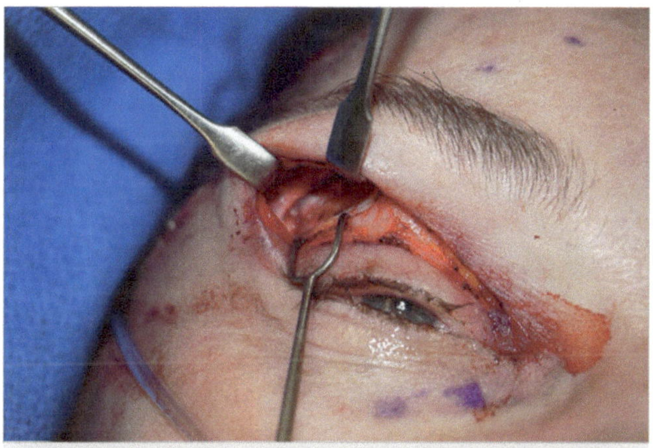

Fig. 36.6 Lateral upper blepharoplasty dissection. Subperiosteal dissection is performed and the lateral orbital thickening is released.

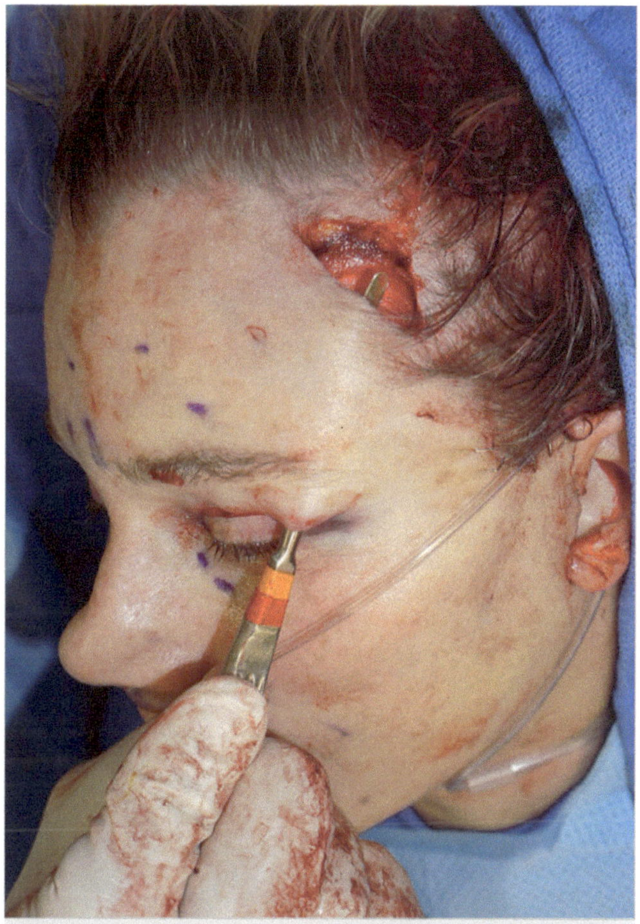

Fig. 36.7 Continuity between the temporal and upper blepharoplasty subperiosteal dissection planes is demonstrated.

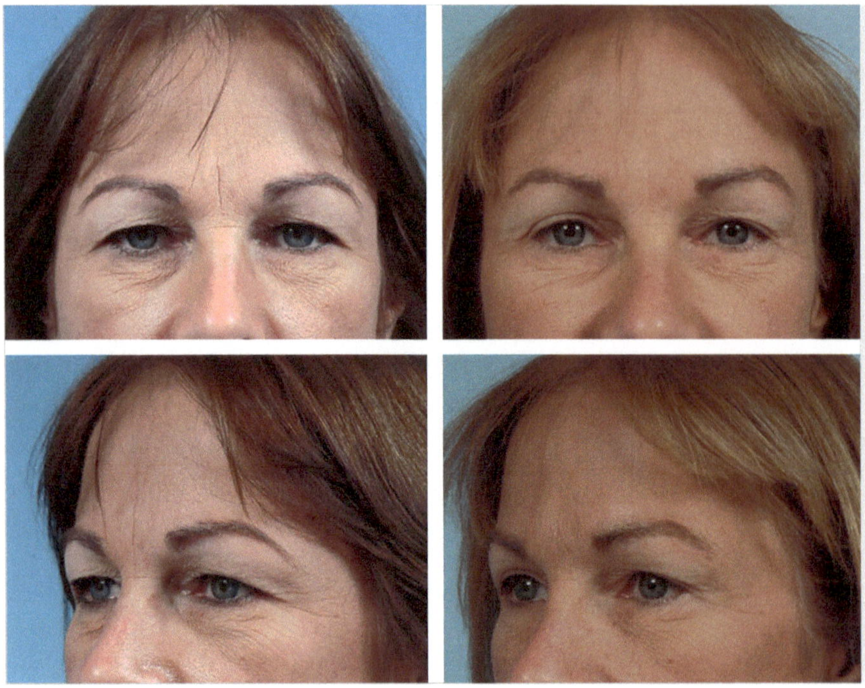

Fig. 36.8 Preoperative and postoperative photos of a 51-year-old woman at 1-year follow-up after upper and lower blepharoplasty and lateral brow lift bilaterally.

36.5 Conclusion

This procedure is a comprehensive treatment for lateral brow hooding and can be performed under local anesthesia. The results are natural and reliable in the long term using a combined lateral and upper blepharoplasty approach.

Further Readings

Codner MA, Kikkawa DO, Korn BS, Pacella SJ. Blepharoplasty and brow lift. Plast Reconstr Surg. 2010; 126(1):1e–17e

Drolet BC, Phillips BZ, Hoy EA, Chang J, Sullivan PK. Finesse in forehead and brow rejuvenation: modern concepts, including endoscopic methods. Plast Reconstr Surg. 2014; 134(6):1141–1150

Knize DM. Anatomic concepts for brow lift procedures. Plast Reconstr Surg. 2009; 124(6):2118–2126

Turin SY, Vaca EE, Cheesborough JE, Sinno S, Mustoe TA. Simplified lateral brow lift under local anesthesia for correction of lateral hooding. Plast Reconstr Surg Glob Open. 2019; 7(6):e2098

Warren RJ. The modified lateral brow lift. Aesthet Surg J. 2009; 29(2):158–166

37 Brow and Forehead: Subcutaneous Temporal Brow Lift

Sammy Sinno and Charles H. Thorne

Abstract

For patients with thin skin and lateral brow ptosis, a subcutaneous temporal brow lift employing a zig-zag hairline incision is an extremely effective technique to improve brow position and shape.

Keywords: Brow ptosis, temporal brow lift, zig-zag incision, brow laxity, subcutaneous dissection

Key Points

- This technique does not address the medial brow. Most patients require lateral brow elevation only.
- The ideal candidate is one with significant brow laxity and thin skin.
- The forehead skin is redraped in the vertical direction along the incision, making sure to preserve the zig-zag nature of the closure.

37.1 Preoperative Steps

- The ideal patient is an elderly patient with Fitzpatrick skin type I or II.
- The procedure is performed via a zig-zag incision along the vertical portion of the temporal hairline. The technique requires excision of dog-ears along the transverse portion of the temporal hairline and along a portion of the frontal hairline (▶ Fig. 37.1).
- The technique does not address the medial brow.
- The goal is to elevate the lateral brow to a level approximately equal to that of the medial brow.
- Elevating the medial brow necessitates an even greater degree of lateral brow elevation to achieve an aesthetically pleasing brow shape.
- The technique is often performed in combination with standard upper blepharoplasty.
- If a facelift is performed concomitantly, the brow and face incisions are not continuous unless a prehairline incision is used for the face.

37.1.1 Temporal Access and Dissection

- Local anesthesia is infiltrated in all areas of planned dissection.
- After 10 minutes, a #15 blade is used to make the zig-zag incision.
- The skin and subcutaneous tissue are raised off the superficial surface of the frontalis muscle for several centimeters using a #10 blade.
- When convenient, a lighted retractor is inserted, and the dissection is continued inferiorly to the region of the brow using scissors.
- Dissection is lateral to the supraorbital nerve branches.
- The elevation is complete when the entire lateral brow is freely mobile. Typically, dissection just below the lateral brow is required (▶ Fig. 37.2).

37.1.2 Skin Redraping

- The forehead skin is redraped in a vertical direction along the vertical portion of the temporal hairline.
- The excess skin is excised along with dog-ears along the frontal hairline and horizontal portion of the temporal hairline, taking care to preserve the zig-zag nature of the incision/closure (▶ Fig. 37.3).

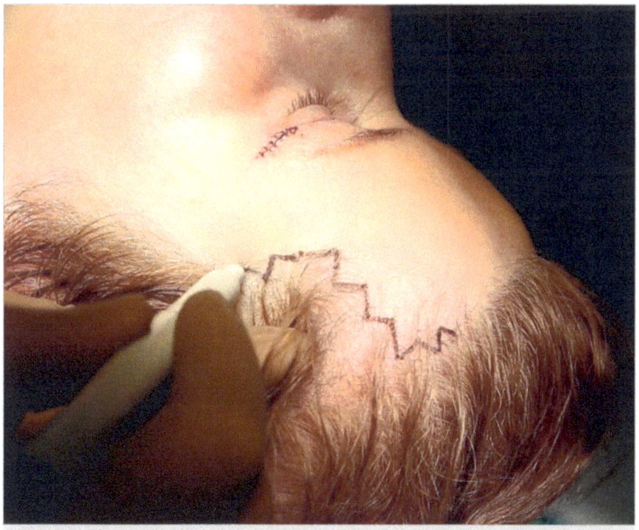

Fig. 37.1 Incision markings.

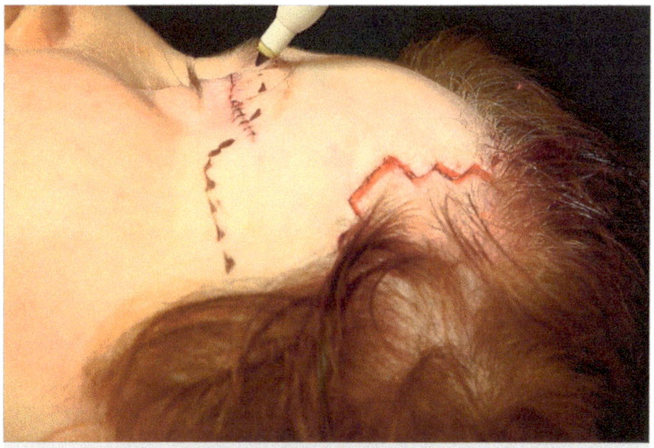

Fig. 37.2 Extent of dissection (*dashed black line*).

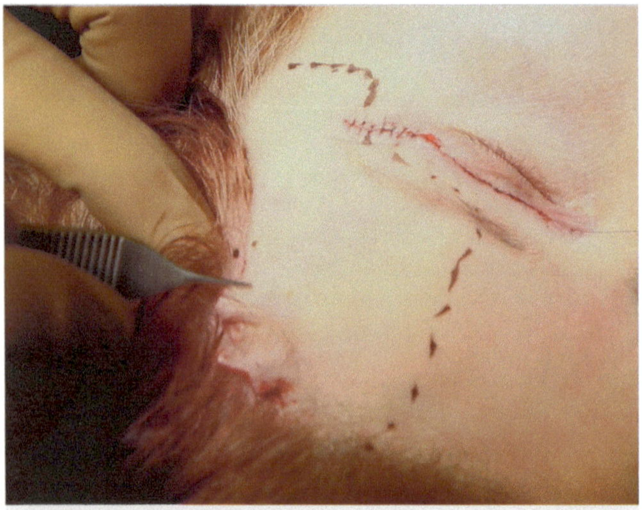

Fig. 37.3 Redraping of skin.

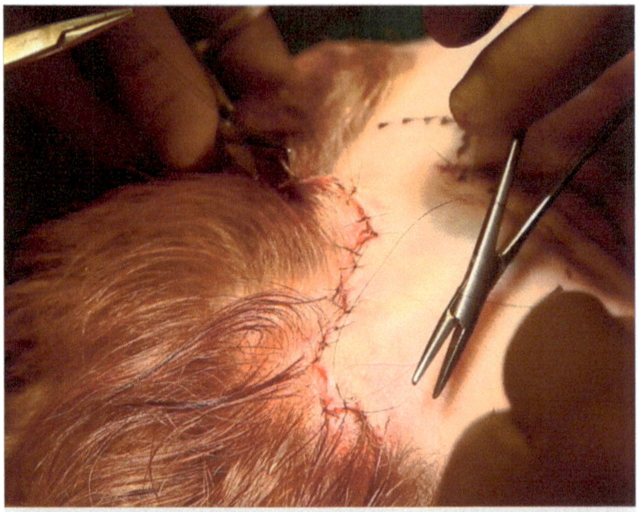

Fig. 37.4 Closure.

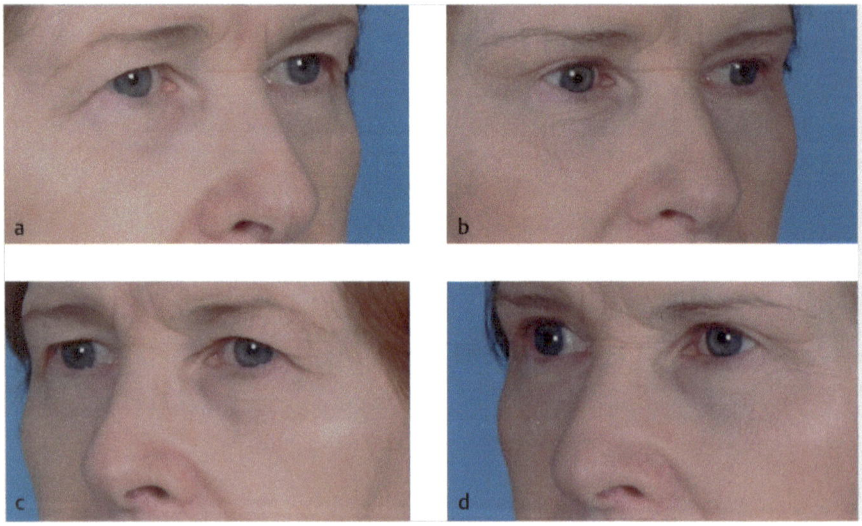

Fig. 37.5 (a, c) Preoperative and (b, d) postoperative photos of a 68-year-old patient 1 year following the subcutaneous temporal brow lift technique.

37.1.3 Closure

- A 7 mm Jackson-Pratt (JP) drain is placed through a posteriorly placed stab incision in the hair and is frequently removed before the patient leaves the facility an hour or two later.
- The closure is performed using only 5–0 nylon sutures (▸ Fig. 37.4).

37.2 Postoperative Care

- Every other suture is removed after 4 to 5 days with the remainder removed in 7 days.
- Silicone ointment can be used on the incisions for the first 6 to 9 months.

37.3 Case Example

Preoperative and postoperative photos of a 68-year-old patient 1 year following the subcutaneous temporal brow lift technique (▸ Fig. 37.5).

37.4 Conclusion

Since the point of fixation is close to the lateral brow, this procedure is an effective technique for lateral brow elevation. The best candidates are those who have significant brow laxity and thin skin, which is unlikely to develop significant scars.

See **Video 37.1.**

Further Readings

Bidros RS, Salazar-Reyes H, Friedman JD. Subcutaneous temporal browlift under local anesthesia: a useful technique for periorbital rejuvenation. Aesthet Surg J. 2010; 30(6):783–788

Connell BF, Lambros VS, Neurohr GH. The forehead lift: techniques to avoid complications and produce optimal results. Aesthetic Plast Surg. 1989; 13(4): 217–237

Miller TA. Lateral subcutaneous brow lift. Aesthet Surg J. 2003; 23(3):205–210

Ullmann Y, Levy Y. In favor of the subcutaneous forehead lift using the anterior hairline incision. Aesthetic Plast Surg. 1998; 22(5):332–337

Wolfe SA, Baird WL. The subcutaneous forehead lift. Plast Reconstr Surg. 1989; 83(2):251–256

Part IV

Otoplasty

IV

38 Otoplasty

Sammy Sinno, Joshua M. Cohen, and Charles H. Thorne

Abstract

Prominent ears and other ear deformities affect over 10% of the general population. For most patients with prominent ears, otoplasty provides consistent results. Excessively large ears or ears with undesirable contours (Stahl's ears, underdeveloped helical rims, etc.) will require additional maneuvers.

Keywords: Otoplasty, prominent ears, conchal setback, antihelical fold, auricular cartilage

Key Points

- Assessment of the ear should be performed in thirds and not all patients will require surgical modification of all "thirds."
- Soft tissue must be removed from deep to the concha to facilitate conchal setback.
- Placement of Mustarde sutures is important to help with upper third setback and creation of an antihelical fold.

38.1 Preoperative Steps

- Each third of the ear is assessed for prominence (upper, middle, and lower) (▶ Fig. 38.1 and ▶ Fig. 38.2).
- Not all patients will require surgical modification of all three "thirds" of the auricle.
- The procedure is performed under local anesthesia in adults and adolescents and general anesthesia in children.

38.1.1 Incision and Exposure

- An incision is made in the retroauricular sulcus.
- The medial surface of the auricular cartilage is exposed.
- Soft tissue is removed from deep to the concha to facilitate conchal setback.
- A triangle of skin is excised from the medial surface of the lobule in anticipation of lobular setback.

38.1.2 Combination of Small Conchal Excision and Setback

- A crescent of cartilage of no more than 3 mm is excised from the concha at the junction of the floor and the posterior wall.
- The conchal defect is approximated with PDS sutures.
- A conchal mastoid suture of 3–0 PDS is placed (▶ Fig. 38.3).

38.1.3 Lobule Repositioning

- Soft tissue is removed from the retrolobular sulcus to expose the caudal aspect of the concha.
- Three sutures of 5–0 PDS are used to not only approximate the skin but also include a bite of cartilage on the deep surface of the concha in order to correct lobular prominence.

38.1.4 Upper Third Setback and Creation of Antihelical Fold

- A series of mattress sutures of 4–0 clear nylon are placed between the scapha and the concha and between the scapha and triangular fossa, beginning caudally and progressing toward the upper third of the auricle (Mustarde sutures) (▶ Fig. 38.4).
- Some patients will require one to two sutures in the upper third while others will require six to seven sutures in the middle and upper thirds.

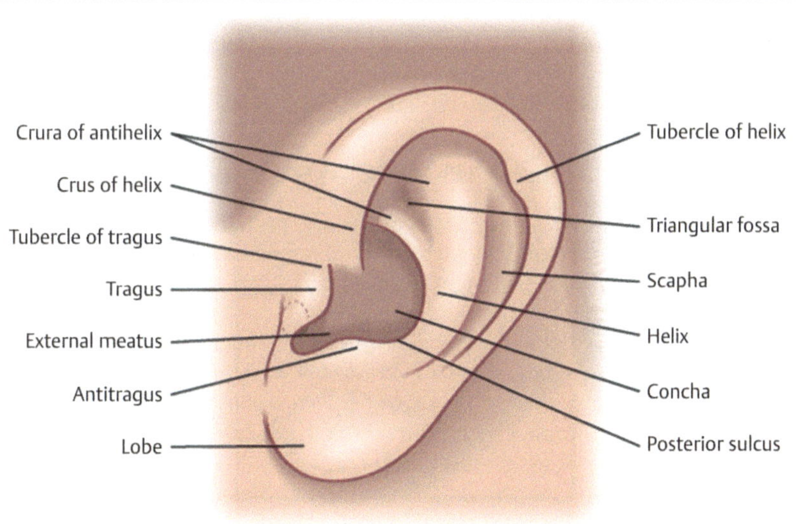

Fig. 38.1 Landmarks of an aesthetic ear. (Reproduced with permission from Mesa J, Buchman S, Mackay D, et al, eds. Atlas of Operative Craniofacial Surgery. 1st ed. Thieme; 2019.)

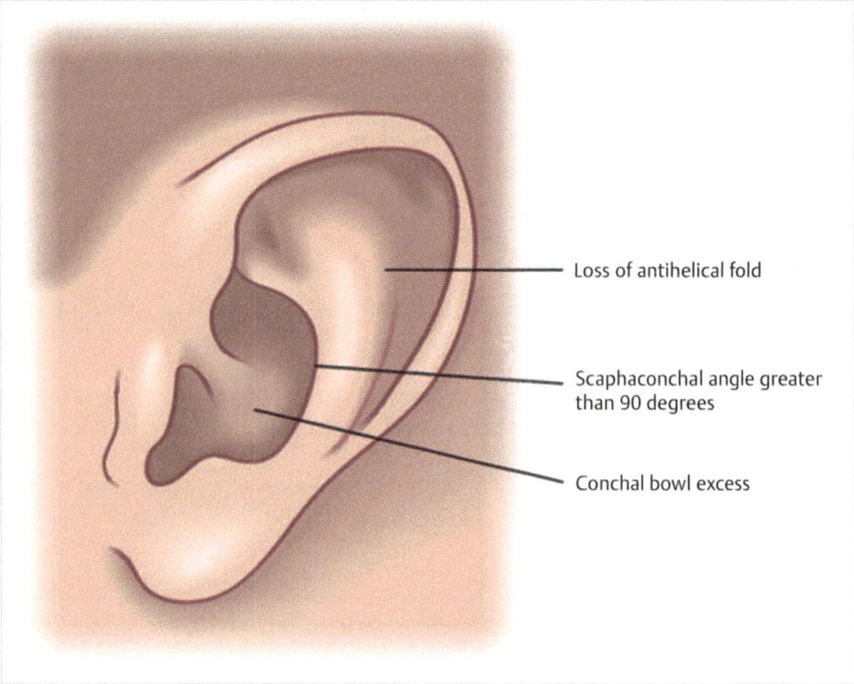

Fig. 38.2 Morphology and proportions of the prominent ear. (Reproduced with permission from Mesa J, Buchman S, Mackay D, et al, eds. Atlas of Operative Craniofacial Surgery. 1st ed. Thieme; 2019.)

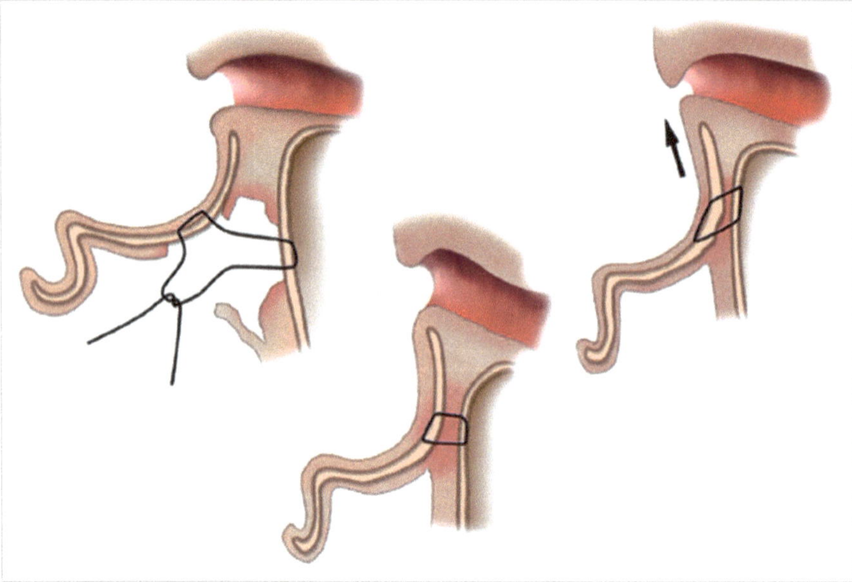

Fig. 38.3 Conchal mastoid sutures to correct conchal excess. (Reproduced with permission from Pu L, ed. Aesthetic Plastic Surgery in Asians: Principles & Techniques. 1st ed. Thieme; 2015.)

38.1.5 Hatch-Hitch

- For patients in whom the angle created by the temporal scalp and the ascending helix is excessively large, a 1.5 cm incision is made at the cranial end of the retroauricular sulcus and a 3–0 PDS suture is placed between the temporalis fascia and the cartilage in the ascending helix.

38.1.6 Lateral Incision

- For patients who require scapha reduction to shorten the ear or an increase in helical rim definition, a lateral incision is added just inside the helical rim.

38.2 Postoperative Care

- A soft, bulky dressing is wrapped as loosely as possible around the patient's head.
- The dressing is removed 3 to 5 days later.
- No sutures require removal.
- The patient may shower and shampoo after the dressing is removed and is instructed to wash in the retroauricular sulcus with a soapy Q-tip when showering.
- Some patients feel more secure with a headband for a week or so, but this is not required.
- If the patients insist on wearing a headband, they are cautioned that headbands should be as loose as possible without falling off.

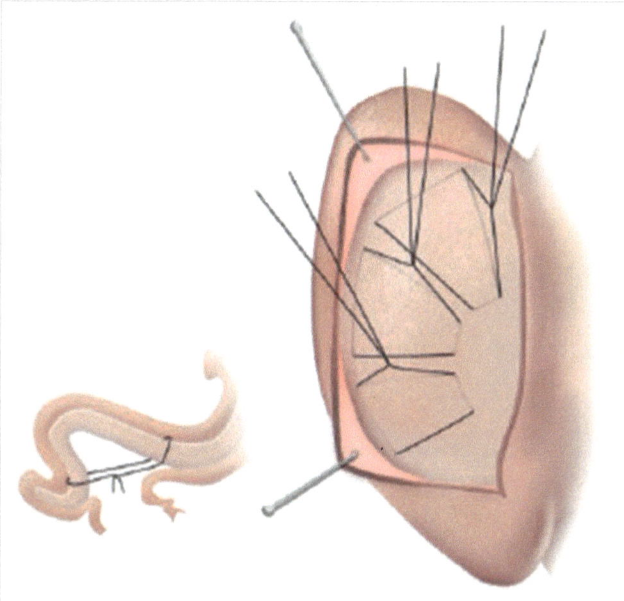

Fig. 38.4 Mustarde mattress suture technique to create the antihelical fold. (Reproduced with permission from Pu L, ed. Aesthetic Plastic Surgery in Asians: Principles & Techniques. 1st ed. Thieme; 2015.)

38.3 Case Example

Preoperative and postoperative photos of a patient 2 months following the otoplasty technique in (a) preoperative anteroposterior (AP), (b) preoperative oblique, (c) preoperative lateral, (d) postoperative posteroanterior (PA), (e) postoperative oblique, (f) postoperative lateral, and (g) postoperative close up PA views (▶ Fig. 38.5a–g).

38.4 Conclusion

One of the most critical aspects of the procedure is judging the endpoint; the helical rim should be a straight line when viewed from posterior. This technique will result in an occasional undercorrection but will rarely result in an overcorrection. Skin excision, except as described for lobule repositioning, is usually not necessary except in cases of extreme setback where redundant skin is unsightly. Some patients may return with protruding clear nylon sutures that require removal. This may occur months to years later.

See **Video 38.1.**

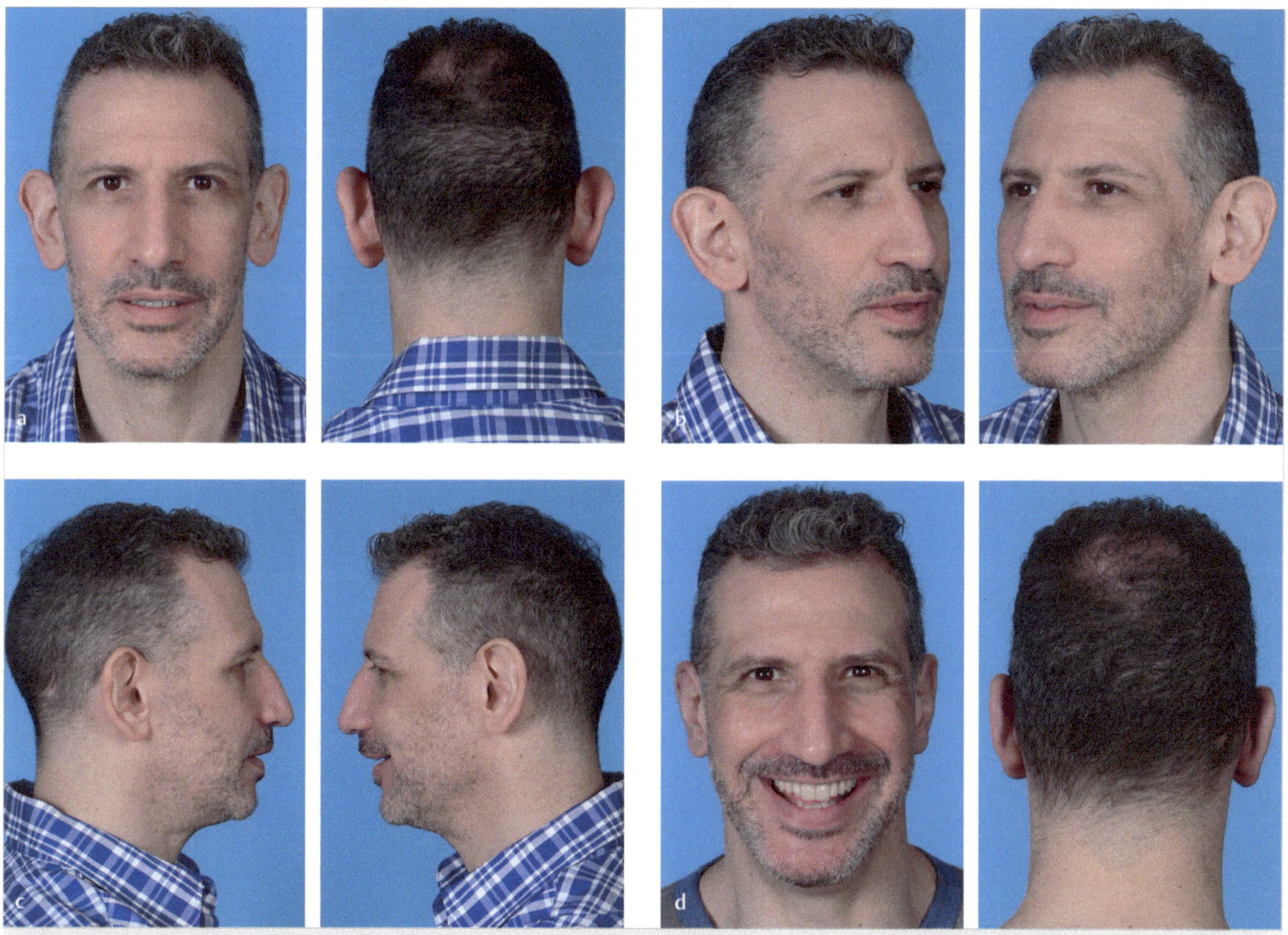

Fig. 38.5 Preoperative and postoperative photos of a patient 2 months following the otoplasty technique in **(a)** preoperative anteroposterior (AP), **(b)** preoperative oblique, **(c)** preoperative lateral, **(d)** postoperative posteroanterior (PA),

(Continued)

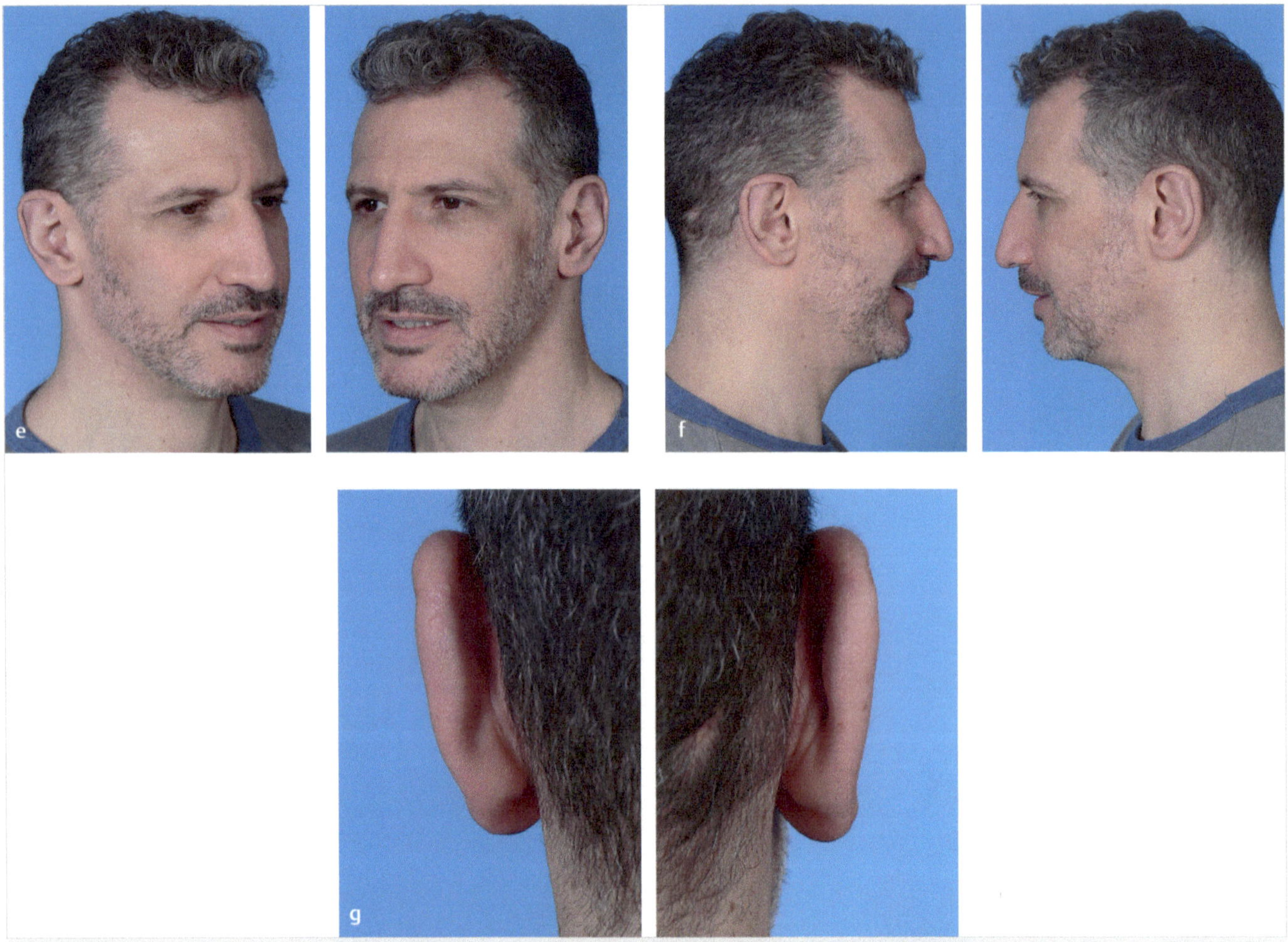

Fig. 38.5 (*Continued*) **(e)** postoperative oblique, **(f)** postoperative lateral, and **(g)** postoperative close up PA views.

Further Readings

Janis JE, Rohrich RJ, Gutowski KA. Otoplasty. Plast Reconstr Surg. 2005; 115(4): 60e–72e

Pawar SS, Koch CA, Murakami C. Treatment of prominent ears and otoplasty: a contemporary review. JAMA Facial Plast Surg. 2015; 17(6):449–454

Sinno S, Chang JB, Thorne CH. Precision in otoplasty: combining reduction otoplasty with traditional otoplasty. Plast Reconstr Surg. 2015; 135(5):1342–1348

Thorne CH. Otoplasty. Plast Reconstr Surg. 2008; 122(1):291–292

Thorne CH, Wilkes G. Ear deformities, otoplasty, and ear reconstruction. Plast Reconstr Surg. 2012; 129(4):701e–716e

39 Otoplasty with Anterior Scoring

Ira L. Savetsky, Yash J. Avashia, and H. Steve Byrd

Abstract

Prominent ears and other ear deformities are quite common. Understanding the underlying anatomy and associated anatomical anomalies causing ear deformities will help guide surgical technique. Otoplasty procedures aim to restore an abnormal appearing ear into a natural appearing ear without evidence of surgical intervention.

Keywords: Otoplasty, prominent ears, ear deformity, conchal excess, antihelical fold, conchoscaphal angle, conchal-mastoid sutures

Key Points

- A thorough understanding of the anatomy of the normal and prominent ears is key to correct and precise analysis of ear deformities.
- Otoplasty techniques aim to correct ear deformities without evidence of surgical intervention.

39.1 Anatomy

- The ear is a composite of cartilage and skin with five key elements—concha, helix, antihelix, tragus, and lobule. Additional structures are antitragus, intertragic notch, and Darwin's tubercle (▶ Fig. 39.1).
- The cartilage of a neonatal ear is softer and more malleable whereas the cartilage become stiffer and more calcified as aging advances.
- The ear is 85% of its adult size by the age of 3 years and reaches its mature size in boys in 7 years and in girls in 6 years.
- Ear length matures in boys in 13 years and in girls in 12 years.
- The vascular supply to the ear is from branches of the external carotid artery, primarily the posterior auricular and the superficial temporal arteries.
- Innervation of the ear is supplied by the anterior and posterior branches of the great auricular nerve, the auriculotemporal nerve, and branches of the vagus and glossopharyngeal nerves.

39.2 Anatomy of the Prominent Ear

- Conchal hypertrophy or excess.
- Inadequate antihelical fold.
- Conchoscaphal angle greater than 90 degrees.
- Combination of conchal hypertrophy and underdeveloped antihelical fold.
- Cranial abnormalities.
- Lobular protrusion.
- Anterolateral displacement of the tail of the helix.

39.3 Goals of Otoplasty

- All upper third ear protrusion must be corrected.
- The helix of both ears should be seen beyond the antihelix from the front view.
- The helix should have a smooth and regular line throughout.
- The postauricular sulcus should not be markedly decreased or distorted.
- The helix to mastoid distance should fall in the normal range of 10 to 12 mm in the upper third, 16 to 18 mm in the middle third, and 20 to 22 mm in the lower third.
- The position of the lateral ear border of the head should match within 3 mm at any point between the two ears.
- Production of a smooth, rounded, and well-defined antihelical fold.
- A conchoscaphal angle of 90 degrees.
- Conchal reduction or reduction of the conchomastoidal angle.
- Lateral projection of the helical rim beyond the lobule.

39.4 Preoperative Steps

- Age 6 or 7 years is appropriate for surgical correction given that the ear is nearly fully developed.
- Assess the degree of antihelical folding.

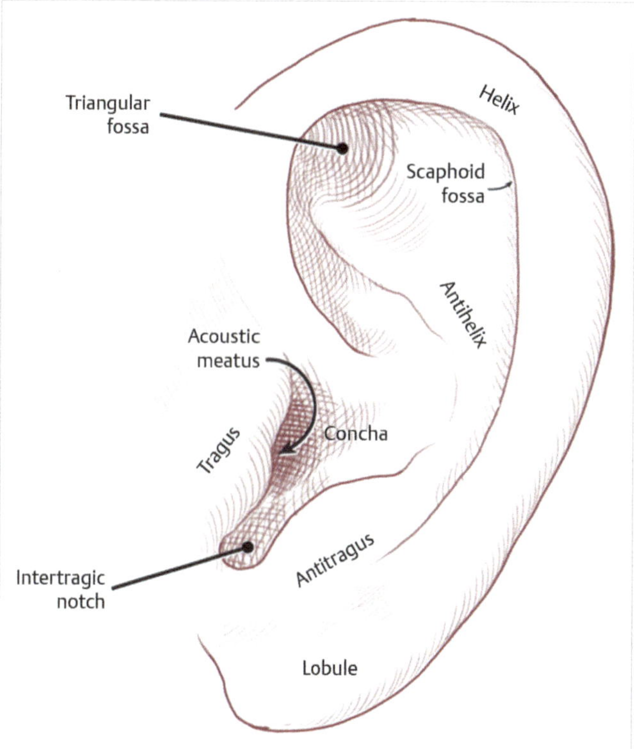

Fig. 39.1 Ear anatomy. (Reproduced with permission from Ali K, Meaike J, Maricevich R, Olshinka A. The Protruding Ear: Cosmetic and Reconstruction. Semin Plast Surg 2017;31(3): 152–160.)

- Assess the depth of the conchal bowl.
- Determine the plane of the lobule and deformity.
- Determine the angle between the helical rim and the mastoid plane.
- Assess the quality and spring of the auricular cartilage.

39.5 Operative Steps

- Measurements and markings (▶ Fig. 39.2):
  - Set vertical height at 7 mm (children of 5–6 years of age).
  - Set vertical height at 9 mm (teenagers/adults).
  - It is important to mark the antihelix in a curvilinear manner.
  - Incision is marked in a curvilinear manner from the inferior to the superior sulcus.
- Skin is incised with a #15 blade.
- Posterior skin flap is elevated in a subcutaneous plane using electrocautery.
- A portion of the posterior auricular muscle is excised to make room for the cymba concha setback.
- Anterior skin flap is elevated in a subcutaneous plane using scissors.
- The anterior cartilage is approached through a window made between the interface of the antitragus and the cavum concha (▶ Fig. 39.3). A traditional anterior approach is performed in select cases (i.e., Stahl's deformity).
- A subperichondrial plane is elevated anteriorly using a small Joseph elevator.
- The anterior cartilage is then scored.
- The cartilage is then fractured, and the malleability of the cartilage is assessed.
- The concha is then incised and elevated using a #15 blade.
- To prevent a telephone deformity, the intertragal cartilage is divided inferiorly and at the root of the helix superiorly.
- Excision of the curved cymba concha is performed.
- Suturing of the concha is performed using a 4–0 clear nylon from the mastoid fascia to the concha.
- The soft tissue is then sutured over the cartilage using a 5–0 Vicryl suture.
- Horizontal mattress sutures are placed using 4–0 clear nylons to recreate the antihelical fold.
- Concha-mastoid sutures are placed using 4–0 clear nylons to setback the ear.
- Earlobe is setback and sutured down using 5–0 Vicryl suture.
- The skin is redraped and the excess skin is excised.
- Skin closure is performed using 4–0 Vicryl sutures placed in a buried deep dermal fashion.
- Skin glue is then placed over the incision.
- Ear molding is prepared using 1:1 DETAX® addition A and B and allowed to harden followed by placement of EAR BAND-IT®.

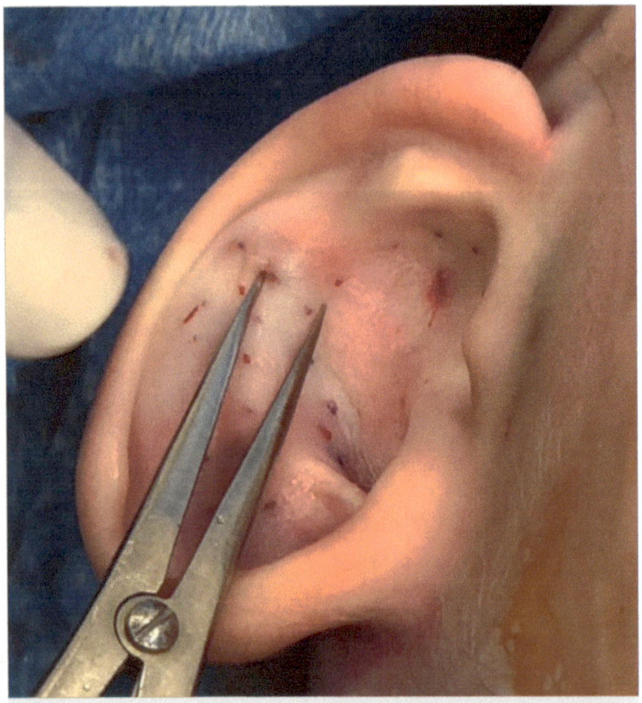

Fig. 39.2 Vertical height is set at 7 mm in children.

39.6 Case Example

A 7-year-old boy presented to the senior author (H. Steve Byrd) with prominent ears. Preoperative (left) anteroposterior (AP), posteroanterior (PA), and lateral views of the patient are shown. Postoperative (right) views at 3-month follow-up are shown (▶ Fig. 39.4a–c).

39.7 Conclusion

A thorough understanding of the anatomy of the normal and prominent ear is crucial for surgical success. The goal of otoplasty is to correct ear deformities without evidence of surgical intervention.

See **Video 39.1.**

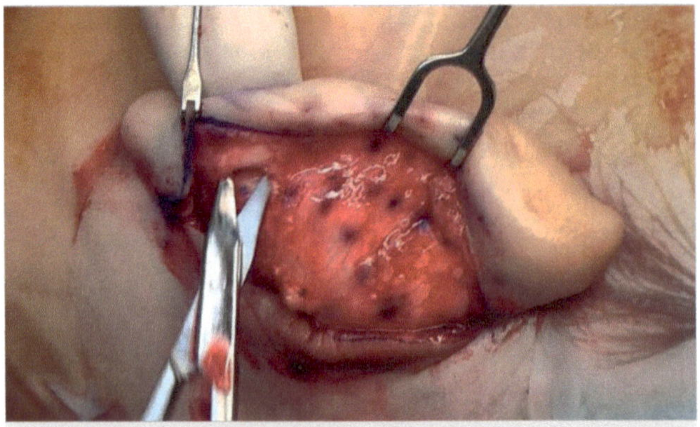

Fig. 39.3 A window is made between the interface of the antitragus and the cavum concha to access the anterior cartilage.

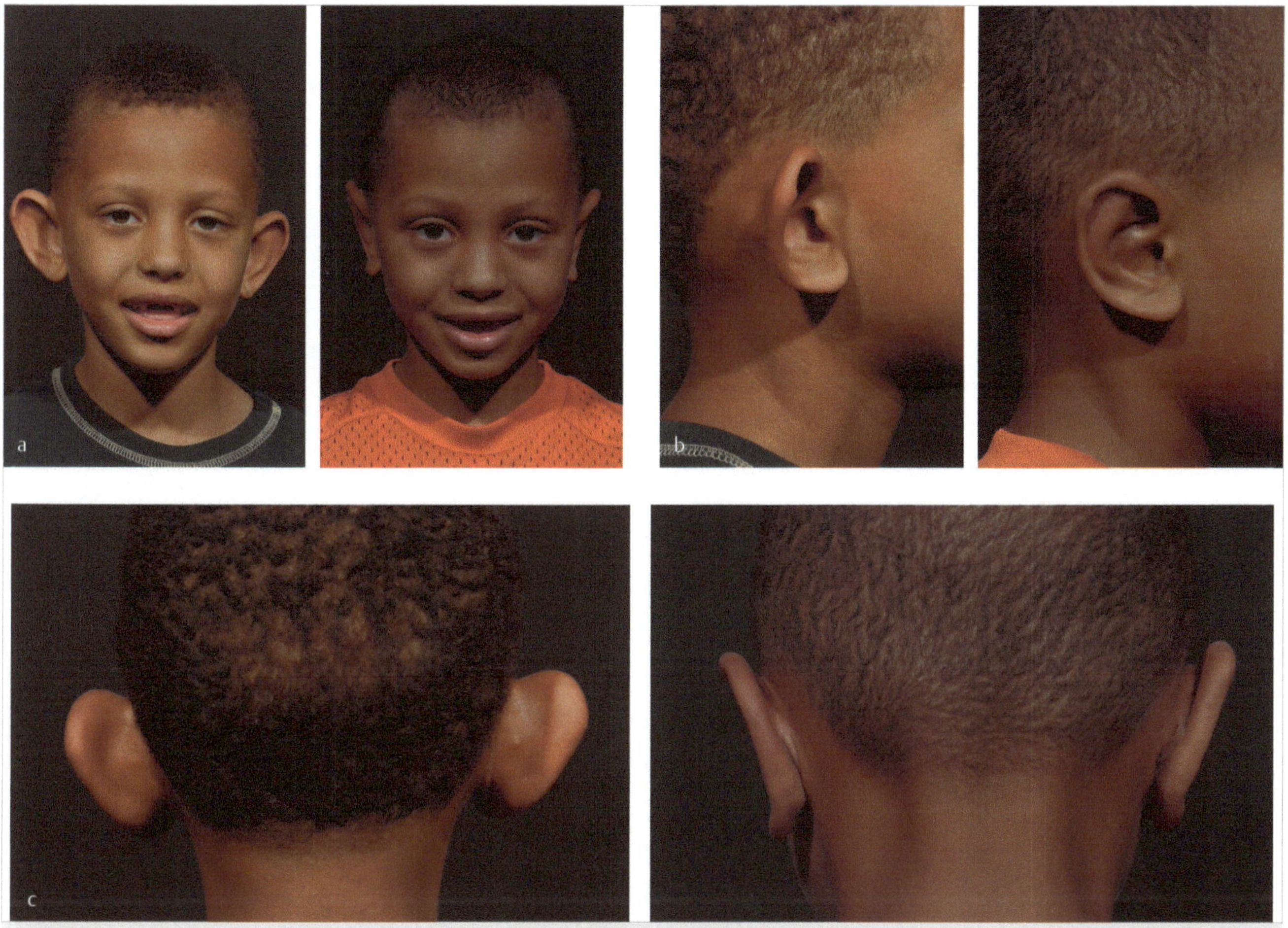

Fig. 39.4 (a–c) A 7-year-old boy presented to the senior author (H. Steve Byrd) with prominent ears. Preoperative (left) anteroposterior (AP), posteroanterior (PA), and lateral views of the patient are shown. Postoperative (right) views at 3-month follow-up are shown.

Further Readings

Furnas DW. Otoplasty for prominent ears. Clin Plast Surg. 2002; 29(2):273–288, viii

Janis JE, Rohrich RJ, Gutowski KA. Otoplasty. Plast Reconstr Surg. 2005; 115(4):60e–72e

Thorne CH, Wilkes G. Ear deformities, otoplasty, and ear reconstruction. Plast Reconstr Surg. 2012; 129(4):701e–716e

Tuncer S, Demir Y, Atabay K. A simple surgical technique for correction of macrotia with poorly defined helical fold. Aesthetic Plast Surg. 2010; 34(2):136–140

Yuen A, Coombs CJ. Reduction otoplasty: correction of the large or asymmetric ear. Aesthetic Plast Surg. 2006; 30(6):675–678

Part V

Perioral Rejuvenation

V

40 Lip Lift

Rod J. Rohrich, Stephanie E. Farber, and Paul N. Afrooz

Abstract

Perioral aesthetics play a central role in creating a youthful facial appearance. For this reason, interest in perioral rejuvenation has been growing. Lip lift is a surgical procedure intended to decrease lip ptosis, increase eversion of the vermilion, and increase incisal show—all characteristics of a youthful periorbital region. The operation involves the excision of a strip of skin and muscle just inferior to the nose at the superior-most aspect of the upper lip. This intervention effectively rotates and raises the upper lip for an improved facial aesthetic. Here, we characterize the appearance of a youthful lip and perioral region and discuss technical variations of the lip lift procedure.

Keywords: Lip, lip lift, periorbital rejuvenation, facial aging, facial rejuvenation, lip augmentation

Key Points

- The periorbital region is not adequately addressed by other commonly performed surgical or nonsurgical procedures that aim to create a more youthful appearance.
- Lip lift is a surgical procedure intended to treat periorbital aging by decreasing upper lip ptosis, increasing vermilion eversion, and increasing incisal show.
- Noninvasive procedures such as lip augmentation and skin resurfacing can be combined with lip lift to act as a comprehensive perioral rejuvenation strategy.

40.1 Preoperative Steps

40.1.1 Anatomy of the Youthful Lip

- The upper lip aesthetic unit includes the dry vermilion and cutaneous upper lip bordered by the nasal base and nasolabial folds.
- An attractive upper lip subunit is characterized by a short philtrum, a prominent cupid's bow, and a full, everted vermilion.
- Philtral height should be approximately 18 to 20 mm, with an upper lip height of 7 to 8 mm, or about 25% of total upper lip height.
- The upper to lower lip relationship is characterized by an upper lip that protrudes 1 to 2 mm past the lower lip and is 75 to 80% of the volume.
- Other characteristics of the youthful upper lip include a slight superior tilt to the commissure and 1 to 3 mm of incisal show.

40.1.2 Characterizing the Aging Lip

- The aging lip is characterized by elongation of the upper lip, flattening of the vermilion, descent of the commissures, and loss of definition of cupid's bow.
- Patients who have undergone a facelift, necklift, or other facial rejuvenation operation may complain of a persistent, aged appearance that can sometimes be attributed to the lips and perioral region. Therefore, lip procedures can more thoroughly address facial aging.
- Other procedures in the perioral region can impact upper lip aesthetics and result in a more aged appearance. For example, fillers injected into the nasolabial folds and piriform aperture can cause lengthening and stiffening of the upper lip due to the downward push of the filler on the lip tissue.

40.1.3 Determination of Surgical Plan

- A systematic approach can be used to classify senile deformities of the upper lip and determine the best suited interventions by measuring philtral height, labial height, and dental show.
- An abnormal philtral height can be corrected with lip lift, while an abnormal labial height can be corrected with lip augmentation. If both measures are abnormal, a combined procedure should be used.

40.2 Operative Approaches

See **Video 40.1** and **Video 40.2**.

40.2.1 Central Lip Lift

- The central lip lift is performed most commonly.
- Markings are designed in a bull's horn pattern with the superior border drawn just inferior to the columellar base and nostril sill and extending along the alae to the alar-facial grove, allowing for more lift laterally (▶ Fig. 40.1). The inferior border is marked based on the amount of desired tissue excision, keeping in mind the aforementioned aesthetic ideals (lip length, incisal show, etc.) and noting any asymmetries.
- A full-thickness excision is made including skin and subcutaneous tissue with or without partial thickness excision of the orbicularis (▶ Fig. 40.2).

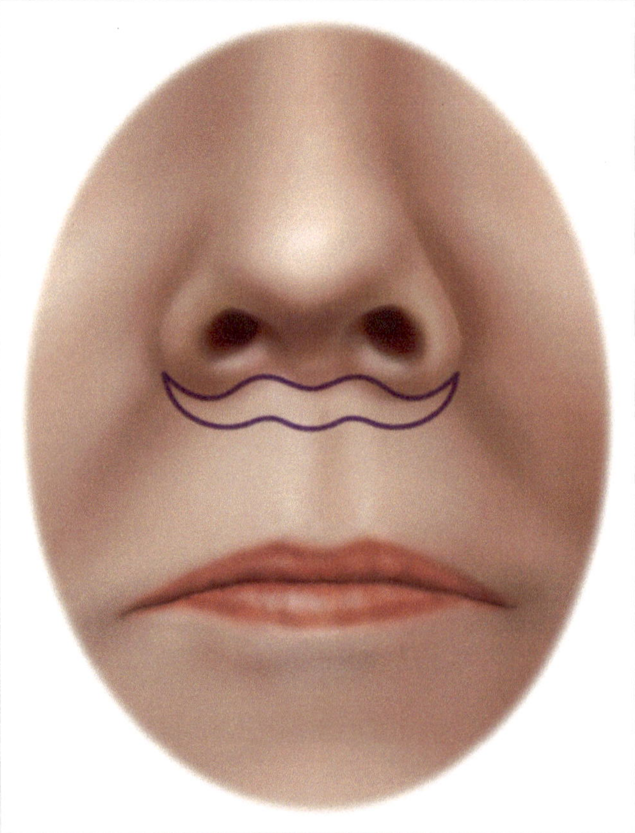

Fig. 40.1 Markings are designed in a bull's horn pattern with the superior border drawn just inferior to the columellar base and nostril sill and extending along the alae to the alae-facial grove, allowing a for more lift laterally.

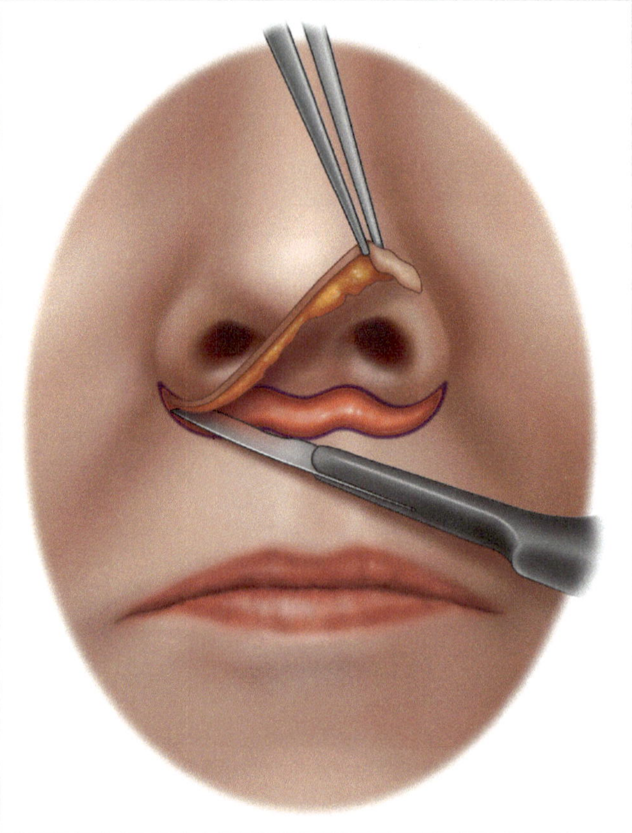

Fig. 40.2 A full-thickness excision is made including skin and subcutaneous tissue with or without partial thickness excision of the orbicularis.

- The incision is closed in layers and any autologous fat or fillers are injected at this time (▸ Fig. 40.3).

40.2.2 Adjunctive Procedures

- Lip resurfacing addresses the radially oriented fine rhytides surrounding the upper and lower lips and can be performed using dermabrasion, laser, or chemical peels.
- Lip augmentation increases lip volume, eversion, and cupid's bow definition and can be performed with autologous materials (i.e., fat grafting) or alloplastic materials (i.e., hyaluronic acid).

40.3 Postoperative Care

- Patients are instructed to maintain head elevation.
- Sutures are removed in 5 to 7 days postoperatively.
- Sun protection and avoidance are critical to maintaining an inconspicuous scar.

40.4 Case Example

Preoperative and postoperative photos of a patient following the lip lift procedure both in repose and smiling (▸ Fig. 40.4a, b).

40.5 Conclusion

Of the noninvasive and invasive procedures that plastic surgeons offer to patients seeking facial rejuvenation, lip lift is the only technique that addresses the philtral lengthening, vermilion inversion, and decreased incisal show that occur with aging.

Lip lift can be combined with skin resurfacing to address upper lip skin changes and lip augmentation to increase vermilion fullness and will thereby serve as a comprehensive perioral rejuvenation strategy.

In a climate in which multiple providers and specialties are able to offer noninvasive interventions for facial rejuvenation, plastic surgeons are uniquely qualified to perform the lip lift operation.

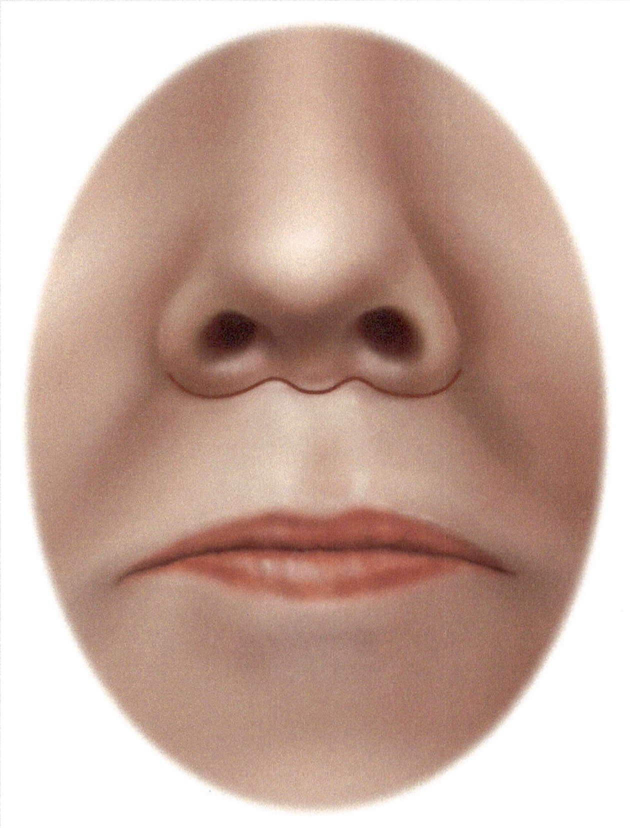

Fig. 40.3 The incision is closed in layers and any autologous fat or fillers are injected at this time.

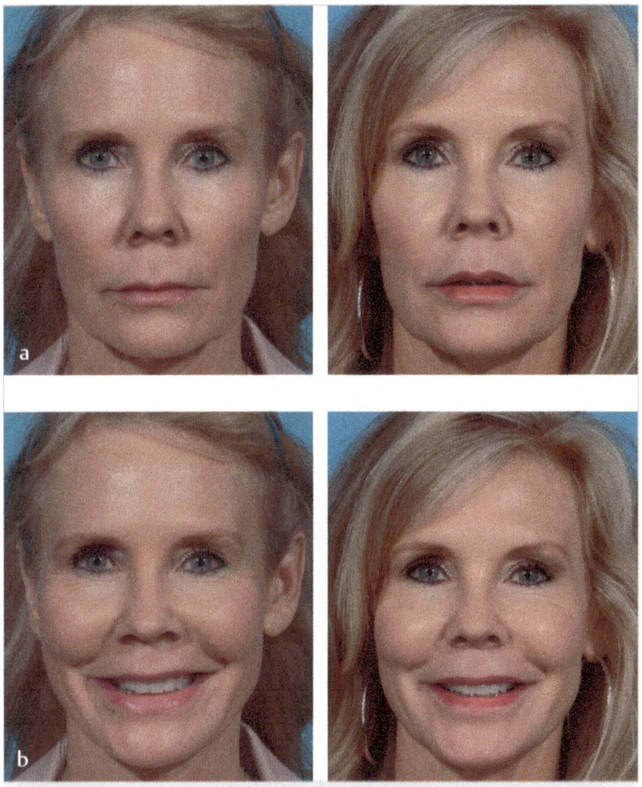

Fig. 40.4 **(a)** Preoperative and **(b)** postoperative photos of a patient following the lip lift procedure both in repose and smiling.

Limitations of the lip lift include its preferential impact on the central two-thirds of the upper lift and inability to significantly raise the commissures. Patients should be counseled preoperatively about these limitations.

Further Readings

Austin HW. The lip lift. Plast Reconstr Surg. 1986; 77(6):990–994

Haworth RD. Customizing perioral enhancement to obtain ideal lip aesthetics: combining both lip voluming and reshaping procedures by means of an algorithmic approach. Plast Reconstr Surg. 2004; 113(7):2182–2193

Lee DE, Hur SW, Lee JH, Kim YH, Seul JH. Central lip lift as aesthetic and physiognomic plastic surgery: the effect on lower facial profile. Aesthet Surg J. 2015; 35(6):698–707

Raphael P, Harris R, Harris SW. The endonasal lip lift: personal technique. Aesthet Surg J. 2014; 34(3):457–468

Santanchè P, Bonarrigo C. Lifting of the upper lip: personal technique. Plast Reconstr Surg. 2004; 113(6):1828–1835, discussion 1836–1837

41 Lip Enhancement with Filler Injection

Christopher C. Surek and Roy Kim

Abstract

This chapter provides a succinct and high-yield approach to comprehensive lip enhancement with filler injection.

Keywords: Philtrum, cupid's bow, white roll, dry vermilion, lip tubercles, wet vermilion, wet–dry junction, oral commissure

Key Points

- A comprehensive understanding of lip anatomy, specifically subunits and vascular architecture, is paramount prior to performing lip injection.
- Age, gender, and ethnic considerations must be noted and discussed in preinjection consultation.
- The "youthful" lip and the "aging" lip have unique morphology characteristics that often require customized approaches.
- A reproducible and safe algorithm is critical to address the philtrum, white roll, dry vermilion, and wet vermilion in lip enhancement procedures.
- A filler injection "crash kit" must be assembled and accessible in your office in the event a vascular occlusion occurs following lip injection.

41.1 Preoperative Steps

41.1.1 Lip Anatomy (▶ Fig. 41.1)

Upper Lip (Formed by the fusion of two lateral tubercles with a central tubercle)

- Subunits:
  - Philtrum.
  - Cupid's bow and white roll (aka vermilion–cutaneous junction).
    - Corresponds with the insertion of the pars marginalis leaflet of the orbicularis oris muscle.
  - Dry vermilion.
  - Wet vermilion.

Lower Lip (Formed by the fusion of two lateral tubercles)

- Subunits:
  - White roll.
  - Dry vermilion.
  - Wet vermilion.

Vascular Anatomy (▶ Fig. 41.2)

- Inferior labial artery (ILA):
  - It is supplied by the main facial artery.
  - It most commonly travels medially near the lower lip vermilion border. *However, in 10 to 15% of patients the main ILA branch can traverse as low as the labiomental crease.*
  - Caution should be taken when approaching for labiomental crease augmentation in any patient as it is possible the ILA may be in close proximity.
- Superior labial artery (SLA):
  - Supplied by the main facial artery.
  - Typically branches off the facial artery within an area 1.5 cm lateral to the oral commissure.
  - Travels superior to the white roll for the lateral two-thirds of the lip and then traverses inferior to white roll at medial third of the upper lip toward the central tubercle.

41.1.2 Treatment Plan with Patient

- Contraindications:
  - Pregnancy.
  - Current cold sore outbreak.
  - History of sensitivity to hyaluronic acid filler.
- The youthful lip (▶ Fig. 41.3a–f):
  - The youthful lip is often a true "enhancement" procedure.
  - There are minimal aging changes of the skin, orbicularis, fat, and alveolus.
  - Objectives are often to create additional shape and volume.
- The aging lip (▶ Fig. 41.3a–f):
  - The aging lip is often a true "restoration" procedure.
  - Depending on the patient, there are various levels of bony and soft tissue loss accompanied by a lengthening and flattening of the orbicularis oculi muscle.

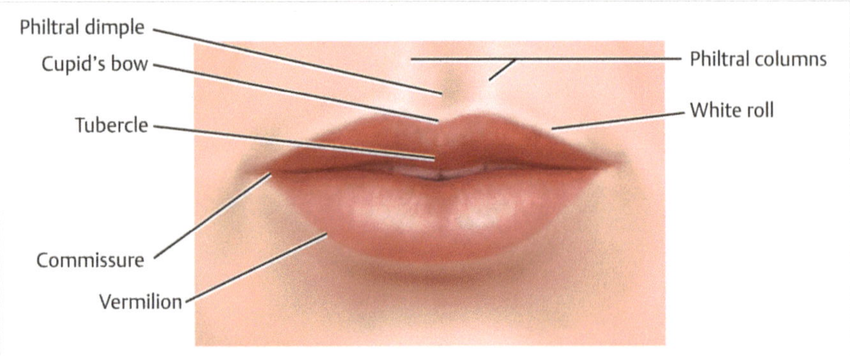

Fig. 41.1 The anatomical subunits of the lip: philtrum, cupid's bow, white roll, dry vermilion, and oral commissure.

- Objectives are often toward restoration of definition, volume, and shape that have been diminished during the aging process.
- Expectations:
  - It is important to discuss with the patients their goals and expectations to ensure there is understanding between the patients and the injector.

41.2 Operative Steps

See **Video 41.1** and **Video 41.2.**

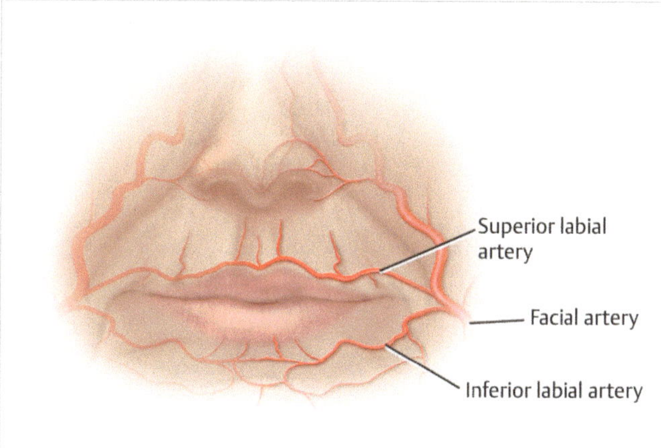

Fig. 41.2 Vascular anatomy of the perioral region: facial artery, inferior labial artery, and superior labial artery.

41.2.1 Aseptic Technique

- Proper aseptic technique is paramount to help prevent adverse sequela.

41.2.2 Anesthesia

- Topical anesthetic.
- Local anesthetic injections.
  - Field block: Infraorbital nerve, mental nerve.
  - Direct injection into planned cannula port sites.

41.2.3 Product Selection

- Hyaluronic acid is the most common filler injected in the lip.
- Particle size, G-prime, and product cohesivity must all be taken into consideration when selecting filler product.
  - Decide if the fine lines of the lip, the lip itself, or both will be injected.
  - Typically, a lower G-prime filler is used for fine lines around the lips and a higher G-prime filler is used for the defining border and body.

41.2.4 Lip Injection Algorithm

- Definition (this can be explained to the patient as the "outline"):
  - Philtrum.

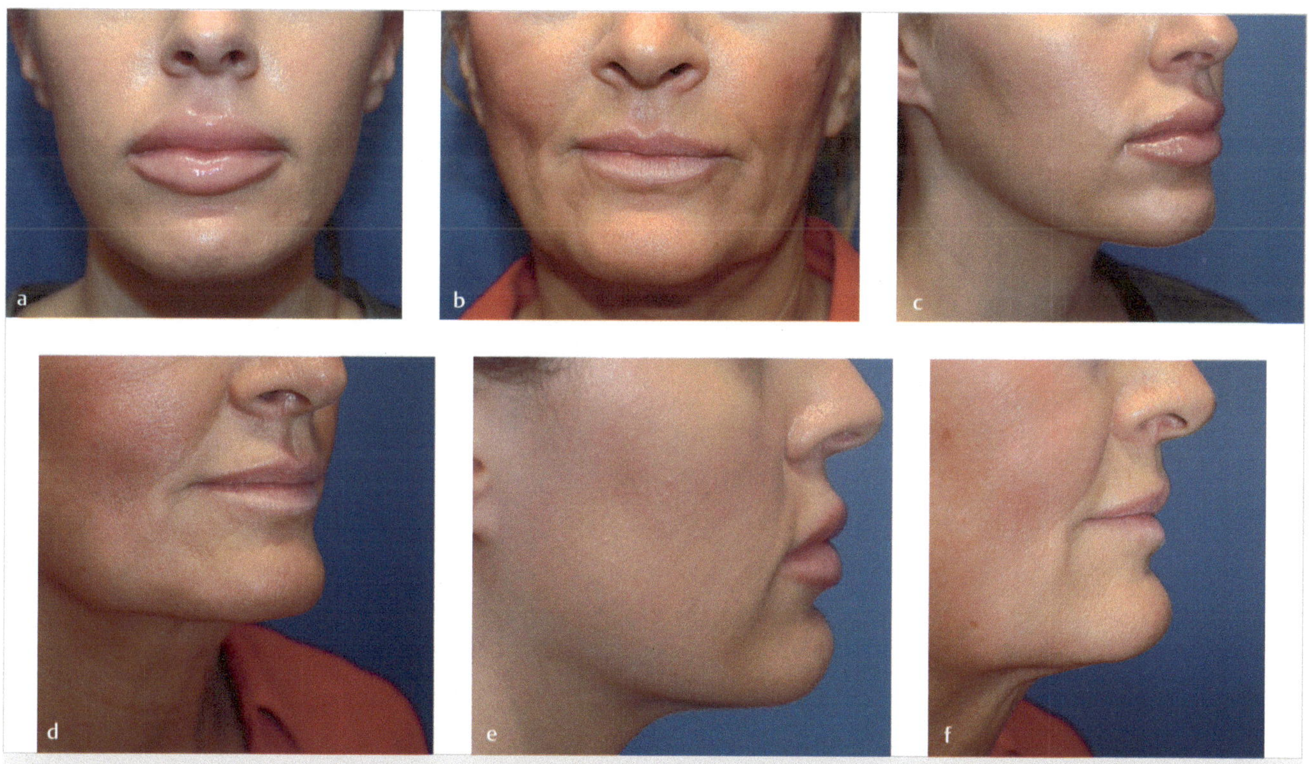

Fig. 41.3 "Mother–daughter" comparison: These models are mother and daughter. The following set of images will demonstrate the unique differences between the youthful and the aging lip. **(a)** Anteroposterior (AP) view of the daughter representing a youthful lip. **(b)** AP view of the mother representing an aging lip. **(c)** Oblique view of daughter representing a youthful lip. **(d)** Oblique view of the mother representing an aging lip. **(e)** Lateral view of the daughter representing a youthful lip. **(f)** Lateral view of the mother representing an aging lip.

- White roll and cupid's bow.
- Commissure.
- Shape (this can be explained to the patient as the "lipstick show"):
  - Dry vermilion.
- Proportion (this can be explained to the patient as maintaining "balance"):
  - Volume comparison between upper and lower lips.
  - Traditional teaching suggests a ratio of 1:1.6; however, patient-specific morphology and ethnicity should be taken into consideration.

41.2.5 Special Considerations

- Aspirate at all times if indicated.
- Adjunctive methods such as vertical suture, dental floss, or other modalities may be considered if indicated to help with shape creation.
- Keyhole effect—the ability to see a slight hole in the central portion of the upper and lower lips—is considered the aesthetic ideal by most patients.
- Direct pressure at all times to ensure less bleeding and bruising.
- Filler crash kit: All injectors should have proper supplies in the event of inadvertent vascular occlusion. This should always include hyaluronidase. Other recommended products include, but are not limited to, aspirin, nitroglycerin paste, and supplemental oxygen.

41.2.6 Adjunct Aesthetic Considerations

- Lower facial proportions should be maintained; therefore, consideration should be given to simultaneous chin enhancement if needed following lip enhancement (▶ Fig. 41.4a, b).

41.3 Postoperative Care

- Direct pressure to areas of bleeding or oozing.
- Apply ice.
- Monitor for signs of vascular compromise.
- Consider antiviral prophylaxis, especially for patients with a history of cold sores.

41.4 Case Example

This is a 34-year-old female patient who has never undergone a filler injection procedure. She desires enhancement of her philtrum, white roll, and red vermilion. We performed injection with hyaluronic acid filler. Needle injection was performed for the philtrum, cupid's bow, and white roll. Cannula injection

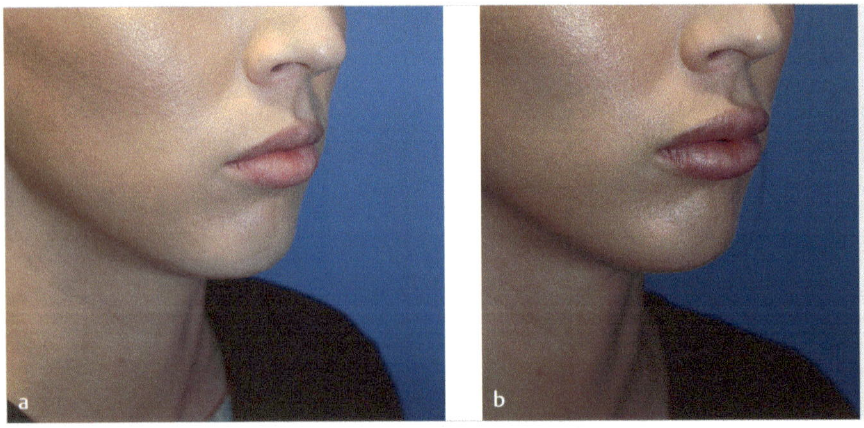

Fig. 41.4 **(a)** Oblique view preprocedure: The patient has lip asymmetry as well as chin recession; therefore, both should be treated. **(b)** Oblique view postprocedure: The patient has undergone lip enhancement as well as chin enhancement to maintain lower facial proportions.

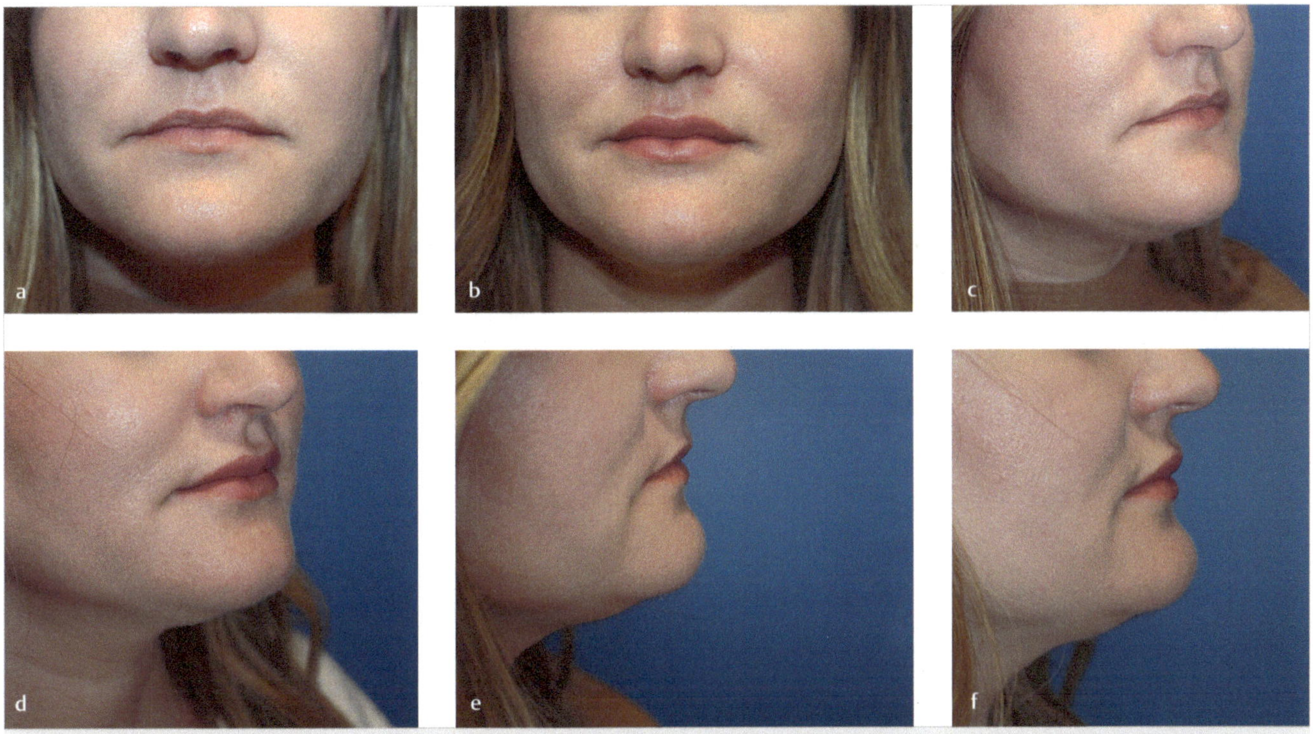

Fig. 41.5 Before and after case example. **(a)** Anteroposterior (AP) view prior to lip enhancement procedure. **(b)** AP view following lip enhancement procedure. **(c)** Oblique view prior to lip enhancement procedure. **(d)** Oblique view following lip enhancement procedure. **(e)** Lateral view prior to lip enhancement procedure. **(f)** Lateral view following lip enhancement procedure.

from lateral port site was used to volumize the red vermilion in the pre-orbicularis oris plane (▶ Fig. 41.5a–f).

41.5 Conclusion

Lip enhancement with filler injection is a common procedure that can help improve contour and shape in the "youthful" lip and/or restore volume and shape in the "aging" lip. The injector must have a good knowledge and respect for lip vascularity and subunit anatomy. The injectors should develop a reproducible and safe algorithm to approach lip injection procedures and equip themselves with the proper tools to treat potential complications.

Further Readings

de Maio M, Wu WTL, Goodman GJ, Monheit G, Alliance for the Future of Aesthetics Consensus Committee. Facial assessment and injection guide for Botulinum toxin and injectable hyaluronic acid fillers: focus on the lower face. Plast Reconstr Surg. 2017; 140(3):393e–404e

Ramaut L, Tonnard P, Verpaele A, Verstraete K, Blondeel P. Aging of the upper lip: Part I: A retrospective analysis of metric changes in soft tissue on magnetic resonance imaging. Plast Reconstr Surg. 2019; 143(2):440–446

Rohrich RJ, Bartlett EL, Dayan E. Practical approach and safety of hyaluronic acid fillers. Plast Reconstr Surg Glob Open. 2019; 7(6):e2172

Snozzi P, van Loghem JAJ. Complication management following rejuvenation procedures with hyaluronic acid fillers-an algorithm-based approach. Plast Reconstr Surg Glob Open. 2018; 6(12):e2061

Surek CC, Guisantes E, Schnarr K, Jelks G, Beut J. "No-touch" technique for lip enhancement. Plast Reconstr Surg. 2016; 138(4):603e–613e

42 Fat Grafting to the Perioral Region

Rod J. Rohrich and Raja Mohan

Abstract

One major adjunct in facial rejuvenation is autologous fat transfer or facial fat grafting to various facial fat compartments of the face. An important region to consider is the perioral region where deep and fine perioral rhytides are visible. Autologous fat grafting to this region adds volume to areas that are hollow or have become deflated secondary to aging and skin laxity.

Keywords: Fat grafting, perioral rejuvenation, facial aging, fat transfer

Key Points

- Fat grafting to the perioral region is a useful adjunct in facial rejuvenation.
- Autologous fat grafting to the superficial fat compartments of the perioral region (▶ Fig. 42.1) is meant to address volume deflation and deep rhytides that cannot be addressed with a facelift.
- Other modalities such as chemical peels, microdermabrasion, and laser resurfacing induce dermal regeneration but do not add volume to the perioral region.
- Fat injections are not recommended for the white roll. Injections into the white roll are unpredictable and asymmetric secondary to movement.

42.1 Preoperative Steps

42.1.1 Analysis

- A thorough preoperative analysis of the lower third of the face to identify areas of volume deflation and tissue laxity is performed.
- Areas of volume deflation as well as deep rhytides are marked preoperatively in the perioral region to determine areas requiring volumization.
- The lips become thin with age and subcutaneous fat atrophies. In addition, the nasolabial folds and marionette lines become more prominent with deflation and descent of fat.

42.2 Operative Steps

See **Video 42.1** and **Video 42.2**.

42.2.1 General Technique of Autologous Fat Harvest and Transfer

- Adipose tissue is harvested from the medial thighs using a 10-mL syringe with a 14-gauge (3 mm multihole) cannula.
- No wetting or infiltration solution is used for the harvest.
- The harvested lipoaspirate is centrifuged at 2,250 rpm for 1 minute followed by removal of the infranatant and supernatant to isolate the fat meant for transfer.

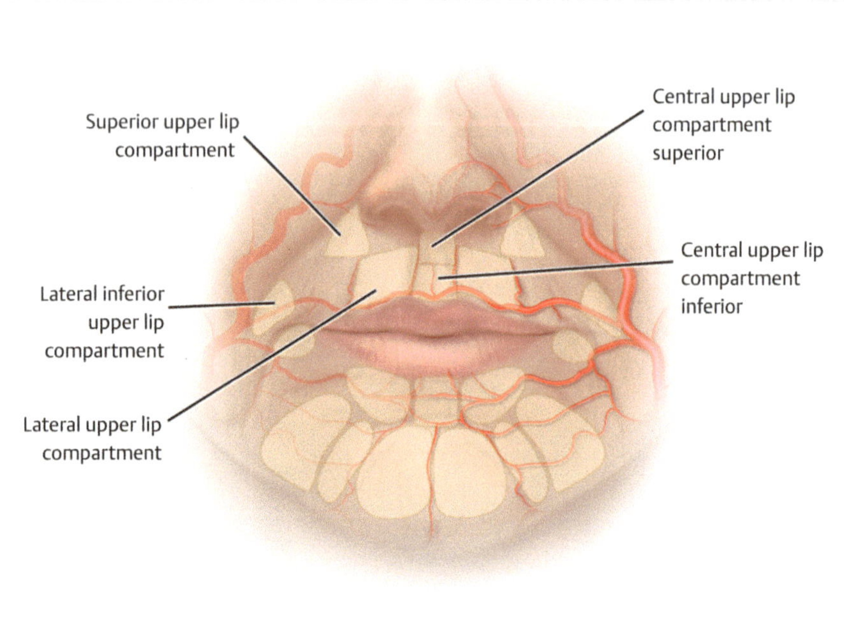

Fig. 42.1 Superficial fat compartments of the perioral region.

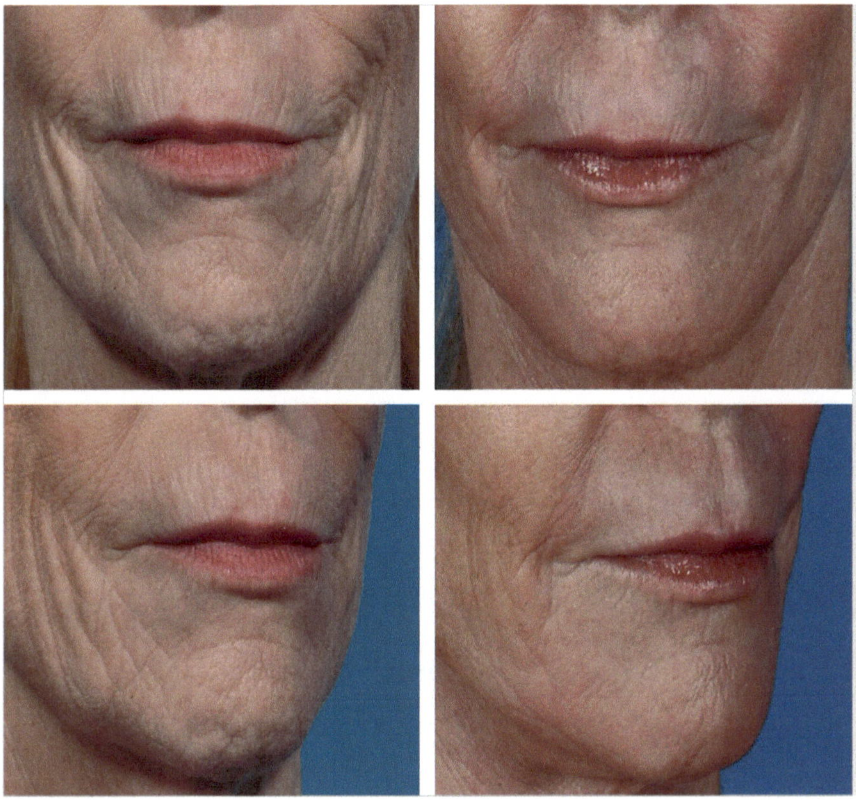

Fig. 42.2 Preoperative and postoperative photographs of a woman who underwent rhytidectomy with perioral rejuvenation using autologous fat. The perioral regions appear more youthful. The deep rhytides are less visible and the perioral and mental regions are blended with a smoother transition.

- The harvested fat is collected in 1-mL syringes.
- For any facial fat compartment, the 1-mL syringe with the harvested fat is connected to a blunt cannula and injected at a low pressure with anterograde and retrograde motions.

42.2.2 Injection Technique for Mental Region

- Using a 1-cc syringe attached to a 22-gauge, 1.5-cm blunt cannula, small aliquots of fat are transferred to areas of the perioral region requiring volumization.
- Autologous fat is transferred to areas of lateral hollowing, the upper lip, and marionette lines.
- In general, fat concentrate of 1 to 2 mL is placed in each superficial fat compartment of the perioral region.
- Areas of fat transfer should be massaged and molded to achieve uniformity and symmetry.

42.3 Postoperative Care

- Cold compresses are used over the face intermittently for the first 72 hours postoperatively.
- Patients are encouraged to avoid head turning and limit facial movements for the first week.
- Patients rest with head elevated to 45 degrees without the use of pillows to avoid flexion of the neck.

42.4 Case Example

Preoperative and postoperative photographs of a woman who underwent rhytidectomy with perioral rejuvenation using autologous fat. The perioral regions appear more youthful. The deep rhytides are less visible and the perioral and mental regions are blended with a smoother transition (▶ Fig. 42.2).

42.5 Conclusion

Fat augmentation to the perioral region can restore volume loss associated with aging that other modalities are unable to address. Fat augmentation to the perioral region can soften the superficial fat compartments of the perioral region.

Further Readings

Pezeshk RA, Stark RY, Small KH, Unger JG, Rohrich RJ. Role of autologous fat transfer to the superficial fat compartments for perioral rejuvenation. Plast Reconstr Surg. 2015; 136(3):301e–309e

Rohrich RJ, Afrooz PN. Finesse in face lifting: the role of facial fat compartment augmentation in facial rejuvenation. Plast Reconstr Surg. 2019; 143(1):98–101

Rohrich RJ, Ghavami A, Constantine FC, Unger J, Mojallal A. Lift-and-fill face lift: integrating the fat compartments. Plast Reconstr Surg. 2014; 133(6):756e–767e

Rohrich RJ, Pessa JE. The anatomy and clinical implications of perioral submuscular fat. Plast Reconstr Surg. 2009; 124(1):266–271

Rohrich RJ, Pessa JE. The fat compartments of the face: anatomy and clinical implications for cosmetic surgery. Plast Reconstr Surg. 2007; 119(7):2219–2227, discussion 2228–2231

43 Neuromodulation for Perioral Rejuvenation

Steven Fagien and Yash J. Avashia

Abstract

Neuromodulation for perioral rejuvenation requires a particular understanding of the function and complexity of the perioral muscular anatomy and function. Unlike the upper face where muscle groups can be more easily isolated, the lower facial region muscles are uniquely intertwined making specific isolation to a target area more challenging. Optimum technique and dosing as well as appropriate patient selection are therefore required to deliver predictable and consistent results.

Keywords: Perioral rejuvenation, orbicularis oris, depressor anguli oris, botulinum toxin type A, neuromodulation, perioral rhytides

Key Points

- Lips are the central focus to lower face aesthetics.
- Vertical perioral rhytides can be a result of aging, smoking, and frequent mimetic expressions.
- Fine wrinkles of the perioral region are often addressed with filler, but controlled use of neuromodulators can be used separately or in combination.
- Complex functions of the perioral region deserve careful attention. Neuromodulation in the lower facial regions should be practiced by experienced injectors.

43.1 Anatomy

- Perioral musculature includes the orbicularis oris, depressor anguli oris, and the mentalis.
- The orbicularis oris is the sphincteric muscle of the mouth.
- The origin of depressor anguli oris is in the lower jaw and it inserts into the angle of the mouth. The function is to depress the angle of the mouth and pull it backwards (posteriorly).
- The mentalis raises the skin over the chin and can create surface dimpling.

43.2 Perioral Injection Technique

43.2.1 Orbicularis Oris (▶ Fig. 43.1)

- The average number of injection points is a total of two to seven for the upper and lower lips.
- The average total starting dose for the perioral area is 2 to 6 U with 1 U per injection point.
- Conservative techniques recommend 0.5 to 0.75 U per point and will be dictated by the number of injection points and desired results.
- Areas to avoid injection include the midline upper lip at the philtrum and both commissures.
- Injections usually should be kept superficial and symmetrical. Symmetry is a critical component to perioral neuromodulation unless one is attempting to treat pre-existing asymmetry.
- Injections should be just above the vermilion border, and no higher than 5 mm above the border to avoid inversion, eversion, or lip ptosis.
- The use of ice for topical anesthetic effect is beneficial for enhanced patient comfort.
- The initial approach is to begin with one site per quarter lip (quadrant) and reassess in 2 weeks. Lower doses usually have shorter duration and this as well as the potential for temporary lip dysfunction (overly weak "pursing" or "difficulty using a straw") should be explained to the patient prior to treatment (▶ Fig. 43.1).
- Injection sites should be 0.5 to 1 mm above the vermilion border. Injections are superficial.

43.2.2 Depressor Anguli Oris

- The depressor anguli oris muscles are treated with low doses of 2 to 5 U per side.
- Potential complications:
  - Overtreatment of the perioral area can result in difficulty in pursing the lips, speech impairments (inability to pronounce "b" and "p"), and difficulty in eating and using a straw.
  - Unintentional overtreatment of the depressor anguli oris muscles may result in involvement of other muscles resulting in oral incompetence, drooping, and lower lip asymmetry.

43.3 Case Example

This is a young, 34-year-old female presenting with the desire for improvement in upper lip eversion. She has not had any prior soft tissue filler to her upper lip and similarly, did not want any filler at the time of consultation. Hence, 2 units of onabotulinum toxin A was injected 1 mm above the vermilion border, laterally on both sides at a midpoint between the lateral commissure and cupid's bow. Care was taken not to inject centrally

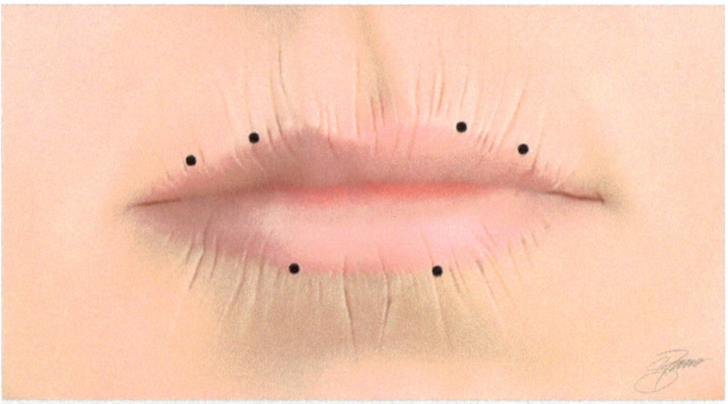

Fig. 43.1 Perioral neuromodulator injection.

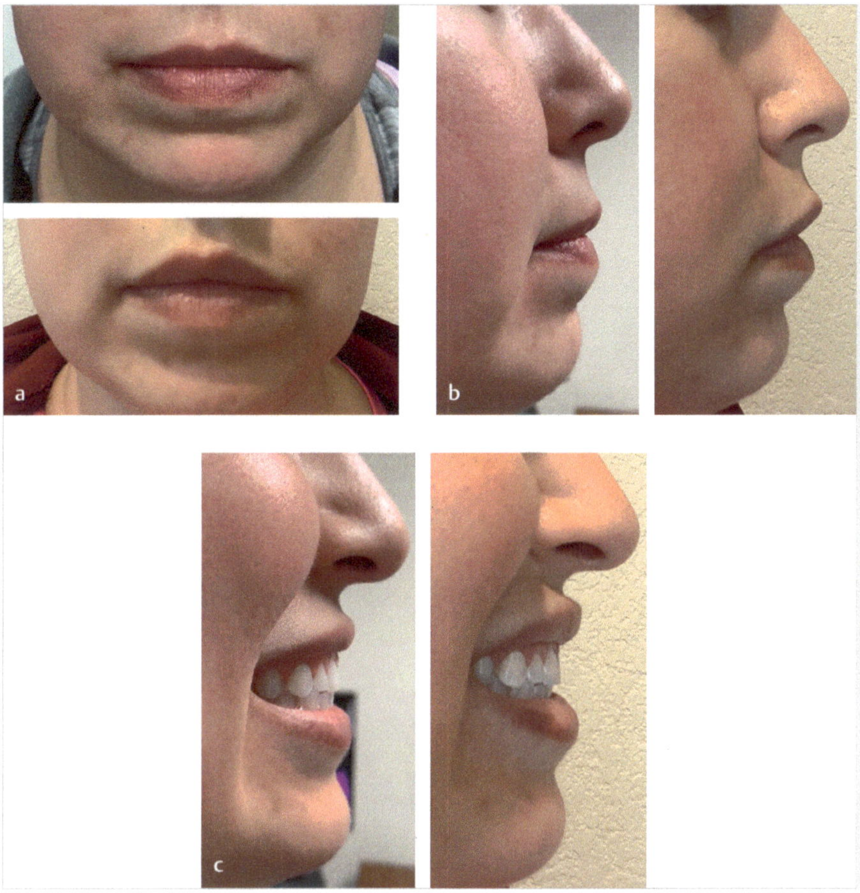

Fig. 43.2 (a–c) This is a young, 34-year-old female presenting with the desire for improvement in upper lip eversion. She has not had any prior soft tissue filler to her upper lip and similarly, did not want any filler at the time of consultation. Hence, 2 units of onabotulinum toxin A was injected 1 mm above the vermilion border, laterally on both sides at a midpoint between the lateral commissure and cupids bow. Care was taken not to inject centrally or higher than 1 mm above the vermilion border, which has the risk of loss of the orbicularis oris sphincteric function. The case images demonstrate before and 2 weeks after injection. Take note of the slight eversion of the upper lip on repose and upon animation (smile).

or higher than 1 mm above the vermilion border, which has the risk of loss of the orbicularis oris sphincteric function. The case images demonstrate before and 2 weeks after injection. Note the slight eversion of the upper lip on repose and upon animation (smile) (▶ Fig. 43.2a–c).

43.4 Conclusion

Patient selection and optimum injection technique are paramount. Patients who depend on perioral function (musicians, singers, speakers) are not optimal candidates. Conservative treatment is recommended for first-time treatments with reassessment at 2 weeks. Avoid treating the corners of the lips, which could result in drooping and drooling. Avoid the midline of the upper lip to avoid flattening the lip. Avoid treating too distantly from the lip margin.

Keep injections superficial and massage laterally. Injections into the lower lip area are more likely to affect function; therefore, treat conservatively, if at all. Consider using botulinum toxin type A in conjunction with resurfacing procedures and fillers. Use ice liberally to anesthetize the area, as injections in the perioral area can be painful.

See **Video 43.1**.

Further Readings

Carruthers J, Fagien S, Matarasso SL, Botox Consensus Group. Consensus recommendations on the use of botulinum toxin type a in facial aesthetics. Plast Reconstr Surg. 2004; 114(6) Suppl:1S–22S

Fagien S. Botulinum toxin type A for facial aesthetic enhancement: role in facial shaping. Plast Reconstr Surg. 2003; 112(5) Suppl:6S–18S, discussion 19S–20S

Fagien S, Raspaldo H. Facial rejuvenation with botulinum neurotoxin: an anatomical and experiential perspective. J Cosmet Laser Ther. 2007; 9 Suppl 1:23–31

Fagien S, Carruthers A, Carruthers J. Expanded uses of BTX-A for facial aesthetic enhancement. In: Fagien S, ed. Cosmetic Oculoplastic Surgery. 4th ed. London UK: Elsevier Publishers; 2007:303–336

Fagien S, Brandt FS. Primary and adjunctive use of Botox in facial aesthetic surgery: beyond the glabella. In: Matarasso A, Matarasso SL, eds. Clinics in Plastic Surgery. Philadelphia: W. B. Saunders Co.; 2000:127–148

Part VI

Chin Augmentation and Jaw Rejuvenation

VI

44 Jaw Fillers

K. Kay Durairaj, Vivian N. Nguyen, and Omer Baker

Abstract

A defined jawline gives strength, character, and beauty to the face. The jawline elegantly enhances the face and gives a distinctive border between the face and neck. Nonsurgical interventions with injectable fillers such as hyaluronic acid (HA) fillers and non-HA fillers are an excellent tool for beauty enhancement and rejuvenation of lower face aging changes. The use of fillers to improve mandible projection and reduce jowl heaviness has become more popular as more people are seeking the means to combat signs of facial aging.

Fat atrophy, dermal collagen breakdown, subcutaneous volume loss, and bone resorption are the culprits that change the lower face. HA-based fillers are beneficial for jawline augmentation, as they have a medium to high G-primes and are used to reverse blunting of the angle of the mandible and lower face jowling. Non-HA fillers such as calcium-based fillers are useful to achieve more pronounced projection and support of bone resorption changes around the mandibular ligaments. Nonhyaluronic fillers have among the highest G-primes and act as biostimulators. Because of their unique biostimulatory properties and chemical composition, non-HA fillers cannot be dissolved and demand experienced injectors with comprehensive anatomical knowledge.

A stepwise approach to jawline contouring gives the best results. The areas which give the most effective jawline sculpting include four primary injection sites: the mandibular angle, the antegonial notch, the prejowl sulcus, and the junction of the anterior end of the mandibular body with the mentum. The volumizing lift of high-density fillers in these locations improves herniation of fat around the mandibular ligaments.

The ability of injectable fillers to alleviate subcutaneous volume loss and reduce tissue laxity has revolutionized medical aesthetics. Lower face and jawline fillers are minimally invasive procedures that reliably improve the jawline with excellent safety and efficacy.

Keywords: Jawline filler, jawline, jowls, mandible, facial aging, bone resorption, G-prime, biostimulator, HA filler, non-HA

Key Points

- Treatment of facial aging changes must address the maintenance of youthful jawline projection and correction of its volume changes. Jawline aging changes include skin with dermal collagen breakdown, fat pads with subcutaneous fat atrophy, and bone resorption.
- Hyaluronic gel fillers and nonhyaluronic acid (non-HA) biostimulator injections are highly effective for correcting jawline aging changes. HA-based fillers are beneficial for moderate soft tissue augmentation, as they have a moderate to high G-prime, indicating the filler's elastic ability to resist compression and improve volumization. Non-HA-based fillers help to achieve more robust augmented facial features because of their higher G-primes, ability to contour bone density changes, and ability to act as biostimulators to induce secondary neocollagenesis.

44.1 Preoperative Steps

44.1.1 Background Knowledge

- Mandibular bone resorption is most prominent in locations with muscle attachments and vascular structure crossings, requiring correction. Changes in bone density contribute to jowling by causing bone to remodel in a convex configuration, causing retraction of the facial ligaments and muscles.
- Assessment of the aging changes of the mandible should involve inspection of the retaining ligaments, the bony mandible, the prejowl sulcus, the masseter muscle, and the skin changes.
- There are two key retaining ligaments within the jowl: the platysma mandibular ligament and the mandibular osseocutaneous ligament. Both of these ligaments work together to maintain tissue and muscle stability in the lower face. Filler injections supporting these ligaments will treat bone resorption changes by helping facial ligaments retain their mechanical effect on surrounding tissues. Myomodulation of lower face muscles by accurate filler placement around the mandibular ligaments also contributes to their improved function and lift.
- Fillers can alleviate the appearance of jowls by improving bone projection of the mandible and maxilla, allowing for increased support of the drooping tissues in the prejowl area of the mandible and the mentum.

44.1.2 Preoperative Clinical Understanding

- Patients should be counseled at least 7 days prior to injection to avoid any agents that could cause blood thinning such as aspirin, ibuprofen, Motrin (or any other nonsteroidal anti-inflammatory drugs [NSAIDs]), fish oils, or vitamin E. Alcohol consumption 7 days before and after injection is not advised, as this increases the risk of bruising and swelling.

44.1.3 Day of Procedure

- Conduct a detailed health history assessment on patient's known allergies, medical conditions or contraindications to potential fillers, prior filler, facial surgery, trauma, and implant history.
- Makeup should be removed, and the face should be cleansed with 70% alcohol, chlorhexidine, or betadine to ensure sterile conditions.
- Pretreatment pictures for photographic documentation should be taken for pre- and postprocedural comparisons.

44.1.4 Filler Selection

- Patients exhibiting heavy jowling benefit most from high G-prime products such as calcium hydroxyapatite and high G-prime hyaluronic gel fillers. These dense fillers have viscoelastic properties that can mimic the support and contours of periosteum. Patients with superficial subcutaneous dermal thinning will benefit most from medium hyaluronic gel fillers, as their G-prime properties allow for plumping and hydration of dermal thinning.

- Patients who are new to injectables, indecisive, or nervous about filler reversibility should be treated with hyaluronic fillers. Those with facial scar tissue changes who may have abnormal lymphatic and vascular supply after surgical procedures are also advised to use hyaluronic gel fillers. The effects of HA gel fillers can be reversed and dissolved with hyaluronidase (unlike non-HA fillers). Both HA fillers and non-HA fillers have a 12- to 24-month duration.
- The sculpted and contoured aesthetic that often appeals to younger patients can be best achieved through non-HA fillers such as calcium hydroxyapatite. This is an implant composed of carboxymethylcellulose and calcium hydroxyapatite. Additionally, it is a biostimulator that can induce primary and secondary neocollagenesis wherever it is placed. Through neocollagenesis, the effects of these fillers continue post injection, and is unable to be reversed or dissolved.
- Patients who are highly sensitive or have proven to be allergic or reactive to other injectables should consider non-HA calcium hydroxyapatite over HA, as it is biocompatible with human tissues and is nonantigenic. It is advisable that novice injectors start with HA fillers because of their reversibility and shorter duration.

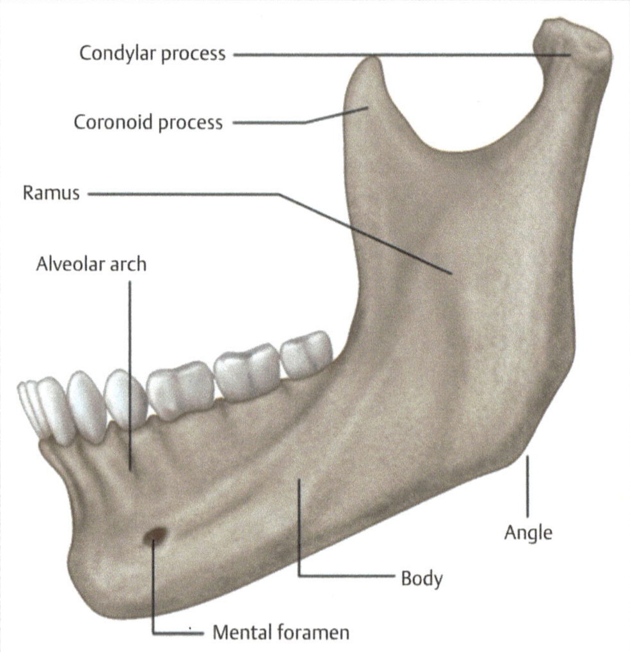

Fig. 44.1 Side-view depiction of the three-dimensional structure of mandible, the angle of the mandible, and the ramus of mandible. (Reproduced with permission from Watanabe K, Shoja MM. Anatomy for Plastic Surgery of the Face, Head, and Neck. Thieme; 2016.)

44.1.5 Anatomy Assessment and Markings

- Evaluate the medial and lateral malar fat pads for any deflation or descent, as it is important to determine if drooping and the weight of the cheek are contributing to jowling and jawline changes. It is important to revolumize the lateral maxillae and maxillary eminence.
- Assess the ideal mandible angle (▶ Fig. 44.1). This gonial angle is formed by the junction at the midpoint of the posterior border of the ramus and the inferior border of the body of the mandible (▶ Fig. 44.1 and ▶ Fig. 44.2). This varies between gender, but a good standard for women to adhere to is 120 to 125 degrees and 130 to 140 degrees for men.
- Evaluate the deep lateral chin compartment (▶ Fig. 44.3). As described by Lamb and Surek in their textbook, *Facial Volumization: An Anatomic Approach*, this region contains a fat pad that is integral for providing volume to the prejowl sulcus. The fat pad can be located deep to the depressor anguli oris (DAO) muscle. This fat layer protects the mental nerve and because it is located close to the inferior labial artery, injecting filler into here requires caution.
- Evaluate muscles that also influence jawline contours, such as the masseter muscle, which can make the jawline appear bulky. In addition to this, the DAO muscle contributes to the downwards pull around the mouth and the deep groove of the prejowl sulcus (▶ Fig. 44.4). The DAO contributes to fat tissue descent in the prejowl sulcus region, the region directly inferior to the commissure and is in association with the mandibular ligament. The mandibular ligament suspends the sagging tissue that contributes to jowling from behind the marionette furrow and with filler correction, tissue suspension will be enhanced.
- The masseter muscle is a two-layer structure, with a superficial and deep component located at the lateral surface of the ramus and mandibular angle (▶ Fig. 44.5). Injections into the masseter muscle will cause the appearance of hypertrophic masseter muscles and must be avoided. Palpating the anterior border of the masseter muscle leads to the antegonial notch. It is important to know that the presence of a large mandibular antegonial notch is indicative of mandibular resorption changes, which should be addressed with filler to correct the contour deformity. From a point anterior to the prejowl sulcus, a cannula can be used with retrograde threading technique to place a high density, integrated hyaluronic filler.
- At the junction of the anterior end of the mandibular body and mentum, linear retrograde threads of filler can be placed in several directions to support the oral commissure and lip and to extend contouring to the chin and mental crease. This increases maximum mandibular projection.
- Placement of fillers surrounding the supportive mandibular ligaments is critical to alleviate the herniation of fat that creates jowls (▶ Fig. 44.6). As described by Lamb and Surek in their textbook *Facial Volumization: An Anatomic Approach*, the platysma mandibular ligament can be found roughly 5 cm distal to the gonial angle, superior to the mandibular border. Injections here are beneficial, as this is a point of muscular stability for the platysma. The mandibular osseocutaneous ligament can be found by palpating between the anterior jowl

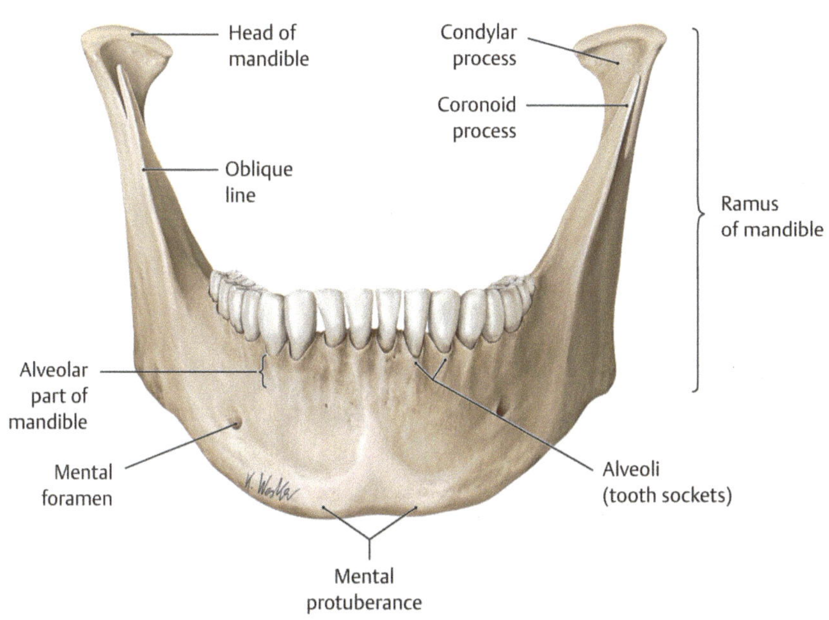

Fig. 44.2 Front-view depiction of the three-dimensional structure of mandible, the angle of the mandible, and the ramus of mandible. (Reproduced with permission from Watanabe K, Shoja MM. Anatomy for Plastic Surgery of the Face, Head, and Neck. Thieme; 2016.)

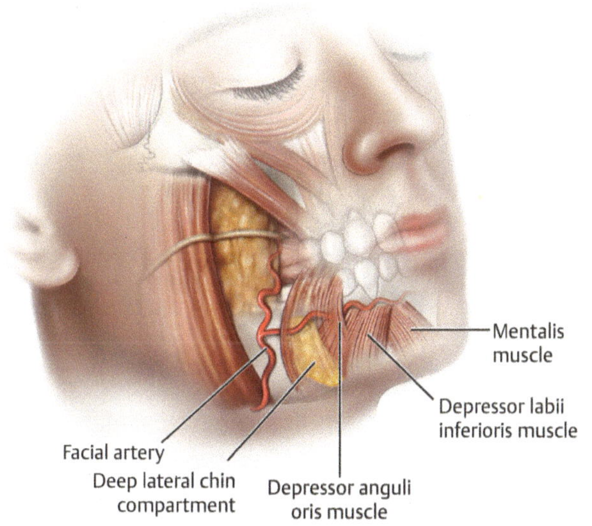

Fig. 44.3 Deep lateral chin compartment and inferior labial artery anatomical locations.

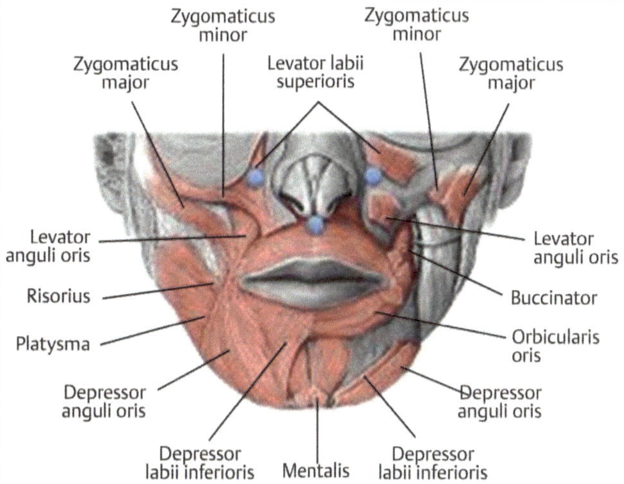

Fig. 44.4 Depressor anguli oris muscle location and structure. (Reproduced with permission from Benson BE, Blitzer A. Botulinum Neurotoxin for Head and Neck Disorders. Thieme; 2012.)

and marionette line. It is located approximately 1 cm superior to the mandibular border and 5.5 cm from the gonial angle. Injections here will provide structural support and lift to sagging tissue, to create a youthful jawline.

44.1.6 Anatomical Danger Zones and Markings

- The antegonial notch can be found by palpating just anterior to the masseter, at the lower border of the mandibular ramus. The facial artery branch can be avoided with deep palpation and feeling for the slight bounding pulse. The inferior labial artery is another branch of the facial artery that is in the injection plane and should be avoided. The inferior labial artery is located deep to the platysma, in a region about 2.5 cm from the labial commissure and another 2.5 cm inferior to the ramus of the mandible.
- The parotid gland and branches of the facial nerve are located in the preauricular area (▶ Fig. 44.7). Injections into the parotid salivary gland tissue can cause problems with salivation, mastication, or facial nerve injury if they are in the incorrect plane. The facial nerve branches exit in the preauricular area including the frontal, zygomatic, buccal, marginal mandibular, and cervical branches (▶ Fig. 44.8).

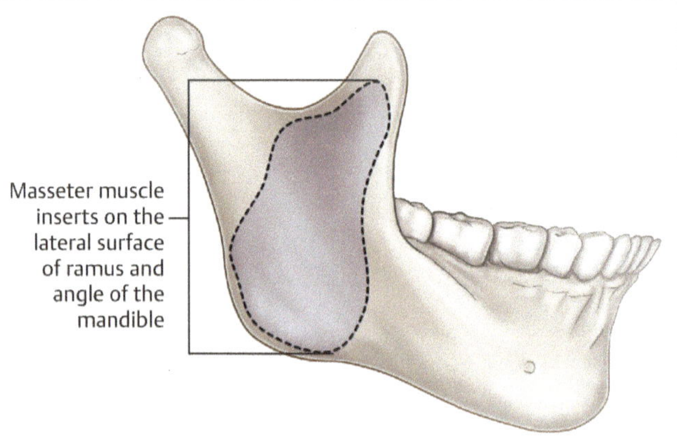

Fig. 44.5 Masseter anatomy.

Caution must be exercised around the mental foramen as this cavity contains dense vasculature and the mental nerve.

- The marginal mandibular nerve branches toward the DAO and should be avoided (▸ Fig. 44.9). This nerve exits the parotid masseteric fascia and courses through the sub-superficial muscular aponeurotic system (sub-SMAS), about 3 mm anterior to the facial vessels and 2.2 cm distal to the gonial angle. Furthermore, this nerve has a branch that typically spans 1 cm superior to the mandibular osseocutaneous ligament.

44.2 Operative Steps

44.2.1 Choice of Filler

- Determine which filler is best for the patient's skin quality and laxity. Either moderate or high G-prime hyaluronic gel fillers or nonhyaluronic filler can be used individually or together.

44.2.2 Syringe Preparation: Dr. Kay's Recommended Calcium Hydroxyapatite Reconstitution

- Calcium hydroxyapatite—recommended to mix with red adapter 1 syringe (1.5 cc) with 0.3 to 0.5 cc lidocaine with 1:100,000 epinephrine.

44.2.3 Needle Selection

- The general rule of thumb is to use the smallest needle gauge that can still efficiently deliver the product.
- A 27-gauge, 1 to 1.5″ long needle is recommended.

44.2.4 Sterility

- Cleanse the skin with betadine and remove all makeup.

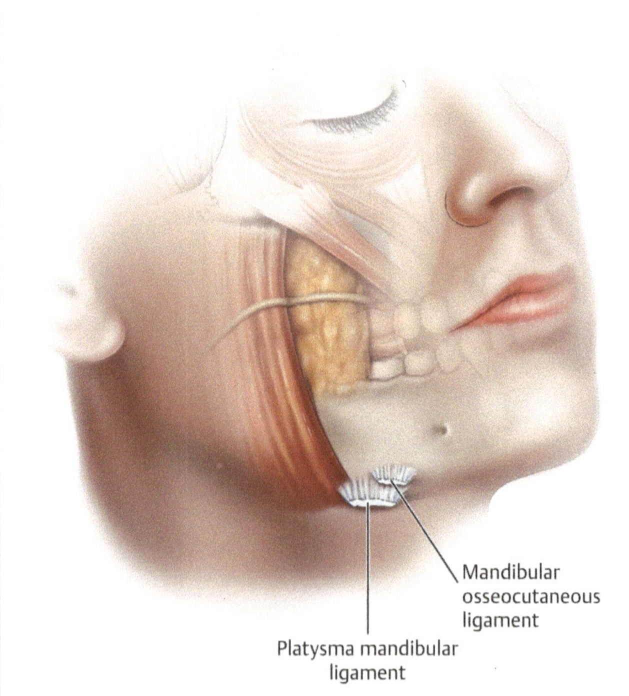

Fig. 44.6 Retaining ligaments within the jaw.

44.2.5 Injecting

- The angle of the mandible is first addressed using a high G-prime structural filler. The first step is to create an entry point using a 27-gauge needle. The needle should enter the skin in a perpendicular orientation with attention to point the needle bevel in the direction of the deepest area to fill. An ideal entry point would be one that is superomedial and about 0.5 cm from the apex of the mandibular angle. A bolus of approximately 0.3 cc should be delivered to this injection site. Filler is used to create a sharp contour of the angle and deep boluses are injected in the preauricular area.
- The ideal mandible angle for each patient will vary, but typically for females the ideal angle is 120 to 125 degrees and for males it is 130 to 140 degrees. Injections should be strictly performed on periosteum, with the intent of recreating the posterior and anterior aspects of the angle. The needle should be advanced from the dermal-subdermal junction into the preauricular area, to create a linear ridge of filler that mimics the edge of the mandible.
- Moving anteriorly on the mandible, the next injection site is the antegonial notch. Palpate for the facial artery first and place the nondominant hand on the artery to lightly retract it posteriorly out of the direction of injection. Keep this hand placement to ensure a safe injection away from the artery and inject a bolus of 0.2 to 0.3 cc into the antegonial notch.
- Further down the mandible is the jowl fat compartment region that should not be injected as this can cause additional swelling, bruising, and more jowling. Anterior to the jowl fat compartment is the prejowl sulcus fat pad injection. This

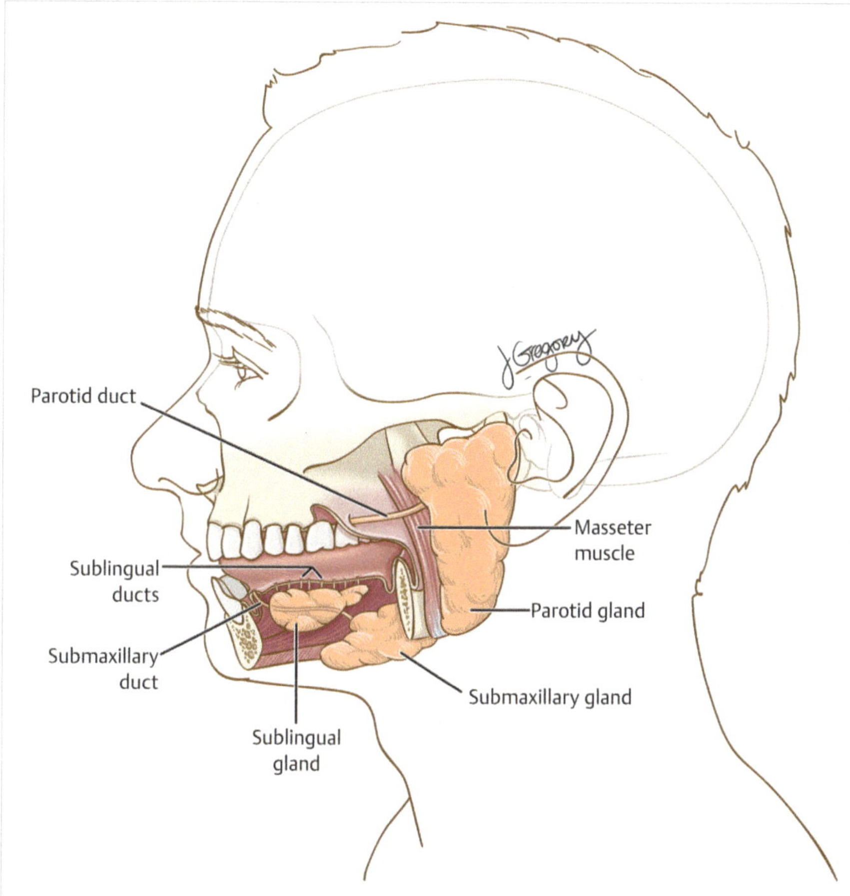

Fig. 44.7 Parotid duct/gland location. (Reproduced with permission from Anthony P. Sclafani. Total Otolaryngology—Head and Neck Surgery. Thieme; 2104.)

region contains another branch of the facial artery that requires additional palpation and posterior retraction in order to safely inject a bolus of 0.1 to 0.2 cc into this site. The next injection site to target is located at the anterior end of the mandibular body and mentum. Again, palpating for another branch where the facial artery crosses and retracting it is necessary in order to successfully deliver a bolus of 0.1 to 0.2 cc.

- Next, the fat pads surrounding the two retaining ligaments, the platysma mandibular and mandibular osseocutaneous, should be injected with small boluses of 0.1 to 0.2 cc of filler. This helps to support areas of fat herniation over the mandibular ligaments.
- The final injections should be delivered into the subcutaneous plane via subcutaneous threading in between these four injection points, totaling 0.2 to 0.3 cc. The subcutaneous plane is a safe plane to inject. Immediate molding of the product is advised in order to ensure the filler is placed smoothly to ensure the jawline exhibits the sculpted angle and shape desired.

44.3 Possible Side Effects and Complications

- Improper filler injection techniques can lead to vascular obstruction and serious complications such as visual compromise, blindness, stroke, necrosis, vascular occlusion, etc., and will need immediate intervention. Other delayed signs of vascular occlusion include ecchymosis, neovascularization, bruising, skin blanching, pain, long-term erythema, scarring, and pigment changes.
- Injecting a filler with higher G-prime and viscoelasticity has a higher risk of vascular occlusion. Non-HA fillers like calcium hydroxyapatite are not readily dissolvable because of their mineral content, other than experimentally with sodium thiosulfate. In order to prevent vascular occlusion, a complete understanding of the anatomical locations of critical facial vessels and danger zones is needed.

44.4 Postoperative Care

- Typically, effects of the treatment will begin presenting immediately after treatment. The filler is typically fully settled in 14 days. Avoid putting pressure on the mandible area, sleeping directly on the face, or getting facial treatments for 7 days. Use face masks for 1 to 2 weeks post treatment. Minimize exposure of the treated area to the sun or heat for at least 24 hours after treatment and if possible, until swelling and redness disappears. Note that salt, alcohol, and heat worsen possible swelling effects.

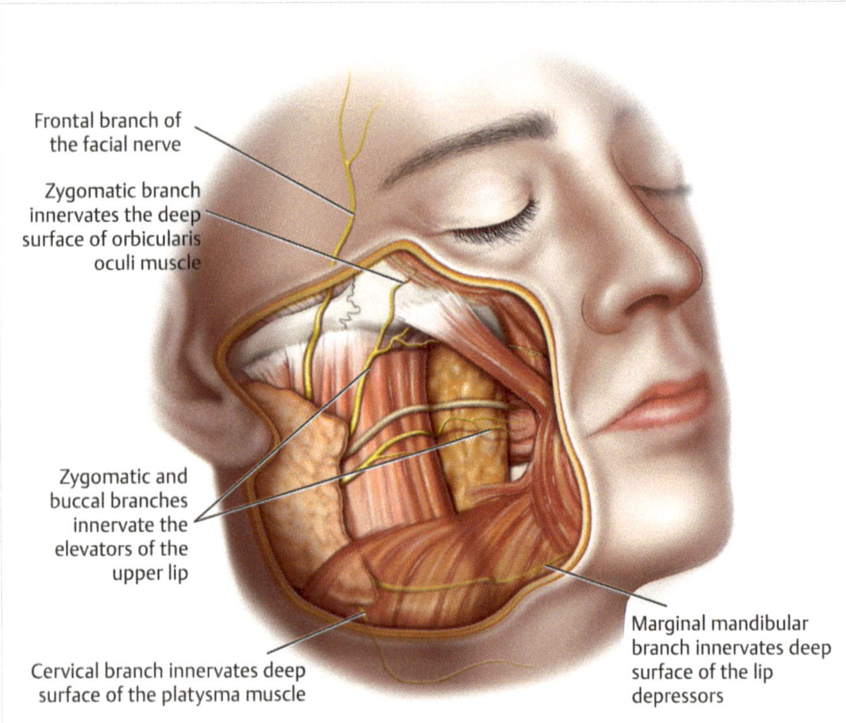

Fig. 44.8 Facial artery anatomy.

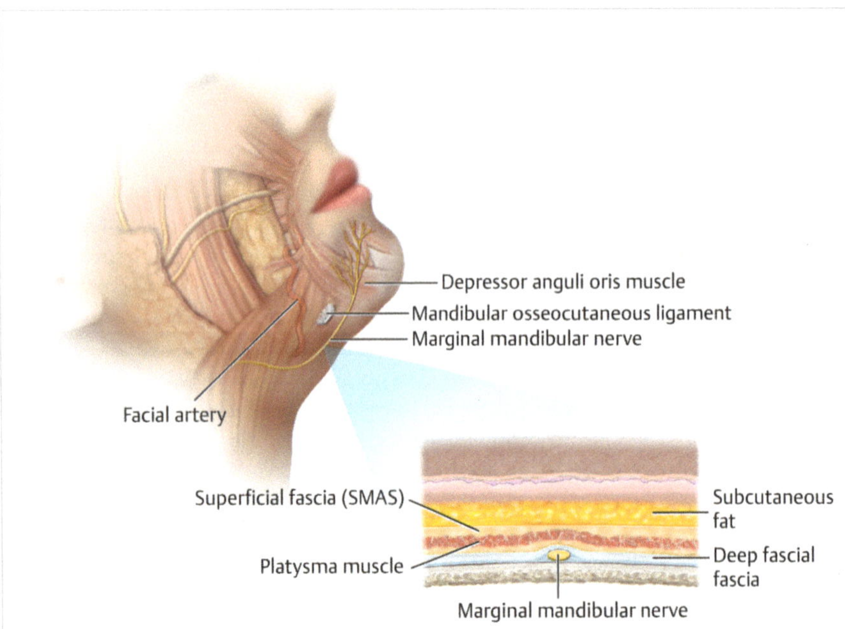

Fig. 44.9 Location of the marginal mandibular branch of the facial artery.

- Some swelling and bruising can occur within the first 3 to 4 days of treatment. This swelling and bruising can lead to asymmetry, which is normal. If the asymmetry persists, a follow-up appointment can be made to re-evaluate. Massaging the area and applying ice to it can help alleviate swelling, but make sure to massage and apply ice gently.

44.5 Case Example

Case Study: Left panel: Picture of a 30-year-old female prior to receiving any jawline filler. Right panel: Photo of the same female after receiving 1 syringe of calcium hydroxyapatite injection to the jaw (▶ Fig. 44.10a, b).

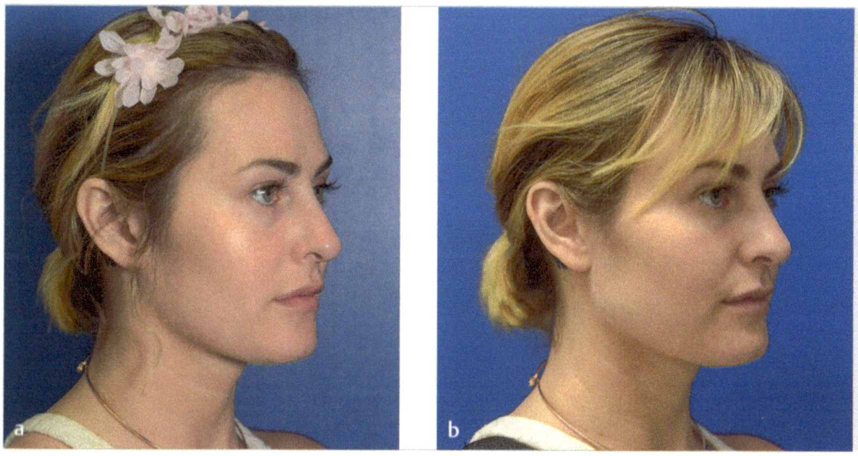

Fig. 44.10 (a, b) Left panel: Picture of a 30-year-old female prior to receiving any jawline filler. Right panel: Photo of the same female after receiving 1 syringe of calcium hydroxylapatite injection to the jaw.

44.6 Conclusion

An individualized approach is important in selecting the product best suited to patient's anatomy. Using a nonhyaluronic filler is beneficial for patients who have significant drooping and sagging. The non-HA fillers are more contouring, more supportive, and can promote natural collagen growth post injection, whereas HA fillers are more beneficial for patients who want a more subtle, natural look.

A stepwise approach to jawline contouring provides the best results. The areas that yield the most effective jawline sculpting include four primary injection sites: the mandible angle, the antegonial notch, the prejowl sulcus, and the junction of the anterior end of the mandibular body with the mentum. The volumizing lift of high-density fillers in these locations improves herniation of fat around the mandibular ligaments.

Overall, jawline fillers help patients achieve more youthful contours by reducing jowling and sagging to create a more sculpted and defined look.

See **Video 44.1**.

Further Readings

Alghoul M, Bitik O, Mcbride J, Zins JE. Relationship of the zygomatic facial nerve to the retaining ligaments of the face. Plast Reconstr Surg. 2012; 130:42

Brennan C. Avoiding the "danger zones" when injecting dermal fillers and volume enhancers. Plast Surg Nurs. 2014; 34(3):108–111, quiz 112–113

Jacovella PF. Use of calcium hydroxylapatite (Radiesse) for facial augmentation. Clin Interv Aging. 2008; 3(1):161–174

Lamb J, Surek C. Facial Volumization. 1st ed. New York: Thieme Medical Publishers; 2018:37–47

Salti G, Rauso R. Facial rejuvenation with fillers: the dual plane technique. J Cutan Aesthet Surg. 2015; 8(3):127–133

45 Chin Implant

Rod J. Rohrich and Erez Dayan

Abstract
Chin implants are a useful method to consistently achieve increased projection of the mentum in the anteroposterior direction. This technique is particularly useful in patients who require >2 mm of projection. The authors prefer using smooth silicone implants placed through a submental approach.

Keywords: Microgenia, chin implant, silicone chin implant, chin augmentation

Key Points

- In women, the chin should be approximately 2 mm posterior to the upper lip line. In men the chin should align with the upper lip line vertical.
- Chin projection is a key component of the lateral facial assessment and can be corrected with fat grafting alone if microgenia is <2 mm, or with a chin implant if >2 mm projection is required.
- Smooth silicone implants are preferable to porous materials (i.e., porous polyethylene).

45.1 Preoperative Steps

- A detailed medical history and physical are obtained for all patients prior to treatment. Exclusion criteria include: open wounds, active infection, dermatologic conditions, bleeding disorders, immunocompromised state, or the need for orthognathic correction of the maxillary–mandibular relationship.
- Consultation with the patient should be used to establish realistic expectations as well as to educate the patient on important perioperative care instructions for optimal results.

45.2 Operative Steps (▶ Fig. 45.1 and ▶ Fig. 45.2)

- See **Video 45.1**.
- A submental incision is marked and infiltrated with local anesthesia.
- Using a #15 blade, a 2 cm incision is made through the subcutaneous tissue. Next, a periosteal elevator is used to develop a precise subperiosteal pocket for placement of the silicone anatomic chin implant sizer. The area is undermined from the menton laterally along the lateral mandibular border to preserve the mental nerves bilaterally.
- After ascertaining the correct size and projection based upon the preoperative markings and discussion with the patient, the silicone chin implant size/projection is chosen and precisely placed on the menton.
- The implant is stabilized in the midline to the periosteum with a 3–0 Vicryl (Ethicon Inc., Somerville, NJ) suture.
- The mentalis muscle and subdermal area are closed with 4–0 Vicryl (Ethicon Inc., Somerville, NJ) deep interrupted suture.
- The skin is closed with simple interrupted 6–0 nylon sutures.

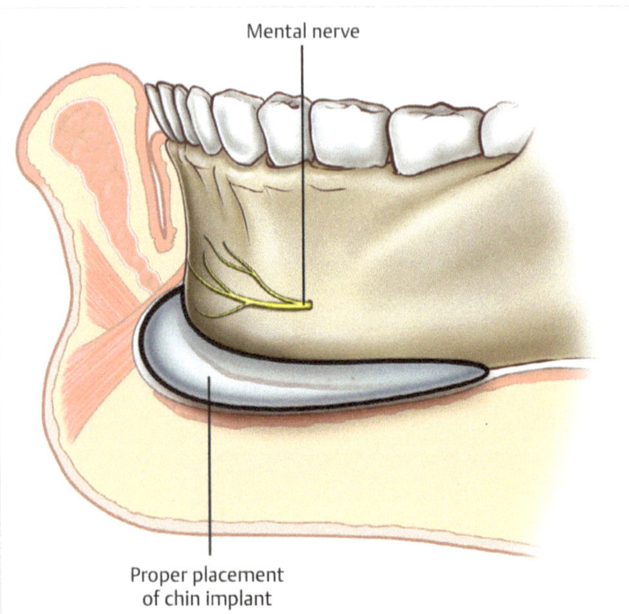

Fig. 45.1 Proper placement of chin implant relative to menton and mental neurovascular bundle.

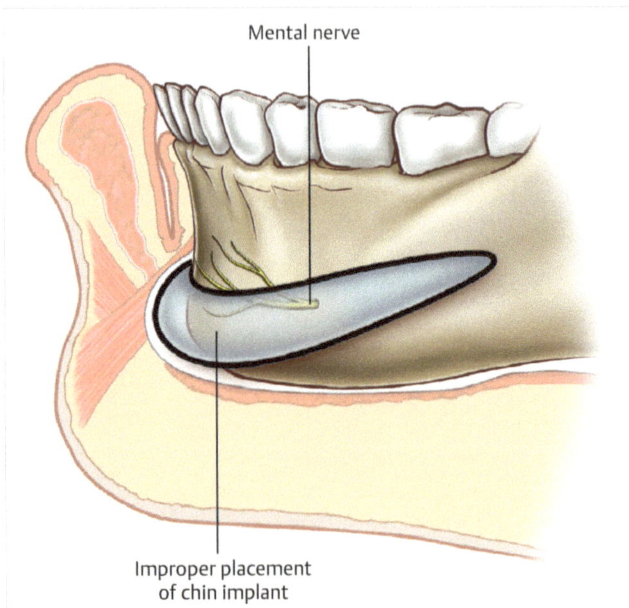

Fig. 45.2 Incorrect placement of chin implant, showing compression of mental nerve.

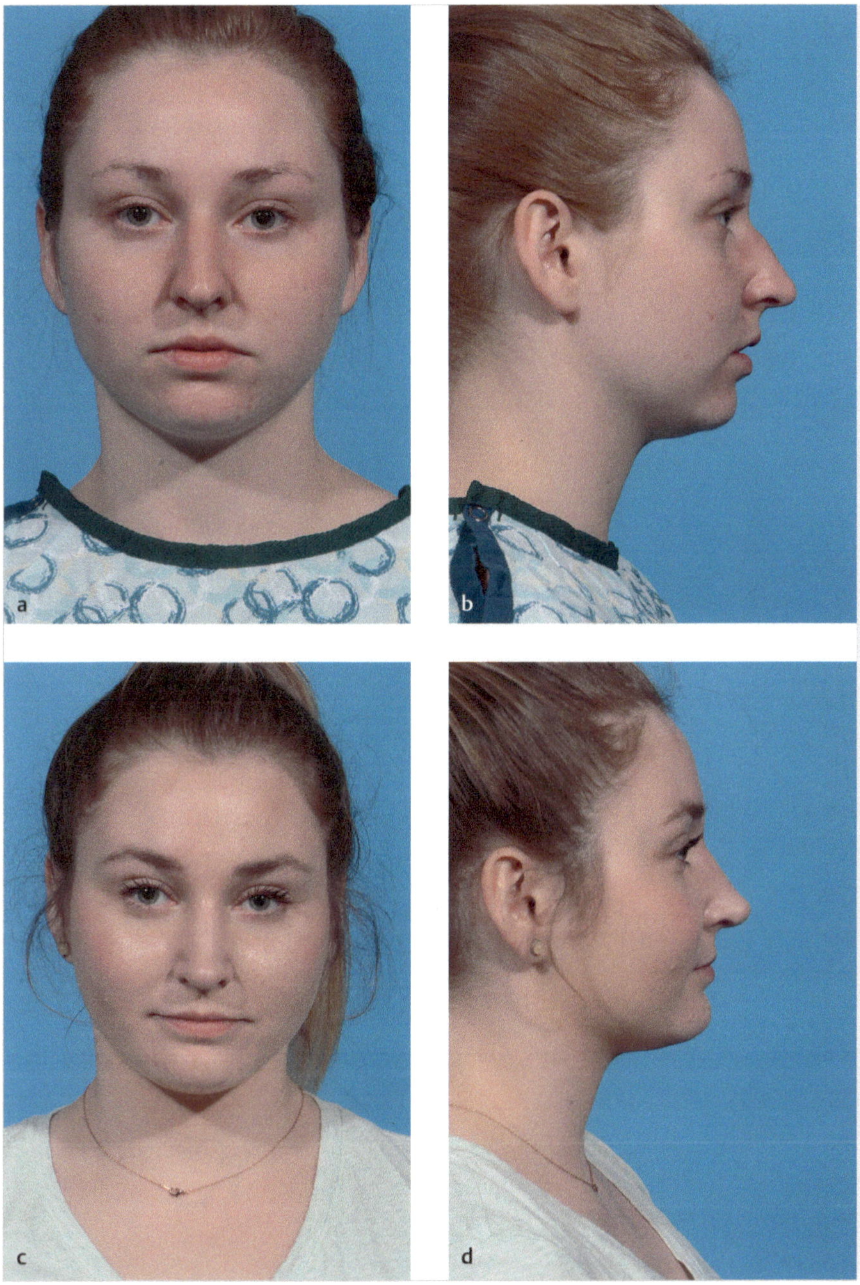
a
b
c
d

Fig. 45.3 (a–d) A 22-year-old female with a notable microgenia who underwent a combined rhinoplasty and chin augmentation with a small silicone implant. Postoperative images show improved harmony of the nose–lip–chin.

45.3 Postoperative Care

- Patients are instructed to refrain from strenuous activity for 2 to 3 weeks.
- On occasion the chin is taped to maintain soft tissue envelope position and obliterate dead space.

45.4 Case Example

A 22-year-old female with notable microgenia who underwent a combined rhinoplasty and chin augmentation with a small silicone implant. Postoperative images show improved harmony of the nose–lip–chin (▸ Fig. 45.3a–d).

45.5 Conclusion

For patients with microgenia > 2 mm, a chin implant is the procedure of choice to improve projection and harmony of the lower face in both men and women. Precise pocket formation and implant selection are critical to avoid undesirable implant migration and step-offs. Precise reapproximation of the mentalis is necessary to avoid a witch's chin deformity.

Further Readings

Flowers RS. Alloplastic augmentation of the anterior mandible. Clin Plast Surg. 1991; 18(1):107–138

McCarthy JG, Ruff GL, Zide BM. A surgical system for the correction of bony chin deformity. Clin Plast Surg. 1991; 18(1):139–152

McCarthy JG, Ruff GL. The chin. Clin Plast Surg. 1988; 15(1):125–137

Michelow BJ, Guyuron B. The chin: skeletal and soft-tissue components. Plast Reconstr Surg. 1995; 95(3):473–478

Zide BM, Longaker MT. Chin surgery: II. Submental ostectomy and soft-tissue excision. Plast Reconstr Surg. 1999; 104(6):1854–1860, discussion 1861–1862

46 Fat Grafting to the Chin

Rod J. Rohrich and Raja Mohan

Abstract

One major adjunct in facial rejuvenation is autologous fat transfer or facial fat grafting to various facial fat compartments of the face (▶ Fig. 46.1). One important region to consider is the chin where deep rhytides are often seen in the aging face. Some patients may have mild microgenia. Autologous fat grafting to this region adds volume to areas that are hollow or have become deflated. It can also add volume to patients who have microgenia.

Keywords: Fat grafting, chin augmentation, facial aging, fat transfer

Key Points

- Fat grafting to the chin is a useful adjunct in facial rejuvenation and does not carry the risks of implant-based or osseous genioplasty.
- Autologous fat grafting to the chin is indicated in patients with mild microgenia or facial rhytides requiring volumization.
- This technique also helps to address asymmetries and contour irregularities that cannot be adequately corrected by chin implants.

46.1 Preoperative Steps

46.1.1 Analysis

- A thorough preoperative analysis of the lower third of the face to identify areas of volume deflation and tissue laxity is performed.

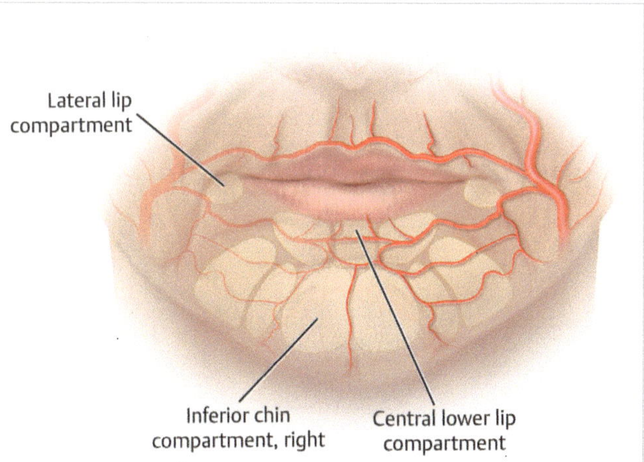

Fig. 46.1 Fat compartments of the lower face. (Reproduced with permission from Pessa JE. Facial Topography. Thieme; 2012.)

- Areas of volume deflation as well as deep rhytides are marked preoperatively in the mental region to determine areas requiring volumization.
- Microgenia is assessed based on a plumb line drawn from the upper lip to the menton.
- When analyzing the lip–chin relationship with this plumb line, patients with mild underprojection (<5 mm) are good candidates for autologous fat grafting to the chin.

46.2 Operative Steps

See **Video 46.1** and **Video 46.2**.

46.2.1 General Technique of Autologous Fat Harvest and Transfer

- Adipose tissue is harvested from the medial thighs using a 10-mL syringe with a 14-gauge (3 mm multihole) cannula.
- No wetting or infiltration solution is used for the harvest.
- The harvested lipoaspirate is centrifuged at 2,250 rpm for 1 minute followed by removal of the infranatant and supernatant to isolate the fat for transfer.
- The harvested fat is collected in 1-mL syringes.
- For any facial fat compartment, the 1-mL syringe with the harvested fat is connected to a 16-gauge blunt cannula and injected at a low pressure with anterograde and retrograde motions.

46.2.2 Injection Technique for Mental Region

- Using a 1-cc syringe attached to a 16-gauge blunt cannula, small aliquots of fat are transferred to areas of the mental region requiring volumization.
- Common areas to address are the labiomental sulcus, lateral chin hollowing, and midline cleft.
- The access sites are the midline to address a midline cleft or bifid chin. Two lateral sites are used to address lateral chin hollowing. One site laterally is used for the labiomental crease.
- To treat the midline, augmentation is performed by depositing fat (approximately 1–2 cc) above the periosteum. The cannula is then pointed laterally to treat areas lateral to the midline and approximately 1 to 2 cc is deposited.
- The lateral chin hollows are accessed laterally and 2 to 3 cc of fat is transferred to these areas in a radial and longitudinal manner.
- For a deep labiomental sulcus, 1 to 2 cc is injected to fill this depression.
- Autologous fat can also be transferred along the inferior and lateral mandibular border if needed.

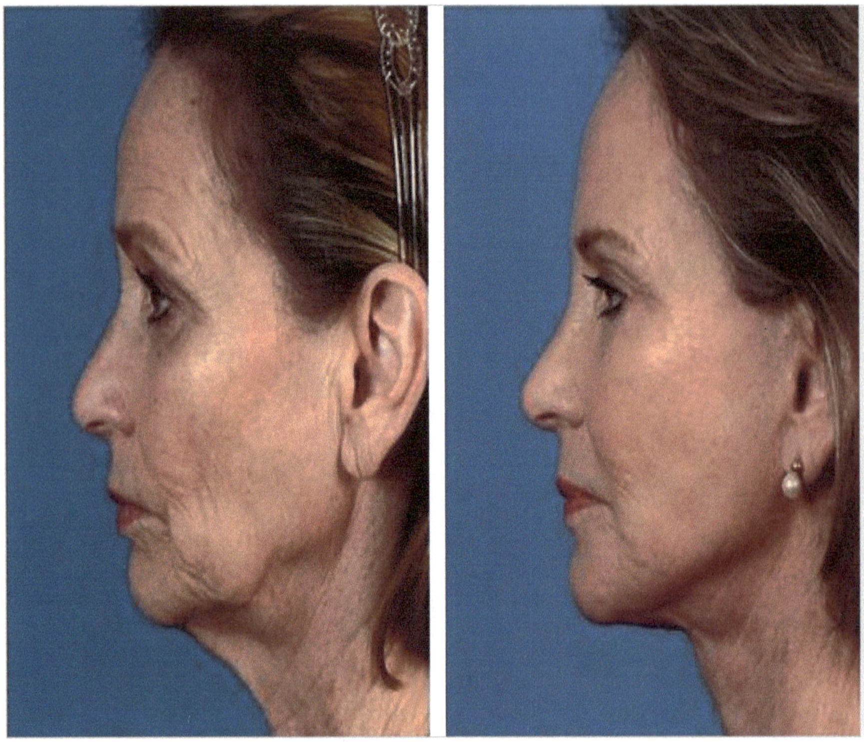

Fig. 46.2 This patient underwent a lift-and-fill facelift and as an adjunct, also had chin augmentation with autologous fat. The facelift helped to improve her cervicomental angle and eliminate jowling that was present preoperatively. In addition, her mild microgenia was corrected with facial fat augmentation. She has an improved lip–chin relationship postoperatively, which makes her appear more youthful.

- In general, fat concentrate of 1 to 2 mL is placed in each region and overcorrected by 50% in women and 100% in men.
- Areas of fat transfer should be massaged and molded to achieve uniformity and symmetry.

46.3 Postoperative Care

- Cold compresses are used over the face intermittently for the first 72 hours postoperatively.
- Patients are encouraged to avoid head turning and limit facial movements for the first week.
- Patients rest with head elevated to 45 degrees without the use of pillows to avoid flexion of the neck.

46.4 Case Example

This patient underwent a lift-and-fill facelift and as an adjunct, also had chin augmentation with autologous fat. The facelift improved her cervicomental angle and eliminated jowling that was present preoperatively. In addition, her mild microgenia was corrected with facial fat augmentation. She has an improved lip–chin relationship postoperatively, which makes her appear youthful (▶ Fig. 46.2).

46.5 Conclusion

Fat augmentation to the chin can restore volume loss associated with aging. Fat augmentation to the chin can soften marionette lines and deep rhytides in this region. The most commonly treated sites are the midline cleft, lateral hollows, and labiomental sulcus. This technique avoids the risks of implant-based or osseous genioplasty and is appropriate for patients with mild microgenia. We recommend overcorrection in men and undercorrection in women.

Further Readings

Pezeshk RA, Small KH, Rohrich RJ. Filling the facial compartments during a face lift. Plast Reconstr Surg. 2015; 136(4):704–705

Rohrich RJ, Afrooz PN. Finesse in face lifting: the role of facial fat compartment augmentation in facial rejuvenation. Plast Reconstr Surg. 2019; 143(1):98–101

Rohrich RJ, Ghavami A, Constantine FC, Unger J, Mojallal A. Lift-and-fill face lift: integrating the fat compartments. Plast Reconstr Surg. 2014; 133(6):756e–767e

Rohrich RJ, Sanniec K, Afrooz PN. Autologous fat grafting to the chin: a useful adjunct in complete aesthetic facial rejuvenation. Plast Reconstr Surg. 2018; 142(4):921–925

Rohrich RJ, Pessa JE. The fat compartments of the face: anatomy and clinical implications for cosmetic surgery. Plast Reconstr Surg. 2007; 119(7):2219–2227, discussion 2228–2231

47 Buccal Fat Pad Excision

Rod J. Rohrich, Yash J. Avashia, Ira L. Savetsky, and Nikhil A. Agrawal

Abstract

The buccal fat pad can be a cause of excess facial width and can blunt the jaw line. Excision of this fat is a great option for patients who would like a slimmer lower face. If there is excess excision of the fat pad, then premature aging will occur. The fat pad is broken up into lobes and through a small intraoral incision and gentle traction, excision can be limited to the buccal extension of the buccal fat pad. This will lead to nice contour of the lower face without the complication of premature aging.

Keywords: Fat pad excision, fat compartments, buccal fat, facial analysis, cheek fullness, masseter hypertrophy, mandibular definition

Key Points

- Buccal fat pad excision is an excellent procedure to narrow the width of the lower face.
- The fat pad is split into four main lobes that are separated by a thin fibrous layer.
- Excess traction or dissection of the fat pad can lead to excision of too many lobes of the fat pad and premature aging.

47.1 Preoperative Steps

47.1.1 Anatomy and Analysis (▶ Fig. 47.1a, b)

- The buccal fat pad consists of a main body and four extensions:
  - Buccal extension.
  - Pterygoid extension.
  - Superficial temporal.
  - Deep temporal.
- Examine the patient and the source of the buccal and mandibular contour:
  - Anterior buccal fullness can be treated by buccal fat removal.
  - Posterior buccal fullness can be treated by Botox injections to the masseter.
  - Mandibular border definition is best augmented by filler.

47.1.2 Managing Expectations

- Define where the patient would like the width of the face reduced.

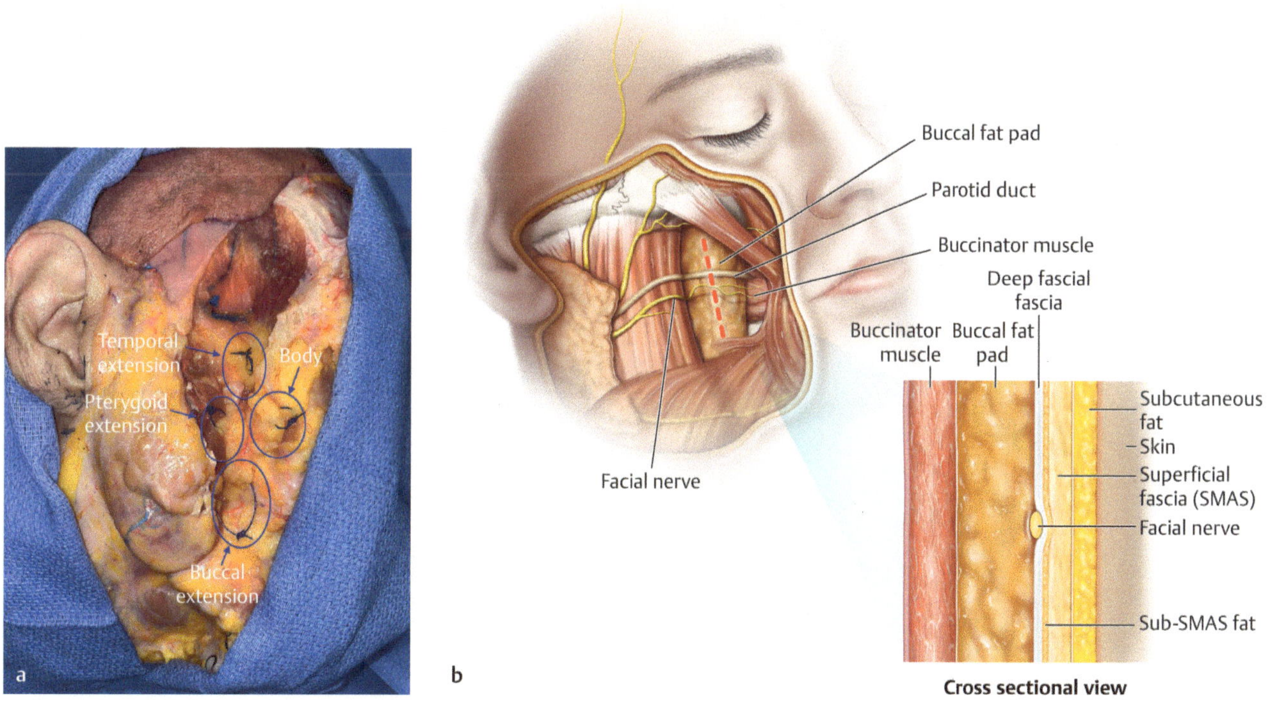

Fig. 47.1 **(a)** The lobes of the buccal fat pad are displayed here. The superficial and deep temporal extensions are superior. The body is anterior. The pterygoid extension is seen posteriorly and the buccal extension is seen inferiorly. **(b)** The body of the buccal fat pad is adjacent to the buccal branches of the facial nerve, which can be injured if excess traction is provided during surgery.

- Discuss the risk of premature aging and need for fat grafting of the face when the patient is older for facial rejuvenation.
- In the right patient, this surgery can be done in the office under local anesthesia.

47.2 Operative Steps

See **Video 47.1**.

47.2.1 Markings and Anesthesia

- The horizontal 2 cm incision is marked 2 cm inferior to Stensen's duct.
- For hemostasis and anesthesia, 4 mL of 1% lidocaine with epinephrine is injected.
- Two intraoral Obwegeser retractors are utilized for visualization.
- The incision is made with Bovie electrocautery to prevent any bleeding that may obstruct visualization (▶ Fig. 47.2).

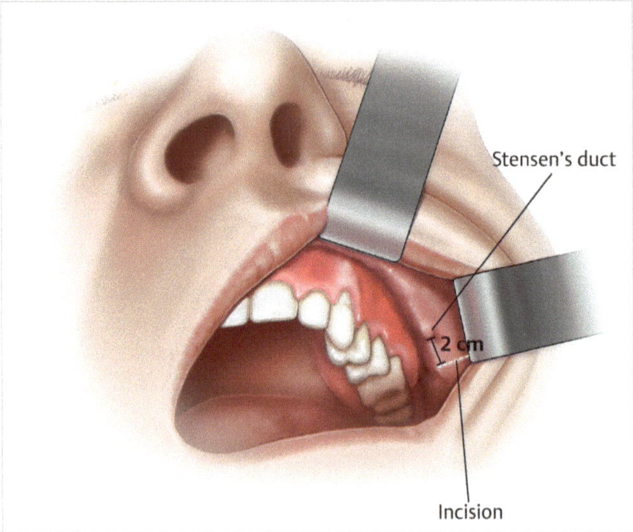

Fig. 47.2 Stensen's duct is identified and a transverse incision is made 2 cm inferior to this.

47.2.2 Dissection and Excision

- Dissection then proceeds bluntly with scissors.
- The fat pad is encountered and grasped with smooth forceps.
- The fat is gently teased out of the incision.
- Over-aggressive dissection will cause the fibrous layers between the lobes of the fat to be violated and more than just the buccal extension will be removed.
- Excision of fat should be done entirely with Bovie.
- It is also important to note that the volume of the buccal fat pad is not symmetrical so excision should be asymmetric as well.

47.2.3 Closure and Postoperative Care

- Close incision with 4–0 Vicryl sutures in a simple interrupted fashion.
- The patient is placed on a soft diet for 1 week.
- Perform 1-week long oral rinse course with 0.12% chlorhexidine.

47.3 Complications

- Dehiscence can generally be managed by secondary healing.
- Although hematoma is unlikely, it would need to be drained acutely.
- The fat pad is in close proximity to the buccal branches of the facial nerve so this carries a theoretical risk.

47.4 Case Example

Example of preoperative and postoperative buccal fat pad excision. Preoperative photos on the left, and 6 months post-operative photos on the right (▶ Fig. 47.3a–c).

47.5 Conclusion

Buccal fat excision is reliable for removing fullness from the anterior cheek. The procedure can be done in the office or in the operating room. Benefits must be weighed against the risk of premature aging.

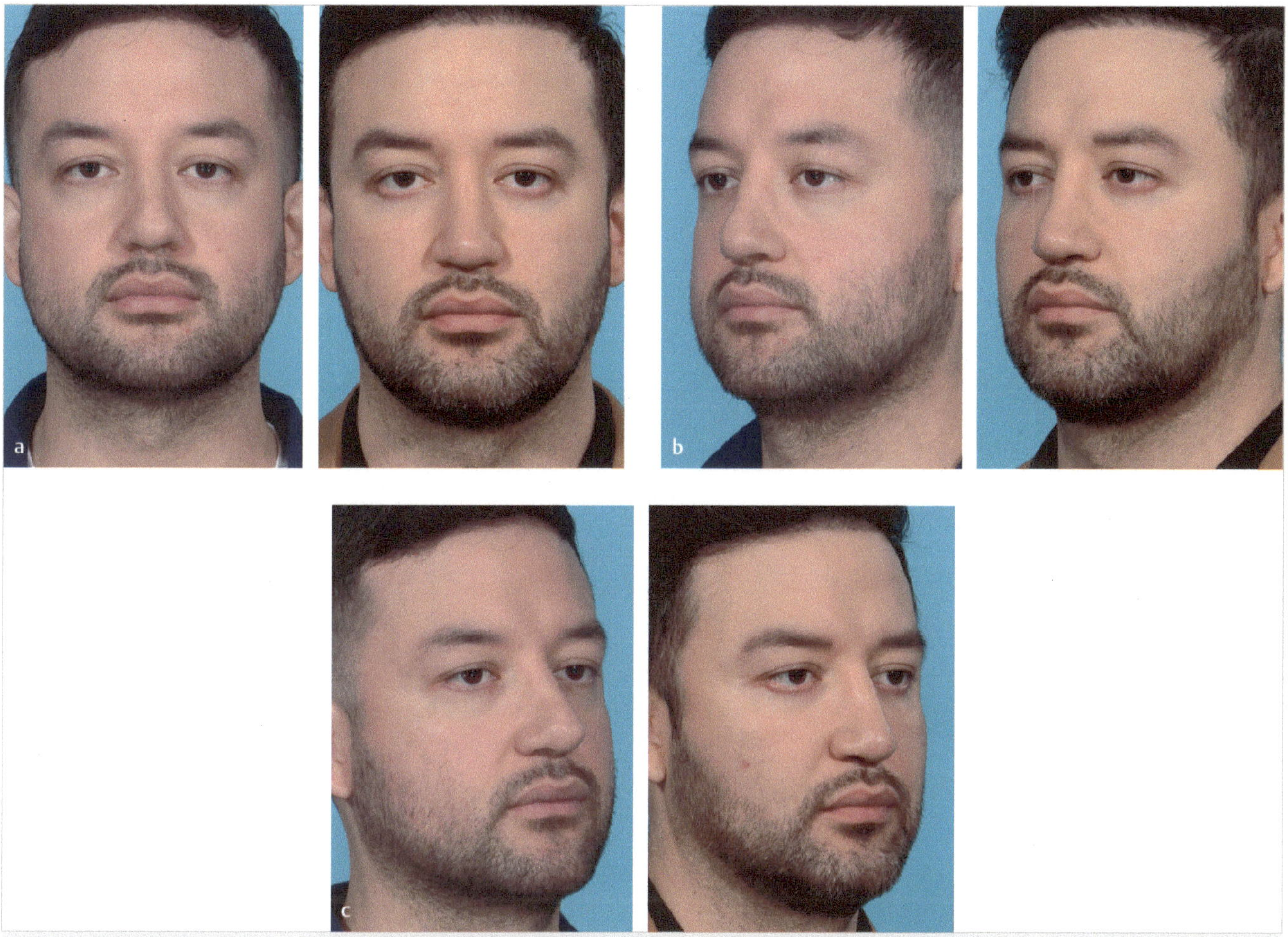

Fig. 47.3 (a–c) Example of preoperative and postoperative buccal fat pad excision. Preoperative photos on the left, and 6 months postoperative photos on the right.

Further Readings

Benjamin M, Reish RG. Buccal fat pad excision: proceed with caution. Plast Reconstr Surg Glob Open. 2018; 6(10):e1970

Sezgin B, Tatar S, Boge M, Ozmen S, Yavuzer R. The excision of the buccal fat pad for cheek refinement: volumetric considerations. Aesthet Surg J. 2019; 39(6): 585–592

Matarasso A. Buccal fat pad excision: aesthetic improvement of the midface. Ann Plast Surg. 1991; 26(5):413–418

Stuzin JM, Wagstrom L, Kawamoto HK, Baker TJ, Wolfe SA. The anatomy and clinical applications of the buccal fat pad. Plast Reconstr Surg. 1990; 85(1): 29–37

Zhang HM, Yan YP, Qi KM, Wang JQ, Liu ZF. Anatomical structure of the buccal fat pad and its clinical applications. Plast Reconstr Surg. 2002; 109(7):2509–2518

Part VII

Neuromodulators Finesse

VII

48 Neuromodulation of Glabella and Forehead

Steven Fagien and Yash J. Avashia

Abstract

Injectable neuromodulators are the most popular of all facial aesthetic procedures due to their relative ease of use, minimal downtime, and predictability. With the improvements in injection techniques, an enhanced understanding of the functional facial muscular anatomy, and the introduction of new products, neuromodulators can be selected based on their individual performance and injector preferences. Furthermore, additional facial areas are now amenable to nonsurgical intervention. Understanding the effects of these drugs, the target anatomy, and optimized injection techniques allow us to deliver safe and consistent results. Detailed assessment and focused neuromodulation of the muscles of the forehead and glabella can achieve temporary improvement in upper facial shape and reduction/elimination of rhytides of these regions.

Keywords: Neurotoxin, forehead, frontalis, glabella, procerus, depressor supercilia, corrugator supercilia, Botox

Key Points

- The lower frontalis muscles primarily function as elevators of the eyebrows and contribute to dynamic horizontal forehead rhytides.
- The upper frontalis can function as a hairline depressor.
- The glabellar complex includes procerus, corrugator supercilii, and depressor supercilii muscles, which contribute to vertical and horizontal frown lines, respectively.
- The lateral orbital portion of the orbicularis oculi muscle functions in part, as a lateral eyebrow depressor, and contributes to crow's feet, which are dynamic rhytides along the lateral orbit during squinting and smiling.
- Focused assessment and neuromodulation of these muscles are the objectives of this chapter.

48.1 Neuromodulators

- The neurotoxin for cosmetic neuromodulation is derived from *Clostridium botulinum*, a spore-forming, gram-positive anaerobe.
- The Type A subtype is most widely studied and acts its mechanism of preventing presynaptic release of acetylcholine at the neuromuscular junction.
- Five commercially available preparations of neurotoxin have been approved by the U.S. Food and Drug Administration (FDA), each with a similar yet unique performance profile. Units of each neurotoxin are not interchangeable:
  - Botox Cosmetic (onabotulinumtoxinA).
  - Dysport (abobotulinumtoxinA).
  - Jeuveau (prabotulinumtoxinA).
  - Xeomin (incobotulinumtoxin A).
  - Myobloc (botulinum toxin type B).
- Indications:
  - FDA approved facial regions.
  - Improvement in dynamic facial rhytides and facial shape is widely off-label.
- Contraindications (as indicated on the package insert):
  - Active infection or hypersensitivity.
  - Patients with neuromuscular disorders such as amyotrophic lateral sclerosis (ALS), myasthenia gravis, and Lambert-Eaton syndrome.
  - Coadministration with aminoglycoside antibiotics that interfere with neuromuscular transmission.
  - Pregnant women (Category C).
  - Lactating patients.
  - Inflammatory skin conditions.

48.2 Preoperative Evaluation

48.2.1 Forehead Anatomy

- Frontalis muscle:
  - Sole brow elevator and upper forehead depressor that originates from the galea aponeurotica and inserts into the superciliary ridge of the frontal bone.
- Glabellar muscles:
  - Procerus: The muscle originates from the inferoanterior surface of the paired nasal bones and inserts into the skin of the nasal root.
  - Corrugator supercilii: They lie deep to the frontalis and procerus muscles. The oblique head originates at the superciliary arch, and the transverse head inserts into the skin right above the brow-lash line, which is approximated by a vertical extension from the medial corneoscleral limbus.
  - Depressor supercilii: This muscle immediately inferior and superficial to the corrugator is, by some, considered as a component of the orbicularis oculi complex and part of a functional group together with the corrugators, which also depress the medial/central brow. This muscle originates at the medial orbital rim and extends to the medial aspect of the bony orbit.

48.2.2 Upper Facial General Assessment

- The upper face should be evaluated by a general assessment that considers deficiencies that might benefit by treatment from both a surgical, filler, and neuromodulator approach.
- The temple should be flat or slightly convex, without any significant concavity, depression, or hollowing (see *Chapter 53 Filler Finesse: Forehead*).
- The aesthetically desirable female eyebrow should be over the supraorbital margin with the medial aspect slightly lower than lateral aspect.
- In the central aspect, the brow ideally peaks in a vertical line along the lateral limbus of the iris.

- The upper eyelid should have fullness that follows the natural arc of the eyebrow and upper eyelid margin, and there should be no hooding.
- The upper face should be assessed for volume loss in the temples and forehead, position of the eyebrow, and the presence of excess skin in the upper and lower eyelids.
- Presence of static lines at rest and dynamic lines during animation should be evaluated in the forehead, glabella, lateral canthus, and eyebrows.
    - The frontalis muscle elevates the eyebrow and is the only elevator muscle in the upper face.
    - Contraction of the frontalis muscle leads to the development of horizontal forehead lines and can also act as a hairline depressor.
    - Frown lines may develop because of natural aging and ongoing contraction of the procerus, corrugator, and orbicularis oculi muscles.
    - Contraction of the procerus muscle lowers the medial aspect of the eyebrow and is the main contributor to the horizontal lines in this region.
    - Contraction of the corrugator muscle mostly draws down the medial aspect and can centralize the medial brow head of the eyebrow and is primarily responsible for vertical lines.
    - Repeated contraction of numerous facial muscles involved in smiling and squinting, notably the lateral orbicularis oculi muscles, leads to formation of lateral canthal lines, also known as crow's feet lines. These lines start as dynamic only (not present at rest) and eventually become static (present at rest).
    - The orbital part of the lateral orbicularis oculi can affect the position of the eyebrows and primary functions for voluntary eyelid closure.

48.3 Neuromodulation of the Upper Face

48.3.1 Storage and Preparation

- The neurotoxin agent is available in powder form and reconstitution is performed in 0.9% sterile saline. Most injectors prefer to use bacteriostatic saline to reduce injection discomfort but this is considered "off-label."
- Manufacturers recommend using the toxin within 4 hours of reconstitution and storing it at 2 to 8 °C. Experience indicates that the toxin maintains integrity and potency beyond this recommendation.
- Individual preferences regarding reconstitution vary from 1 to 5 mL and were originally felt to have little effect on results, but this concept has been recently challenged and may vary in optimization depending on which neurotoxin is considered and which muscle groups are targeted. Injectors also have varied preferences on syringe and needle types, but most commonly use 1-mL syringes to allow for precise injection of volume with fine tip needles of 30 to 32 gauge.

48.3.2 Anesthesia

- Ice or cold packs.
- Topical and local anesthetic combinations.
- Distraction techniques.

48.3.3 Planning

- Treatment must be individualized based on the patient's individualized desires and preferences, previous experiences, muscle strength, skin thickness, degree of rhytides, and choice of neurotoxin.

48.3.4 Frontalis Injection (▶ Fig. 48.1)

- On-label injections of onabotulinumtoxinA (the only neurotoxin currently "approved" for this region) for treatment of horizontal forehead lines can be performed at five sites, as shown, and this is the "on-label" indication in but this regions FDA approved for the use of onabotulinumtoxinA this area is probably the most varied regarding injector preferences and depends on the choice of neurotoxin and individualized objective analysis.
- Injection techniques are also quite varied and also depend on choice of neurotoxin and desired effects. Intramuscular or intradermal injections are delivered to the target areas that may also be influenced by neurotoxin choice and desired effect.
- The dosing and injection pattern reflect the aesthetic objective of the treatment and degree of muscle activity. For on-label injection with onabotulinumtoxinA, approximately 4 units are given at each injection site (▶ Fig. 48.1).
- Appropriate dosing, regardless of choice of neurotoxin, should be used to avoid a frozen appearance of the forehead, brow asymmetry, or medial and/or lateral eyebrow ptosis.
- Extend the injection sites far enough laterally to avoid excessive elevation of the lateral part of the eyebrow ("Mephisto" or "Spock" appearance).

48.3.5 Glabellar Complex Injection (▶ Fig. 48.2)

- To avoid eyebrow ptosis, in some individuals while treating the frontalis muscles, it can be important to also treat the depressors of the glabellar complex and the lateral canthus to minimize the tendency towards brow ptosis in some individuals.
- Injections to the glabellar region are primarily performed for the elimination or reduction of vertical "frown lines" that are dynamic but can also reduce static lines over time and serve to shape the medial eyebrow and prophylaxis.
- Injections of any of the neurotoxins for treatment of glabellar lines have traditionally involved five injection sites (▶ Fig. 48.2) but vary depending on the choice of drug and patient presentation that might vary from two to more than eight injection points depending on the patient presentation and desired effects. Additional treatment / injections to the medial orbicularis muscle/depressor supraciliaris muscles can be beneficial in some individuals.
- On-label injections are made into the procerus muscle (one site) and the medial and lateral corrugator muscles (two sites per side), which may also vary.
- For injections into the procerus muscle, pinching the skin can help guide the injection and it can be either intramuscular or intradermal (to avoid bleeding/bruising).
- Injection into the medial corrugator muscle is made by gently pinching the skin and inserting the needle to full depth while angled laterally upward. This is typically a deep injection just

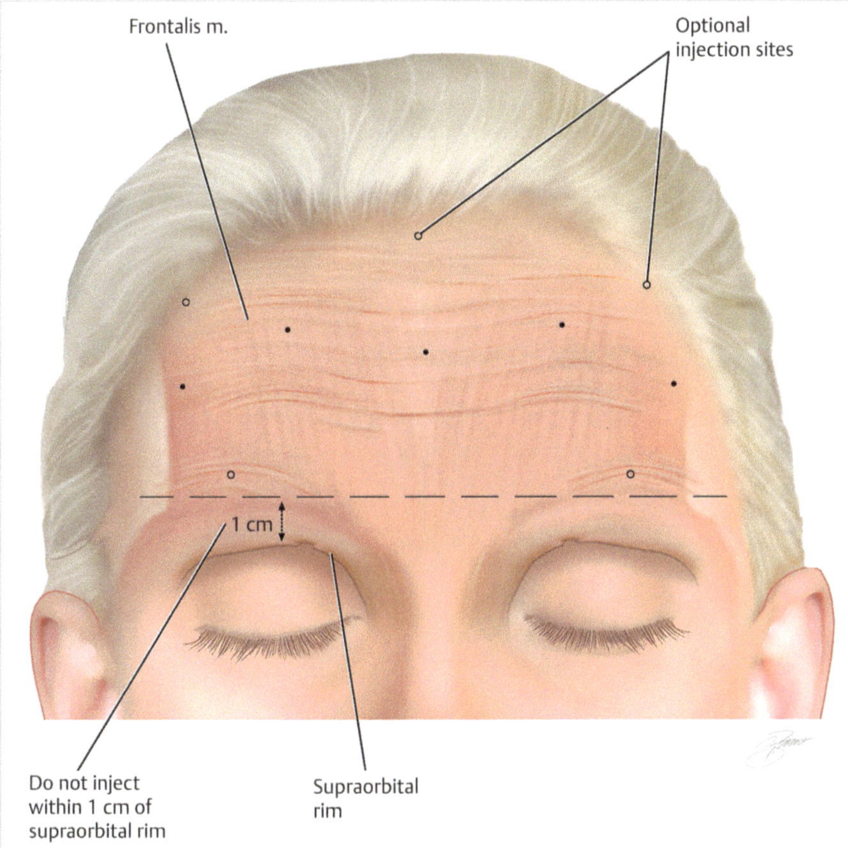

Fig. 48.1 Frontalis neuromodulator injection. (Reproduced with permission from Kontis T, Kacombe V. Cosmetic Injection Techniques: A Text and Video Guide to Neurotoxin Fillers. 2nd ed. Thieme; 2019.)

above the medial eyebrow lateral to the most medial wrinkle or fold, which is the location of the supratrochlear artery (to avoid).

- Because of its more superficial location, injection into the lateral corrugator muscle can be facilitated by pinching the skin and inserting the needle to one-third of its depth while angled laterally upward; however, if the injection is too superficial, the frontalis in this region can be more affected.

48.3.6 Crow's Feet and Other Effects with Orbicularis Muscle Injection

- Successful treatment of crow's feet lines in most situations can be accomplished by injections at three (on-label) or more sites per side.
- Two different patterns have been recommended depending on whether the lateral eyebrow position is low or high and the pattern of crow's feet that might involve a more medial aspect of the lateral lower eyelid.
- In those individuals who desire or benefit from a more elevated lateral eyebrow, an additional injection point can be administered just beneath the lateral brow cilia for enhanced brow lift effects.
- Insert the needle just subdermal and inject the neurotoxin superficially and subdermally into the lateral fibers of the orbicularis oculi muscle usually is most effective.
- Keep the patient's eyes closed. Use a finger to protect the upper eyelid and it is always best to inject with the direction of the needle and needle tip away from the eye. This area is prone to bleeding because of its high vascularity, and more superficial placement (creating a "wheel") can minimize bruising.
- Optional and advanced pretarsal orbicularis muscle injection (▸ Fig. 48.3) can also be administered for those individuals with mild to moderated degrees of blepharoptosis. Doses must be reduced to 1 U per injection point to avoid lagophthalmos.
- Total dosing depends on the severity of rhytides. Dynamic rhytides are well treated with neuromodulation. Often, static rhytides will not be completely addressed.
- Dosing per each injection is approximately 1 to 4 units.

48.4 Case Examples

48.4.1 Case 1

This example demonstrates the efficacy of forehead neuromodulation with neurotoxin. With a systematic approach to forehead neuromodulation, both dynamic horizontal and vertical rhytides can be treated and many patients benefit from a combination of neuromodulation and fine-line filling (▸ Fig. 48.4). *See Chapter 53 Filler Finesse: Forehead.*

48.4.2 Case 2

This example demonstrates the efficacy of periorbital neuromodulation of the orbicularis oculi muscle. A systematic approach to the lateral orbicularis oculi muscle helps to remove crow's feet lines which are more prominent on animation (▸ Fig. 48.5).

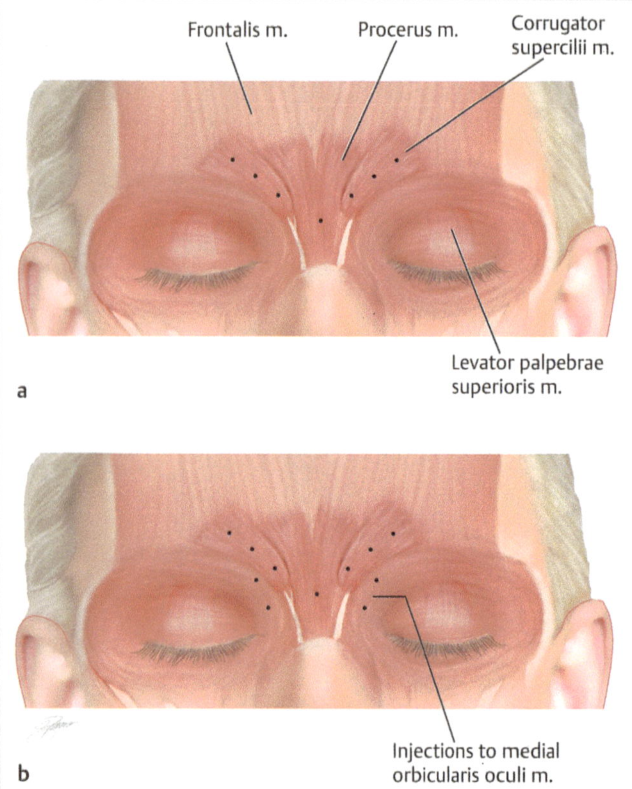

Fig. 48.2 (a, b) Glabellar complex neuromodulator injection. (Reproduced with permission from Kontis T, Kacombe V. Cosmetic Injection Techniques: A Text and Video Guide to Neurotoxin Fillers. 2nd ed. Thieme; 2019.)

48.5 Conclusion

Safe and consistent neuromodulation entails: (1) understanding the patient's desires and prior experiences; (2) knowledge of the regional muscle anatomy; (3) assessment for facial asymmetry, severity of rhytides, and dynamic nature of the muscles; (4) understanding the individual performance profiles for each of the neurotoxins; and (5) safe/effective techniques for injection

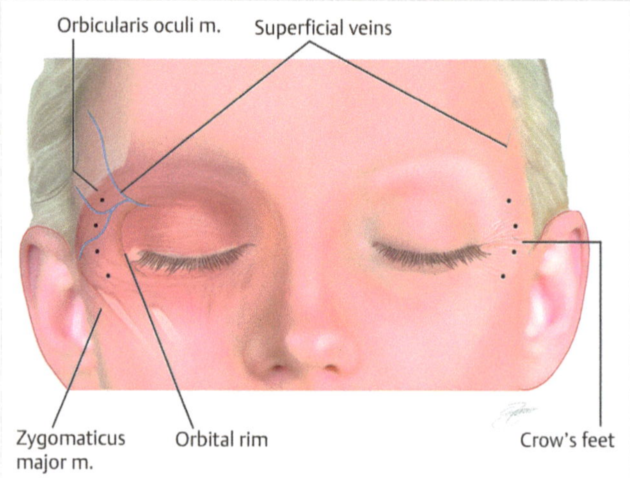

Fig. 48.3 Crow's feet neuromodulator injection. (Reproduced with permission from Kontis T, Kacombe V. Cosmetic Injection Techniques: A Text and Video Guide to Neurotoxin Fillers. 2nd ed. Thieme; 2019.)

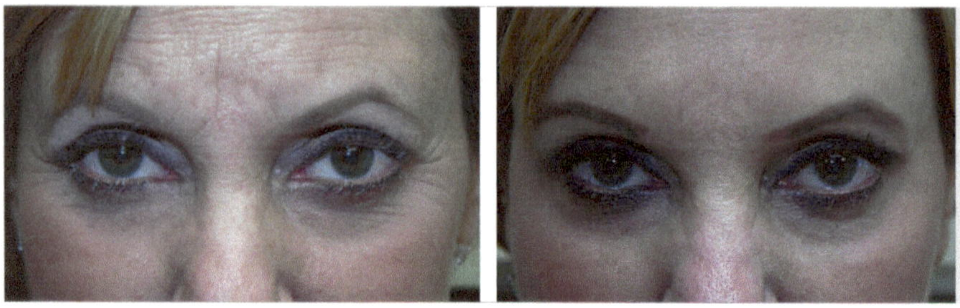

Fig. 48.4 Case 1. This example demonstrates the efficacy of forehead neuromodulation with neurotoxin. With a systematic approach to forehead neuromodulation, both dynamic horizontal and vertical rhytides can be treated.

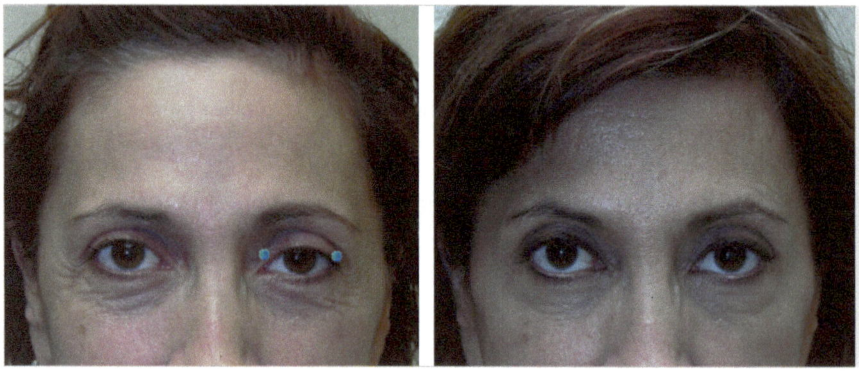

Fig. 48.5 Case 2. This example demonstrates the efficacy of periorbital neuromodulation of the orbicularis oculi muscle. A systematic approach to the lateral orbicularis oculi muscle helps to remove crow's feet lines which are more prominent on animation.

to avoid or reduce discomfort, unwanted side effects. and delivering the best results for each patient.

See **Video 48.1**.

Further Readings

Carruthers J, Fagien S, Matarasso SL, Botox Consensus Group. Consensus recommendations on the use of botulinum toxin type a in facial aesthetics. Plast Reconstr Surg. 2004; 114(6) Suppl:1S–22S

de Maio M, Swift A, Signorini M, Fagien S, Aesthetic Leaders in Facial Aesthetics Consensus Committee. Facial assessment and injection guide for botulinum toxin and injectable hyaluronic acid fillers: focus on the upper face. Plast Reconstr Surg. 2017; 140(2):265e–276e

Fagien S. Botulinum toxin type A for facial aesthetic enhancement: role in facial shaping. Plast Reconstr Surg. 2003; 112(5) Suppl:6S–18S, discussion 19S–20S

Fagien S, Carruthers A, Carruthers J. Expanded uses of BTX-A for facial aesthetic enhancement. In: Fagien S, ed. Cosmetic Oculoplastic Surgery. 4th ed. London UK: Elsevier Publishers; 2007:303–336

Fagien S, Cox SE, Finn JC, Werschler WP, Kowalski JW. Patient-reported outcomes with botulinum toxin type A treatment of glabellar rhytids: a double-blind, randomized, placebo-controlled study. Dermatol Surg. 2007; 33(1 Spec No.):S2–S9

Fagien S. Temporary management of upper lid ptosis, lid malposition, and eyelid fissure asymmetry with botulinum toxin type A. Plast Reconstr Surg. 2004; 114(7):1892–1902

49 Botulinum Toxin Injection to Crow's Feet

Joshua M. Cohen and Sammy Sinno

Abstract
Repeated contraction of numerous facial muscles involved in smiling and squinting, most notably the orbicularis oculi, leads to the formation of canthal lines. These lines initially appear only during animation but over time can become static due to age-related skin changes. Lateral canthal lines, or "crow's feet," are one of the FDA approved indications for botulinum toxin.

Keywords: Botulinum toxin, Botox, canthal lines, crow's feet, lateral canthus

Key Points

- Lateral canthal lines may be due to contraction of the orbicularis oculi during animation. Botulinum toxin injection reduces the orbicularis oculi contraction, thereby reducing the appearance of lines in the lateral canthal region.
- The number of botulinum toxin units needed and/or injection points is variable based on the activity of the orbicularis oculi.
- A lateral "brow lift" can be achieved by injection of a few units at the tail of the lateral brow.

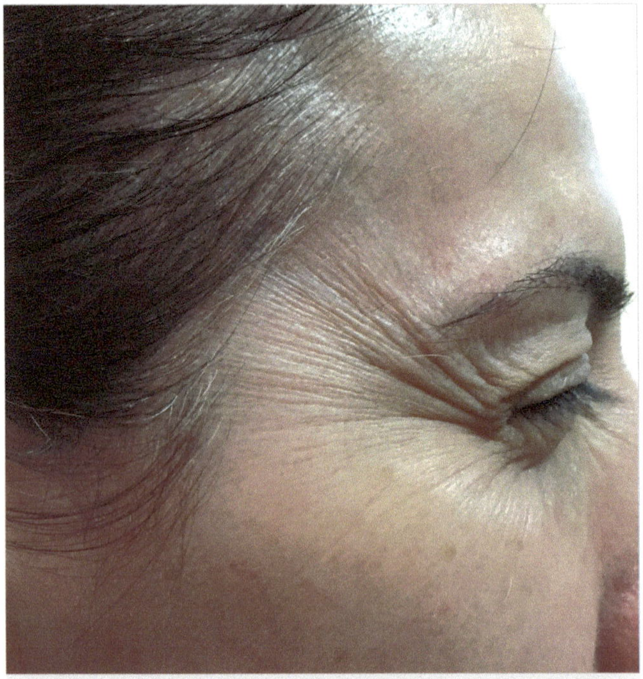

Fig. 49.1 Patient demonstrating lateral canthal lines during animation.

49.1 Preprocedural Steps

- Patients who present for treatment of crow's feet vary in age, typically starting in their 20s.
- Canthal lines have two etiologies:
  - Contraction of the orbicularis oculi muscle during animation such as smiling or squinting (▶ Fig. 49.1).
  - Excess skin laxity that causes an excess of tissue hanging over the lateral canthal area; these patients commonly have significant wrinkles at rest and will not have significant improvement with botulinum toxin and are candidates for a surgical brow lift.
- Asymmetries between the two sides are noted.
- It is not uncommon for the eye with more lateral canthal lines or a smaller palpebral aperture to require more neurotoxin.

49.2 Procedural Steps

See **Video 49.1**.

49.2.1 Botulinum Toxin Administration to the Crow's Feet

- The patient is prepped with an alcohol swab.
- Any large veins in the canthal area are noted and avoided to prevent bruising (▶ Fig. 49.2).

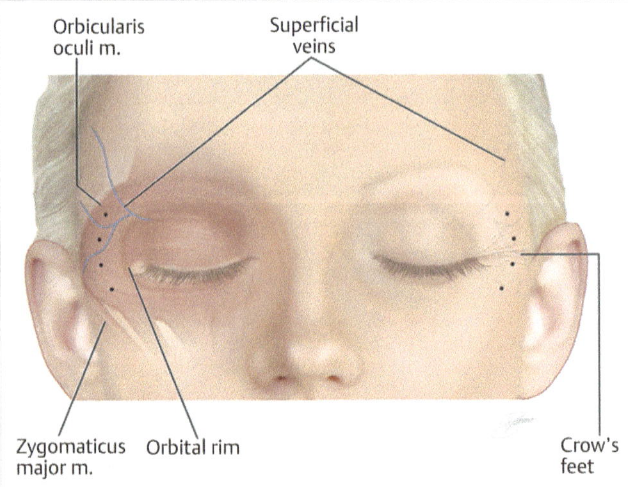

Fig. 49.2 Standard injection points with anatomical outline and observance of superficial veins.

- In patients with significant wrinkles in this area, 12 to 15 units of botulinum toxin are used per side.
- Three injection points are standard. Treatment starts at the level of the lateral canthus, and then one injection above and one below (▶ Fig. 49.3).

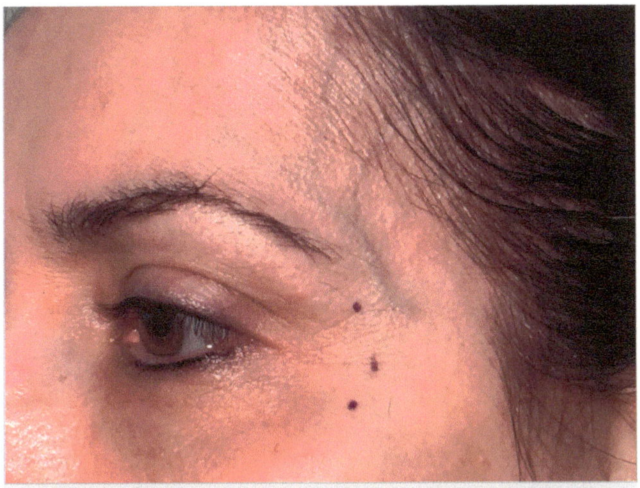

Fig. 49.3 Standard injection points on patient with visible large superficial vein.

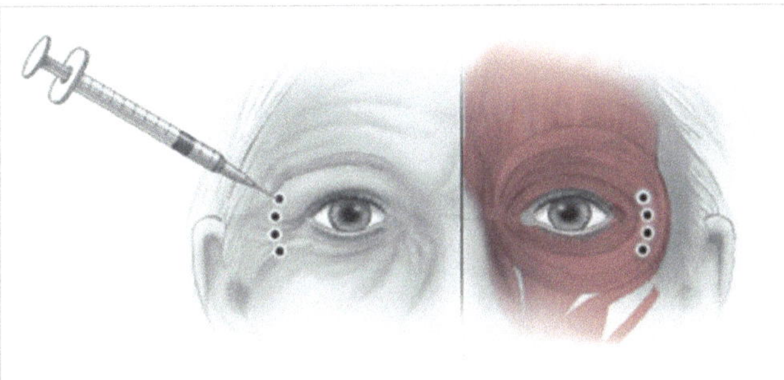

Fig. 49.4 Additional injection point just caudal to the tail of the brow for a "lifting" effect.

- A second "double row" can be injected for a more active orbicularis oculi with peripheral wrinkles.
- A lateral "brow lift" can be achieved by injecting an additional 3 to 4 units superiorly just caudal to the tail of the brow (► Fig. 49.4).

49.3 Postprocedure Care

- Ice can be used to minimize bruising and swelling.
- Patients are asked to refrain from exercise and alcohol for one evening following injections.
- Patients should avoid tight-wearing hats or headbands.
- Results begin to take effect in 1 week.

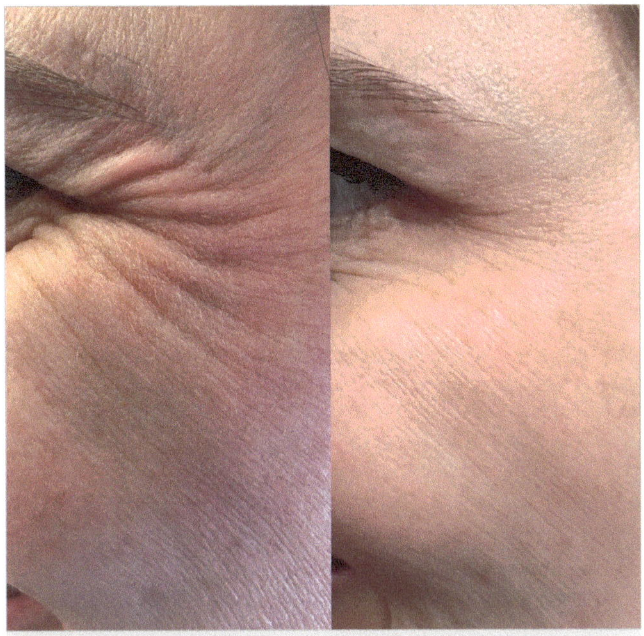

Fig. 49.5 Preprocedure and postprocedure photos of a patient 1 month following injection of 15 units of botulinum toxin per side.

49.4 Case Example

Preprocedure and postprocedure photos of a patient 1 month following injection of 15 units of botulinum toxin per side (► Fig. 49.5).

49.5 Conclusion

The use of botulinum toxin is an effective modality for treatment of dynamic lines surrounding the lateral canthus.

Further Readings

Carruthers J, Carruthers A. Botulinum toxin type A treatment of multiple upper facial sites: patient-reported outcomes. Dermatol Surg. 2007; 33(1 Spec No.):S10–S17

Carruthers J, Fagien S, Matarasso SL, Botox Consensus Group. Consensus recommendations on the use of botulinum toxin type a in facial aesthetics. Plast Reconstr Surg. 2004; 114(6) Suppl:1S–22S

de Maio M, Swift A, Signorini M, Fagien S, Aesthetic Leaders in Facial Aesthetics Consensus Committee. Facial assessment and injection guide for botulinum toxin and injectable hyaluronic acid fillers: focus on the upper face. Plast Reconstr Surg. 2017; 140(2):265e–276e

Monheit G. Neurotoxins: current concepts in cosmetic use on the face and neck—upper face (glabella, forehead, and crow's feet). Plast Reconstr Surg. 2015; 136(5) Suppl:72S–75S

Sykes JM, Trevidic P, Suárez GA, Criollo-Lamilla G. Newer understanding of specific anatomic targets in the aging face as applied to injectables: facial muscles—identifying optimal targets for neuromodulators. Plast Reconstr Surg. 2015; 136 5:56S–61S

50 Microbotox of the Face, Neck, and Scars

Woffles T. L. Wu

Abstract

Microbotox is a technique where microdroplets of onabotulinumtoxinA are injected into the superficial layers of the skin and soft tissues of the face and neck as a superficial carpet of tiny drops to reduce fine lines and wrinkles, improve skin texture, and sheen and improve lower face and cervicomental contouring without compromising muscle function or mobility. Droplet size and not the dose is the most important consideration when injecting botulinum toxin into the face and neck.

Microdroplets have a limited diffusion capacity with the result that the injected onabotulinumtoxinA remains more targeted at the deep dermal level or where the superficial fibers of the facial muscles are inserted into the undersurface of the dermis. As a result, deeper muscular activity is retained and patients look and feel more natural.

Three mixtures of microbotox are employed: Microbotox-20 which contains 20 units of onabotulinumtoxinA in a 1-mL syringe of diluted toxin (used for pores and fine lines) over the infraorbital and central T-zone areas, Microbotox-24 which contains 24 units in 1 mL solution that includes lidocaine and is used for upper and lower face and neck in thin-skinned individuals such as females, and Microbotox-28 which contains 28 units in 1 mL solution and is used for upper and lower face and neck in those with thicker skin such as males. Effects last for 3 to 4 months.

Keywords: Microbotox, microdroplets, droplet size, diffusion, skin texture, cervicomental contouring

Key Points

- Microbotox, which was developed by this author in 2000, is a microdroplet technique of administering microdoses of onabotulinum toxin into the face and neck to achieve a reduction of lines and creases, improve skin texture, sheen, and appearance, and better cervicomental and jawline contouring with a decrease of horizontal neck lines, without the complications and stiff, rigid appearance that often accompanies the use of standard macrodroplet injections of full strength onabotulinum toxin in these areas.
- The microdroplets are injected as tiny blebs into the dermis or the interface between the dermis and the upper fibers of the facial and neck muscles at approximately 1 cm intervals, creating a superficial "carpet" of tiny onabotulinum toxin droplets. These muscles are unique in that some of their superficial fibers are attached to the undersurface of the dermis, thereby creating the active and passive crease lines of the face and neck that we are familiar with. Weakening of these superficial muscle fibers decreases lines and wrinkles without compromising the integrity and strength of the deeper muscle layers, which are unaffected and can still actively contract. This confers a more natural facial appearance.
- Microbotox also has an effect on skin by reducing sweat and sebaceous gland activity that in turn decreases the visibility of facial pores, improves its texture and sheen as well as decreases acne.
- Microbotox is also useful in speeding up the healing of fresh surgical wounds by acting as a chemical splint to decrease skin tension across the wound edges, reducing the red/brown phase of wound healing, and preventing keloid formation.
- The microbotox technique was developed by this author using primarily Onabotulinum Toxin Type A (Botox, Allergan Pharmaceuticals Ireland, Westport, Co. Mayo, Ireland) and for this reason, the toxin will be referred to in the text as Botox or microbotox.

50.1 Underlying Principle and Concepts

- With the advent of onabotulinum toxin and its popularization since the mid-1990s, on-label indications for the drug around the world include a five-point injection technique for the glabellar frown lines (20 units), a six-point injection technique for the crow's feet (24 units), and a five-point technique for the forehead (20 units).
- Each of these points is a droplet of 0.1 mL containing 4 units of standard onabotulinum toxin. A standard bottle of onabotulinum toxin is usually prepared with 2.5 mL of saline to make the calculation of dose administration easier to understand: 0.5 mL is 20 units, 0.6 mL is 24 units, and 0.7 mL is 28 units. A 1-mL syringe of standard onabotulinum toxin therefore contains 40 units.
- Doctors have largely followed these on-label guidelines with the consequence that patients often return complaining that their forehead feels stiff, eyebrows are immovable and at a lower position than before injection, and they also notice deeper infraorbital and cheek creases appearing below the region of crow's feet blockade, thereby conferring an unwanted, unnatural "Botoxed" appearance. In some cases, they may experience upper eyelid ptosis due to diffusion of the toxin into the levator muscles.
- This author realized that too much toxin was being administered and that the most important consideration when injecting onabotulinum toxin was not the dose but the droplet volume. Large droplets of 0.1 or 0.05 mL have a much wider three-dimensional diffusion radius, which not only affects an area beyond the point of injection but also the entire depth of the soft tissue envelope.
- Microbotox on the other hand uses microdroplets of 0.01 mL or less (▶ Fig. 50.1).

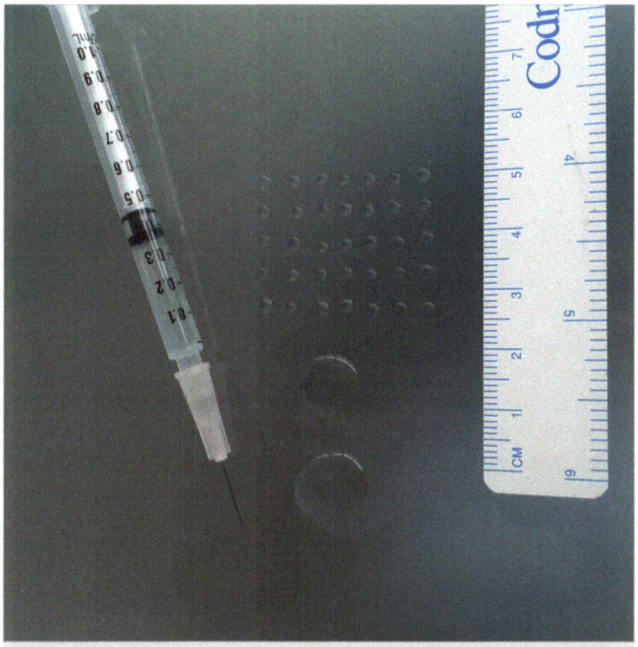

Fig. 50.1 Comparison between volume and size of a 0.1 or 0.05 cc droplet and a cluster of microbotox microdroplets all of which add up to 0.05 cc.

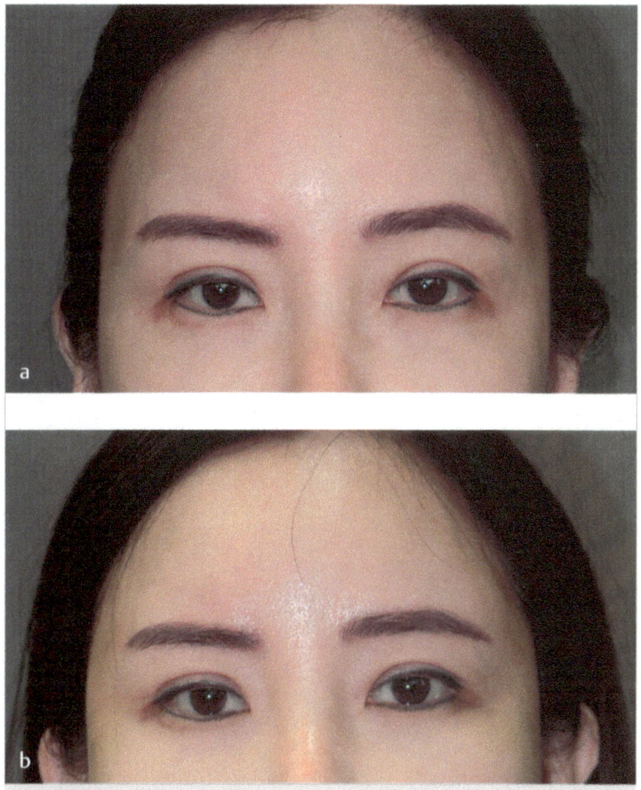

Fig. 50.2 (a, b) Microbotox of the upper facial third (forehead, glabellar, crow's feet areas) showing a bright, lifted appearance of the eyebrows, smoothening of frown lines and improved skin appearance and reflectance.

50.2 Microbotox of the Facial Upper Third

- There are some patients who request and like a totally smooth and immovable forehead without a trace of movement in the glabella region and certainly no crow's feet lines. Standard doses of Botox can achieve this.
- For those patients who want a more natural or refined appearance, with some movement of all the muscles, the microbotox technique is extremely useful as this does not paralyze the muscles completely (▶ Fig. 50.2a, b).
- A third category is those patients who may need some standard macrodroplets into specific muscles such as the medial glabellar frown (corrugator origin) or the central crow's feet region just lateral to the lateral canthus but a microbotox technique to the forehead. Here, the author uses both standard as well as microbotox techniques in combination.
- Each patient has to be individually assessed as different patterns of eyebrow elevation exist. Some patients are central "pullers" where the medial eyebrow is more elevated than the lateral aspect, some are lateral "pullers" where the eyebrow has a greater lateral elevation than medially and some are uniform "pullers" where the eyebrow elevates without any distortion in its shape. Microbototox-24 is used for females whilst Microbotox-28 is used in males with thicker skin and more active glabellar muscles.
- As aesthetic trends have changed through the years and the emphasis is now on a more natural appearance, this author prefers to employ microbotox droplets for the entire facial upper third. There are much fewer complications and fewer complaints. Patients are informed that the effect will last from 3 to 4 months.

50.3 Microbotox of the Facial Middle Third

- The middle third of the face includes the lower eyelids, bunny lines and the skin over the nose and cheeks which may have prominent pores, oily skin, rosacea or acne.
- Standard doses of onabotulinum toxin can be used to treat lower eyelid lines and hypertrophic tarsal muscle rolls but this can be fraught with some complications such as lower eyelids that do not move at all on smiling or worse, an over relaxation of the orbital portion of the orbicularis oculi muscle allowing eyebags to become more noticeable. Patients can be very discerning and will not hesitate to voice their displeasure with such an appearance.
- Microbotox injections in the skin of the middle facial third can more effectively smoothen and tighten the skin (due to the neurochemically induced bulk atrophy of the sweat and sebaceous glands) as well as by decreasing the subtle pulling and tethering effects of the facial muscles where they are attached to the skin (▶ Fig. 50.3a, b).

50.4 Microbotox of the Lower Face and Neck

- The area of the lower face and neck that benefits from microbotox injections is defined as a zone bounded by a line three

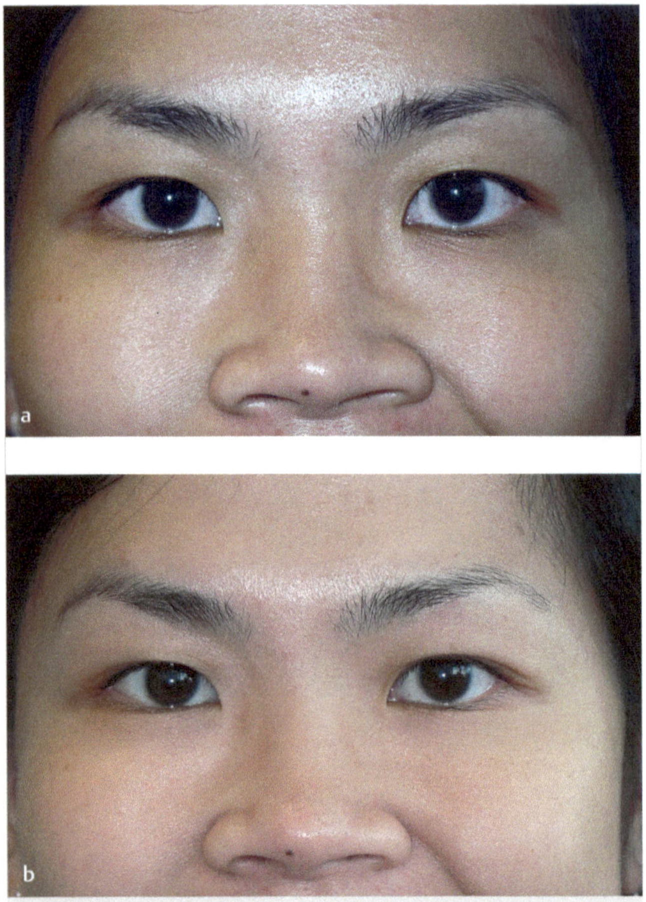

Fig. 50.3 (a, b) Before and after microbotox of the infraorbital and mid cheek zones with reduction of fine lines, smoothening of skin surface and decreased pore visibility.

fingerbreadths above and parallel to the lower border of the mandible, one fingerbreadth posterior to the lateral edge of the depressor anguli oris and all the way down over the cervicomental angle and anterior neck to the upper border of the clavicle, in front of the anterior border of the sternocleidomastoid. This corresponds with the anatomical extent of the platysma as it sweeps up from the clavicle over the jawline to blend in with the superficial musculoaponeurotic system (SMAS) of the face (▶ Fig. 50.4a–c).

- Injections are only delivered outside of this area over and posterior to the sternocleidomastoid if there are horizontal neck lines that extend far laterally or if there are particularly strong lateral platysmal bands. The intent of delivering microbotox into this area is not only to improve neck skin texture, color and smoothness (▶ Fig. 50.5a–c) but also to decrease the activity of the superficial fibers of the platysma muscle that in turn creates a lifting effect of the jowls and jawline as well as better cervicomental contouring.

50.5 The Platysma Effect

- When a muscle contracts, it shortens in length and its diameter or girth increases. The axial contraction creates an outward lateral force or shift (bulging) on either side of the muscle. If only one side of the muscle is weakened, then upon activation, the muscle will contract on the side that is normal, causing a movement vector away from the weakened side.
- The platysma muscle is a large sheet of subcutaneous muscle whose superficial fibers insert into the undersurface of the overlying skin. As it contracts it shortens the distance between the chin and the clavicle with blunting of the cervicomental angle. This can be easily seen by contracting the muscle.

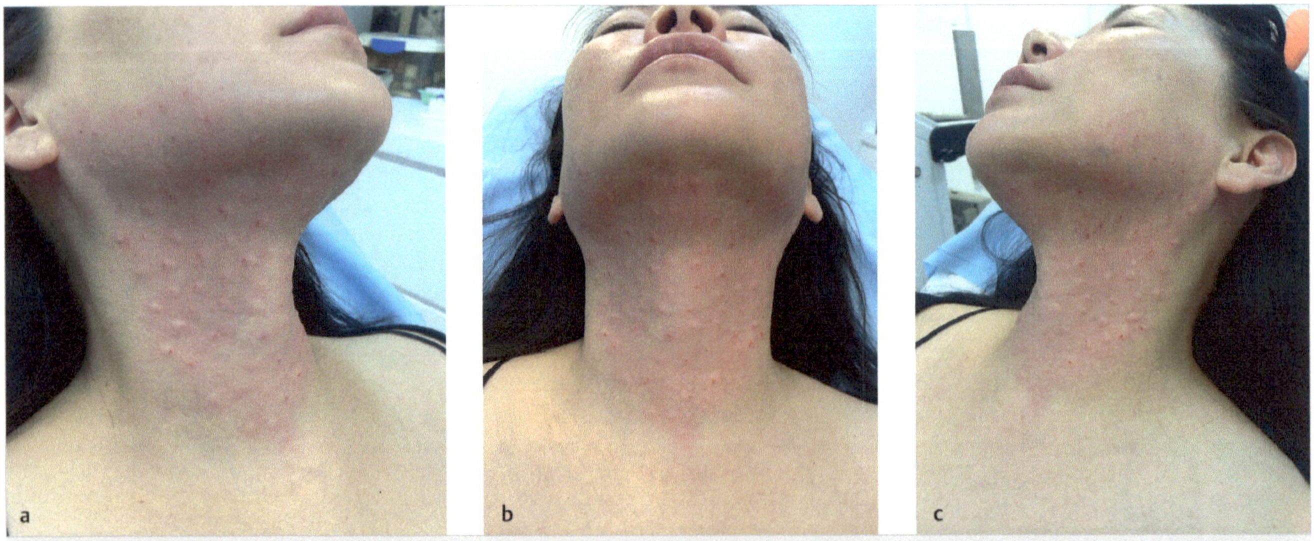

Fig. 50.4 (a–c) Distribution of over 200 microdroplets over the lower face and neck regions as delineated by a continuous line three fingerbreadths above the mandibular border, posterior to the depressor anguli oris, over the entire neck and cervicomental region anteriorly and limited posteriorly by the border of the sternocleidomastoid. This corresponds to the extent of the platysma muscle.

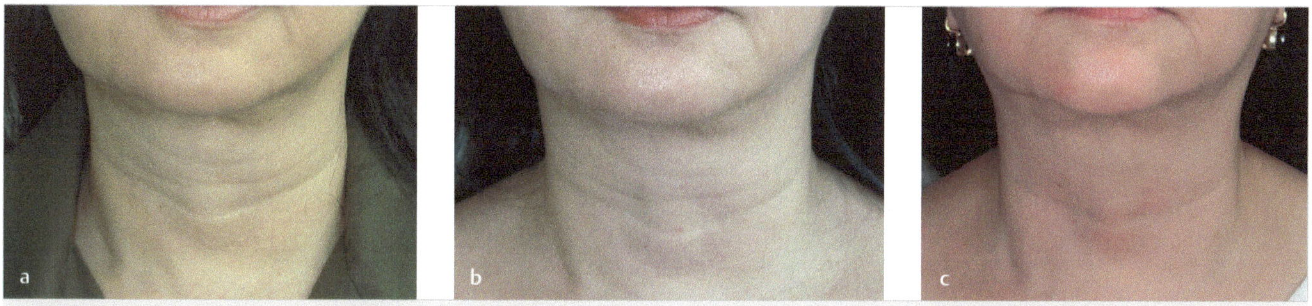

Fig. 50.5 (a–c) Microbotox of horizontal neck lines seen pre injection and 2 weeks and 2 months post injection showing a visible smoothening of the anterior neck.

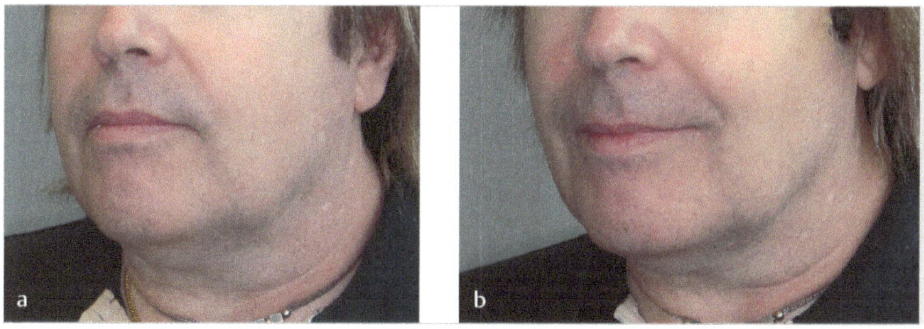

Fig. 50.6 (a, b) A 65-year-old man with complaints of a heavy neck and sagging jawline received 3 syringes (3 cc) of Microbotox-28 with a total of 84 units. Before and 2 weeks post injection, the tightening of the jawline and better cervicomental contouring is noticeable.

- Weakening the superficial fibers of the platysma muscle with microbotox injections decreases the appearance of horizontal neck lines and vertical bands whilst the deeper muscle fibers continue to function and exert their muscle pull inwards and upwards creating a more snug apposition of the platysma to the underlying neck structures. This creates a more defined cervicomental angle as well as the illusion of lifting of the jowls and jawline (▶ Fig. 50.6a, b). This mechanism of action is called the platysma effect.
- Microbotox over the surface of the chin mound reduces the effect of a popply chin without the complications of a lopsided smile due to unwanted diffusion of the toxin to the depressor labii or the depressor anguli oris muscles (▶ Fig. 50.7a, b).
- Microbotox of the lower face and neck is a simple nonsurgical solution that is ideal for patients who seek improvement of mild neck laxity and jowling, crepey neck skin with a rough texture, horizontal neck lines and vertical banding but do not wish to undergo surgery.
- It can be used in conjunction with other skin tightening devices and therapies. Effects do not last more than several months and the procedure needs to be repeated periodically. Loss of result is therefore not considered a failure.

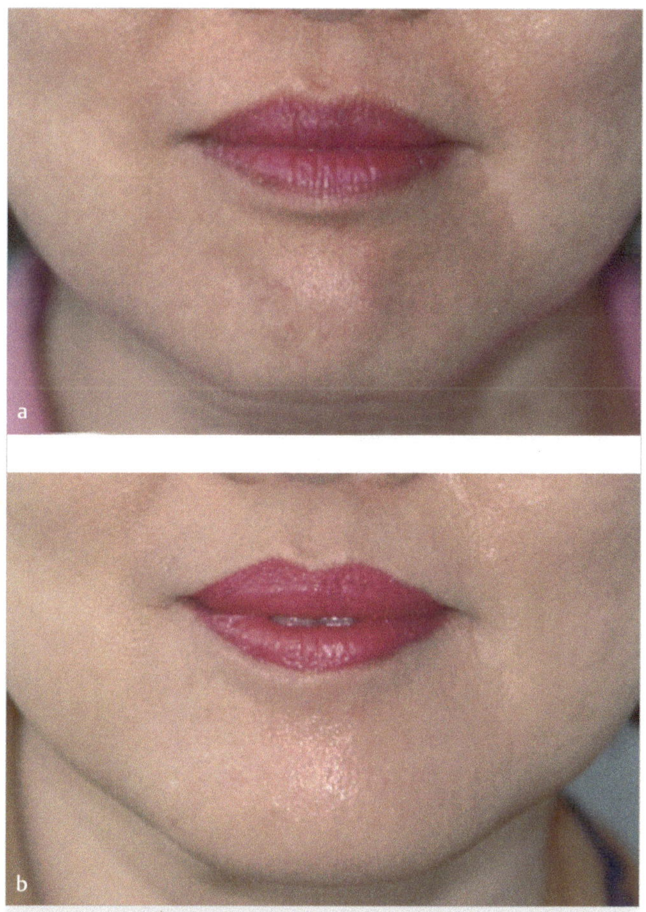

Fig. 50.7 (a, b) Before and after microbotox of the chin mound, upper facial third (glabella, crow's feet, forehead) and cheeks. Note the elevated smoothened brow, reduction of popply chin and overall improvement of facial texture and sheen.

50.6 Microbotox for Scars and Keloids

Microbotox injections are administered to fresh surgical wounds just prior to the removal of stitches on the 7th or 8th postoperative day. There is a reduction of skin tension across the wound, decreasing the incidence of hypertrophic or keloid scars and the early redness of these scars fades more rapidly. This is beneficial for Asian patients who have a higher tendency to have hypertrophic scars and keloids. The author uses this

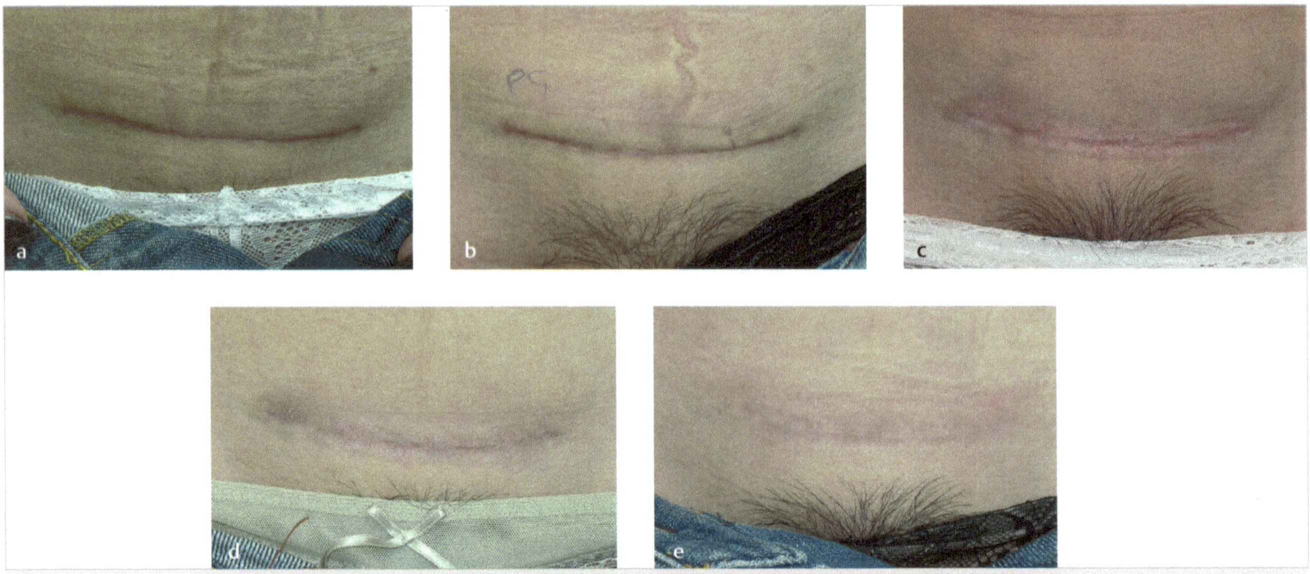

Fig. 50.8 A 3-week-old Cesarian scar with early hypertrophy seen at: (a) pre injection with 1 syringe of Microbotox-24, (b) 1 month later, (c) 2 months later, (d) 3 months later, (e) 5 months later. The injection was repeated at each session.

technique routinely in all patients with facial or body lacerations, breast augmentation or reduction, Cesarian, abdominoplasty or CABG scars (▶ Fig. 50.8a–e). The technique is clearly shown in the video.

50.7 Case Example

A 3-week-old Cesarian scar with early hypertrophy seen at: (a) pre injection with 1 syringe of Microbotox-24, (b) 1 month later, (c) 2 months later, (d) 3 months later, (e) 5 months later. The injection was repeated at each session (▶ Fig. 50.8a–e).

50.8 Conclusion

Microbotox has proven to be an effective and versatile technique that can be used to improve: (1) Facial and neck lines and wrinkles without compromising natural muscle movements; (2) skin texture, pores, rosacea, and acne; (3) lower face tightening and cervicomental contouring; (4) fresh postoperative scar recovery; and (5) treatment of hypertrophic or keloid scars.

See **Video 50.1**.

Further Readings

Wu WTL. Non surgical facial rejuvenation with the 4R principle: innovative uses of Botox and facelifting with the Woffles lift. In: Panfilov D, ed. Aesthetic Surgery of the Facial Mosaic. Berlin: Springer; 2006:636–649

Wu WTL. Skin resurfacing with Microbotox and the treatment of keloids. In: Benedetto Anthony V, ed. Botulinum Toxins in Clinical Aesthetic Practice. 2nd ed. New York: Informa Healthcare; 2011:190–205

Wu WTL. Botulinum toxin A injections for facial rejuvenation and reshaping. In: Lee P, Chen YR, Li QF, Park DH, Takanayagi S, Wu TL, Woffles, Wei FC, eds. Aesthetic Plastic Surgery in Asians: Principles and Techniques. Vol. I and II. 1st ed. CRC Press; 2015:149–169

Wu WTL. Microbotox of the lower face and neck: evolution of a personal technique and its clinical effects. Plast Reconstr Surg. 2015; 136(5) Suppl:92S–100S

Wu WTL. The microbotox technique. In: Tonnard P, Verpaele A, Bensimon R, eds. Centrofacial Rejuvenation. Thieme; 2017:289–310

51 Neck Bands

Rod J. Rohrich and Ira L. Savetsky

Abstract

A comprehensive and systematic facial analysis is critical in establishing goals and formulating a precise plan for neuromodulator facial rejuvenation. The degree of preplatysmal and subplatysmal lipodystrophy is noted and recorded. The presence of anterior platysmal banding and whether the bands are partial or full in relation to the mandibular border are also noted.

Keywords: Neck bands, platysma, mandibular contouring, botulinum toxin, neurotoxin

Key Points

- A comprehensive and systematic facial analysis is critical in establishing goals and formulating a precise plan for neuromodulator facial rejuvenation.
- Setting realistic expectations with the patient is critical in achieving high patient satisfaction.

51.1 Preprocedural Steps

51.1.1 Facial Analysis

- The initial consult begins with a thorough facial analysis including facial proportions, identification of areas with volume deflations, rhytides, and tissue laxity.
- The degree of preplatysmal and subplatysmal lipodystrophy is noted.
- The extent of the jowls that extend into the neck and obscure the mandibular contour must be noted.
- The presence of anterior platysmal banding and whether the bands are partial or full in relation to the mandibular border is also noted.

51.1.2 Criteria of a Youthful Neck (Ellenbogen and Karlin) (▶ Fig. 51.1)

- Distinct inferior mandibular border.
- Visible subhyoid depression.
- Visible thyroid cartilage bulge.
- Visible anterior border of the sternocleidomastoid muscle.
- Cervicomental angle of 105 to 120 degrees.

51.1.3 Stigmata of the Aging Neck

- Obtuse cervicomental angle (skin laxity, preplatysmal fat, subplatysmal fat, low position of hyoid bone).
- Platysmal bands.
- Aging lower face/chin.
- Indistinct mandibular border.

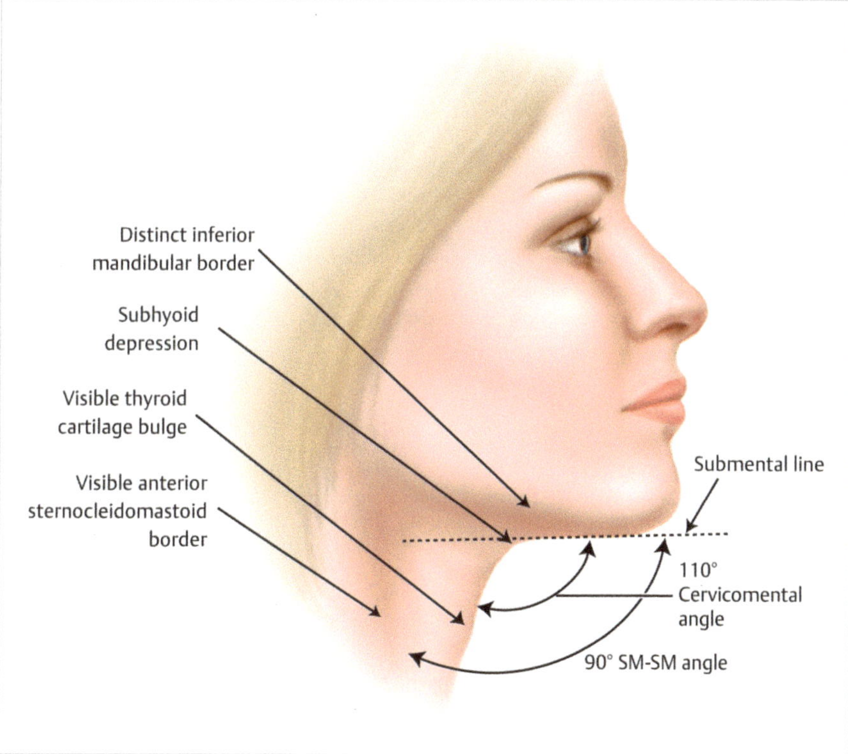

Fig. 51.1 Criteria of a youthful neck.

51.1.4 Platysmal Bands

- Pathogenesis likely related to age-related weakening of the cervical fascia resulting in a bulge from deeper neck structures thus creating bands.
- Evaluate for static (passive) or dynamic (active) central and/or lateral platysmal banding.
- The location, course, and distance between bands are noted.

51.2 Procedural Steps

See **Video 51.1**.

51.2.1 Botulinum Toxin

- Effective in treating platysmal bands, particularly dynamic bands.
- Can be used to delay or supplement surgical intervention in a case of postoperative persistent banding or in patients who are reluctant to undergo surgery.
- Toxin is injected directly superior and lateral (▸ Fig. 51.2) to the band as well as directly into the platysmal band (▸ Fig. 51.3) but only when grasped and distracted away from the neck to avoid potential complications such as dysphagia.
- Starting dose is 10 to 30 units in women and 10 to 40 units in men; however, there is variability depending on the thickness of the band.
- Inject 10 units along the mandibular border to improve jaw contour (Nefertiti effect).
- Perform 2 to 12 injections per band, approximately 1 to 2 units every centimeter.
- A total of approximately 40 to 100 units are used.
- The best results are seen in patients with minimal skin laxity and active bands.

51.3 Postprocedural Care

- Avoid Aspirin, Motrin, Advil, Aleve, vitamin E (>400 units per day), and fish oil at least 7 to 10 days prior to your appointment and for 5 days following treatment.
- Apply covered ice packs to the treated area for the first 24 hours.
- Avoid strenuous exercise such as running, yoga, and weightlifting for 24 hours.

51.4 Case Example

Anterior views of a 63-year-old woman before (left) and 1 week after (right) botulinum toxin injection for platysmal bands (▸ Fig. 51.4a, b).

51.5 Conclusion

Accurate systematic facial analysis is crucial for facial rejuvenation success. The surgeon's goals and patient's expectations must be aligned. Use of botulinum toxin is an effective method for platysmal banding particularly in patients with active bands and minimal skin laxity.

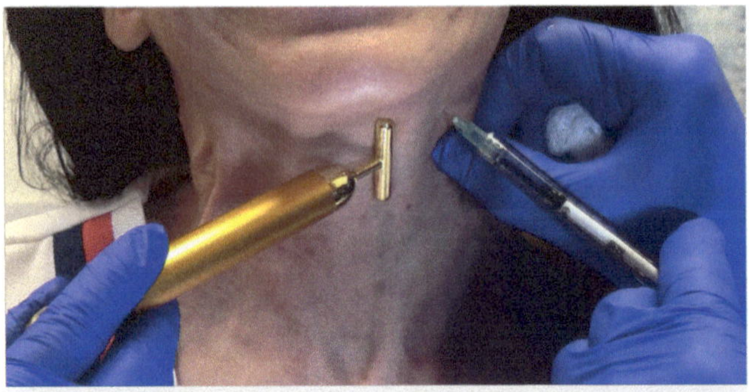

Fig. 51.2 Toxin is injected directly superior and lateral to the band.

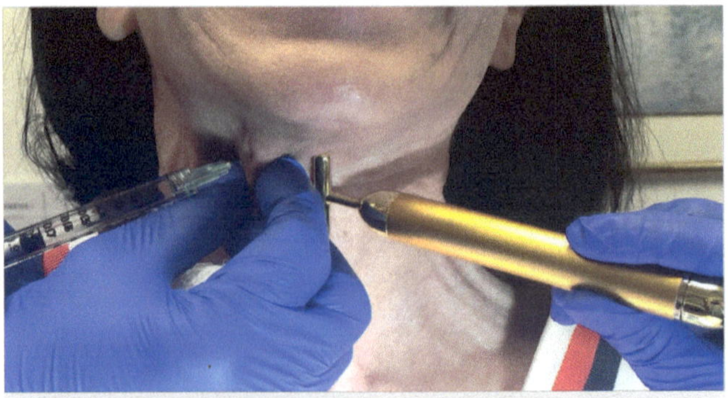

Fig. 51.3 Toxin is injected directly into the platysmal band but only when grasped and distracted away from the neck.

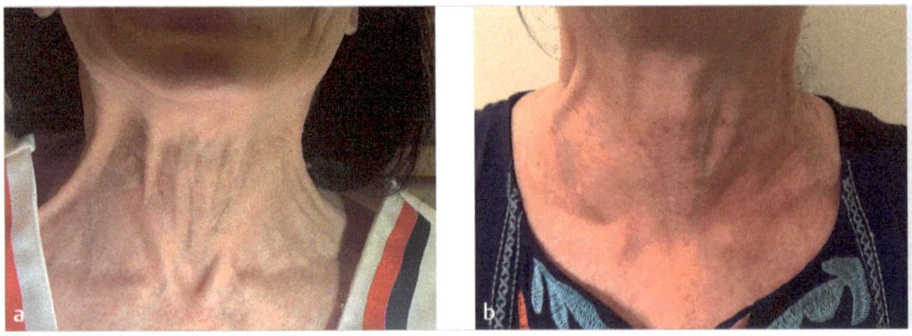

Fig. 51.4 (a, b) Anterior views of a 63-year-old woman before (left) and 1 week after (right) botulinum toxin injection for platysmal bands.

Further Readings

Brandt FS, Bellman B. Cosmetic use of botulinum A exotoxin for the aging neck. Dermatol Surg. 1998; 24(11):1232–1234

de Castro CC. The anatomy of the platysma muscle. Plast Reconstr Surg. 1980; 66(5): 680–683

Ellenbogen R, Karlin JV. Visual criteria for success in restoring the youthful neck. Plast Reconstr Surg. 1980; 66(6):826–837

Kane MA. Nonsurgical treatment of platysmal bands with injection of botulinum toxin A. Plast Reconstr Surg. 1999; 103(2):656–663, discussion 664–665

Matarasso A, Matarasso SL, Brandt FS, Bellman B. Botulinum A exotoxin for the management of platysma bands. Plast Reconstr Surg. 1999; 103(2):645–652, discussion 653–655

52 Neurotoxins: Masseter Hypertrophy

Heather J. Furnas and Grace J. Graw

Abstract

Masseter hypertrophy can be successfully treated nonsurgically with neurotoxin. The condition can result in a square, boxy face in women, giving them a masculine appearance. Bruxism and clenching can result in masseter hypertrophy. Three injections into the central, inferior, and posterior portion of the muscle, where it is the thickest, can result in improvement in 2 weeks. Noting anatomic landmarks while planning the injections minimizes complications.

Keywords: Masseter hypertrophy, bruxism, clenching, boxy face, square face, neurotoxin, neuromodulator

Key Points

- Masseter hypertrophy can cause both functional impairment (i.e., bruxism and pain) and aesthetic dissatisfaction (i.e., wide, boxy contour of lower face).
- Neurotoxin treatment can improve patient's functionality and cosmesis, and offer an effective, alternative mode of management to surgical reduction for masseter hypertrophy.
- Almost all non-East Asian patients present with masseter hypertrophy associated with bruxism, whereas hypertrophy in the East Asian population is almost universally benign.
- Masseter hypertrophy can occur unilaterally as well as bilaterally.

52.1 Preoperative Steps

52.1.1 Analysis

- To evaluate, inspect the lower face for a boxy or square-shaped appearance.
- Palpate for masseter hypertrophy and rule out bony contours, overdeveloped parotid, and thick adipose tissue as the cause of the widened lower face.
- Assess skin laxity, as injections in patients with poor skin tone may cause exacerbation of jowls for up to 2 months after treatment.
- To assess muscle bulk, palpate the masseter during both relaxation and contraction.
- Use standard frontal view photographs for preoperative and postoperative analysis, with optional lateral views to note muscle contraction changes.

52.2 Procedural Steps

See **Video 52.1**.

52.2.1 Anatomical Considerations

- The masseter is a three-layer masticatory muscle arising from the zygomatic arch and inserting on the lateral ramus and angle of the mandible.
- Branches of the masseteric nerve are most commonly found in the lower middle third of masseter muscle.
- The facial vein usually runs anterior to the muscle, and the facial artery usually runs anterior to the facial vein.
- The parotid duct usually runs superior to a line drawn between the earlobe and oral commissure.
- The risorius muscle may partially cover the anterior masseter.
- Safety zone (▸ Fig. 52.1):
  - Superior border: Imaginary line drawn between earlobe and oral commissure.
  - Inferior border: Mandibular border.
  - Anterior border: 1 cm posterior to the anterior edge of the masseter muscle.
  - Posterior border: Posterior masseter muscle.

52.2.2 Injection Technique

- Dosage of onabotulinum toxin A is divided equally among three injections per single masseter muscle.
- Masseteric thickness determines the total dosage of onabotulinum toxin A per muscle:
  - Mild hypertrophy: 20 to 25 U
  - Moderate hypertrophy: 25 to 30 U
  - Severe hypertrophy: 30 to 40 U
- Inject using a 30-gauge needle with a 1-mL syringe.
- Injection sites:
  - Usually three injection sites per side (▸ Fig. 52.2):

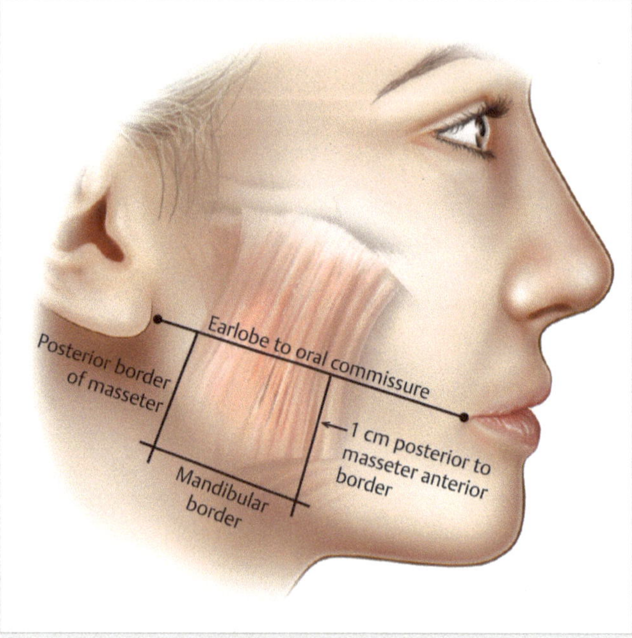

Fig. 52.1 Safety zone: **Superior border**: Earlobe to oral commissure. **Posterior border**: Posterior border of masseter. **Anterior border**: 1 cm posterior to masseter's own anterior border. **Inferior border**: Mandibular border.

- First injection: Thickest, central region of the muscle bulge, usually 1.5 cm superior to mandibular angle.
- Second and 3rd injections: Distribute equidistant from the 1st across the bulging surface to form a triangle, staying inferior and posterior on the muscle to prevent inadvertent paralysis of the pterygoids and to prevent diffusion to the mimetic muscles.

  - For severe hypertrophy, total dosage may be divided into 4 + injection sites, distributed evenly to prevent post-treatment muscle bulging.
- Technical tips:
  - To prevent inadvertent diffusion and paralysis of the medial and lateral pterygoids, stay below the sigmoid notch of the mandible.
  - Stay posterior on the muscle to avoid anterior diffusion of botulinum toxin into the risorius, the zygomaticus major and minor, and the levator anguli oris muscles to prevent facial expression and smile asymmetry.

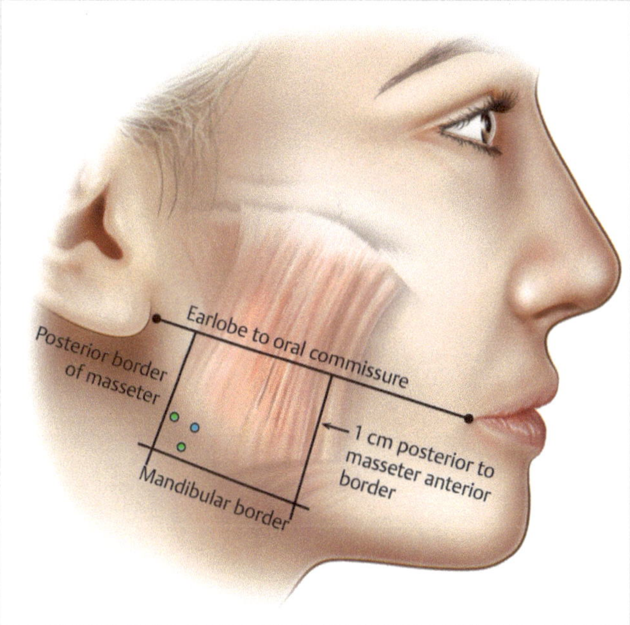

Fig. 52.2 Injection sites: 1st injection (blue) in thickest, central region of the muscle bulge, usually 1.5 cm superior to the mandibular border. Second and third injections (green) equidistant from the first site, evenly distributed over the bulge, staying inferior and posterior on the masseter.

52.3 Postprocedural Care

- Masseter atrophy typically begins to be noticeable in 1 to 2 weeks.
- Patients showing a minimal response may return for booster injections at 1-month intervals until the desired endpoint is achieved.
- Endpoint: Lack of palpable masseter muscle movement upon clenching.
- Booster injections to maintain the endpoint may be performed at 6-month intervals, though results may last for 12 months or longer.
  - Rapid reduction of masseter bulk may cause cheek hollowing and jowling.
  - To prevent cheek hollowing and jowling, perform injections with a smaller dosage over a longer period of time rather than a larger dosage over a shorter period of time.
- For maintenance of appearance, patients usually undergo injections one to two times per year.

52.4 Case Example

A 29-year-old woman presented for facial slimming as well as pain of the temporomandibular joint. She had 20 U of onabotulinum toxin A injected into each masseter, divided into equal amounts for three injections, for a total treatment of 40 U. Postoperative photos were taken 2 weeks later (▶ Fig. 52.3a, b). She experienced no complications. The treatment resulted in full relief of her jaw pain, fewer headaches, and a slimmer jawline. The results have persisted for 14 months, during which time she became pregnant and delivered her baby. However, when she weans, she plans to return for booster treatments every 6 months.

52.5 Conclusion

Botulinum toxin injection is an effective, nonoperative tool used to achieve aesthetic contouring of a wide, square-shaped lower face caused by masseter hypertrophy. Knowledge of important landmarks is important to achieve favorable results and to avoid complications affecting appearance and function. Optimal outcomes with neurotoxin use are achieved when masseter muscle movement is no longer palpable upon jaw clenching. Sustained appearance of a slimmer lower face may require maintenance injections every 6 to 12 months, depending on the patient's response.

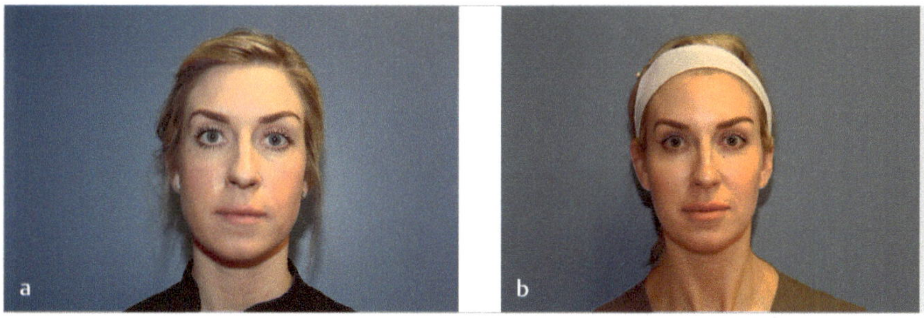

Fig. 52.3 **(a)** Preoperative and **(b)** postoperative photos of a patient 2 weeks after undergoing botulinum toxin injection for masseter hypertrophy.

Further Readings

Almukhtar RM, Fabi SG. The masseter muscle and its role in facial contouring, aging, and quality of life: a literature review. Plast Reconstr Surg. 2019; 143(1): 39e–48e

Kim NH, Chung JH, Park RH, Park JB. The use of botulinum toxin type A in aesthetic mandibular contouring. Plast Reconstr Surg. 2005; 115(3):919–930

Kim NH, Park RH, Park JB. Botulinum toxin type A for the treatment of hypertrophy of the masseter muscle. Plast Reconstr Surg. 2010; 125(6):1693–1705

Liew S, Dart A. Nonsurgical reshaping of the lower face. Aesthet Surg J. 2008; 28(3): 251–257

Wu WTL. Botox facial slimming/facial sculpting: the role of botulinum toxin-A in the treatment of hypertrophic masseteric muscle and parotid enlargement to narrow the lower facial width. Facial Plast Surg Clin North Am. 2010; 18(1):133–140

Part VIII

Filler Finesse

VIII

53 Filler Finesse: Forehead

Steven Fagien, Rod J. Rohrich, and Yash J. Avashia

Abstract

Prior to a greater understanding of the aging forehead, neurotoxins had been the main focus for the elimination of forehead lines and glabellar furrows. A youthful forehead exhibits certain qualities that include smooth contours. Current applications of forehead rejuvenation include addressing these contours of the forehead including the temple region and improvement or elimination of static rhytides with the combined use of neurotoxins and fillers. A review of the relevant anatomy is essential so that one is aware of the best target regions as well as to avoid inadvertent injection into regional arteries, veins, and nerve bundles. Slow, smooth, and careful injection technique with appropriate volumes is critical. Detailed assessment of areas of soft tissue paucity will aid in tailoring volume restoration technique.

Keywords: Hyaluronic acid filler, intravascular injection, augmentation, temporal volumization, forehead filler

Key Points

- Filler products illustrated here will include Juvederm® Ultra (Allergan plc, Dublin, Ireland) but similar results can be obtained with other hyaluronic acid filler products from both Vycross or Hylacross technologies, the Restylane® (Galderma) family of products, Belotero® (MERZ) and the RHA products (Revance).
- Understanding relevant anatomy is essential to achieve optimal results and to avoid inadvertent injection into regional arteries, veins, and nerve bundles with subsequent adverse events.
- Slow, smooth, and careful injection technique is critical.
- Injection technique may vary but must consider ways to maximize results while avoiding complications.
- Aspiration does not guarantee extravascular location, but is advised in many situations to ensure proper placement of needle or cannula.
- Injection volume should be tailored to achieve desired treatment effect and avoid potential complications.

53.1 Upper Facial Assessment

- The temple should be flat, slightly concave, or slightly convex, without any significant concavity, depression, hollowing, or marked step-off from the lateral zygoma posteriorly.
- Age-related volume loss in the upper face can result in hollowing of the temples. Youthful temples are typically flat or slightly convex; temple volumization is indicated for temples that have become overly concave.
- The aesthetically desirable female eyebrow should be over the supraorbital margin with middle aspect slightly lower than lateral aspect.
- The position and/or shape of the eyebrow may change with aging. Fillers can enhance eyebrow contour and volume, and may be used for improving the elevation of the eyebrow tail in cases where onabotulinumtoxinA provides insufficient eyebrow lifting.
- The upper face should be assessed for volume loss in the temples and forehead, position of the eyebrow, and the presence of excess skin in the upper and lower eyelids.
- Dynamic forehead lines are usually treated with a neuromodulators, but hyaluronic acid fillers can be safely used to treat deep horizontal (static) wrinkles (or horizontal lines that treated with neuromodulators induces brow ptosis) to create a smooth contour across the forehead.
- Most hyaluronic acid fillers are not designed for fine-line filling, as is the case with Juvederm® Ultra that must be reconstituted to a lower concentration to be optimal for superficial dermal injection/placement.

53.2 Upper Facial Filler

53.2.1 Preparation

- Makeup and other contaminants on the face should be removed before the injection and should be avoided on the day of the procedure.
- Aseptic technique should be used, which includes thorough hand washing and wearing gloves, and sterile technique with needle transfer or when reconstituting product.
- Skin site preparation for Vycross® products should include either chlorhexidine, povidone-iodine, or similar and for Hylacross® products alcohol will suffice.
- The skin should be visibly assessed for local dermatologic disorders (comedones, acne), active bacterial or viral infections, or inflammatory disease processes.
- Treatment in irritated or inflamed skin should be avoided.

53.2.2 Technical Aspects

- For fine-line filling, 30- or 32-gauge, 0.5-inch needles are suggested depending on product used or method of reconstitution.
- The injection needle should be changed regularly to minimize the risk of infection and increased discomfort from blunting.
- A slow injection speed with smaller needles is essential for avoidance of product spread when the needle is inadvertently placed intravascularly.
- Smaller needles also tend to cause less bruising and limit volumes, reducing local adverse events.
- In treatment areas with challenging anatomy or a higher risk of complications, it may be advisable to use blunt cannulas instead of needles; however, these do not guarantee against complications.

53.2.3 Forehead Line Filling (▶ Fig. 53.1)

- Static forehead lines that are not appropriate for chemodenervation of the frontalis are best treated with reconstituted Juvederm® Ultra.
- Reconstitution is variable and depends on the skin thickness and rhytid depth but usually is accomplished by (author Steven Fagien's preference) mixing, blending, or "dilution" of the products to approximately 50% of the packaged concentration of 24 mg/mL to around 12 mg/mL by adding equal amounts of anesthetic solution (i.e., add 1 mL of lidocaine with epinephrine to 1 mL of Juvederm® Ultra, yielding 2 mL of reconstituted product).
- A 32-gauge needle is used and rhytid reduction/elimination is accomplished by serial threading or serial puncture with the needle nearly parallel to the skin surface with particular caution to inject intradermally.
- Injections proceed to full correction without overcorrection.
- Blanching from epinephrine is expected and looks completely different from an inadvertent arteriolar injection.

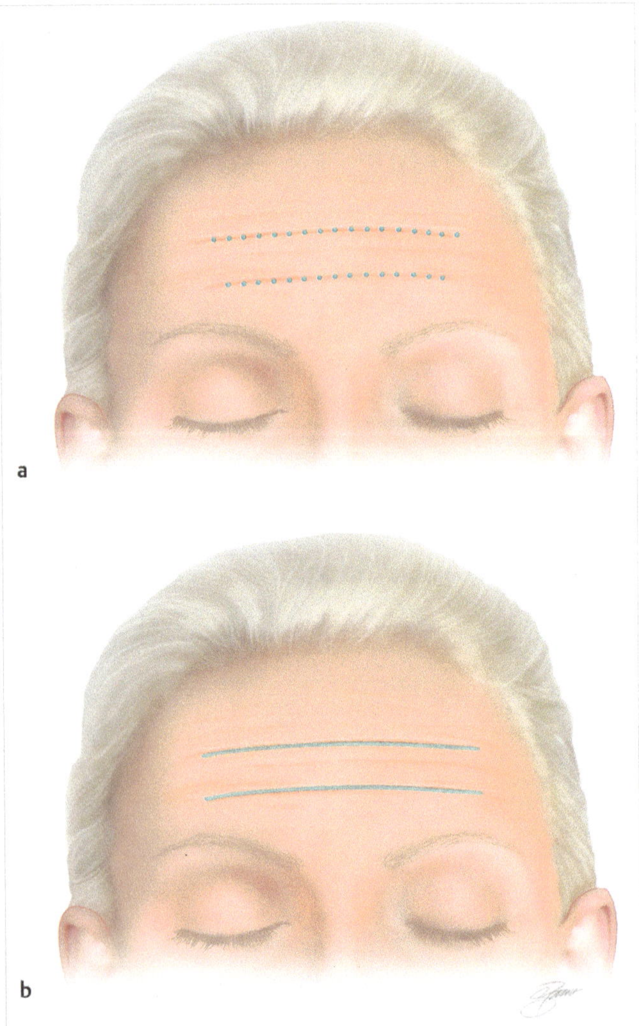

Fig. 53.1 **(a, b)** Horizontal rhytid correction with fillers.

53.2.4 Volumization of Temples (▶ Fig. 53.2)

- Voluma is more often preferred for moderate-to-severe volume deficiency in the temple when injected into the supraperiosteal space (deep to the temporalis muscle) of the temporalis fossa while an alternate method using reconstituted Juvederm® Ultra Plus may be indicated or preferred for mild to moderate volume deficiency and is injected subcutaneously (superficial to the temporalis muscle). Both have their advantages. The deep plane is typically devoid of vessels and can be safely applied using the Swift method. While safer, this technique typically requires larger volumes to achieve the designated end-point. The sub-cutaneous plane is more efficient (more lift per volume of injectant as in most areas) but it closer to vessels that could be problematic.
- Identify temporal artery by palpation or direct visualization and the network of temporal veins by inspection, as well as the junction of the temporal crest or fusion line with the orbital rim. It can be helpful to mark both areas as well as visible subcutaneous veins to steer clear of and landmarks for injection.
- Identify area of greatest volume loss.
- For the deep plane/supraperiosteal injection technique: Needle should be positioned 1 cm superior to the lateral orbital rim along the temporal fusion line and 1 cm lateral to the temporal crest and away from the identified vessels.
- Insert the needle perpendicularly down to bone, aspirate, and then inject very slowly using a supraperiosteal bolus injection. Injection volumes vary depending on a host of factors including severity.
- Pressure with the free hand superiorly at the level of the hairline will avoid unwanted spread superiorly and posteriorly.
- After removing the needle, apply pressure on the injection site for several minutes to tamponade bleeding from any venous puncture and avoid late-onset bruising.

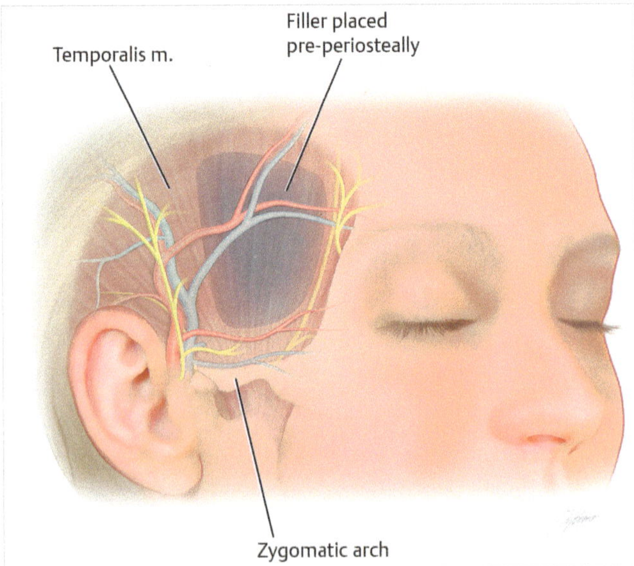

Fig. 53.2 Safe temporal augmentation with fillers.

- Gentle molding of the temporal region may be required after injection of typical volumes in the 0.3 to 1.0 mL range for most temporal hollows.
- Severe volume loss may require up to 2 mL of Voluma per side.
- If using Juvederm® Ultra Plus, a second injection should be made along the lateral edge of the frontozygomatic arch, medial to the first injection, or convert to an ultra-dilute reconstituted Juvederm® Ultra by mixing 1 mL of product to injector's preferred diluent (either local anesthetic, saline, or combination) to (up to) a total of 5 mL, injecting approximately 1.5 to 2.5 mL per temple in the subcutaneous plane. Particular attention is needed with this technique to avoid vessels and observe immediate soft tissue/temple reflation. Reflation is immediate in this superficial plane and lack of this observation should prompt immediate cessation (could possibly be in a blood vessel) and moving the needle to a near/ adjacent location and reinjection.

53.2.5 Safety Points

- Visual inspection and palpation to avoid the superficial temporal artery and vein that lie in the subcutaneous tissue.
- Select a supraperiosteal location high in the temporal fossa to minimize the risk of intravascular events.
- The deep temporal arteries and the middle temporal artery are commonly located more posteriorly to this point, and the calibers of these arteries are small in this region; however, aspiration before injection is always warranted.
- Avoid deep needle injections into the lower or posterior fossa above the zygomatic arch, which pose a potential risk of palate necrosis from injections into branches of the internal maxillary artery.

53.2.6 Eyebrow Filler

- Eyebrow shaping can be achieved using Juvederm® Ultra Plus.
- Identify the orbital rim to avoid inadvertent injection into the orbital cavity.
- Position the needle and aspirate before injection.
- Insert the needle at the lateral end of the eyebrow, inject horizontally in the direction of the eyebrow and very slowly using a supraperiosteal bolus injection, and then massage upward to shape. Injections in the lateral aspect of the eyebrows are intended to promote support of the roof.
- Remember to palpate the orbital rim and protect with a finger to avoid migration of the filler into the upper eyelid.
- Avoid overcorrection of the eyebrow with filler, because it can result in an unduly prominent eyebrow appearance or cause eyelid edema.
- The second injection should be made in the same manner medial to the first injection along the eyebrow.
- Be careful to avoid the supraorbital foramen when injecting lateral to it.

53.2.7 Forehead Filler

- Position the needle near the lateral end of the horizontal rhytid, at least 2 cm above the eyebrow.
- Insert the needle fully, inject very slowly using a supraperiosteal bolus injection, and inject deeply to avoid the forehead and temporal vessels and nerve.
- The needle tip must be on the bone beneath the galea to access this avascular plane. Moving medially along the forehead, the second and third injections are given on the same facial side at least 2 cm above the eyebrow.
- Inject very slowly using a supraperiosteal bolus injection, and inject deeply to avoid the supraorbital and supratrochlear vessel bundles.

53.2.8 Safety Points

- Inject at least 2 cm above the eyebrow, and supratrochlear and supraorbital vessels.
- Maintain deep injection to avoid the subcutaneous vessel bundles.

53.3 Complications

- Common early and self-limited complications include erythema, edema, pain, and bruising.
- Lumps and bumps or bluish-gray discoloration under the skin caused by the Tyndall effect may occur with injection of fillers when injected too superficially and usually can be managed by massage, passage of time, or the use of hyaluronidase.
- Allergic reactions (very rare with hyaluronic acid fillers) typically occur within several hours and can be avoided, in most cases, by careful pretreatment interview of patients.
- If vascular compromise or compression caused by hyaluronic acid fillers occurs or is suspected, it will typically be evident by skin or reticular changes, pallor, blanching, and pain along the distribution of the artery that is distinguishable from blanching from epinephrine and if diagnosed, must be treated aggressively with injection of hyaluronidase into the area which in most situations of impending skin compromise can be completely reversed.
- Late filler complications including delayed onset of nodules, which are fortunately rare and can occur months after treatment, can be treated with oral corticosteroids and other anti-inflammatory agents.
- Please refer to manuscripts regarding current and more comprehensive methods of treatment of complications should they arise.

53.4 Case Example

This example demonstrates a middle-aged female with deep forehead rhytides that had been sub-optimally treated with neuromodulation causing both ineffectivity and brow ptosis. Intradermal

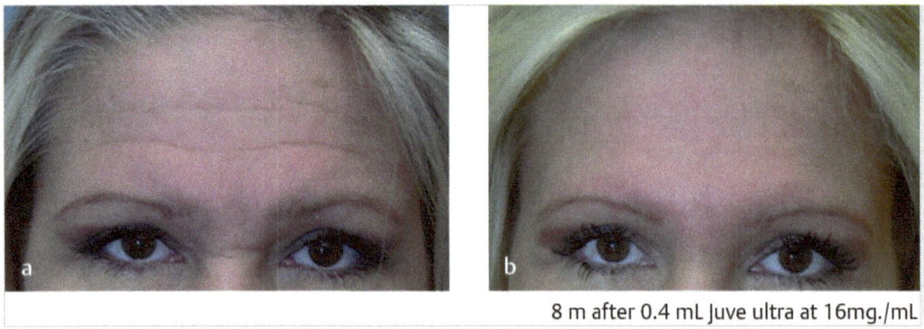

Fig. 53.3 (a, b) This example demonstrates a middle-aged female with deep forehead rhytides. Intradermal injection of hyaluronic acid with the techniques described were performed. Postprocedural image demonstrates removal of the horizontal rhytides.

injection of hyaluronic acid with the techniques described above were performed. Postprocedural image demonstrates removal of the (static) horizontal rhytides (▶ Fig. 53.3).

53.5 Conclusion

The use of hyaluronic acid fillers is helpful to provide correction of volume loss, structural support, and improvement of upper facial rhtyides. The upper face has been considered a basic area for exclusive use of botulinum toxin but has now become an area that is best and more comprehensively addressed using a combination of neurotoxins and fillers. The use of fillers to the upper facial regions remains challenging due to risks of potential intravascular complications, and a complete understanding of the anatomy and management of complications, should they arise, is paramount.

See **Video 53.1**.

Further Readings

Carruthers J, Humphrey S, Beleznay K, Carruthers A. Suggested injection zone for soft tissue fillers in the temple? Dermatol Surg. 2017; 43(5):756–757

Carruthers JD, Fagien S, Rohrich RJ, Weinkle S, Carruthers A. Blindness caused by cosmetic filler injection: a review of cause and therapy. Plast Reconstr Surg. 2014; 134(6):1197–1201

de Maio M, Swift A, Signorini M, Fagien S, Aesthetic Leaders in Facial Aesthetics Consensus Committee. Facial assessment and injection guide for botulinum toxin and injectable hyaluronic acid fillers: focus on the upper face. Plast Reconstr Surg. 2017; 140(2):265e–276e

Sclafani AP, Fagien S. Treatment of injectable soft tissue filler complications. Dermatol Surg. 2009; 35 Suppl 2:1672–1680

54 Filler Finesse: Temples

Val Lambros

Abstract

In many faces, the temples will hollow, making the face look gaunt and older as well as making it look longer and narrower. This may be remedied by filling the temples with injectable products. A method of doing so is described as well as a method of previewing the results of the procedure so the patient may know what he or she may expect.

Keywords: Aging face, hollow temples, HA filler injections of temples, cannula injection, dilution of fillers, gaunt face, narrow face

Key Points

- Hollowing of the temples is a powerful indicator of aging. Treatment can make a profound difference in the overall perception of the face.
- Correction may be accomplished with relatively simple injections.
- In the subcutaneous and subfascial planes the correction can last several years with hyaluronic acid (HA) fillers.

54.1 Preoperative Steps

- Analysis is the key to successful treatment. Understand the course of the facial nerve (▶ Fig. 54.1a, b).
- Aging frequently results in hollowing of temples with exposure of the lateral orbit and visibility of the temporal fusion line, which gives the head and face a gaunt narrow look. The tails of the brows appear short and low as they follow the reduced radius of curvature of the temple.
- One of the major effects of filling the temple is the lengthening and apparent elevation of the tail of the brow.
- Ideally temples should be flat, neither concave nor convex.
- It is important to note the position of the temporal artery, which can often be seen and confirmed by palpation. If there is doubt, a Doppler is useful to map out any branches traversing the temple (▶ Fig. 54.2a–c).
- The decision to inject the temples is based on whether the patient likes the look of fuller temples.
- Because the benefit of temple injection is a visual concept, not easily understood when described verbally, I like to inject the temple with a few cubic centimeters of dilute local anesthetic to show the patient and myself the desired effect (and for pain and hemostasis as well). This is like trying on clothes before buying them and patients uniformly like the idea of being able to see the result before committing to the injection; moreover, the patient now gets to make the decision about the procedure in a truly informed way. The injection of product follows this "preview." Typically, 1.5 to 2 cc of the product is used per side.
- At the time of writing this, I prefer Juvederm Ultra.
- The success of any filler treatment depends on careful and thoughtful distribution.
- The temple has three distinct areas: the main hollow of the temple, the tail of the brow, and a small vertical hollow frequently seen inferior to the tail of the brow.
- There are two main methods for injecting temples: a periosteal transmuscular approach and a subcutaneous/subgaleal (subtemporoparietal fascia) approach, which I prefer for its smoothness and longevity.

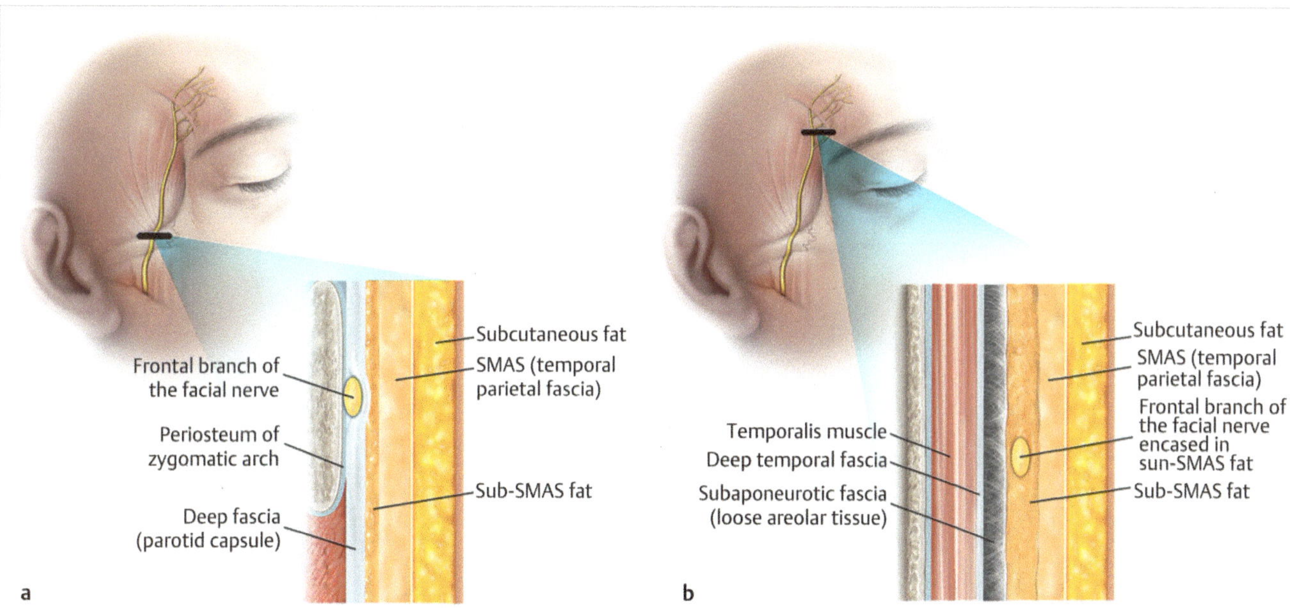

Fig. 54.1 The course of the facial nerve **(a)** inferiorly and **(b)** superiorly.

- The periosteal transmuscular approach places the filler in a single bolus placed on the periosteum 1 cm posterior and 1 cm superior to the inferior origin of the temporal fusion line at the lateral orbit. This approach, although easy, direct, and convenient, only addresses the superior portion of the temple hollow and tail of the brow. Duration of HA fillers with this approach is around 6 months in my experience, considerably shorter than the subcutaneous/subgaleal approach.
- Longevity of effect in the subcutaneous/subgaleal plane is almost always greater than 2 years; 3 years is not uncommon. Since the product is distributed over the whole temple and lateral brow, it covers a wider area very smoothly.

54.2 Operative Steps

- See **Video 54.1**.
- Distributing a concentrated filler evenly over a broad area is technically difficult, a task made much easier by reconstituting the product.

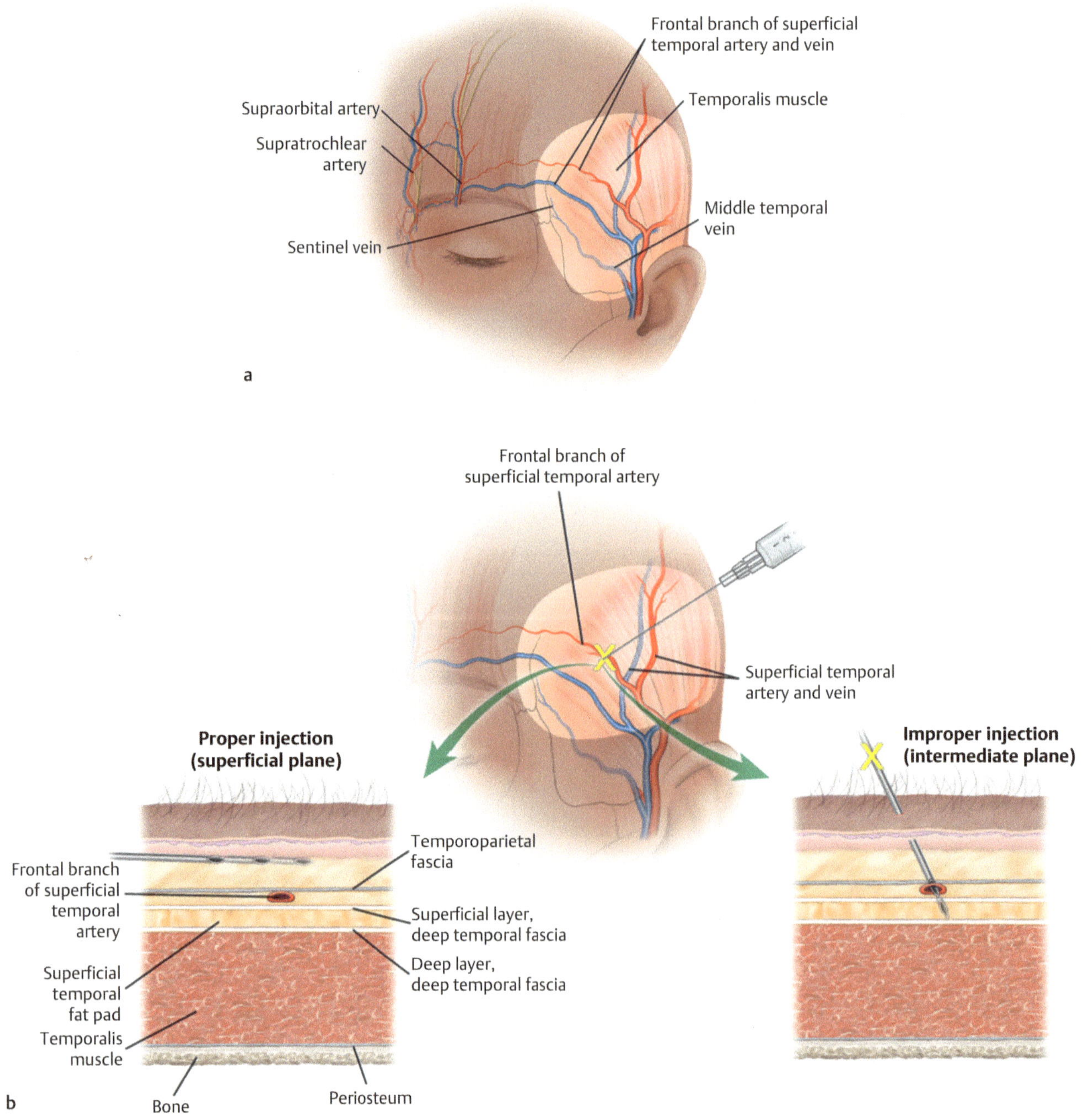

Fig. 54.2 **(a)** Relevant vascular anatomy and proper injection depth in the **(b)** superficial plane.

(Continued)

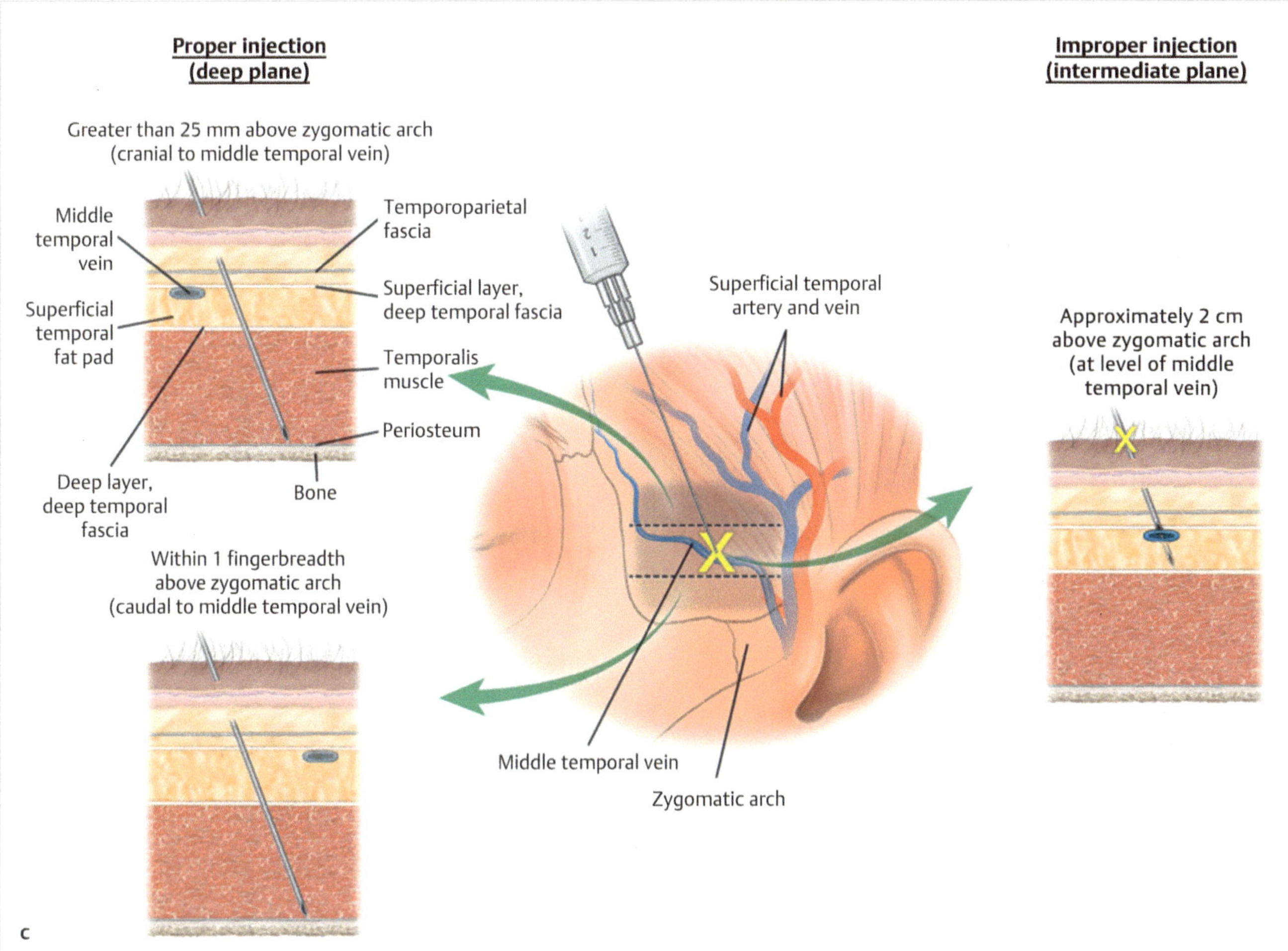

Fig. 54.2 *(Continued)* (**c**) Proper injection depth in the deep plane.

- An analogy might be trying to paint a wall evenly with a small can of concentrated paint. It is much easier to paint the wall evenly with dilute paint; then the diluent evaporates.
- The product is reconstituted with one part of product to two parts saline, so an injection of 1 cc of product would consist of 3 cc total injectate. Using a transfer hub, it is mixed between two syringes and injected through a 22-gauge, 2-inch cannula. Because the product is viscous when rehydrated, injection through a 25-gauge cannula can be difficult.
- The tail of the brow is injected in the subcutaneous plane and the remainder of the injection is between the deep and superficial fascia (i.e., subgaleal). If the cannula is introduced at a shallow angle from inferior to the temple hollow it will flex and glide on the deep temporal fascia and follow the plane deep to the temporal arteries.
- Multiple passes are made to spread the mixture as evenly as possible. The product tends to flow backwards along the shaft of the cannula rather than spread radially from the tip and will make a bolus close to the injection site unless finger pressure is applied over the proximal cannula to guide the flow distally.
- The superficial temporal veins will likely be enlarged for up to a few weeks after the injection; the patients should be informed.
- The reconstituted product makes an alarmingly large temporary saline bulge, which mostly dissipates in the first half hour. The dilution of the product along with even injection is responsible for the very smooth contouring that this method produces.

54.3 Postoperative Care

- There is little to do post injection. There may be small residual swelling for a day or so.
- Ice is used for the first few hours, though bruising with a cannula is uncommon; if it occurs, it will appear in the lower eyelid.

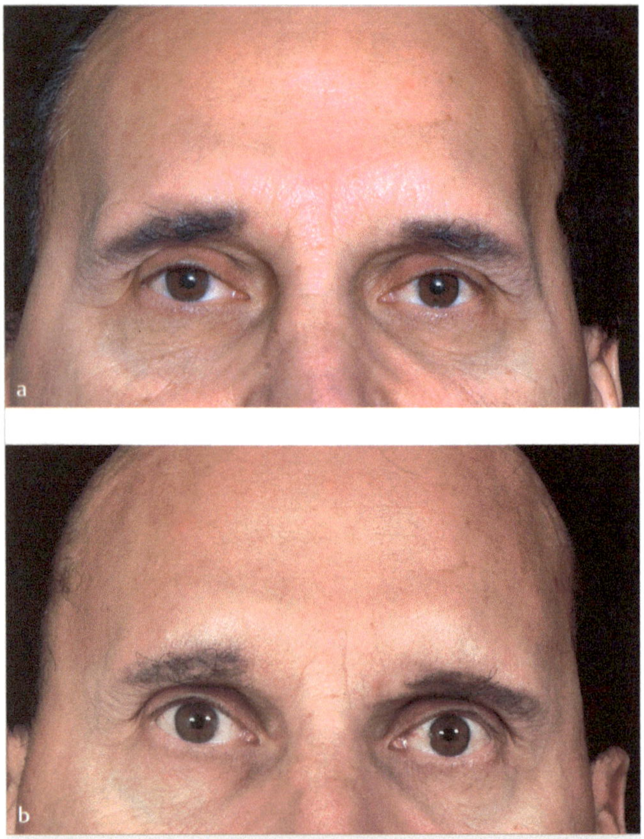

Fig. 54.3 (a, b) A 65-year-old male seen before and 2 years after temple injections of 2 cc per side.

- Since the patient has in effect seen and approved the results of the procedure with the local anesthetic preview, complaints about the aesthetic effects of the injection are very rare. To date, I have not had to dissolve product in a patient who has seen and approved the result of the "preview" with the local anesthetic.

54.4 Case Example

A 65-year-old male seen before and 2 years after temple injections of 2 cc per side (▶ Fig. 54.3a, b).

54.5 Conclusion

The power of the treatment to influence the structural background of the face is demonstrated.

Further Readings

Coleman S, Mazzola R, eds. Fat Injection from Filling to Rejuvenation. St. Louis, MO: Quality Medical Publishing; 2009

Fagien S. Variable reconstitution of injectable hyaluronic acid with local anesthetic for expanded applications in facial aesthetic enhancement. Dermatol Surg. 2010; 36 suppl 1:815–821

Lambros V. A technique for filling the temples with highly diluted hyaluronic acid: the "dilution solution." Aesthet Surg J. 2011; 31(1):89–94

Swift A. One Up, One Over Regional Approach in "Upper face: anatomy and regional approaches to injectables" found in supplement issue Soft Tissue Fillers and Neuromodulators: International and Multidisciplinary Perspectives. Plast Reconstr Surg 2015;136(5s):204S–218S

Swift A, DeLorenzi C, Kapoor K. Injection anatomy: avoiding the disastrous complication. In: Jones DH, Swift A, eds. Injectable Fillers: Facial Contouring and Shaping. 2nd ed. Wiley-Blackwell; 2019

55 Part A: Filler Finesse: Cheeks

Rod J. Rohrich, Ira L. Savetsky, and Paul D. Durand

Abstract

The aging midface can be enhanced through volume augmentation. Injections of the arch, malar eminence, and deep medial compartments may result in adjacent hollowing or a noticeable depression in the mature female patient. Our technique addresses these secondary *valleys*. Focus on these areas may improve aesthetic results of malar augmentation.

Keywords: Malar eminence, fat compartment, malar augmentation, cheek filler, peaks, secondary valleys

Key Points

- A comprehensive and systematic facial analysis is critical in establishing goals and formulating a precise plan for malar augmentation.
- A stepwise approach to malar augmentation which addresses secondary valleys restores youthful anatomical landmarks and improves facial aesthetics.

55A.1 Facial Aging

- Facial aging is characterized by collagen loss and thinning of the skin, bone resorption, and lack of soft tissue support and volume.
- The subcutaneous fat of the face is compartmentalized into superficial and deep compartments.
- The malar fat is further divided into medial, middle, and lateral temporal-cheek compartments separated by fascial septae (▶ Fig. 55A.1).
- Loss of fat volume results in atrophy and hollowing of the midface.
- Augmentation of these compartments can be performed to improve facial aesthetics.
- The facial tissues, underlying structures, and fat compartments are independent and must be addressed in an individualized fashion.
- Injection of the deep medial fat compartment increases midface projection.
- Injections of the primary peaks (▶ Fig. 55A.2) in female patients along the zygomatic arch, malar eminence, and

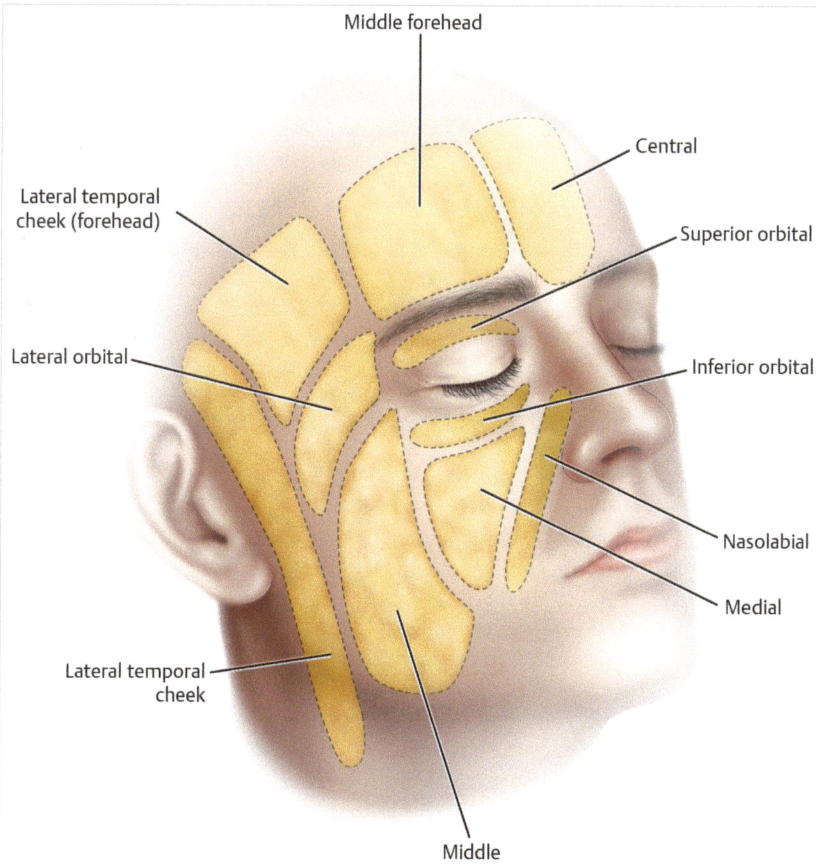

Fig. 55A.1 Malar fat compartments.

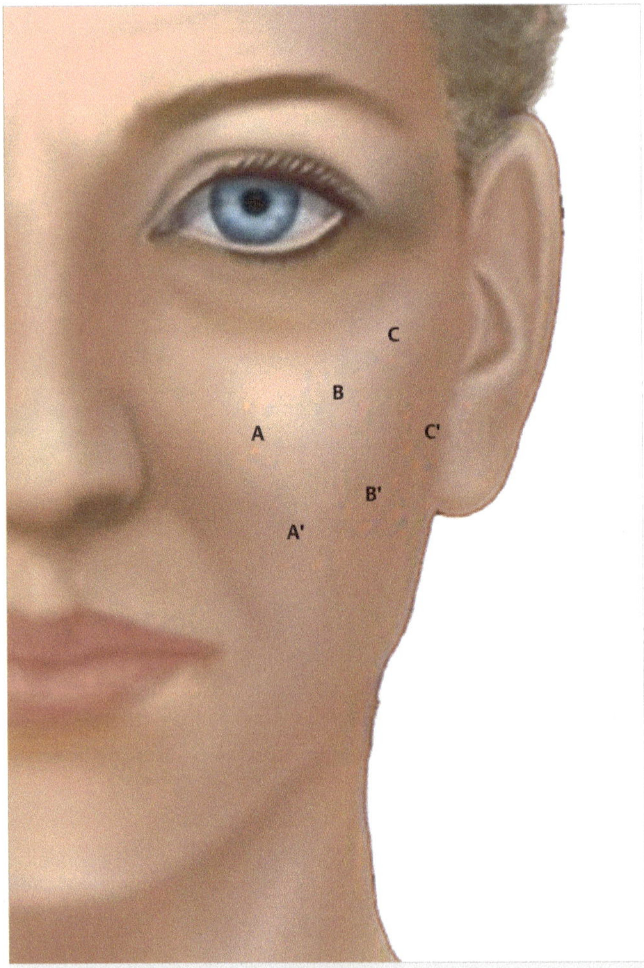

Fig. 55A.2 Malar landmarks in female patient. **Peaks:** Deep malar compartment (A), malar eminence (B), and zygomatic arch (C). **Secondary Valleys:** A', B', and C'.

deep medial compartments will enhance cheek prominence, resulting in an often aesthetically desirable *"high cheek bone"* appearance.

- When the arch, malar eminence, and deep medial compartment are injected in mature female patients, a deepened secondary valley remains (▶ Fig. 55A.2).
- This region of hollowing lies inferior and parallel to the peaks. This area should be filled with volume to improve contour.

55A.2 Planning

- The initial consult begins with a thorough facial analysis including facial proportions, identification of areas with volume deflations, rhytides, and tissue laxity.
- Preparation, dilution, and injection of substances in facial tissues should be performed under sterile technique.
- Properties of fillers including viscosity, stiffness (G´), affinity for water, degree of cross-linking, and concentration of hyaluronic acid (HA) should be considered.
- Generally, it can be advantageous to choose a filler with a higher G´ value and viscosity to provide a lifting effect in midface volumization.
- A 30-gauge needle is used for injections.
- Topical anesthesia is applied and skin cleaned with chlorhexidine.
- Ice rollers and gentle pressure can be used for distraction.
- Lights are utilized for optimal visualization during the procedure.

55A.3 Injecting Secondary Valleys

- The infraorbital rim, malar eminence, and arch are palpated for orientation.
- The superficial medial cheek (lateral to nasolabial fold) and middle cheek compartments (medial to zygomaticus major) are identified.
- The depth and extent of the secondary valley are noted.
- Injections are performed slowly with low pressure and small increments in anterograde/retrograde fashion to maximize safety.
- Injections are performed in the subcutaneous plane along the junction of the medial and middle compartments.
- The infraorbital foramen, which lies approximately a finger breadth below the infraorbital rim in the vertical plane of the medial limbus, should be avoided.
- Additional passes are placed in cross-radial fashion and fanning performed.
- Injections along the lateral compartment can be performed to improve long-standing depressions.
- The goal is to not only correct volume loss but also to improve contour in a smooth, contiguous fashion.
- Gentle massage may be performed to evenly disperse filler material.
- Malar changes should be noted in multiple views (anteroposterior [AP], oblique, lateral) and back lighting is critical to proper assessment.
- Final aesthetic endpoints include lifting of overlying tissues and softening of visible shadows.

55A.4 Aftercare Instructions

- Avoid Aspirin, Motrin, Advil, Aleve, vitamin E (>400 units per day), and fish oil at least 7 to 10 days prior to your appointment and for 5 days following treatment.
- Please contact the office immediately if you experience any of the following:
  - Fever and/or chills.
  - If the treatment area appears red, hot to touch, or "angry" looking.
  - If you experience severe pain or increasing pain.
  - If anywhere at the injection site or surrounding areas discolored blotches develop or the area appears pale.
- Apply covered ice packs to the treated area for the first 24 hours.

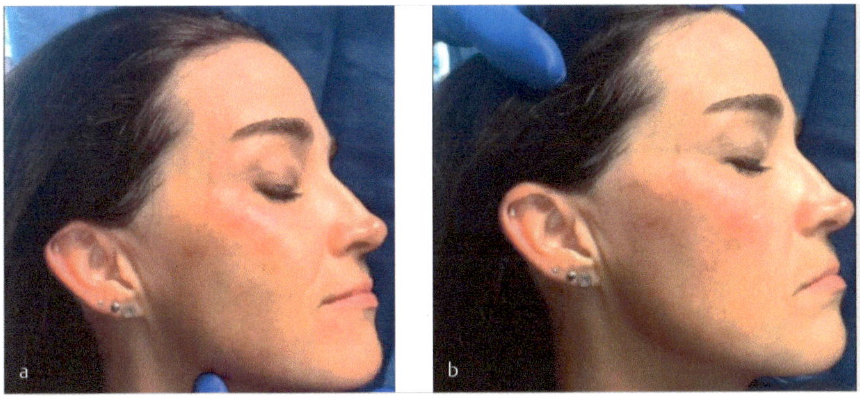

Fig. 55A.3 (a, b) Lateral views before (left) and immediately after (right) malar filler injection.

- Avoid strenuous exercise such as running, yoga, and weightlifting for at least 36 hours and heart rate should to remain below 100 beats per minute.
- The physician will see you in follow-up at 2 weeks and again at 3 months following injections. Call the office to schedule your follow-up appointment at your convenience.

55A.5 Sequela/Complications

- Minor complications include swelling, bruising, or asymmetry and usually subside within a few days.
- Persistent malar edema may require additional time before resolution.
- The most feared complications include tissue necrosis or filler embolization. Acute symptoms may include pain, skin blanching, livedo, or blindness. The patient should be seen in clinic immediately for evaluation. Hyaluronidase should be available and used generously. Other interventions can include massage, warm compresses, topical nitroglycerin, and Aspirin.

55A.6 Case Example

Lateral views before (left) and immediately after (right) malar filler injection (▶ Fig. 55A.3a, b).

55A.7 Conclusion

A stepwise approach to malar augmentation in female patients which addresses secondary valleys is provided. This injection technique restores youthful anatomical landmarks and improves facial aesthetics. Patient satisfaction is high when these secondary endpoints are addressed in malar augmentation.

See **Video 55A.1**.

Further Readings

Cotofana S, Schenck TL, Trevidic P, et al. Midface: clinical anatomy and regional approaches with injectable fillers. Plast Reconstr Surg. 2015; 136(5) Suppl: 219S–234S

Ramanadham SR, Rohrich RJ. Newer understanding of specific anatomic targets in the aging face as applied to injectables: superficial and deep facial fat compartments—an evolving target for site-specific facial augmentation. Plast Reconstr Surg. 2015; 136(5) Suppl:49S–55S

Rohrich RJ, Pessa JE, Ristow B. The youthful cheek and the deep medial fat compartment. Plast Reconstr Surg. 2008; 121(6):2107–2112

Scheuer JF, III, Sieber DA, Pezeshk RA, Campbell CF, Gassman AA, Rohrich RJ. Anatomy of the facial danger zones: maximizing safety during soft-tissue filler injections. Plast Reconstr Surg. 2017; 139(1):50e–58e

Wan D, Amirlak B, Rohrich RJ. The clinical importance of the fat compartments in midfacial aging. Plast Reconstr Surg Glob Open. 2014; 1(9):e92

55 Part B: Filler Finesse: Cheeks

K. Kay Durairaj, Vivian N. Nguyen, Omer Baker, and Simranjit Sidhu

Abstract

The cheek is one of the most important structural features of the facial architecture—signifying youthfulness, fertility, and beauty. It overlies the lateral zygomatic bone, but also encompasses the entire midface, including the tissues below the orbit. Facial fillers should be used in the midface as volumizing agents. Hyaluronic gel fillers can be as effective as fat grafting when used within facial fat pads to augment volume deflation changes. Restoring the volume of the midface is mandatory to improve sagging and drooping and lift central areas of heaviness.

When using facial fillers, we must assess aging in terms of both facial bone changes and fat atrophy. To improve signs of deep bony changes, supraperiosteal injections are placed in areas of bone reabsorption bounded by retaining ligaments and should be done with the highest G-prime fillers. Moderate depth fat pad augmentations are done best by moderate to high G-prime fillers, while more superficial subcutaneous deficiencies are augmented with mild to moderate G-prime fillers.

Targeting the four ligaments within the midface (zygomaticocutaneous, orbital, maxillary, and upper masseteric cutaneous ligaments) improves cheek tissue suspension. The nasolabial, infraorbital, superficial medial cheek, deep medial cheek, and the medial and lateral suborbicularis oculi fat (SOOF) compartments typically undergo volume loss. Boluses delivered along the superior, medial, and inferior border of the zygomatic arch that follow the natural contour of the zygoma enhance projection of the cheek bones. The efficacy of facial fillers to act as volumizing agents enables patients to have long-lasting results that are reliable and minimally invasive.

Keywords: Cheek augmentation, cheek filler, volumizing agents, aging changes, fat atrophy, bone resorption, retaining ligaments, fat pads, zygomatic arch, cheeks

Key Points

- Facial aging is multifactorial and involves a number of changes to the face including gradual loss of dermal collagen and subcutaneous fat occurs, causing subcutaneous volume loss in the nasolabial, infraorbital, superficial medial cheek, deep medial cheek, and the medial and lateral suborbicularis oculi fat (SOOF) compartments are most responsible for sagging and cheek deflation.
- To counteract signs of facial aging, hyaluronic acid (HA) and non-hyaluronic acid (non-HA) injections are both excellent techniques for maintaining youthful projection of the malar fat pads. Both types of fillers differ significantly in terms of G-prime (elastic ability to resist compression), filler longevity, and reversibility. HA fillers have a low-to-high G-prime and are most beneficial to patients who require replacement of fat deflation, who desire a reversible filler, and who prefer a more subtle tissue augmentation. Non-HA fillers have a higher G-prime and can achieve a more contoured look. They are better suited to address deep bone and fat pads changes through their support and ability to induce primary and secondary neocollagenesis.

55B.1 Preoperative Steps

55B.1.1 Background Knowledge

- Several facial retaining ligaments throughout the buccal area anchor and stabilize the superficial and deep fascia, ensuring that the midface fat pads remain in their designated anatomical locations. The retaining ligaments of the midface are the zygomaticocutaneous, orbital, maxillary, and upper masseteric cutaneous ligaments (▸ Fig. 55B.1). Because fat resorption mostly occurs within the bounds of these ligaments, palpating these ligaments at the surface of the skin exposes volume

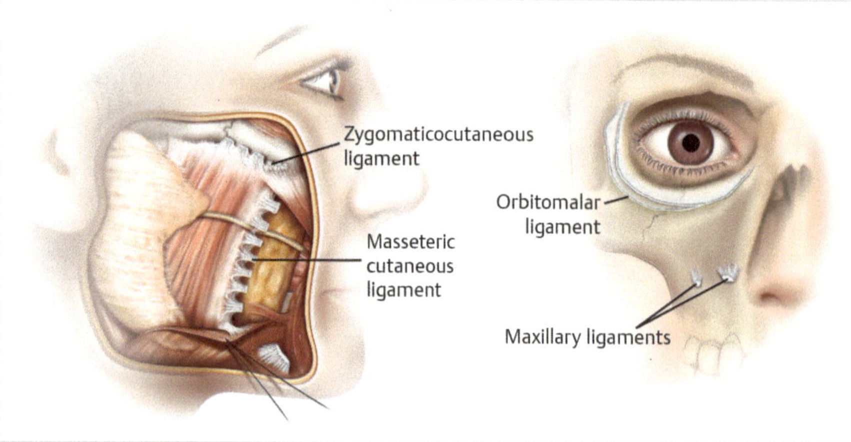

Fig. 55B.1 Facial retaining ligament location and details. The four retaining ligaments of the mid face: zygomaticocutaneous, orbital, maxillary, and upper masseteric cutaneous ligaments form the boundaries that anchor the superficial fat pads and are critical landmarks to understand in order to place fillers for volumetric improvement.

deflation and thinning of the fat pads that will benefit from correction.

- There are superficial and deep fat compartments within the midface that all contribute to malar soft tissue complex descent and lead to distinct morphological changes associated with facial aging such as volume depletion (▶ Fig. 55B.2a–c). The three superficial facial fat compartments are the nasolabial, infraorbital, and superficial medial cheek fat pads. Deep fat regions include the medial and lateral SOOF, buccal, and deep medial cheek fat pads (as described by Wan, Amirlak, Rohrich, and Davis in *The Clinical Importance of the Fat Compartments in Midfacial Aging*).

55B.2 Pretreatment Analysis

55B.2.1 Filler Selection

- Patients new to fillers or concerned about long-term facial structural changes are recommended to use HA fillers, as their effects can be reversed and dissolved. Both HA and non-HA fillers are typically viable for 12 to 24 months. Patients who exhibit soft tissue and subcutaneous changes with dermal thinning benefit from HA fillers, as their variety of G-primes—from low to intermediate to high—enable the filler to better integrate with the tissues to provide a more superficial placement and softening of etched lines. For correction in areas with weakened ligamentous and soft-tissue support, consider using a moderate-to-high G-prime filler in certain areas of the fat compartments and sub-superficial musculoaponeurotic system (sub-SMAS) space.
- The sculpted, contoured aesthetic that often appeals to younger patients can be best achieved with non-HA fillers such as calcium hydroxylapatite. Its high G-prime and viscoelastic properties allow for structural mimicking of the bony zygoma, which ensures maximal projection. Calcium hydroxylapatite is a biostimulator that induces primary and secondary neocollagenesis—the latter facilitates a long-term effect. Patients with sensitive skin or history of reaction to other injectables should consider non-HA over HA, as non-HA is biocompatible with human tissue and is inert and nonantigenic.

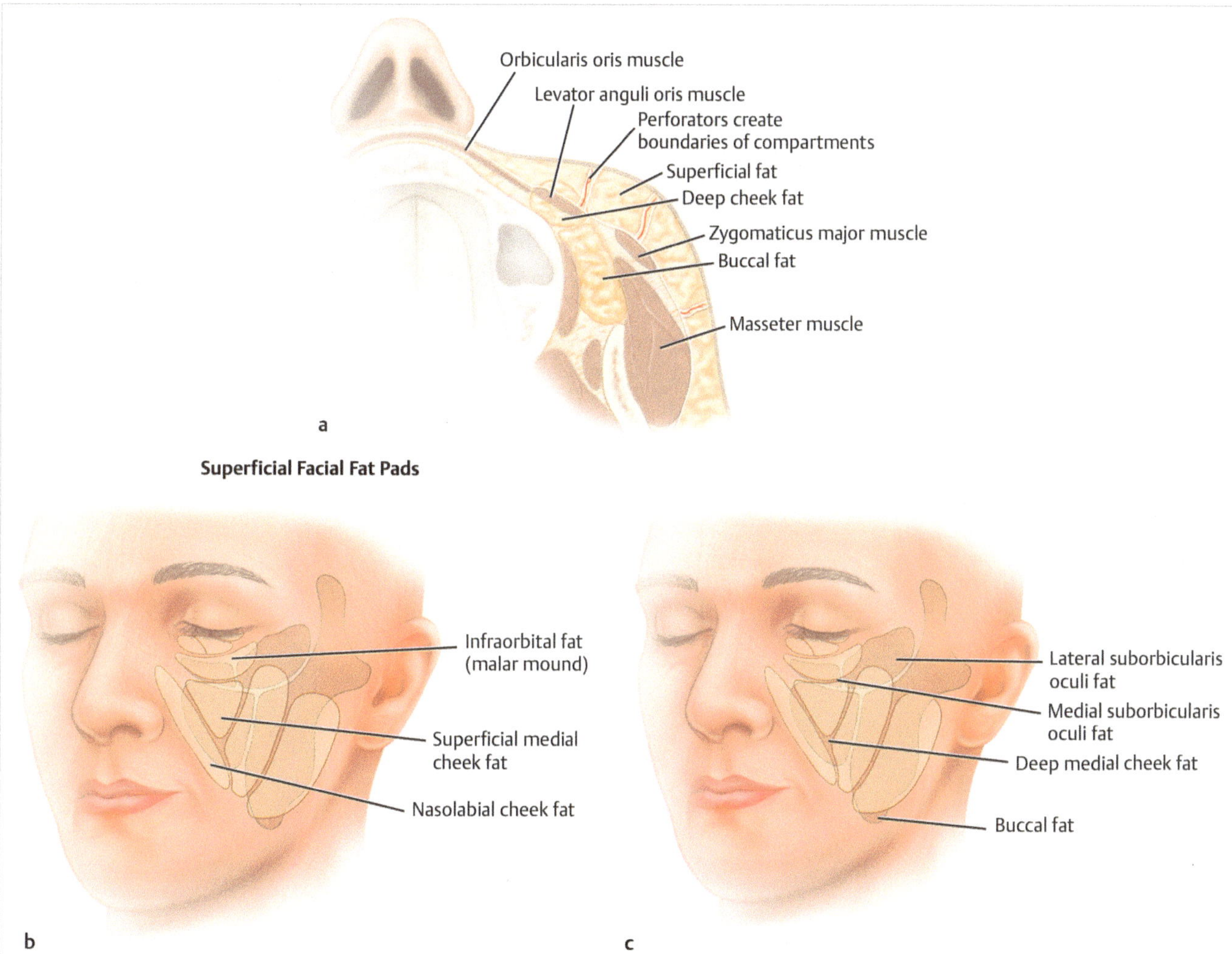

Fig. 55B.2 (a–c) Fat pad compartment locations.

55B.2.2 Anatomy Assessment

- Bisect the face and palpate the zygomatic bone structure bilaterally to assess for asymmetry, deflation, and drooping of the fat pads and jowling.
- Palpate for the zygomaticocutaneous, orbital, maxillary, and masseteric retaining ligaments and assess any weakening connections that affect the ligaments' ability to restrain facial skin against gravitational effects. The zygomaticocutaneous ligament originates from the inferior aspect of the zygomatic arch and expands anteriorly toward the junction between the zygomatic body and arch. The orbital retaining ligament extends along the orbital aperture and terminates where the lateral orbit thickens. The maxillary retaining ligaments are superficial to the maxilla, originating from the masseteric fascia and lying on top of the masseter muscle.
- Evaluate the malar mound and the superficial cheek fat compartments (▶ Fig. 55B.2a–c). The infraorbital fat is located between the orbicularis retaining ligament and the zygomaticocutaneous ligaments at the subcutaneous level and is a continuation of the tear trough. Injections into this area are associated with increased risk of lymphatic damage and edema.
- Nasolabial folds are one of the most prominent signs of facial aging and are best treated by supporting descending malar fat pads to lift their gravitational weight on the nasolabial folds. As described by Lamb and Surek in their textbook, *Facial Volumization: An Anatomic Approach*, volume loss associated with aging is thought to begin in the lateral superficial compartment and progress medially, which correlates with severity of facial aging. Adding volume to these compartments provides support and lift to the cutaneous structures and facilitates proper distribution of tension within the collagenous subdermal fibers. Injecting perpendicular to Langer's lines allows for more natural cheek contouring.
- In older patients, the deep pyriform space (▶ Fig. 55B.3), located deep and anterior to the maxilla requires analysis because the pyriform aperture recesses with age, resulting in enlargement of this hollow. Injecting filler into this site via cannula allows for volumization and lift to the lower midface. Filler can be delivered safely without the risk of intravascular compromise as the angular artery is not within the injection plane and courses laterally and superficially to this space. The deep medial cheek fat pad and Ristow's space are critical to volumize as well in this manner.
- The deep fat pads require evaluation as well because older patients commonly experience deflation in these regions. Deep medial cheek fat consists of medial and lateral components: the medial component is anterior to the premaxillary space and posterior to the deep pyriform space whereas the lateral component neighbors the buccal space and bony maxillary depression (▶ Fig. 55B.4). Filler injection into the medial component and the deep pyriform space achieves effective volume enhancement. These injections should be placed deep and medial in the anterior cheek. The lateral component should not be injected into, as this is a high swelling risk area.
- Injecting into the prezygomatic space (▶ Fig. 55B.5) also allows for enhanced midface volumization. As described by Lamb and Surek in their textbook, *Facial Volumization: An Anatomic Approach*, this space is bounded by the orbital retaining ligaments, deep to the orbicularis oculi muscle and between the SOOF and the preperiosteal fat pad. The SOOF is a narrow fat layer that lies between the orbicularis oculi muscle and the posterior capsule of SMAS. A safe injection can be performed by pinching and retracting the skin and orbicularis upward, while inserting the cannula laterally into the prezygomatic space.
- The premaxillary space should also be analyzed for hollowness. This space expands beneath the posterior capsule of the orbicularis oculi muscle. Great caution should be taken when injecting into this area, as the infraorbital neurovascular

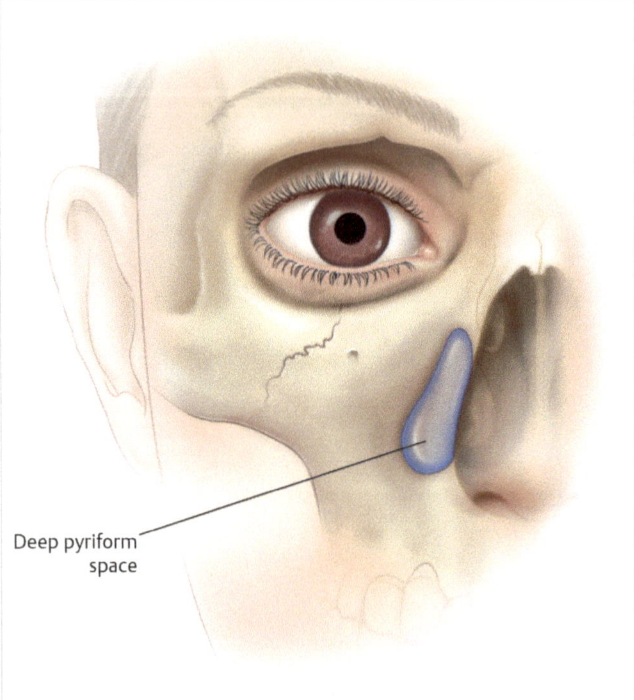

Fig. 55B.3 Anatomical locations of deep pyriform space and platysma.

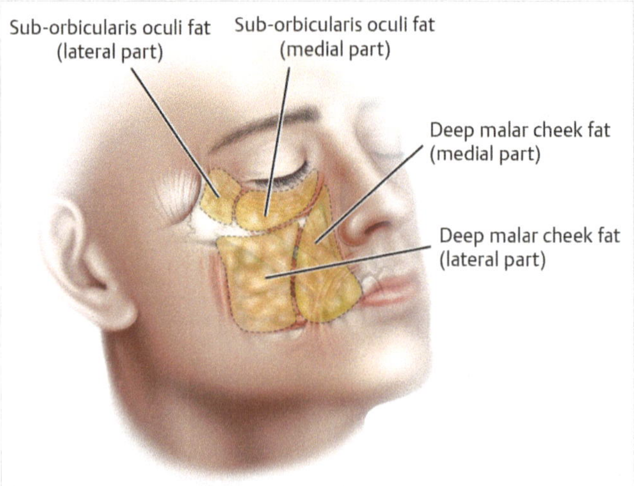

Fig. 55B.4 Anatomical locations of deep medial cheek fat and lateral and medial suborbicularis oculi fat (SOOF).

bundle lies deep to this space near the anterior surface of the levator labii superioris, and the angular vein courses laterally through the border of this space.

55B.2.3 Facial Danger Zones

- The infraorbital nerve foramen (▶ Fig. 55B.6), which lies superficial to the zygomatic process of the maxilla and 1 cm below the orbital rim at the midpupillary line, is within the field of interest and great caution should be taken to avoid nerve damage.

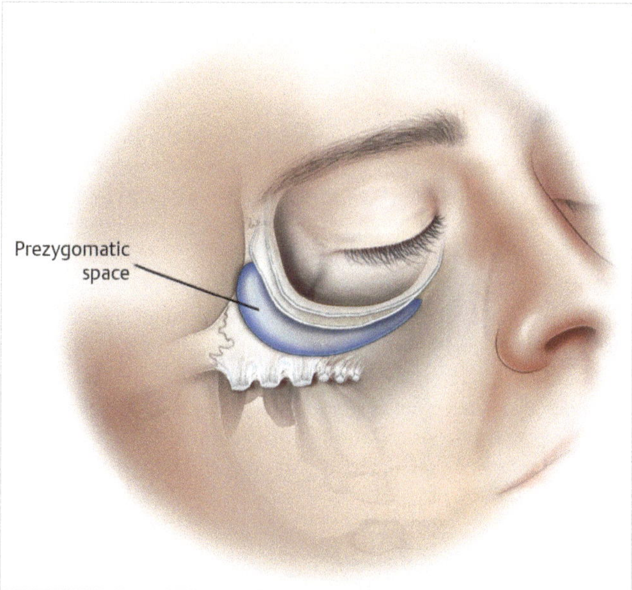

Fig. 55B.5 Prezygomatic space location.

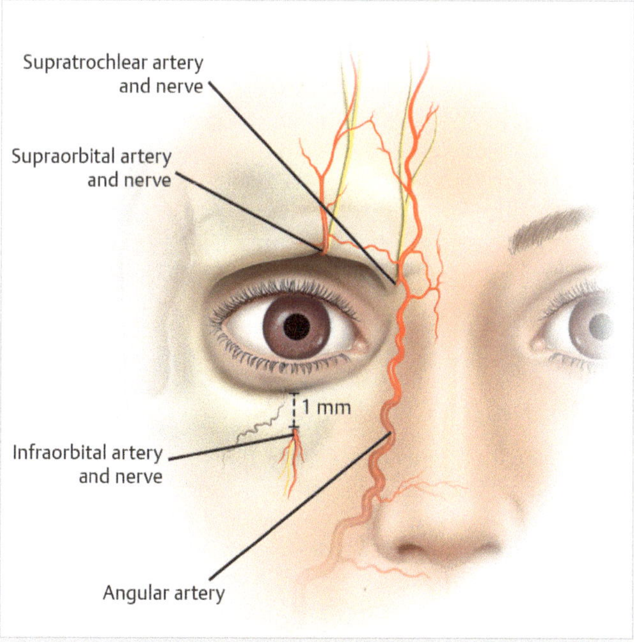

Fig. 55B.6 Location of artery branching and nerves within the midface.

- The zygomatic maxillary vein traverses the zygomatic region horizontally and can be located by bisecting the lateral canthus and moving inferiorly toward the zygoma. Although there is typically some hollowness within this region, this vein needs to be accounted for.
- Five main arteries should be carefully avoided: the facial artery, transverse artery, buccal branch of the maxillary, infraorbital, and zygomatic branch of the lacrimal artery (▶ Fig. 55B.7). The facial artery originates deep to the platysma, coursing deep relative to the posterior belly of the digastric and stylohyoid muscles, and continuing superiorly from the cheek toward the oral commissure, while another branch traverses along the nasal ala to the medial canthus. The transverse facial artery is located on the masseter muscle, inferior to the lower border of the facial nerve's zygomatic branch and superior to the parotid gland. The maxillary artery is located near the parotid gland and traverses from the parotid gland anteriorly toward the neck of the mandible and laterally to the lateral pterygoid muscle. The zygomatic branch of the lacrimal artery enters into the orbit and runs superiorly along the lateral rectus muscle, typically about 0.25 mm down from the lateral canthus.
- The facial artery has a terminal branch called the angular artery (▶ Fig. 55B.7). This specific branch is a significant danger zone as it lies in the field of interest and courses superiorly to the medial commissure of the alar-facial groove and joins with the dorsal nasal branch of the ophthalmic artery. The angular vein should also be accounted for, as it is located lateral to the angular artery and courses laterally through the premaxillary space. When the vein is 5 mm lateral to the medial canthus, it courses along the orbicularis oculi muscle edge.

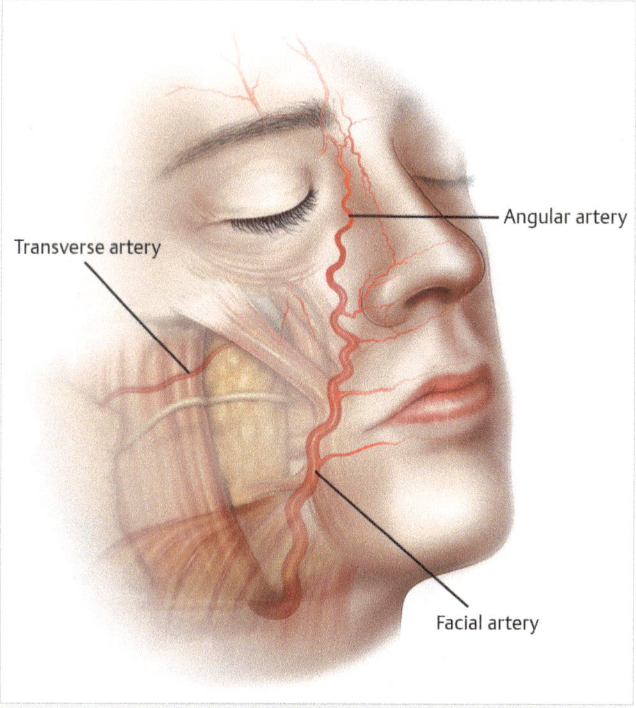

Fig. 55B.7 Facial artery and angular branch location.

- The facial nerve divides into five main branches (frontal, zygomatic, buccal, marginal mandibular, and cervical) that course through the midface and must be avoided. The frontal nerve branching is said to begin 0.5 cm inferior to the tragus and courses 1.5 cm laterally to the supraorbital rim. It is deep within the SMAS and traverses superficially along the temporoparietal fascia approximately 2 cm above the zygomatic arch. The zygomatic branch courses alongside the parotid gland and runs alongside the masseter muscle and transverse facial artery. The buccal branch is located superficial to the upper and lower masseteric ligaments and is within the masseter fascia. The marginal mandibular branch originates from within the platysma-auricular fascia and courses anteriorly along the masseter and toward the level of the mandibular ligament. The cervical branch divides into several other small branches that traverse inferiorly into the neck.

55B.2.4 Facial Markings

- Draw a line from the orbital medial canthus to the oral commissure and another line extending from the malar equator bilaterally. The angle formed by these two lines is a reliable indication of bilateral facial symmetry.
- Bisecting the angle formed from above provides satisfactory directionality for the natural trajectory of the zygomatic bone and where filler can be placed for maximum projection and lift.

55B.3 Operative Steps

55B.3.1 Dr. Kay's Recommended Dilutions

- Calcium hydroxylapatite plain—recommended to mix with luer lock adapter 1 syringe (1.5 cc) with 0.2 to 0.5 cc lidocaine with 1:100,000 epinephrine

55B.3.2 Needle Selection

- A 27-gauge, 1-inch (20-mm) long needle is recommended.

55B.3.3 Sterility

- Makeup should be removed, and the face should be cleansed with 70% alcohol, chlorhexidine, or betadine to ensure sterile conditions.

55B.3.4 Injection Techniques

Malar Contouring

- Always visualize the cheek danger zones and remember to follow the natural borders of the zygoma.
- To maintain safe injections, all injections should stay on periosteum. The use of the cannula is optimal for the volumization of the deep fat pads of the face and periocular areas, providing optimal safety for vascular injury prevention.
- Palpate for the suture holding the temporal bone and the temporal process of the zygomatic bone together. Once this suture is found, continue palpating with two fingers to outline the upper and lower borders of the zygomatic bone.
- The initial injection site is at the apex of the cheek, at the intersection of the lateral and medial portion of the zygoma. This is the most important injection site because if the apex is drooping, tissues will deflate over the zygoma. Injecting a 0.3 cc bolus into this site helps to lift and elevate the fat pad.
- Moving inferiorly along the lower border of the zygoma, deliver three boluses of 0.1 to 0.2 cc about 1 cm apart from one another, tapering upwards. It is important to have at least one of these boluses delivered, supporting the upper masseteric cutaneous ligaments and possibly another bolus delivered at the zygomatic cutaneous ligaments. A good landmark for the lower border is the line previously drawn from the malar equator.
- Travel superiorly along the upper border of the zygoma. At the junction of the orbit and cheek, there is a small flat area on the zygomatic bone at the prezygomatic space. Injecting a 0.2 cc bolus into this site provides maximum projection of the upper cheek bone.
- Continue to move superiorly along the upper border of the zygomatic bone, while being mindful and palpating for the zygomaticofacial foramen. Two more boluses of 0.1 to 0.2 cc should be delivered about 1 cm apart on this upper border, specifically where the zygomaticocutaneous ligament lies. The superior border is bounded by the line previously drawn from the lateral canthus to its intersection with the malar equator line.
- The last point of focus should be the mid portion of the zygomatic arch, following the trajectory line formed by bisecting the angle previously found. Small boluses of 0.1 cc should be delivered throughout this line, directly on periosteum.

Addressing Nasojugal Folds

- Make an injection site 1.5 cm inferolateral to the lateral canthus while pinching and retracting the skin to guide the cannula through the prezygomatic space. A popping sound should be audible once the cannula has pierced into this space. Move the cannula within the prezygomatic space along the upper maxilla and feel for the zygomaticocutaneous ligaments and the orbital retaining ligaments. Once within the appropriate location, small boluses totaling 0.6 cc should be delivered within this space to fill the nasojugal folds.

55B.4 Possible Side Effects and Complications

- Improper placement of filler can lead to a number of complications such as vascular obstruction, visual compromise, stroke, necrosis, and vascular occlusion and needs immediate intervention. Common signs and symptoms of vascular occlusion include ecchymosis, bruising, skin blanching, pain, long-term erythema, scarring, and pigment changes.

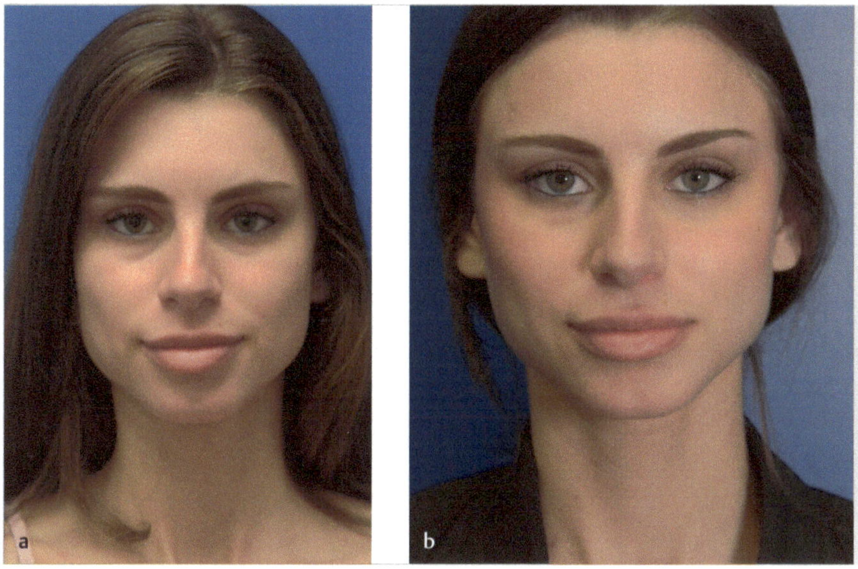

Fig. 55B.8 (a, b) The left panel shows a picture of a 22-year-old patient before she received any filler. The right panel shows the same patient at her follow-up appointment at one month after receiving 1.5 cc total volume of calcium hydroxypatite to her cheeks. The patient's before and after picture illustrates following bony contouring to slim, lift, and sculpt the malar fat pads and alleviate lower face jowling tendencies and heaviness by changing the vector of lift of the midface. The patient does not have the rounded full appearance of malar fat pads typically associated with HA gel fillers.

- Injecting a filler with higher G-prime and viscoelasticity causes a higher risk of vascular occlusion. Because of the chemical composition of non-HA fillers, they are not readily dissolved. Also keep in mind that vascular occlusion can occur even post filler injection. In order to prevent this, a complete understanding of the anatomical locations of critical facial vessels and danger zones is needed.

55B.5 Postoperative Care

- Typically, results of the treatment are effective immediately, but look best 48 hours after treatment has occurred.
- Avoid placing excessive pressure directly on the cheek. Patients should refrain from getting facials or applying face masks to the area for 1 to 2 weeks after treatment.
- Some swelling and bruising can occur within the first 3 to 4 days of treatment and create asymmetry. If asymmetry persists for 2 weeks post injection, schedule a follow-up appointment. Massaging the area and applying ice can help alleviate swelling, but massage and apply ice gently. Prednisone can also be taken as prescribed by a physician.
- Minimize exposure of the treated area to the sun or heat for at least 24 hours after treatment and if possible, until swelling and redness disappears. Note that salt, alcohol, and heat worsen possible swelling effects.

55B.6 Case Example

The left panel shows a picture of a 22-year-old patient before she received any filler on 12/11/2018. The right panel shows the same patient at her follow-up appointment on 01/07/2019 after receiving 1 syringe of calcium hydroxylapatite to her cheeks (▶ Fig. 55B.8a, b).

55B.7 Conclusion

Helping patients to achieve their aesthetic goals require an individualized and stepwise approach to determine the filler best suited for each patient's anatomy. HA fillers help to provide a more natural and moderate cheek augmentation, whereas non-HA fillers and vycross fillers will help to achieve the more contoured and sculpted look with their high G-prime and ability to induce neocollagenesis.

Filler injections targeted at supporting facial retaining ligaments within the midface will help increase tissue suspension and alleviate signs of bone resorption. Evaluation of fat pad changes will help to target areas with volume deflation.

Overall, filler injections into the upper, lower, and middle borders of the zygomatic arch as well as adjacent to facial ligaments and fat pads will help patients to achieve youthful contours within the cheek by allowing for more lift and support within the tissues.

See **Video 55B.1**.

Further Readings

Alghoul M, Bitik O, Mcbride J, Zins JE. Relationship of the zygomatic facial nerve to the retaining ligaments of the face. Plast Reconstr Surg. 2012; 130:42

Allen S. Anatomic danger zones for facial injection of soft tissue fillers. UpToDate. https://www.uptodate.com/contents/anatomic-danger-zones-for-facial-injection-of-soft-tissue-fillers?source=history_widget. Published January 11, 2019. Accessed August 5, 2019

Carruthers A, Carruthers J, Humphrey S. Injectable soft tissue fillers: overview of clinical use. UpToDate. https://www.uptodate.com/contents/injectable-soft-tissue-fillers-overview-of-clinical-use?source=history_widget. Published May 17, 2019. Accessed August 1, 2019

Lamb J, Surek C. Facial columization. 1st ed. New York: Thieme Medical Publishers; 2018:3–23

Maio MD. The 5-point cheek reshape. https://www.mdmaio.com/2018/12/11/the-5-point-cheek-reshape/. Accessed July 14, 2019

56 Filler Finesse: Tear Trough and Upper Eyelid

Patrick Trevidic

Abstract

Aging in the infraorbital area and upper eyelid can be improved using hyaluronic acid. In order to achieve the best results for your patient it is important to have a good knowledge of the anatomy and do a comprehensive patient assessment, and choose the correct technique and product. Here we discuss how to assess your patient's anatomy, and the best technique to use, in order to address a lack of volume in the tear trough, palpebromalar groove, and upper eyelid. When using fillers in this area it is important to ensure that you are injecting into the correct layer and that you are not using too much product.

Keywords: Hyaluronic acid, tear trough, palpebromalar groove

Key Points

- The aging process in the infraorbital area and upper eyelid causes a tired and sad appearance and can be improved by the injection of filler.
- The only useful and long-lasting filler is hyaluronic acid (the injection of fat is not described in this chapter).
- For filler injections, whatever the location, we follow our ATP protocol, which means:
  - First, A: knowledge of the **A**natomy and **A**ssess the patient
  - Second, T: choose the right **T**echnique, and
  - Third, P: use the right **P**roduct
- Make sure you're in the right plane, do not overfill, and do not overpromise results.

56.1 Assessment and Anatomy

56.1.1 Assessment

- Discuss patient's expectations and conduct a patient assessment using historic photos.
- Consider previous treatments or medical diseases that could contraindicate fillers (follow the instructions for use on the leaflet).
- Conduct a clinical examination to determine any other contraindications: eyelid laxity (positive pinch test), malar mounds, positive or neutral vectors, very thin skin, or skin infection.
- If the patient has midcheek depression with a midcheek fold, this needs to be addressed before treating the tear trough and palpebromalar groove.

56.1.2 Anatomy

Infraorbital Rim

- Why do we have a tear trough? The tear tough depression is caused where the orbicularis oculi muscle attaches to the bone. The skin here can have a darker appearance (creating dark circles) and can also be overshadowed by palpebral bags, further causing a tired appearance.
- Why do we have a palpebromalar groove? This is due to the loss of the top of infraorbital fat compartment, creating excessive thinness of the infraorbital lateral orbit.
- What happens during the aging process? Several factors contribute to aging under the eyes: loss of superficial fat (creating and increasing the palpebromalar groove); receding bone at the infraorbital margin deepens the tear trough depression; and increased volume of the palpebral fat pad.
- Where are the anatomical dangers (► Fig. 56.1)? There are none close to the tear trough and palpebromalar groove:
  - The angular artery is superficial in the nasojugal groove, then goes up on the lateral side of the nose.
  - The infraorbital nerve is 3 mm below the orbital margin.

Upper Eyelid: A-Frame Deformity, Sunken or Hollow Eyes

- Why do we age? A-frame deformity or sunken eyes:
  - It could be congenital due to a lack of intraorbital fat or large eye sockets but commonly, post blepharoplasty, it is because the surgeon has removed too much fat. It can also be associated with weakness of the levator palpebrae superioris.
  - During the aging process the depression of hollow eyes is relatively stable with time, but skin laxity increases.
- Where are the anatomical dangers (► Fig. 56.1)?

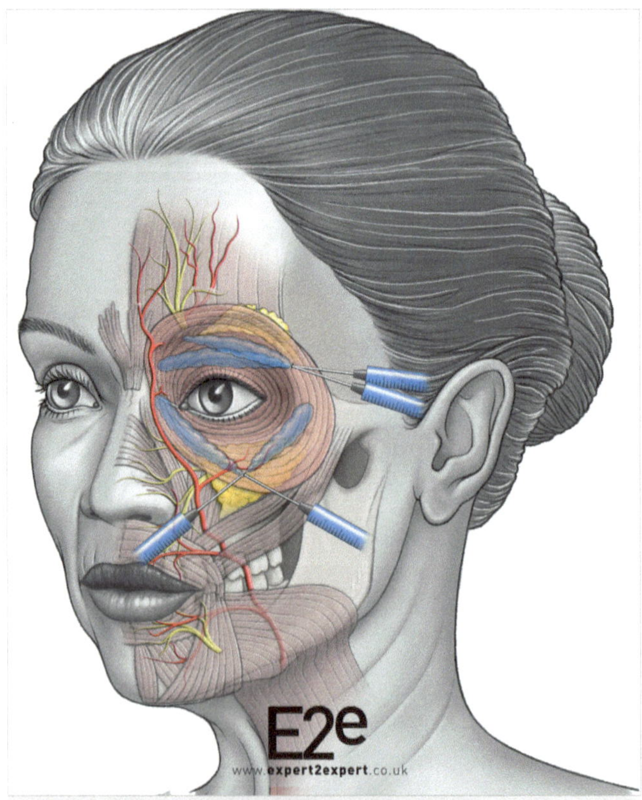

Fig. 56.1 Periorbital injection and anatomical dangers.

- ◦ Anatomical vascular dangers are further away as the deep supraorbital and supratrochlear arteries emerge from the bone foramen.
- ◦ The only theoretical danger is when entering in a retroseptal plane, which can be avoided using a rigid 25-gauge cannula and an entrance point on the orbital rim in the right plane between the bone and the orbicularis oculi.

56.2 Injection Steps

- **Do not forget** to take photos of the face (front and oblique), obtain consent forms, and provide the patient with written information.

56.2.1 Position, Drawing, Disinfection

- Remove patient's makeup.
- The patient is in a sitting position for drawing and injection.
- Keep your elbows at the level of the injection site.
- Mark up the area to correct.
- Disinfect the area.

56.2.2 Equipment

- Use a 25-gauge canula, long enough to reach the top of the tear trough and palpebromalar groove as well as the edge of the hollow eyes from the entrance point; it is between 38 and 55 mm depending on the patient and brand.
- Why use a 25-gauge cannula? In the infraorbital rim it avoids hematoma and bruising (there are no anatomical dangers in this area) and in the supraorbital rim it helps to keep the injection in front of the septum (rather than avoiding the supraorbital and supratrochlear arteries).
- Use a product dedicated to the periorbital area with low cohesivity and low hygroscopic properties to avoid swelling.

56.2.3 Technique

- Start by creating an entrance point with a needle (one gauge more than the cannula's diameter), which will give you the depth and direction of your cannula.
- This entrance point is located as follows:
  - ◦ For the infraorbital rim: At the junction of the tear trough and palpebromalar groove.
  - ◦ For the upper eyelid: A few millimeters under the tail of the eyebrow, medial on the lateral orbital rim.
- Introduce your cannula through the hole so that the blunt tip is on the bone:
  - ◦ For the infraorbital rim it will be inserted into the suborbicularis oculi fat (SOOF) and pushed along the lateral orbital rim under the orbicularis oculi (▶ Fig. 56.2, ▶ Fig. 56.3).
  - ◦ For the upper eyelid, the cannula is introduced through the entrance point, so the plane of introduction will be between the orbicularis oculi muscle and the periosteum.
  - ◦ Gently push the cannula medially.

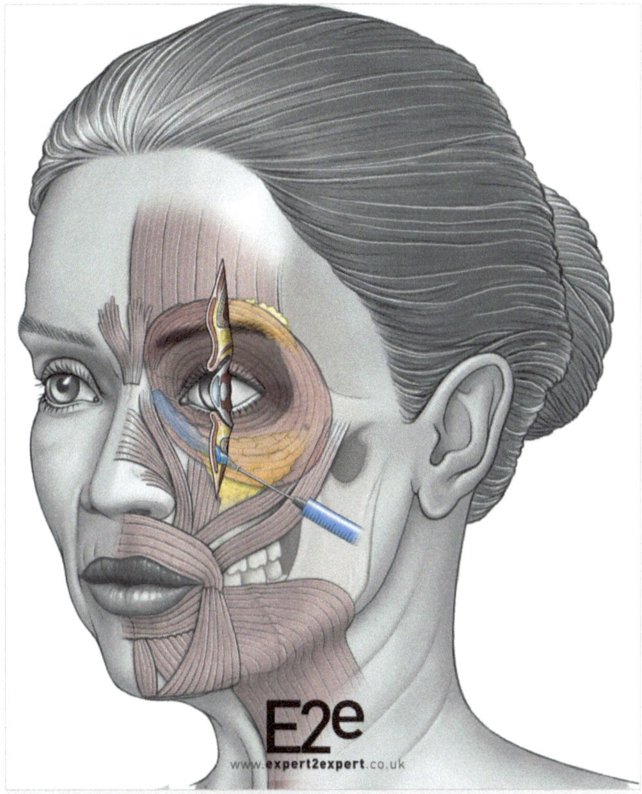

Fig. 56.2 Tear trough injection deep along the bone.

  - ◦ The tip of the cannula will follow the path under the orbicularis oculi and above the septum. This is the anatomical area that must not be crossed.
- Push the cannula horizontally for the best result (▶ Fig. 56.4).
- Push slowly; normally, if you are in the right plane you will feel no resistance.
- If you feel resistance or the patient feels pain, inject a small amount of product (which contains lidocaine) to ease the process and stop the pain.
- Anterograde injection decreases the pain.
- Location of filler deposition: on the bone for infraorbital rim (▶ Fig. 56.2 and ▶ Fig. 56.3) and above the septum for the upper eyelid (▶ Fig. 56.4).
- Average quantity of filler: 0.3 mL for the tear trough, 0.2 mL for the palpebromalar groove, and 0.2 mL for the upper eyelid.
- It is difficult to assess how much filler will be necessary to complete the treatment. A useful hint: always use less rather than more filler. Ask the patients to tell you if they prefer their appearance 2 days (with some swelling) or 3 weeks after treatment; if it is 2 days, they need more filler.
- For the infraorbital rim: Do not massage the area if you get a bump; mold it carefully or you will squeeze the low cohesivity product between your fingers and bone, and push it away from the injection site.
- Duration is very long, with good outcomes.
- If there is any mistake (misplacement or overcorrection) do not wait, use hyaluronidase.

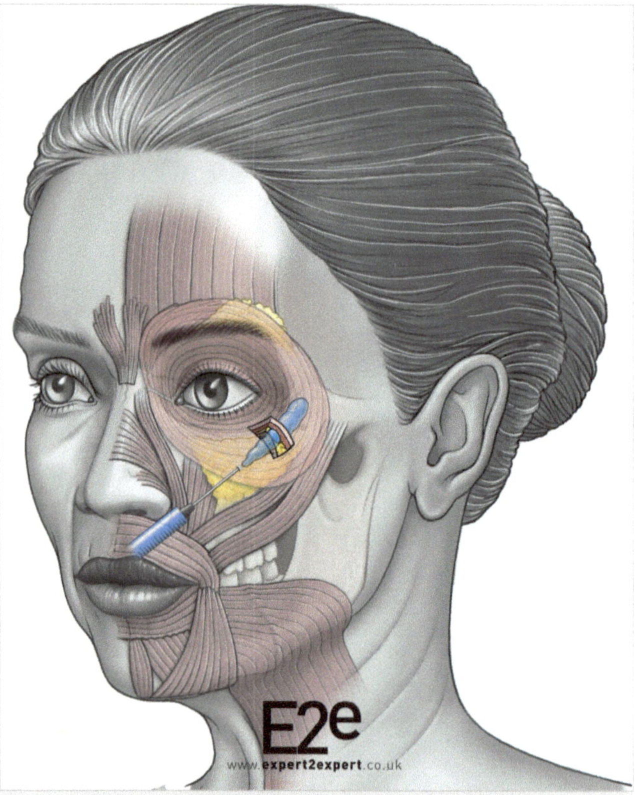

Fig. 56.3 Palpebromalar groove injection deep along the bone.

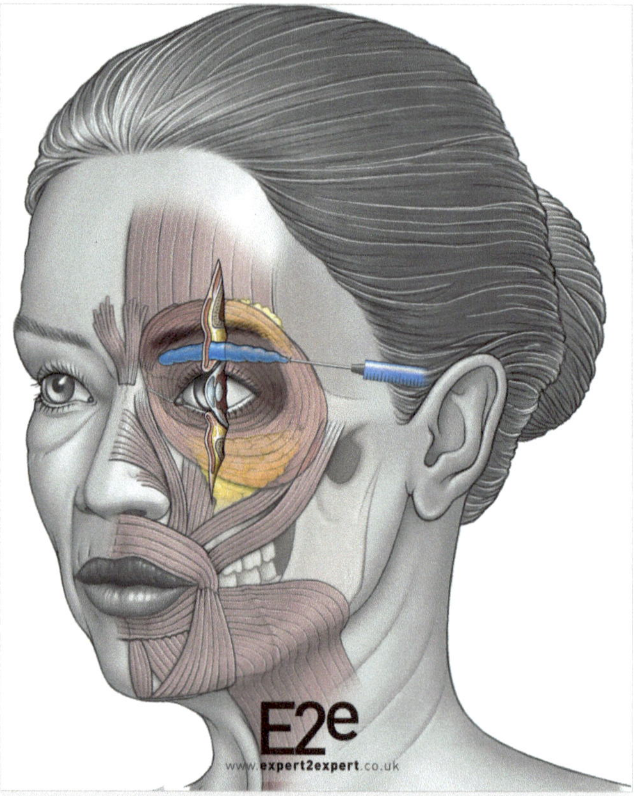

Fig. 56.4 Upper eyelid injection between the orbicularis oculi muscle and the septum.

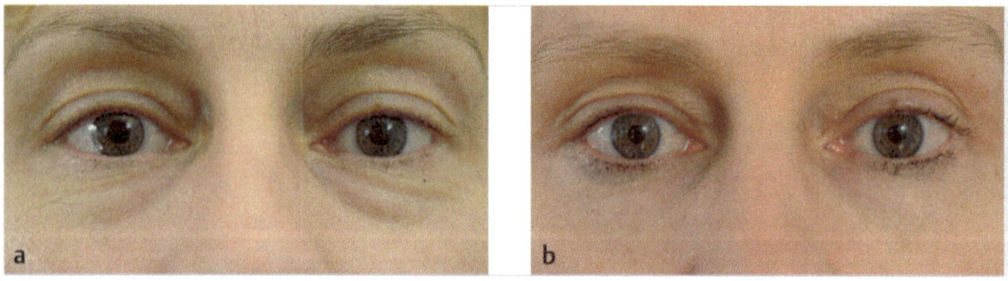

Fig. 56.5 **(a)** Before and **(b)** after photos of a patient 4 months following injection in the tear trough, palpebromalar groove, and upper eyelid.

56.3 Postprocedural Care

- Patients are instructed to rest and sleep with their head elevated, and to take care to avoid applying pressure to the product.
- Postinjection consultation takes place after 3 weeks.

56.4 Case Example

Before and after photos of a patient 4 months following injection in the tear trough, palpebromalar groove, and upper eyelid (▶ Fig. 56.5a, b).

56.5 Conclusion

Hyaluronic acid is a very good option to treat periorbital aging, removing the depressions which create shadows. Make sure you are in the right plane for injection, and do not inject too much filler. Chose the right patient, the right technique, and the right product. Do not forget that you cannot remove all signs of aging in this area with fillers alone; fillers will not address the skin color, palpebral bags, or excess skin.

See **Video 56.1**.

Further Readings

Azib N, Berros P, Braccini F, et al. Anatomy and volumizing injection. Paris: Expert2 Expert Medical Publishing (Oulu); 2013

Cotofana S, Schenck TL, Trevidic P, et al. Midface: clinical anatomy and regional approaches with injectable fillers. Plast Reconstr Surg. 2015; 136(5) Suppl:219S–234S

Criollo-Lamilla G, DeLorenzi C, Karpova E, et al. Anatomy and filler complications. Paris: Expert2Expert Medical Publishing (Oulu); 2017

Farhi D, Trevidic P, Kestemont P, et al. Emervel French Survey Group. The Emervel French survey: a prospective real-practice descriptive study of 1,822 patients treated for facial rejuvenation with a new hyaluronic acid filler. J Drugs Dermatol. 2013; 12(5):e88–e93

Sykes JM, Cotofana S, Trevidic P, et al. Upper face: clinical anatomy and regional approaches with injectable fillers. Plast Reconstr Surg. 2015; 136(5) Suppl: 204S–218S

57 Part A: Filler Finesse: Nose

Rod J. Rohrich and Ira L. Savetsky

Abstract

Soft-tissue fillers are an excellent method to augment or refine nasal irregularities. A systematic and comprehensive nasofacial analysis is critical to ensure soft-tissue filler success. The use of soft-tissue filler has broadened the rhinoplasty surgeon's armamentarium. We review indications of soft-tissue filler injection into the nose as well as injection techniques and pearls.

Keywords: Rhinoplasty, nasofacial analysis, filler, liquid rhinoplasty

Key Points

- Soft-tissue fillers are an excellent modality to augment or refine nasal irregularities.
- A comprehensive and systematic nasofacial analysis is the most critical initial step in establishing goals and formulating a precise injection plan for nasal soft-tissue filler.
- Setting realistic expectations with the patient is critical in achieving high postinjection patient satisfaction.

57A.1 Injection Planning

57A.1.1 Defining Goals

- Have the patients list their top three nasal aesthetic concerns and record them precisely.

57A.1.2 Focused Nasal History

- The patient should be asked about any history of allergic or inflammatory disorders such as hay fever, asthma, rhinitis, and sinusitis.
- Medications and dietary supplements such as acetylsalicylic acid, nonsteroidal anti-inflammatory drugs, and fish oil should be reviewed as they can increase ecchymosis.

57A.2 Nasofacial Proportions and Systematic Nasal Analysis (▶ Table 57A.1)

57A.2.1 "10–7–5" Nasal Analysis

- The frontal view evaluation should include 10 key areas: Facial proportions, skin type/skin thickness, symmetry/nasal deviation, bony vault width, midvault asymmetry, dorsal aesthetic lines, tip shape/tip-defining points, alar rims/base, infratip lobular projection, and periapical hypoplasia/upper lip length.
- In the profile view, 7 areas are evaluated: Radix height and position, dorsal convexity, nasal length, tip projection, tip rotation, alar–columellar relationship, and chin projection.
- Use the base view to assess 5 areas: Nasal projection, nostril shape/symmetry, columella symmetry/width, alar base width, and alar rim flaring.

57A.3 Standardized Photography and Digital Imaging

- Standardized photographs including frontal, lateral, oblique, and basal views should be obtained for every patient.
- Digital imaging is an excellent tool for communicating with the patient and evaluating patient's expectations.

Table 57A.1 Systematic nasofacial analysis

Nasal view	Analysis
Frontal	
1. Facial proportions	Height (thirds), width (fifths), symmetry
2. Skin type/quality	Fitzpatrick type, thin or thick, sebaceous
3. Symmetry/nasal deviation	Midline, dorsal deviation, C-shaped, reverse C-shaped, or S-shaped deviation
4. Dorsal aesthetic lines	Straight, symmetric or asymmetric, well- or ill-defined, narrow or wide
5. Bony vault	Narrow or wide, asymmetric, short or long nasal bones
6. Midvault	Narrow or wide, collapse, inverted-V, saddle deformity
7. Nasal tip	Ideal/bulbous/boxy/pinched, supratip, tip-defining points, infratip lobule
8. Alar rims	Gull-shaped, facets, notching, retraction
9. Alar base	Width
10. Upper lip	Long or short, dynamic depressor septi, upper lip crease
Lateral	
1. Nasofrontal angle and radix	Acute or obtuse, high or low radix, prominent or low nasion
2. Nasal length, dorsum, and supratip	Length: long or short; Dorsum: smooth, hump, scooped out; Supratip: break, fullness, pollybeak, over- or underprojected
3. Tip projection	Over- or underprojected
4. Tip rotation	Over- or underrotated
5. Alar–columellar relationship	Hanging or retracted ala, hanging or retracted columella, maxillary or soft-tissue deficiency
6. Periapical hypoplasia	Maxillary or soft-tissue deficiency
7. Lip–chin relationship	Normal, over- or underprojected chin
Basal	
1. Nasal projection	Over- or underprojected, well- or ill-defined tip-defining points, columellar-to-lobule ratio
2. Nostril	Symmetry, long/narrow or short/wide nostril, nostril–tip ratio, concave or convex ala
3. Columella	Caudal septal deviation, flaring of medial crura
4. Alar base	Width
5. Alar flaring	Type I, II, III, or IV

57A.4 Managing Expectations

- Review all photographic views with the patient.
- It is extremely important to discuss with the patient what can and cannot be achieved with soft-tissue fillers.
- A patient who is focused on minor or uncorrectable problems or with unrealistic expectations despite extensive discussion will likely be disappointed postinjection, regardless of the aesthetic improvement.

57A.5 Soft-Tissue Filler Indications

- Patients who want to “wear a rhinoplasty” before committing to surgery.
- Rhinoplasty patients who do not want to undergo revision surgery to correct a deformity.
- Patients who are not surgical candidates.
- Patients who are awaiting the proper time interval before undergoing a secondary rhinoplasty.

57A.6 Technical Pearls

- Knowledge of nasal anatomy is critical to use soft-tissue fillers accurately and precisely.
- When considering proper application of soft-tissue fillers for nasal contouring, skin thickness is an important consideration. The skin is thinner and more mobile proximally and becomes thicker and more immobile distally (▶ Fig. 57A.1).
- Level of injection is deep dermis or subdermal layers in order to maximize effect while avoiding visibility and Tyndall effect.
- To minimize the risk of intravascular injection, one must take into consideration the subcutaneous location of the nasal vessels superficial to the nasal muscles along with the rich plexus of vessels with contributions from the facial, supraorbital, and supratrochlear arteries (▶ Fig. 57A.2a, b).
- Avoid high-pressure injection, as this has been associated with intravascular injection and emboli to the ocular vessels as well as pressure necrosis.
- Fillers should be injected using the smallest needle possible to maximize control over the volume of injection.

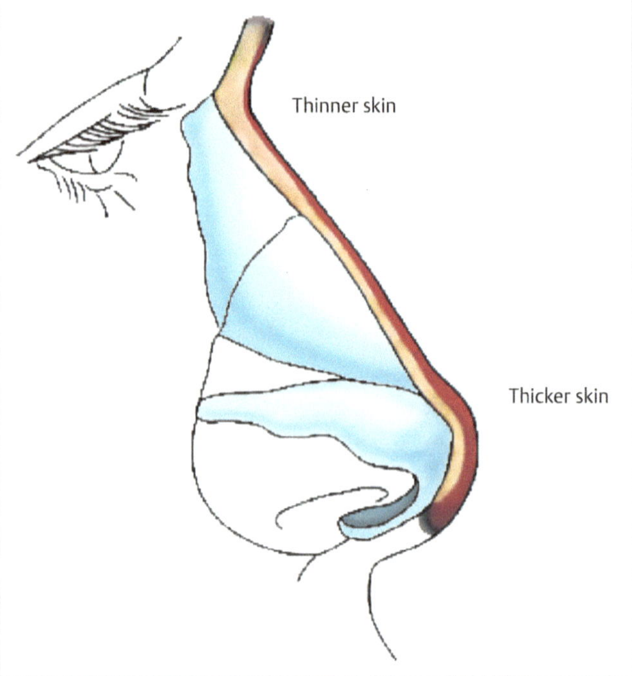

Fig. 57A.1 Injection techniques: nasal dorsum. Voluma is a newer formulation of hyaluronic acid filler with thicker consistency and suitable for volume augmentation when placed in a deep plane along the osteocartilaginous framework. It is subject to postinjection swelling and thus the area should be slightly undertreated. Products with thicker consistency should be avoided in patients with thin skin or decreased soft tissue elasticity after previous rhinoplasty. (Reproduced with permission from Rohrich R, Adams W, Ahmad J, et al, eds. Dallas Rhinoplasty: Nasal Surgery by the Masters. 3rd ed. Thieme; 2014.)

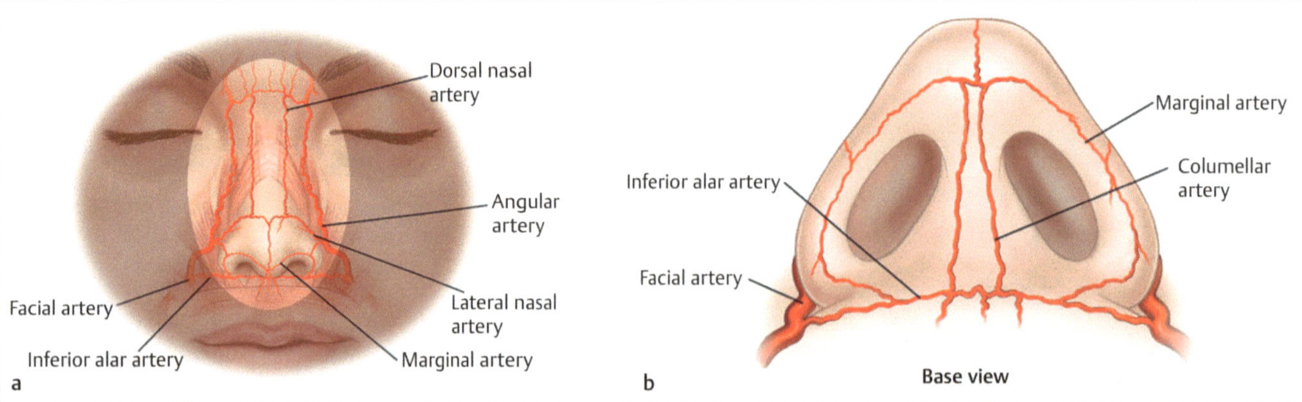

Fig. 57A.2 Vasculature of the nasal aesthetic unit from the anterior view **(a)** and basal view **(b)**. The facial artery travels upward to become the angular artery. Important branches of the facial artery include the lateral nasal artery and inferior alar artery. The paired dorsal nasal arteries are located lateral to the midline along the dorsum of the nose. Intravascular injection into any of these terminal branches of the external carotid system can cause retrograde flow and embolization of the ophthalmic and retinal arteries. (Reproduced with permission from Rohrich R, Stuzin J, Dayan E, et al, eds. Facial Danger Zones: Staying Safe with Surgery, Fillers and Non-invasive Devices. 1st ed. Thieme; 2019.)

57A.7 Site-Specific Injection Technique

57A.7.1 Nasal Dorsum (▶ Fig. 57A.3)

- Best approached using small amounts of hyaluronic acid.
- Restylane is the preferred product to use in this area because of its higher level of cross-linking and lower hydrophilicity.
- After injection, the hyaluronic acid should be gently massaged to help with even distribution, thus avoiding contour irregularities.
- After injection, the surgeon should allow 15 minutes to pass in order to give the soft tissues time to adjust and the product to fully diffuse, which allows for a more accurate assessment of effect before further injection.
- Volume of injection and skin color should be assessed regularly to avoid any compromise of vascular perfusion to the nasal skin.
- Layering the hyaluronic acid from deep to superficial is preferred for volume restoration of the nasal dorsum.
- A threading technique along the long axis of the nasal dorsum should be used to maintain proper nasal shape (▶ Fig. 57A.4).

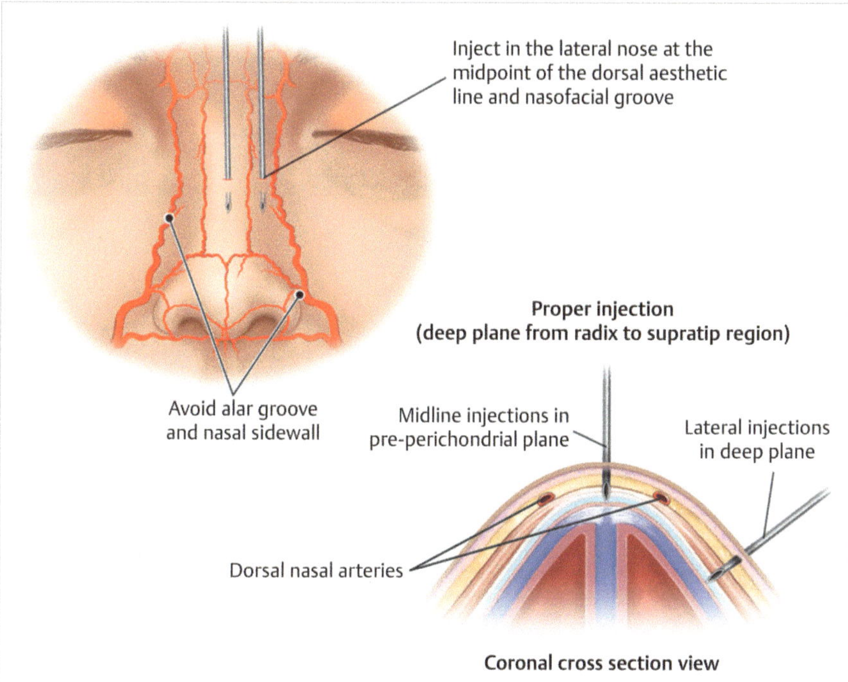

Fig. 57A.3 Schematic of proper injection technique. Injections can be performed deep in the midline from the radix to the supratip break to avoid intravascular injection. If injections are performed laterally, they are performed deeply at the midpoint of the dorsal aesthetic line and the nasofacial groove. (Reproduced with permission from Rohrich R, Stuzin J, Dayan E, et al, eds. Facial Danger Zones: Staying Safe with Surgery, Fillers and Non-invasive Devices. 1st ed. Thieme; 2019.)

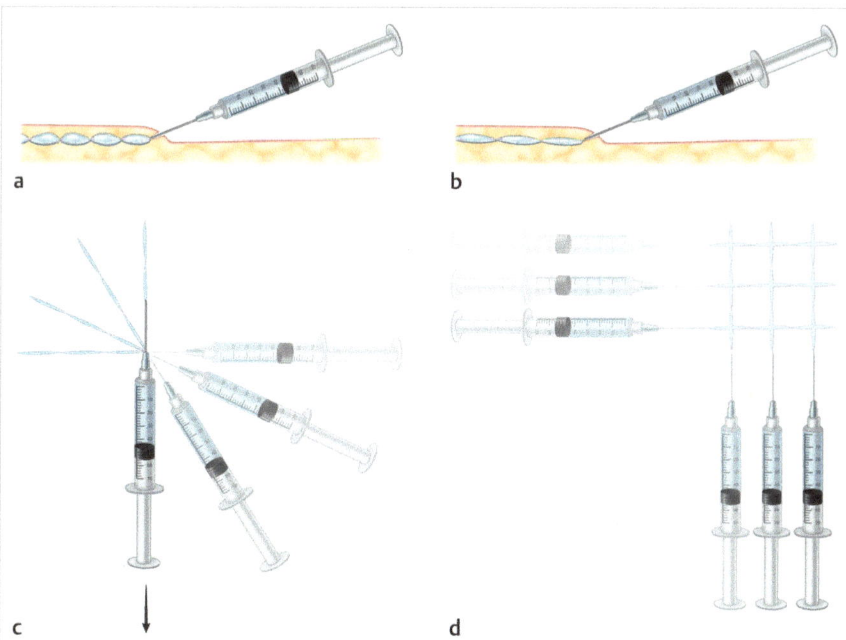

Fig. 57A.4 Injection techniques: **(a)** Serial puncture, **(b)** linear threading, **(c)** fanning, and **(d)** crosshatching/radial. (Reproduced with permission from Rohrich R, Adams W, Ahmad J, et al, eds. Dallas Rhinoplasty: Nasal Surgery by the Masters. 3rd ed. Thieme; 2014.)

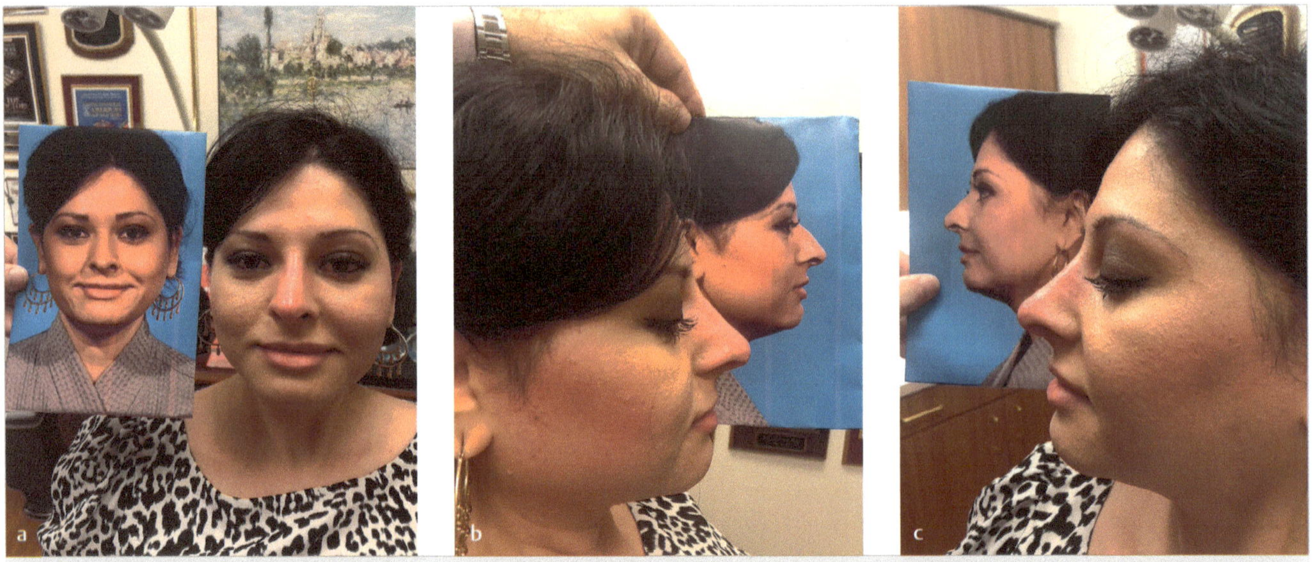

Fig. 57A.5 Anteroposterior views of a 39-year-old woman before and immediately after **(a)** nasal filler injection. **(b, c)** Preinjection and immediate postinjection lateral views.

57A.7.2 Nasal Sidewall (▶ Fig. 57A.3)

- Best addressed using small amounts of hyaluronic acid with postinjection massage and a 15-minute delay before reinjection.
- The skin of the nasal sidewall should also be continually assessed for any evidence of vascular compromise.
- Injection is best performed using a crosshatching technique in order to achieve a uniform volume expansion along the flat plane of the nasal sidewall.
- Restylane is the preferred product to use under the thin skin of the nasal sidewall.

57A.7.3 Nasal Tip and Ala

- Small amounts of hyaluronic acid, postinjection massage, and 15-minute delay before reinjection also apply here.
- The nasal tip skin must be treated with conservative volumes and skin perfusion should be assessed constantly to avoid potentially disastrous sequelae of nasal tip skin compromise.
- Some injectors prefer Juvederm for treatment of the nasal tip and ala because of its malleability several days after injection.
- Considering the aesthetically sensitive contours of the nasal tip and ala, the ability to mold Juvederm after injection proves to be a benefit for the patient and surgeon.
- One should inject via a serial puncture technique to maximize precision and accuracy along this aesthetically critical area.
- Small volumes of hyaluronic acid in the range of 0.1 to 0.2 mL can result in significant contour improvement in the nasal tip.

57A.8 Case Example

Anteroposterior views of a 39-year-old woman before and immediately after (above) nasal filler injection. (Middle, bottom) Preinjection and immediate postinjection lateral views are shown (▶ Fig. 57A.5a–c).

57A.9 Conclusion

Accurate preoperative systematic nasal analysis and evaluation of the nasal airway is crucial for injection success. The surgeon's goals and patient's expectations must be aligned. A complete understanding of the anatomy and key differences between individual product properties will enable selection of appropriate soft-tissue nasal fillers.

See **Video 57A.1**.

Further Readings

Humphrey CD, Arkins JP, Dayan SH. Soft tissue fillers in the nose. Aesthet Surg J. 2009; 29(6):477–484

Kurkjian TJ, Ahmad J, Rohrich RJ. Soft-tissue fillers in rhinoplasty. Plast Reconstr Surg. 2014; 133(2):121e–126e

Rohrich RJ, Ghavami A, Crosby MA. The role of hyaluronic acid fillers (Restylane) in facial cosmetic surgery: review and technical considerations. Plast Reconstr Surg. 2007; 120(6) Suppl:41S–54S

Rohrich RJ, Villanueva NL, Small KH, Pezeshk RA. Implications of facial asymmetry in rhinoplasty. Plast Reconstr Surg. 2017; 140(3):510–516

Villanueva NL, Afrooz PN, Carboy JA, Rohrich RJ. Nasal analysis: considerations for ethnic variation. Plast Reconstr Surg. 2019; 143(6):1179e–1188e

57 Part B: Filler Finesse: Nose

Lara Devgan, Annette K. Kaminaka, and Elizabeth Klein

Abstract

Nonsurgical rhinoplasty can be performed to provide lasting structural and aesthetic changes to the nose. When performed with precise measurement, marking, and injection technique, it is an effective and predictable alternative to surgical rhinoplasty. Nonsurgical rhinoplasties are nonreductive, relying on a change in light and shadows on the nose, rather than a reduction or reshaping of bones or cartilage. As it is not possible to perform narrowing maneuvers, the procedure may be less suitable for wide, overprojected, or very large noses. Results are temporary, lasting 1 to 2 years. Deep periosteal and perichondrial injection in an avascular tissue plane is the safest approach to avoid rare, though serious, vascular complications, including tissue necrosis and permanent blindness.

Keywords: Nonsurgical rhinoplasty, hyaluronic acid, rhinoplasty, filler, injectables, facial optimization

Key Points

- Nonsurgical rhinoplasty is an effective and predictable alternative to surgical rhinoplasty for improving nasal contour in a nonreductive manner.
- Deep periosteal and perichondrial injection in the midline is the safest approach to avoid vascular complications.

57B.1 Preoperative Steps

57B.1.1 Analysis

- A thorough analysis of anatomy, including radix height, dorsal profile alignment, nasofrontal angle, nasolabial angle, ideal tip position, slant of central axis of the nose, dorsal nasal aesthetic lines, tip-defining points, skin thickness, and presence or absence of prior surgical scars. Analysis of front view, profile view, base view, and internal nasal examination are performed on all patients.
- Risk factors for vascular compromise, including prior surgical rhinoplasty, presence of transcolumellar or subnasal scars, medical history, and history of smoking, vaping, or drug use, should be considered.
- Thorough understanding of a patient's goals and expectations is important, as nonsurgical rhinoplasty has significant limitations: it is additive rather than reductive, it is temporary, and it is not possible to perform narrowing maneuvers such as alar base reduction, tip suspension, or cartilage struts.
- A detailed informed consent discussion, including risks of rare but catastrophic complications such as vascular compromise, tissue necrosis, and permanent blindness, must be performed.

57B.2 Operative Steps

See **Video 57B.1**.

57B.2.1 Preparation

- Topical numbing and sterilization of the nose are performed.
- A high viscosity, high density, high G′ hyaluronic acid filler is prepared. Prior to any hyaluronic acid filler injection, a full complement of emergency supplies, including 20,000 IU of hyaluronidase, nitropaste, aspirin, hot compresses, and an on-call ophthalmologist prepared to perform retrobulbar injection, must be secured.

57B.2.2 Injection Technique

- Upon needle entry, aspiration of the syringe is performed to assess for safety of the intended augmentation site.
- Filler is injected deeply and in the midline using a microdroplet injection technique, injecting on withdrawal of the needle and continuously moving to mitigate concerns about intravascular injection.
- Injection is carried out in the avascular tissue plane immediately overlying the periosteum or perichondrium.
- Injection is carried out deep and in the midline of the nose for highest likelihood of avoiding the variant and complex vasculature of the nose.
- In performing nonsurgical rhinoplasty, I think of the injectable filler as if it were a surgical cartilage graft, using the lifting vector of the filler to perform a tip flip or elevation of the nasolabial angle.

57B.2.3 Dorsal Straightening

- To create the illusion of a straightened dorsum, injection may need to be performed in the radix, as well as below a dorsal hump.
- Raising the height of the supratip break will create a straighter appearing nose, but will also lengthen the appearance of the nose. Mitigating straightness with perceived tip angle relies on the injector's aesthetic judgment.
- When straightening the dorsum, it is important not to overbuild the nose, lest the injector creates a bulky or leonine appearance of the nose.

57B.2.4 Tip Refinement

- To create the appearance of a more delicate nasal tip, I inject filler laterally, over the domes of the lower lateral cartilages, immediately above the perichondrium.
- I visualize the filler as if it were a liquid shield graft in order to conceptualize the placement of product for the most desirable aesthetic appearance of the nose.
- It is important to inject the nasal tip judiciously, not only in order to avoid vascular compromise and nasal tip necrosis, but also to avoid making the nasal tip appear more bulbous or bulky.

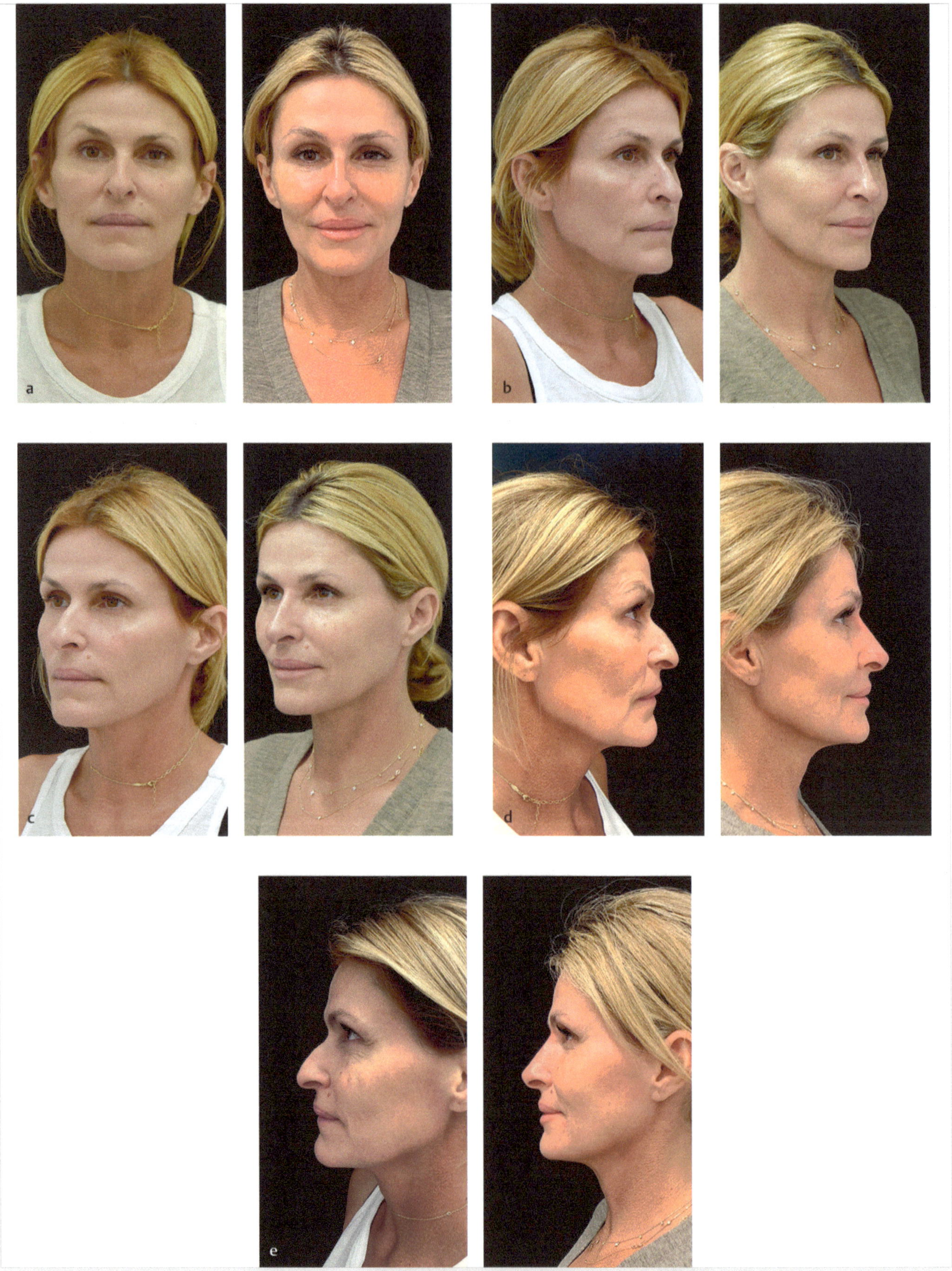

Fig. 57B.1 (a–e) This is a 50-year-old woman who desired nonsurgical improvement of the contour of her nose, with specific reference to her dorsal hump, bulbous nasal tip, and acute nasolabial angle. After consultation and analysis, I performed nonsurgical rhinoplasty using hyaluronic acid based filler to soften her deep radix, straighten her dorsum, elevate her nasal tip, and add definition to her tip-defining points. The patient was very satisfied with her outcome.

57B.2.5 Correction of Asymmetry

- Filler may be injected off-midline to create a feeling of improved symmetry in some cases, but surgical judgment is needed to assess the safety of this maneuver on a case by case basis.

57B.2.6 Correction of Postsurgical Nasal Deformities

- Alar notching, pollybeak deformity, pinched tip, saddle nose, and irregularity of the contour of the nose may all be addressed using these guiding principles.
- Risks are greater in postsurgical noses due to compromised blood supply and the presence of scar tissue.

57B.3 Postoperative Care

- Patients are instructed to avoid alcohol and other blood thinners for several days before and after any injectable procedure.
- Avoidance of strenuous activity for 1 day and head elevation are recommended.
- Avoidance of direct pressure on the nose, such as with heavy eyeglasses or sleeping face down, is advised.
- Cold compresses are possible, but they may promote deformation of carefully placed filler, and are not routinely recommended for this procedure in my practice.
- Filler may last 6 months to 2 years, depending on the amount and type of product used, as well as the patient's metabolic rate and anatomic characteristics. Patients are advised to follow-up when they notice filler regression, but prior to complete dissolution of product. Subsequent sessions of filler have been noted to last longer than the initial sessions, and can also achieve more dramatic results, perhaps owing to the pre-existing lattice of tissue support from the initial session.

57B.4 Case Example

This is a 50-year-old woman who desired nonsurgical improvement of the contour of her nose, with specific reference to her dorsal hump, bulbous nasal tip, and acute nasolabial angle. After consultation and analysis, I performed nonsurgical rhinoplasty using hyaluronic acid based filler to soften her deep radix, straighten her dorsum, elevate her nasal tip, and add definition to her tip-defining points. The patient was very satisfied with her outcome (▶ Fig. 57B.1a–e).

57B.5 Conclusion

Nonsurgical rhinoplasty is a predictable and effective alternative to surgical rhinoplasty for many patients. Nonsurgical rhinoplasty relies on a change in light and shadows on the nose, rather than a reduction or reshaping of bone or cartilage, so it may be less suitable for wide, overprojected, or very large noses. Deep perichondrial and periosteal injection in an avascular tissue plane in the midline of the nose is the safest way to avoid vascular compromise.

Further Readings

Bray D, Hopkins C, Roberts DN. Injection rhinoplasty: non-surgical nasal augmentation and correction of post-rhinoplasty contour asymmetries with hyaluronic acid: how we do it. Clin Otolaryngol. 2010; 35(3):227–230

Humphrey CD, Arkins JP, Dayan SH. Soft tissue fillers in the nose. Aesthet Surg J. 2009; 29(6):477–484

Jasin ME. Nonsurgical rhinoplasty using dermal fillers. Facial Plast Surg Clin North Am. 2013; 21(2):241–252

Kim DW, Yoon ES, Ji YH, Park SH, Lee BI, Dhong ES. Vascular complications of hyaluronic acid fillers and the role of hyaluronidase in management. J Plast Reconstr Aesthet Surg. 2011; 64(12):1590–1595

58 Filler Finesse: Upper Eyelid Sulcus

Val Lambros

Abstract

In many patients the superior orbital rim and brow deflate with age, and it makes sense to fill the area to regain the sense of a young eye. To show the patient the effect of the procedure, the area is filled with local anesthetic before injection.

Keywords: Orbit hollowing, HA fillers, orbital and brow injections, aging eyes, local anesthetic preview, facial harmony, eye lifts

Key Points

- In youth the periorbital area is characterized by abundant subcutaneous tissue with elastic overlying skin. Young upper eyelids are long and full. With time, the soft tissues of the eyebrow and orbit may thin and hollow, the orbital rim becomes apparent, and the eye looks shorter, rounder, and gaunt.
- This latter contour is often seen after upper eyelid surgery. Though orbits like these can appear highly defined and dramatic with considerable acreage for makeup, they can also make the eye and face look older in general.
- In some people, reinflation of the brow and superior orbit looks better.
- This is a visual concept, which is not intuitive for many patients; simply describing it does not let a patient understand how treatment will appear.
- My practice for decades has been to "preview" the effect of the treatment by injecting the brows with dilute local anesthetic to duplicate the effect of the filler.
- Patients uniformly like this idea. Just like trying clothes on before buying, patients can see and understand the desired result before actually doing a potentially expensive procedure, which they might not like. It lets the patient make the most informed decision possible. In addition, the injector can look at the preview and decide whether and where to modify the injection for maximum benefit. The patient is now numb from the anesthetic and vasoconstricted as well.
- Placing the local anesthetic precisely is more difficult than the injection of the product. It is easy to make blobs in the skin. Doing the previews makes the clinician a better injector.

58.1 Injection

- As can be seen in ▶ Fig. 58.1, the brow region contains numerous large arteries. As can also be seen, the arteries course deep to the orbicularis and frontalis at the level of the brow. The key to filling the brow safely is to inject precisely into the subcutaneous brow fat pad, an area clearly absent of vessels as pictured.
- This is analogous to other parts of the face such as the lips, nose, or glabellar frown lines, where the location of the arteries is known and avoided. The "local preview" not only vasoconstricts the area, but by expanding the volume of the brow region, gives the injector a larger target volume for needle placement adding to safety. I believe (but cannot prove) that injecting HA filler into an area which has been expanded with saline leads to better diffusion of product and more even distribution. This injection has been remarkable smooth perhaps because of this effect.
- This is not an injection for beginners; the injector needs to have the ability to confine the depth of the needle to the subcutaneous plane. It is probably not suited for bolus injection and finger smoothing. I believe that linear injections work best. The injection should be as smooth as possible before using some finger pressure to finalize the distribution evenly.
- For cost reasons, the typical injection is usually ½ cc of product per side. This amount may underdo some brows, but will improve all the correctly chosen patients. I prefer particulate HA products.
- The injection of product is done immediately after the patients approves the preview.
  - Product placement is partly visual, which is apparent through the local anesthetic and partly tactile. I prefer to use a 30g ½ inch needle to inject across the brow.
- Cannulas may be used, but they are whippier than needles. In some orbits the globe sits immediately adjacent to the superior orbital rim and could be injured. The curvature of the brow is difficult to follow with a cannula.
- With this technique the amount of filler per pass is tiny, about 3 hundredths of a cc per pass. Perhaps most importantly the needle is always kept moving.
  - Starting laterally, for each entrance of the needle, superiorly, neutral, and inferiorly slanted passes are made. The injections then march across the brow in the subcutaneous plane. The injections are kept at or above the inferior margin of the superior orbital rim except for a small amount medially.
- In the soft tissue of the medial orbit, tiny injections are made to fill the delicate curves there. A needle offers considerably more precision in this location than a cannula. Tiny passes of product are used in the subcutaneous space.
- Intra-arterial injection of product, though very rare, should always in the back of one's mind.
- As would be expected a needle produces more bruising in the brow than a cannula would be expected to. This is discussed with the patients beforehand. For this procedure, I think more precision is worth the bruising.
- In some patients, a small amount of lax eyelid skin may be filled and expanded. There may be some real or apparent elevation of the brow. Since the primary function of brow filling is expansion of the skin, if the injector attempts to elevate the

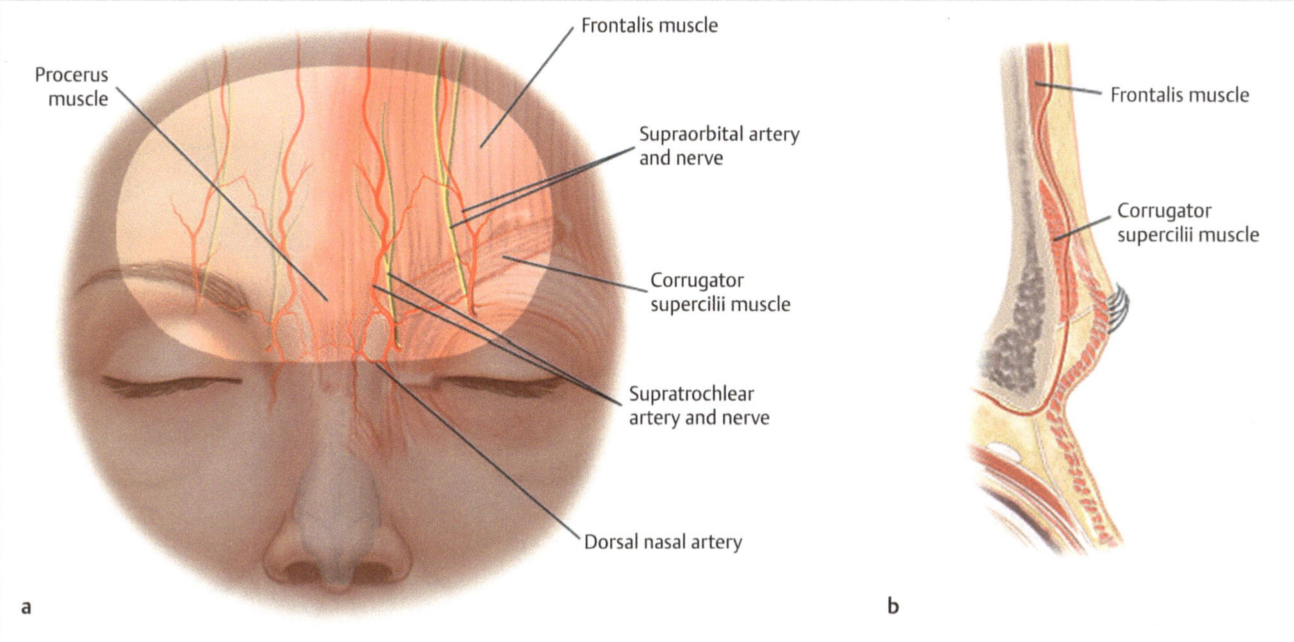

Fig. 58.1 (a) Diagram showing the mimetic muscles in the glabellar and forehead region. The corrugator supercilii muscle is responsible for vertical and oblique glabellar frown lines. The procerus muscle is responsible for transverse dorsal nasal rhytides. The frontalis muscle is responsible for transverse forehead rhytides. **(b)** Cross section demonstrating the deep-to-superficial path of the supratrochlear and supraorbital artery as it exits the supraorbital rim.

brows or fill in a large amount of extra upper lid skin, the brows will likely appear unnaturally large.

- There are many patients who, from age or excisional eyelid surgery look quite hollow (the "nursing home eye") and are not candidates for further traditional surgery. Also, there are patients who exhibit flat non-projecting negative vector superior orbital rims. Both these groups have the potential for very attractive improvement from brow filling and consequent visual shrinking of a large depleted orbit.
- Some of the best lid results I have seen have been in patients who had some brow fill and a small removal of eyelid fat and skin.

58.2 Postoperative Care

- Ice is really all that is done for the first day. Most patients have some bruising initially, with the final result becoming visible in a week or two.
- Since patients who had the local anesthetic preview know what results to expect from the injection, unhappiness with the procedure is distinctly uncommon. Minor touch-ups are sometimes necessary and hyaluronidase in small doses will fix small irregularities. The brows are usually slightly underdone with this amount of product but patients infrequently want more.
- Duration of particulate HA fillers in this location is upwards of 2 years; 3 years is common.

58.3 Case Example

A 60-year-old female before and 2 years post HA injection of brows. On each side, 1.2 cc was used. This is an interesting configuration. The sloping, medially elevated hollow of the superior orbit imparts a look of anxiety or worry in these patients, perhaps because it resembles an elevated medial brow, which also projects these emotions. Making the medial orbit flatter reduces the emotional projection (▶ Fig. 58.3a, b).

58.4 Conclusions

In the carefully selected and prepared patients, brow (and temple) filling can make the patients look considerably better than before. This procedure is particularly useful for patients with age deflation or after excisional surgery of the upper orbit. The results can last for 2 to 4 years.

See **Video 58.1**.

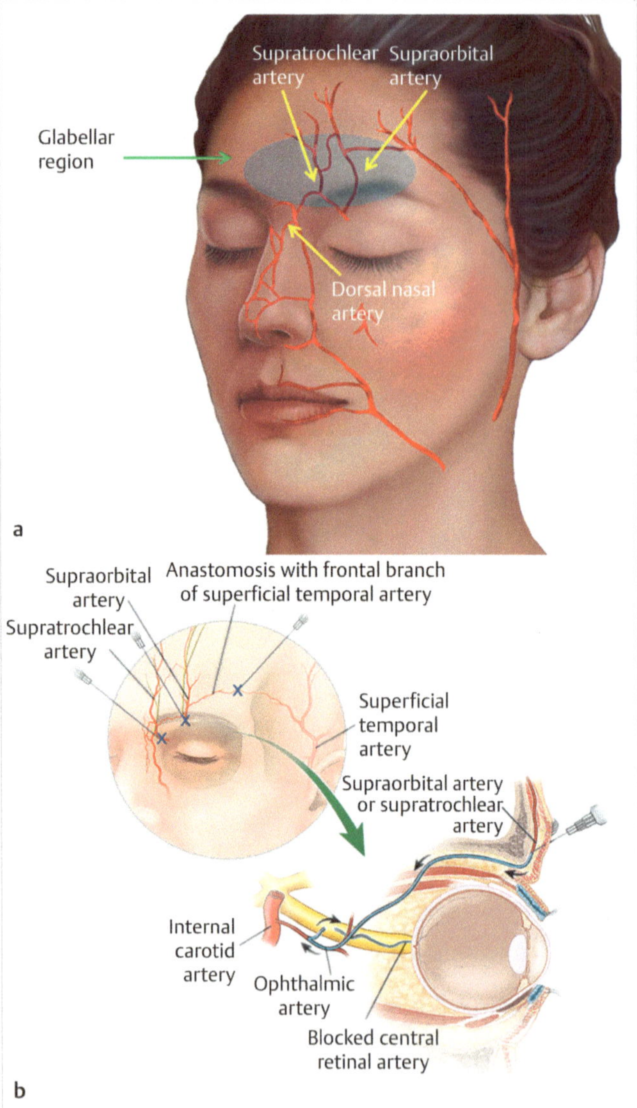

Fig. 58.2 **(a)** Rich anastomoses between the supratrochlear, supraorbital, and dorsal nasal arteries in the glabellar region create potential routes for retrograde embolization to the ophthalmic artery. **(b)** Inadvertent intravascular injection into the supraorbital or supratrochlear artery can create retrograde propagation of foreign material into the ophthalmic artery. Subsequent distal embolism from the ophthalmic artery into the central retinal artery can cause vision loss. (Reproduced with permission from Rohrich R, Stuzin J, Dayan E, et al, eds. Facial Danger Zones: Staying Safe with Surgery, Fillers and Non-invasive Devices. 1st ed. Thieme; 2019.)

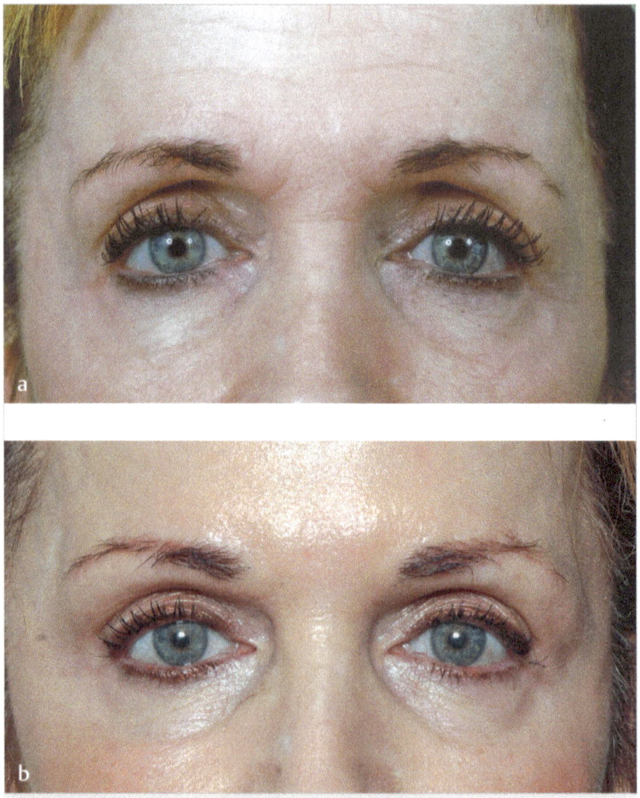

Fig. 58.3 A 60-year-old female **(a)** before and **(b)** 2 years post hyaluronic acid (HA) injection of brows, 1.2 cc per side. This is an interesting configuration. The sloping, medially elevated hollow of the superior orbit imparts a look of anxiety or worry in these patients, perhaps because it resembles an elevated medial brow, which also projects these emotions. Making the medial orbit more flat reduces the emotional projection.

Further Readings

Coleman SR. Structural fat grafting. St. Louis, MO: Quality Medical Publishing; 2004

Costa CR, Kordestani R, Small KH, Rohrich RJ. Advances and refinement in hyaluronic acid facial fillers. Plast Reconstr Surg. 2016; 138(2):233e–236e

Lambros V. Volumizing the brow with hyaluronic acid fillers. Aesthet Surg J. 2009; 29(3):174–179

Lambros VS. Fat injection for the aging midface. Oper Tech Plast Reconstr Surg. 1998; 5:129–137

Sykes JM, Cotofana S, Trevidic P, et al. Upper face: clinical anatomy and regional approaches with injectable fillers. Plast Reconstr Surg. 2015; 136 Suppl: 204S–218S

59 Filler Finesse: Hands—The Role of Hyaluronic Acid, Calcium Hydroxyapatite, and Autologous Fat

Heidi A. Waldorf, Anup Patel, and Rod J. Rohrich

Abstract

As minimally invasive rejuvenation of the face has become commonplace, awareness of other aging anatomical areas has increased. The discrepancy between a youthful appearing face and aged appearing hands is a particular concern since hands, unlike other parts of the body, are visible in almost all circumstances. Resurfacing techniques, from chemical peels to lasers, can improve skin color and texture, but fail to address contour. In recent years, the injection of autologous fat and off-the-shelf dermal filling agents have become standard of care to restore volume loss. This chapter reviews best practices for hand rejuvenation including how to navigate the complex hand anatomy to provide safe and effective results.

Keywords: Hand, filler, hyaluronic acid, fat, collagen, rejuvenation, calcium hydroxyapatite, hand anatomy

Key Points

- Similar to the face, hand aging is a result of intrinsic and extrinsic factors. However, the tendency for even the aesthetically oriented to ignore hand care and protection means that age tends to show on the hands sooner.
- Intrinsic aging consists of atrophy of the skin dermis, muscles, and subcutaneous fat. Extrinsic aging from photoaging and the use of the hands for activities of daily living like exposure to water, cleansers, and extreme temperatures speed changes in skin texture, density, and color. Thus, aged hands are characterized by lax, wrinkled, and heterogeneously pigmented skin covering hollow dorsal web spaces, prominent bones, tendons, and veins. In addition to discoloration from photoaging, visible veins can produce a blue hue.
- Restoration of a smooth appearing hand requires a combined approach to improve the skin surface and contour. Techniques used include improvement of texture and color utilizing cryosurgery, chemical peels, and energy-based devices. Restoration of a youthful smooth contour include the injection of fat, fillers, biostimulators, and in select cases sclerotherapy to reduce the appearance of prominent vessels.
- The first filler to gain Food and Drug Administration (FDA) approval for hand rejuvenation was Radiesse, calcium hydroxyapatite (Merz, Frankfurt, Germany), in 2015. Calcium hydroxyapatite provides long-term improvement in contour and its opaque nature acts to camouflage prominent veins. Restylane Lyft (Galderma, Texas) became the first hyaluronic acid gel filler approved by FDA for age-related volume loss of the hands in 2018. As a hyaluronic acid, Restylane Lyft can be reversed.

59.1 Pertinent Anatomy (▶ Fig. 59.1)

- Bidic et al described the anatomy of the hand in distinct layers transitioning from superficial to deep: skin, dorsal superficial lamina, dorsal superficial fascia, dorsal intermediate lamina, dorsal intermediate fascia, dorsal deep lamina, and dorsal deep fascia.
- The dorsal superficial lamina is a fatty layer deep to the skin, which lacks sensory nerves and major veins, making it a desirable plane for injections.

59.2 Technique

See **Video 59.1** and **Video 59.2**.

59.2.1 Antiseptic Preparation

- Wipe fingers, web spaces, and dorsal hands and wrists with ChloraPrepTM (70% isopropyl alcohol/3.15% chlorhexidine gluconate) or 70% alcohol followed by LasercynTM Dermal Spray (sodium chloride, sodium sulfate, monobasic sodium phosphate, hypochlorous acid [0.009%], water).

59.2.2 Anesthesia

- Although topical anesthesia with a lidocaine preparation may be used, it is generally not necessary. When using a cannula for injection, small intradermal blebs of 1% lidocaine without epinephrine are placed at the planned insertion sites.

59.2.3 Injection Technique

- When utilizing a disposable blunt tipped cannula, the approach may be distal or proximal. The most common protocols are use of two or three insertion sites between dorsal web spaces or a single insertion site at the junction of the hand and the wrist. Cannula size of 25 gauge, 50 mm or 22 gauge, 70 mm is appropriate and can be passed easily above critical structures.
- When using a needle, filler can be placed via micropuncture of multiple dorsal injections of 0.05 to 0.1 cc, four small bolus injections of 0.2 to 0.5 cc, a single bolus centrally, or by linear threading. Injection is performed by tenting the skin and injecting the filler perpendicular to the skin for bolus technique or parallel for threading technique.

59.2.4 Filling Agent

- Hyaluronic acid does not require specific preparation and can be used out of the box. Alternatively, it may be used off-label, blended with saline for improved malleability or calcium hydroxyapatite to produce opacity.

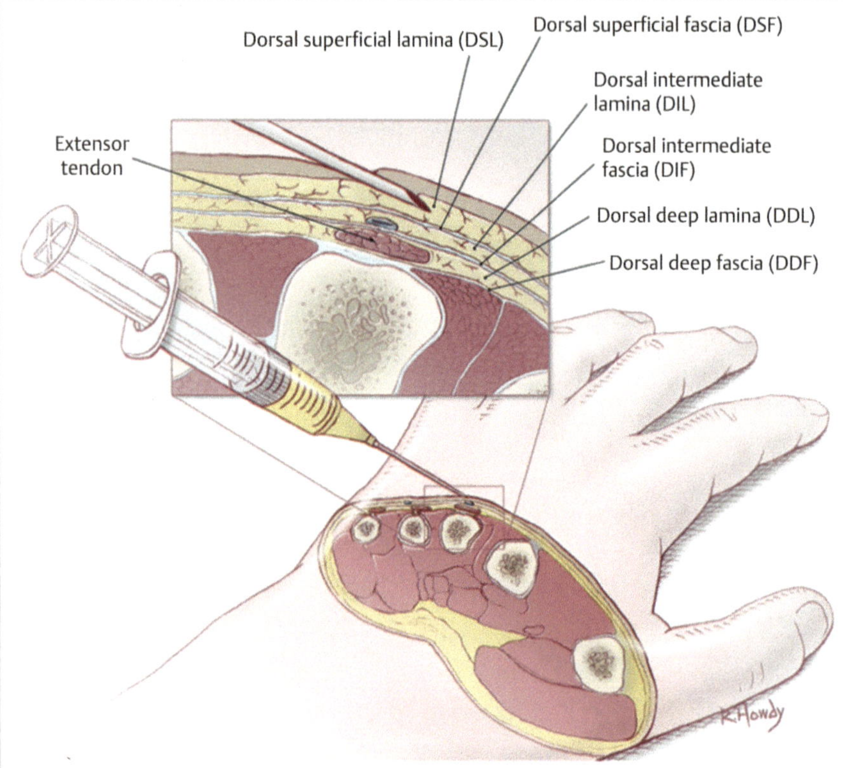

Fig. 59.1 The critical hand anatomy relevant for safe hand rejuvenation.

- Although the on-label indication for calcium hydroxyapatite for hand describes blending 1.5 mL of calcium hydroxyapatite with 0.3 cc of 1% lidocaine, standard usage is a 1:1 dilution of calcium hydroxyapatite with a combination of 1% lidocaine and saline.
- Fat should be harvested from the inner thigh. It must be centrifuged for 1 minute prior to reinjection into the superficial planes of the hand (20–30 cc per side).
- Regardless of the instrument and filling agent used, proper placement in the dorsal superficial and dorsal intermediate layer is important to avoid the dorsal deep layer, veins, and tendons. It is also critical to add filler or fat gradually and reassess both hands during treatment. Massage of the treatment areas between injections is helpful to evaluate progress.
- Once symmetry is achieved, the dorsal hands may be massaged with ultrasound gel, glycerin serum, or other lubricant across the dorsal hands to create a smooth contour. Treatment may be completed in one session as long as hand function is not compromised. It should be noted that patients with smaller hands and/or slimmer wrists may still complain of enough edema and discomfort to limit their activity. Splitting the treatment into two sessions, 2 to 4 weeks apart, is an option that provides gradual improvement without edema or discomfort.
- A vinyl glove without fingers can be slipped over each hand and an ice pack slipped underneath.

59.3 Postinjection Instructions

- After calcium hydroxyapatite injection, your physician may ask you to gently massage the tops of your hands for several minutes a day (3 minutes, three times a day for 3 days).
- To reduce bruising and swelling, patients should avoid all anticoagulants not prescribed by a physician including alcohol, aspirin, nonsteroidal anti-inflammatory drugs (NSAIDs), vitamin E, supplements containing fish oil, St John's wort, gingko, ginseng, and garlic at least 7 to 10 days prior to and for 3 to 5 days following treatment. No medication should be stopped without the express consent of the prescribing physician.
- To reduce swelling, it is helpful to apply covered ice packs to the treated areas 10 to 20 minutes per hour while awake for up to first 48 hours. Ice packs may be held in place with vinyl or cotton gloves to allow function.
- Avoid activities that put pressure or increase blood flow to the hands and arms for 1 week.
- For 2 weeks before and after injection, avoid laser and skin treatments of the hands and fingers unless expressly approved by the injecting physician.
- Do not get a manicure for 2 weeks after filler injection.
- Filler injection of the hands is not recommended for patients who have had significant lymph node dissection or have lymphedema of that extremity.

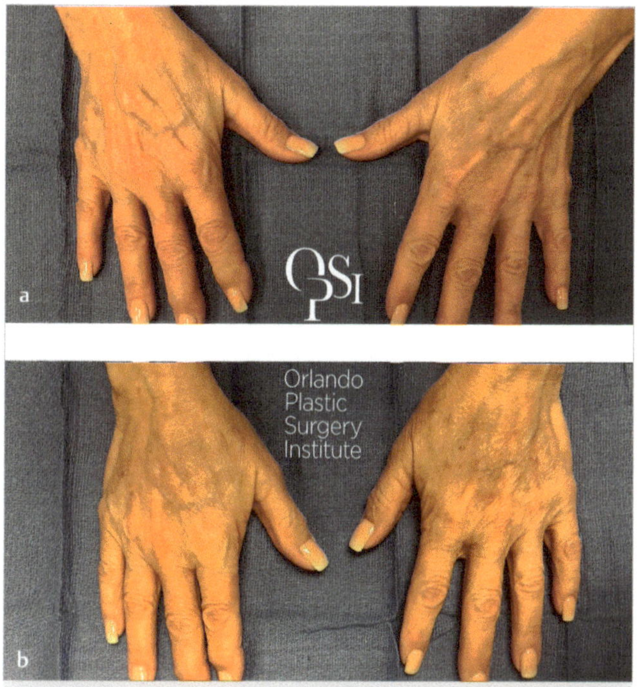

Fig. 59.2 A 60-year-old female presents for hand rejuvenation using hyaluronic acid. **(a)** Preinjection and **(b)** postinjection with Restylane Lyft at 3 months.

- Airplane travel within 2 weeks after filler injection of the hands may cause prolonged and excessive swelling and is not recommended.
- Follow-up at 2 to 3 weeks for any additional treatment. The next follow-up is generally at 4 to 6 months following filler injection.
- The patient should notify the office immediately if any of the following occurs:
  - Fever and/or chills.
  - The treatment area appears red, hot to touch, or "angry" looking.
  - The skin at the injection site or surrounding area develops blisters, scabs, or discolored blotches, or appears pale.
  - Severe or increasing pain or swelling of the extremity.
  - Difficulty moving your hand or fingers.

59.4 Case Example

A 60-year-old female presented for hand rejuvenation using hyaluronic acid. Preinjection and postinjection with Restylane Lyft at 3 months (▶ Fig. 59.2).

59.5 Conclusion

Although facial rejuvenation has become commonplace, treatment of aged hands remains less ubiquitous. Yet, recent FDA approval of two dermal fillers for volume restoration of hands has increased public awareness leading to an increase in demand for hand rejuvenation.

To avoid permanent or temporary disruption of hand function, the injector must have an understanding of the available filling agents, injection tools, and hand anatomy.

This chapter and its associated videos describe standardized filling protocols for the FDA-approved filling agents, calcium hydroxyapatite and hyaluronic acid, and autologous fat. Single and multiple entry, cannula and needle techniques are outlined.

Like their use in the face, fillers and fat in the hands recreate a more youthful contour and are an integral part of combination therapy for hand rejuvenation.

Further Readings

Bidic SM, Hatef DA, Rohrich RJ. Dorsal hand anatomy relevant to volumetric rejuvenation. Plast Reconstr Surg. 2010; 126(1):163–168

Graivier MH, Lorenc ZP, Bass LM, Fitzgerald R, Goldberg DJ. Calcium hydroxyapatite (CaHA) indication for hand rejuvenation. Aesthet Surg J. 2018; 38(1) suppl_1: S24–S28

Hoang D, Orgel MI, Kulber DA. Hand rejuvenation: a comprehensive review of fat grafting. J Hand Surg Am. 2016; 41(5):639–644

Khosravani N, Weber L, Patel R, Patel A. The 5-step filler hand rejuvenation: filling with hyaluronic acid. Plast Reconstr Surg Glob Open. 2019; 7(1):e2073

Riyaz FR, Ozog D. Hand rejuvenation. Semin Cutan Med Surg. 2015; 34(3):147–152

Part IX

Facial Resurfacing

IX

60 Trichloroacetic Acid Peel

Rod J. Rohrich and Erez Dayan

Abstract

Trichloroacetic acid (TCA) is a versatile agent, efficacious in treating a spectrum of facial rhytides and dyschromias at varying concentrations. TCA is commonly used in a 30 to 35% concentration to achieve a medium-depth peel into the upper reticular dermis. The addition of Jessner's solution before the TCA peel application leads to partial removal of epidermis, allowing for deeper penetration of the TCA. This combination is beneficial, as lower concentrations of TCA can be used for the same depth of peel, minimizing complications such as scarring.

Keywords: Chemical peel, TCA, trichloroacetic acid, Jessner's, skin resurfacing

Key Points

- Addition of Jessner's solution to 35% trichloroacetic acid (TCA) improves quality and consistency of the peel while allowing for less TCA to be used for a given effect.
- Preprocedure skin prep is important to avoid complications and optimize results.
- Always ring out gauze or cotton-tip applicators with TCA on it to prevent adverse events.
- Number of passes and pressure are both related to depth of peel.
- Continuously assess color changes to determine depth and efficacy of peel.

60.1 Preoperative Steps

- Consultation with the patient should be used to establish realistic goals and expectations as well as to educate the patient on important perioperative care instructions for optimal results. A careful history and physical examination allow the clinician to determine the patients' candidacy (▶ Table 60.1).
- Our preference is to pretreat all patients for 4 to 6 weeks before chemical peeling. This regimen includes topical tretinoin (0.05–0.1%), hydroquinone (2–4%), sunscreen, and alpha hydroxyl acid (4–10%). Pretreatment improves skin tolerance, regulates fibroblast and melanocyte function, improves dermal circulation, and allows for the treated skin to heal 3 to 4 days faster due to increased cellular division and new collagen formation. Modifications to this preprocedure regimen (dosages and application intervals) are made as needed based on tolerance and skin types. A week before peel, patients are started on a cleansing and toning protocol and are encouraged to maintain adequate hydration and moisture of the skin.
- Acyclovir is initiated 2 days before chemical peel and continued 5 days after the peel in patients with prior history of herpetic lesions.
- Setup is clearly labeled glasses ordered from left to right in the appropriate sequence of usage. The glasses are filled by the practitioner with: (1) 70% ethyl alcohol, (2) acetone, (3) Jessner's solution, and (4) 35% TCA solution.
- In our practice the Jessner's solution is premixed by a pharmacist and contains 100 mg of 95% ethanol, 14 g of resorcinol, 14 g of salicylic acid, and 14 mL of lactic acid. Also, available on this table are 2 × 2 gauze and cotton-tip applicators.

60.2 Operative Steps

- The patient's skin is anesthetized approximately 40 to 60 minutes preprocedure with topical anesthetic (lidocaine/prilocaine cream).
- The procedure begins with cleansing of the skin using a 2 × 2 gauze soaked in 70% ethyl alcohol. Next, acetone is applied in a similar manner as a degreasing agent.
- Jessner's solution is then applied after the skin is air dry to exfoliate and peel the stratum corneum of the epidermis. The depth of the Jessner's peel is controlled by the number of applications. One to four layers of Jessner's solution is applied to the face with the endpoint being uniform areas of erythema with slight areas of frost.
- After the Jessner application is complete, 35% TCA solution is applied. The application of Jessner's solution and TCA is similar, 2 × 2 gauze is saturated and wrung out to avoid any dripping. A three-finger technique is used to allow for a wide and consistent surface area to be covered. A cotton-tip applicator wrung with TCA is used to treat rhytides in the periorbital and perioral region. The skin in these areas is stretched to allow for the peel to reach the bottom of the rhytides. The wooden end of the cotton-tip applicator can be used for selective application of the peel for deeper rhytides. The margin of the area being peeled (typically mandibular border) is lightly feathered to allow for a natural and inconspicuous transition.

Table 60.1 Indications and contraindications for the use of chemical peel

Indications for chemical peel	Contraindications
Superficial or deep rhytides/photoaging	Isotretinoin therapy within last 6 months
Preneoplastic or neoplastic lesions (i.e., actinic keratosis and lentigines)	Absence of pilosebaceous units on face
Underlying skin disease (i.e., acne)	Infection or open wounds (herpes and open acne cysts)
Pigmentary dyschromias	Medium or deep resurfacing procedure within 3 to 12 months
	Recent facial surgery involving undermining
	History of therapeutic radiation exposure
	Fitzpatrick skin types IV, V, and VI

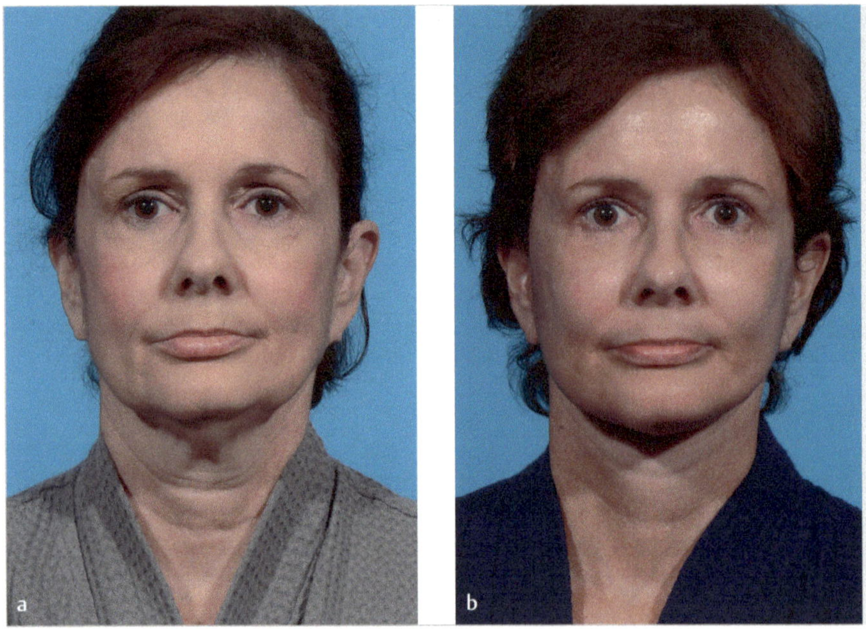

Fig. 60.1 (a, b) A 56-year-old female with notable fine and mild facial rhytides and actinic changes who underwent a lift-and-fill facelift with trichloroacetic acid (TCA) chemical peel. Chemical peel was performed at the completion of the operation following the four-step method: Alcohol, Acetone, Jessner's Solution, and TCA Peel. Postoperative images show the improvement in the patient's fine rhytides, skin tone, and dyschromias.

60.3 Postoperative Care

- Once the peel is complete a thin layer of Bactroban ointment is applied to the treatment areas.
- The patients are instructed not to moisturize the area, as this will impede desired sloughing.
- Typically, 7 to 10 days are needed for skin to slough and re-epithelialize. Dermal regeneration takes up to 6 weeks. Patients may wash their faces daily without scrubbing for the first 3 days. They are instructed to pat the area dry with a soft towel.
- Cold compresses and anxiolytics are used to minimize discomfort and oral narcotics may be used as needed. All patients are given 24 hours of prophylactic antibiotics. Once the skin re-epithelializes (7–10 days) the aforementioned preprocedure regimen is restarted.

60.4 Case Example

A 56-year-old female with notable fine and mild facial rhytides and actinic changes who underwent a lift-and-fill facelift with TCA chemical peel. Chemical peel was performed at the completion of the operation following the four-step method: Alcohol, Acetone, Jessner's Solution, and TCA Peel. Postoperative images show the improvement in the patient's fine rhytides, skin tone, and dyschromias (▶ Fig. 60.1a, b).

60.5 Conclusion

In select patients, combination of Jessner's solution with 35% TCA solution allows for a safe and effective resurfacing of moderate facial rhytides and dyschromias. Preprocedure and postprocedure skin care in addition to systemic application of the chemical peel optimizes results while minimizing potential complications.

See **Video 60.1**.

Further Readings

Glogau RG, Matarasso SL. Chemical peels. Trichloroacetic acid and phenol. Dermatol Clin. 1995; 13(2):263–276

Herbig K, Trussler AP, Khosla RK, Rohrich RJ. Combination Jessner's solution and trichloroacetic acid chemical peel: technique and outcomes. Plast Reconstr Surg. 2009; 124(3):955–964

Matarasso SL, Glogau RG. Chemical face peels. Dermatol Clin. 1991; 9(1):131–150

O'Connor AA, Lowe PM, Shumack S, Lim AC. Chemical peels: a review of current practice. Australas J Dermatol. 2018; 59(3):171–181

Weissler JM, Carney MJ, Carreras Tartak JA, Bensimon RH, Percec I. The evolution of chemical peeling and modern-day applications. Plast Reconstr Surg. 2017; 140(5): 920–929

61 Dermabrasion of the Face

Steven M. Levine and Daniel C. Baker

Abstract

The aging face changes in multiple facets. Although surgery is the gold standard to treat laxity and attenuation of the retaining ligaments, resurfacing techniques can address textural and other surface changes related to aging and environmental damage. Dermabrasion is one highly effective, reliable, and low-cost method to facial resurfacing. It is particularly useful for vertical perioral rhytides.

Keywords: Dermabrasion, resurfacing, perioral rhytides, aging, solar keratosis

Key Points

- The perimeter of any area being treated should be "feathered" to minimize the creation of a transition zone between dermabraded and nondermabraded tissue.
- The key to dermabrasion is to keep the skin on tension at all times.
- The endpoint of dermabrasion is a combination of pinpoint bleeding and visualization of the rhytid effacement. The ideal goal is to completely efface the targeted rhytid before dermabrading too deep and damaging the melanocytes.

61.1 Preoperative Steps

- Indications for dermabrasion are broad and can include desire to improve skin texture, reduce visible fine lines, or reduction in age spots (such as solar keratosis).
- Dermabrasion can be performed on the entire face and neck, or can be isolated to specific aesthetic units such as the glabella or perioral region (▶ Fig. 61.1).
- Dermabrasion can be performed as a stand-alone procedure or in combination with facelift and necklift.
- The primary consideration for preoperative planning is the patient's skin tone. The more pigmentation in the skin, the higher the chance for postdermabrasion complications such as postinflammatory hyperpigmentation or areas of hypopigmentation.
- Some providers choose to pretreat patients with a retinol or bleaching agent for 4 to 6 weeks prior to dermabrasion. The authors do not use pretreatment.
- It is important to elicit a history of oral herpes so that these patients can be pretreated with antiviral medication (▶ Fig. 61.2).

61.2 Operative Steps

61.2.1 Markings and Positioning

- A marker is used preoperatively to stain the fine lines which the dermabrasion is targeting (▶ Fig. 61.3).
- The patient is supine on the procedure table.
- Usually the head of bed is slightly elevated.
- The provider should be sitting for maximum stability.
- The approach can be accomplished using a variety of techniques that yield a controlled, reproducible distribution of mechanical resurfacing in the skin.

61.2.2 Mechanical Dermabrasion

- The face is cleaned with alcohol.

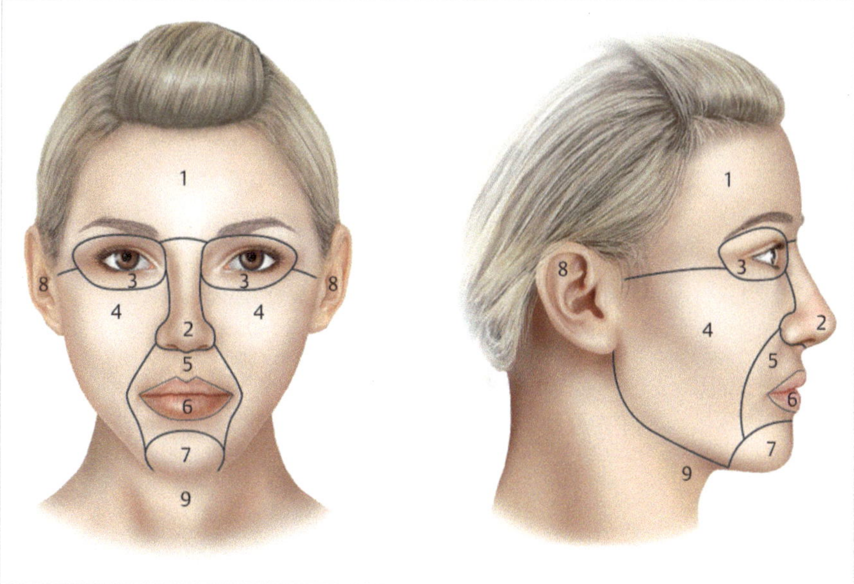

Fig. 61.1 Aesthetic units of the face. (Reproduced with permission from Rohrich R, Stuzin J, Dayan E, et al, eds. Facial Danger Zones: Staying Safe with Surgery, Fillers and Non-invasive Devices. 1st ed. Thieme; 2019.)

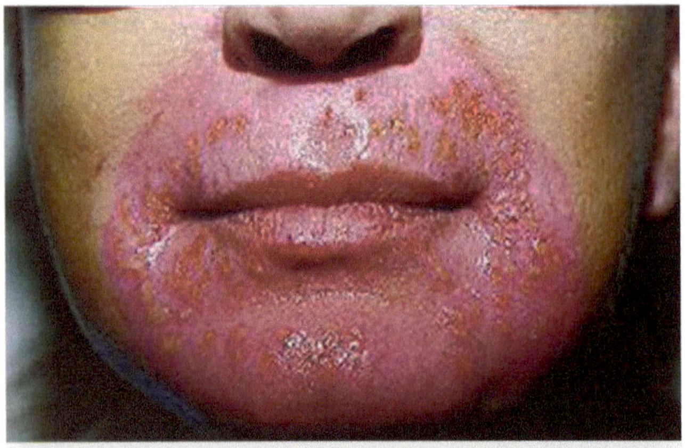

Fig. 61.2 The patient developed a herpes infection after perioral dermabrasion as preprocedure prophylaxis was not done. (Reproduced with permission from Cohen M, Thaller S, eds. The Unfavorable Result in Plastic Surgery: Avoidance and Treatment. 4th ed. Thieme; 2018.)

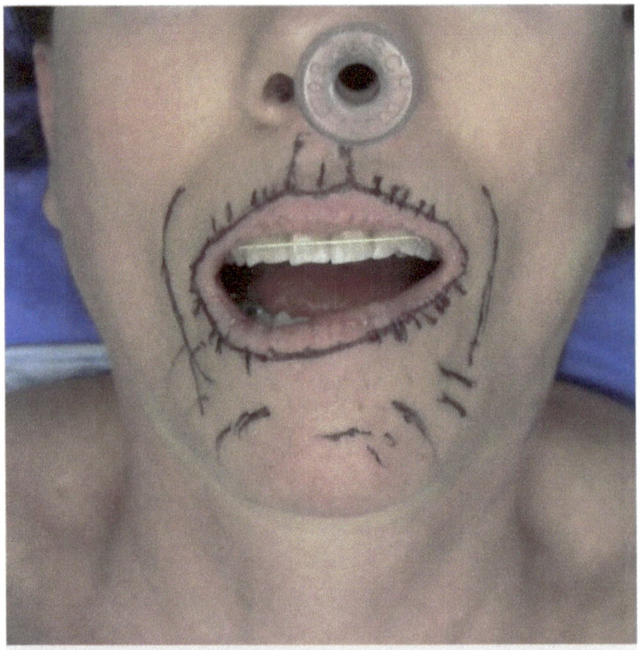

Fig. 61.3 Markings of the fine lines which the dermabrasion is targeting.

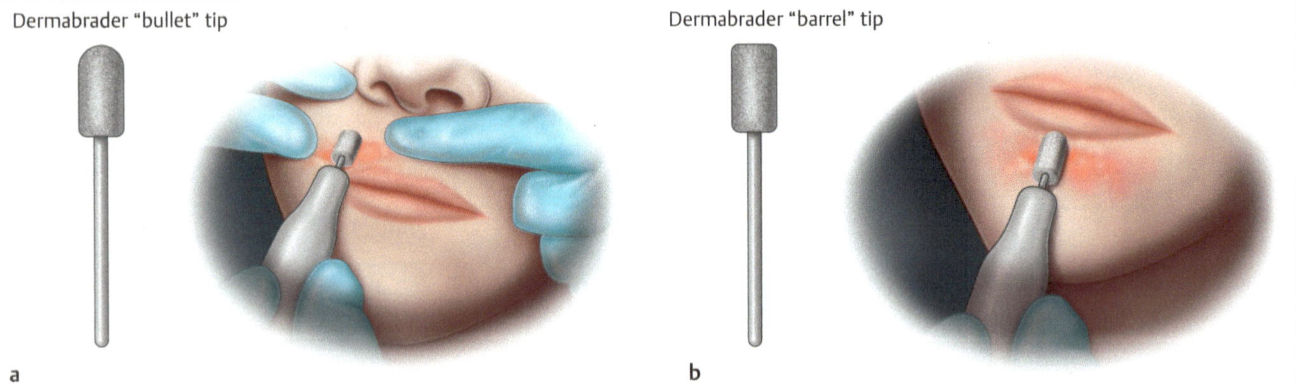

Fig. 61.4 Various dermabrasion tips can be used and include **(a)** bullet for the upper lip and **(b)** barrel for larger areas.

- A small amount (0.1 cc for entire upper lip) of 1% lidocaine with epinephrine is injected into the dermis of the areas to be dermabraded.
- Allow 8 minutes is to pass to obtain the effect of the epinephrine.
- Choose the dermabrasion tip that you feel most comfortable with in a specific area (the authors prefer the "bullet" for areas above the lip and the barrel for larger areas like below the lip) (▶ Fig. 61.4a, b).
- You can effectively dermabrade at a variety of speeds. Start slow (5,000–10,000 rpm) and advance up to 25,000 rpm.
- The key to dermabrasion is to keep the skin on tension and is accomplished with the nondominant hand. Do not attempt to dermabrade an area that is not under tension.
- The endpoint is a combination of pinpoint bleeding and visualization of the rhytid effacement. The ideal goal is to completely efface the targeted rhytid before dermabrading too deep and damaging the melanocytes.
- Keep the dermabrader moving to avoid getting too deep in any particular area.
- The perimeter of any area being treated should be carefully "feathered" to minimize the creation of a transition zone between dermabraded and nondermabraded tissue.
- Always extend the treatment beyond the zone being targeted (i.e., beneath the jaw line if treating the full face).
- It is important to be aware of the entire surgical field. Often a gauze is near the field to aid the provider in wiping blood from the operative field. This gauze can easily get caught in the dermabrader and whip around hitting the patient's face or eye.
- Overaggressive dermabrasion can damage melanocytes and lead to areas of hyperpigmentation.

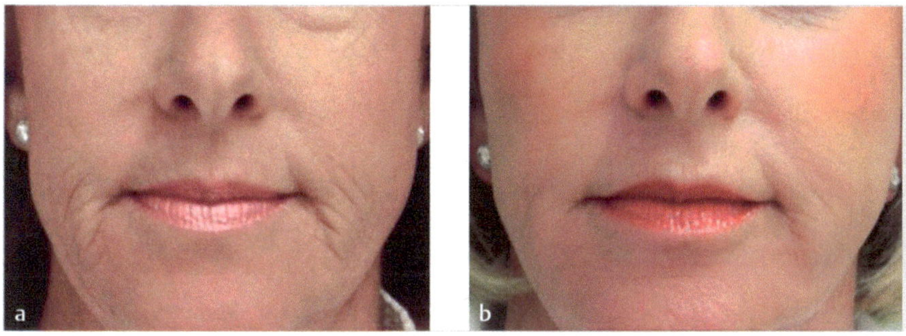

Fig. 61.5 (a, b) Pre- and postoperative photos of a patient at 2-year follow-up after facelift with autologous fat grafting, necklift, 35% trichloroacetic acid (TCA) peel, and perioral dermabrasion.

- Hyperpigmentation can occur which usually resolves on its own. Sun avoidance is paramount. Lightening agents such as topical hydroquinone 4% can be used if necessary.

61.3 Postoperative Care

- This procedure is often combined with a facelift. In this case, the dermabrasion should be performed after the facelift.
- A petroleum-impregnated gauze is applied to the dermabraded areas immediately after the procedure.
- Cool packs are also used to reduce swelling.
- Patients are instructed to use cool compresses at home for the first 24 hours.
- Patients are instructed to remain away from the sun during the acute peeling period (7–10 days postoperatively).
- Sun avoidance should ideally be carried out for several months after dermabrasion.
- Patients should keep the gauze in place for several days. As the skin re-epithializes, the gauze will fall off. When it does, patients should apply a thin layer of petroleum-based ointment three times daily until the skin is re-epithelialized.

61.4 Case Example

Pre- and postoperative photos of a patient at 2-year follow-up after facelift with autologous fat grafting, necklift, 35% trichloroacetic acid (TCA) peel, and perioral dermabrasion in anteroposterior (AP) and oblique views (▶ Fig. 61.5a, b).

61.5 Conclusion

Dermabrasion will predictably improve certain fine lines and reduce the appearance of certain superficial pigmentation issues. The provider needs to start using this technique in a metered fashion to gain comfort with expectations and limitations.

See **Video 61.1**.

Further Readings

Alkhawam L, Alam M. Dermabrasion and microdermabrasion. Facial Plast Surg. 2009; 25(5):301–310

Holmkvist KA, Rogers GS. Treatment of perioral rhytides: a comparison of dermabrasion and superpulsed carbon dioxide laser. Arch Dermatol. 2000; 136(6):725–731

Jared Christophel J, Elm C, Endrizzi BT, Hilger PA, Zelickson B. A randomized controlled trial of fractional laser therapy and dermabrasion for scar resurfacing. Dermatol Surg. 2012; 38(4):595–602

Perkins SW, Sklarew EC. Prevention of facial herpetic infections after chemical peel and dermabrasion: new treatment strategies in the prophylaxis of patients undergoing procedures of the perioral area. Plast Reconstr Surg. 1996; 98(3): 427–433, discussion 434–435

Smith JE. Dermabrasion. Facial Plast Surg. 2014; 30(1):35–39

62 Laser Resurfacing

Pooja Sodha and Paul M. Friedman

Abstract

Fractional ablative and nonablative resurfacing are effective and safe options for the treatment of rhytides, photoaging, scars, and mild laxity. Microscopic thermal zones induce epidermal and dermal remodeling, thereby creating the resurfaced effect. Preoperative evaluation of skin type, isotretinoin use, infections, prior wound healing, and melasma, among other features, is important as this may affect whether treatment should be pursued. Laser settings at time of treatment are determined by the following: the energy, the depth, the density of mircoscopic thermal zones, and the number of passes. Intraoperative skin cooling is important to prevent bulk heating of the skin. Skin of color mandates modifications in the treatment parameters, particularly treatment density. Postoperative care must be instructed in detail to patients, and patients must be diligent to maximize treatment benefits.

Keywords: Resurfacing, laser, ablative, nonablative, rhytides, scar/scarring, photoaging

Key Points

- Fractional ablative and nonablative lasers are effective and safe options for the treatment of rhytides, photoaging, scars, and mild skin laxity due to dermal remodeling as an effect of treatment.
- Nonablative wavelengths create dermal coagulative injury at depths of 1 mm or more, sparing the stratum corneum, while ablative wavelengths induce columns of ablation extending from the stratum corneum to the dermis (up to 4 mm). These noncontiguous injury sites are called microscopic thermal zones. Treatment density (coverage) is 5 to 50% with lower density utilized in darker skin types (▶ Fig. 62.1 and ▶ Fig. 62.2).
- Fractional mode technology affords the ability to treat darker skin types and higher risk anatomic sites albeit with caution.

62.1 Indications

Indications for fractional laser therapy are listed in ▶ Table 62.1.

62.2 Device Selection

- The instructions in this chapter are based on experience with the Solta Fraxel DUAL (1,550 nm/1,927 nm, Erbium/ Thulium) and Solta Fraxel Re:pair (10,600 nm, CO_2). These devices utilize intelligent optical tracking system that distributes the microscopic thermal zones evenly over several passes of the roller accounting for the practitioner's gliding speed, thus reducing risks of bulk heating. The concepts presented in this chapter may be extended cautiously to other infrared nonablative fractional lasers (1,550 nm/ 1,540 nm/1,440 nm) and ablative fractional lasers (2,790 nm/2,940 nm).

62.3 Preoperative Steps

- The facial resurfacing procedure begins with a thorough preoperative analysis to assess the severity of dermatoheliosis, distribution of rhytides, dyschromia, scarring, and overall goals of treatment and patient expectations.
- Patients with concerns about epidermal photoaging, mild rhytides, and scars (atrophic, burn, or traumatic) are good candidates for nonablative fractional resurfacing (NAFR). Younger scars respond better to laser therapy. Patients with deeper rhytides, greater laxity, traumatic scars, burn scars with contractures, and deeper acne scarring are good candidates for ablative fractional resurfacing (AFR). Patients should expect 2 weeks of downtime after AFR.
- Assessment of absolute contraindications, including active infections, pregnancy, and koebnerizing phenomena such as psoriasis and vitiligo.
- Assessment of relative contraindications, including recent tanning or sun exposure, and use of isotretinoin within the last 6 months.
- History of subtle melasma and postinflammatory hyperpigmentation should be assessed as rebound hyperpigmentation may occur after aggressive treatments (high fluence, high coverage). In this case, patients should be counseled on use of fractional nonablative lasers at low fluences and/or low coverage which may necessitate more treatments.
- To avoid pigmentary complications, recommend pretreatment with hydroquinone, retinoic acid, or topical tranexamic acid (such as SkinMedica © Lytera 2.0 or SkinCeuticals © Discoloration Defense) for 2 to 4 weeks prior and photoprotection.
- History of herpes simplex virus (HSV) should be assessed and antiviral prophylaxis should be initiated 1 day prior to treatment and continued for a total of 3 days (nonablative) and 7 days (ablative).
- In our experience, oral antibiotics (Doxycycline 100 mg twice daily started the day before treatment, total 7 days duration) are provided for all patients undergoing AFR.
- In contrast, patients with history of acne undergoing NAFR can be treated with low dose antibiotics (doxycycline 50 mg twice daily started on day of procedure, total 5 days duration) to reduce the risk of acne flare after the procedure.
- Recommend use of Alastin© Regenerating Skin Nectar as pretreatment 2 to 3 weeks prior to procedure to activate dermal remodeling cellular pathways, which will be employed during the postoperative period.
- Topical retinoids should be discontinued 5 days prior to laser treatment.
- Topical anesthesia for 60 minutes prior to procedure is recommended for NAFR (23% lidocaine/7% tetracaine for skin

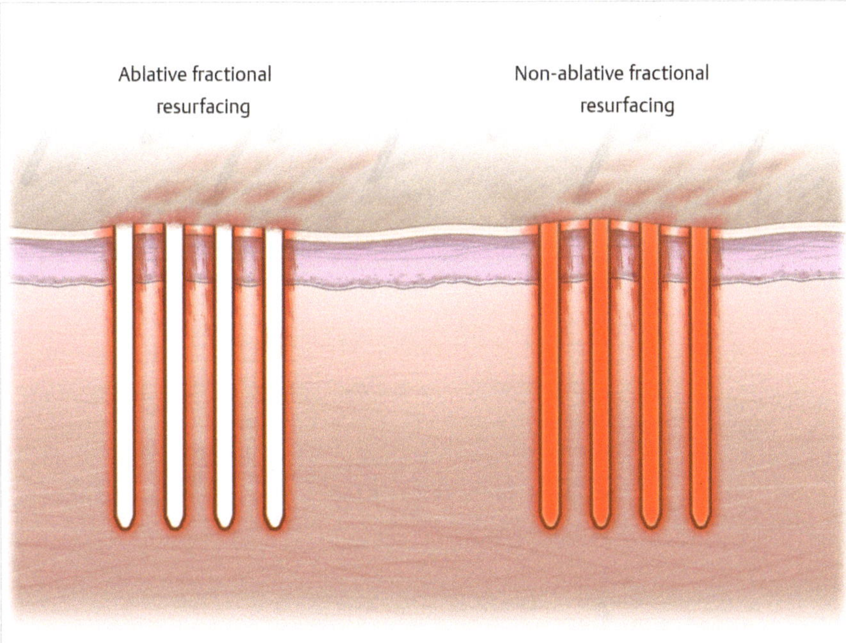

Fig. 62.1 Differences between ablative fractional resurfacing (AFR) and nonablative fractional resurfacing (NAFR).

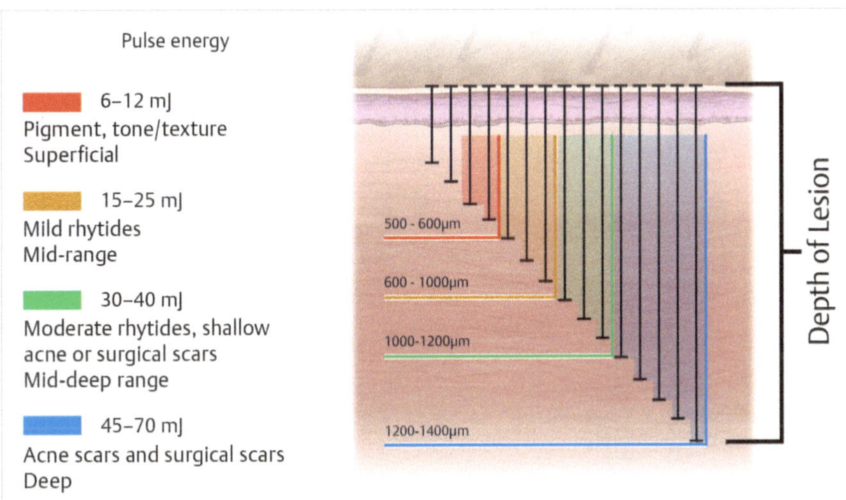

Fig. 62.2 Depth of various lesions and associated pulse energies for the 1550 nm nonablative fractional laser.

Table 62.1 Indications for fractional laser therapy

Nonablative fractional laser therapy	Ablative fractional laser therapy
Photoaging, dyschromia	Rhytides, laxity
Textural changes	Photoaging, dyschromia
Rhytides, laxity	Scars
Scarring: Atrophic, hypopigmented, hypertrophic, burn, postsurgical, mild rhinophyma	Scarring: Atrophic, burn, contractures, postsurgical, traumatic Rhinophyma

types 1–3 and thicker skin; 20% benzocaine/6% lidocaine/6% tetracaine for skin types 4–6, Asian patients, and acne prone skin; EMLA [lidocaine/prilocaine] may also be considered for Asian and sensitive skin types), whereas conscious sedation is recommended for AFR to permit patient comfort.

- Cleanse treatment sites with chlorhexidine liquid to ensure complete removal of topical anesthesia prior to treatment.

62.4 Operative Steps

See **Video 62.1**.

62.4.1 Marking the Treatment Zones

- Mark each of the anatomical regions to be treated, using landmarks such as the temporal region, melolabial fold, melomental fold, zygomatic arch, and mandibular angle to isolate the

treatment zones, such as forehead, cheeks, periorbital skin, nose, upper lip, and chin.
- Recommend caution with reduced density and depth when treating of the face, along the eyelids, and along the jawline and lower neck.

62.4.2 Selecting Treatment Parameters and Intraoperative Measures

- Treatment settings are dictated by four parameters: the energy setting, the depth, the density of microscopic thermal zones, and the number of passes.
- For epidermal indications (such as dyschromia and lentigines), we recommend treatment at superficial, low energy settings with nonablative lasers; for deep lesions (such as acne scarring and rhytides), we recommend treatment at deep, higher energy settings.
- High tension scars should be treated no earlier than 3 months so as to not disrupt wound bed.
- Greater density of microscopic thermal zones improves treatment results for deep lesions as there is greater thermal injury to the dermis; however, this should be minimized in skin of color.
- The number of passes dictates at what rate the microscopic thermal zones are formed. Greater number of passes allows for gradual delivery of the controlled injury and avoids bulk heating. Passes should be oriented in a perpendicular fashion (proximal to distal, then medial to lateral).
- Recommend handheld forced air throughout treatment and between passes to minimize thermal injury, improve patient comfort, and minimize bulk heating.
- If patient discomfort is noted, consider prolonging cooling between passes, decreasing the rate of rolling/stamping, or decreasing energy and/or density of microscopic thermal zones.

62.5 Postoperative Care

- Post-treatment care is a major determinant of postoperative outcomes.

62.5.1 NAFR (▶ Fig. 62.1, ▶ Fig. 62.2, ▶ Fig. 62.3)

- Allow patient to cool for several minutes with cold compress and Zimmer air cooling.
- In skin types 1–3, apply ceramide and growth factor containing moisturizer followed by sunscreen. They may continue treatment with such moisturizer for 1 to 2 weeks after treatment.

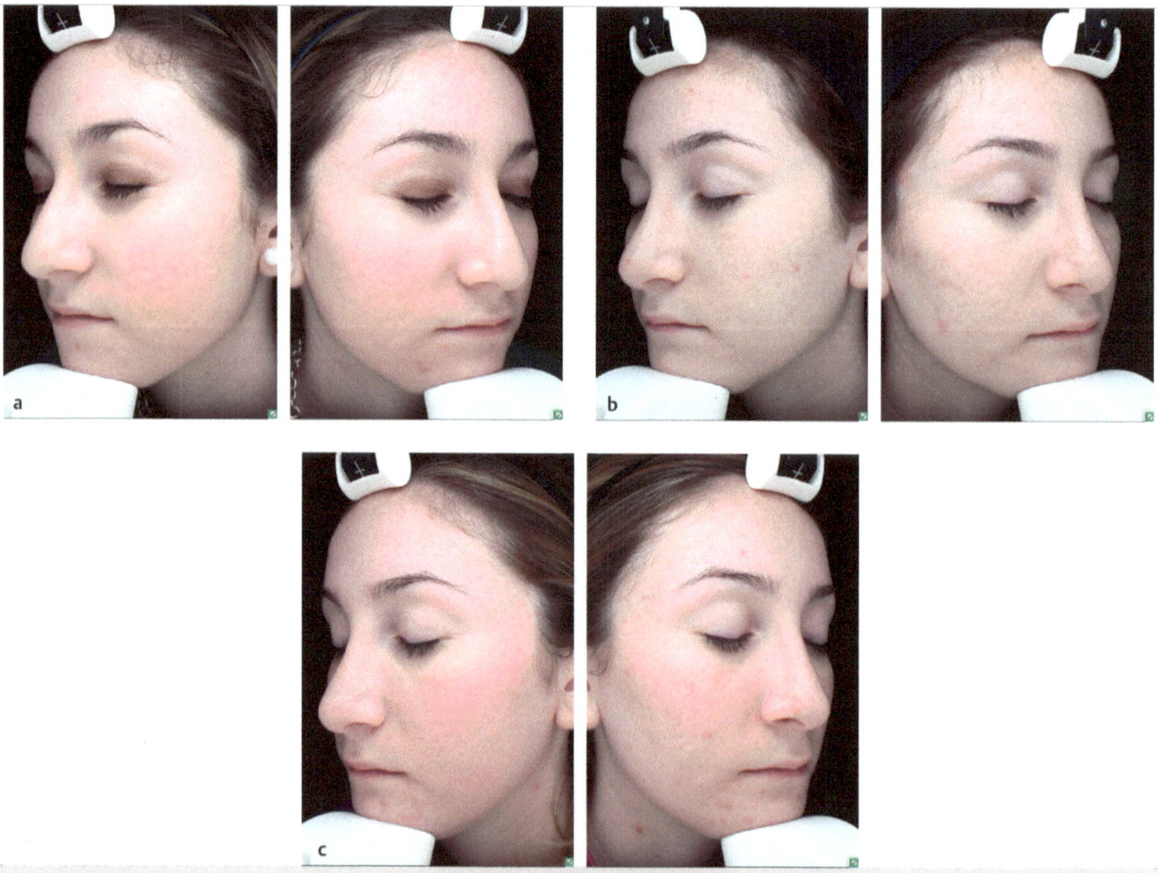

Fig. 62.3 (a) Nonablative fractional resurfacing (NAFR), pretreatment baseline. (b) NAFR, posttreatment, 4 months post seven NAFR treatments for acne scarring. (c) NAFR, 1 year after seven NAFR treatments.

- In skin types 4–6, apply brightening serum (such as SkinCeuticals© Discoloration Defense) to skin prior to application of the moisturizer and sunscreen.
- Patients should be counseled to expect swelling and erythema for 5 to 7 days. If epidermal lesions are treated, a bronze appearance may appear on day 3 and persist for 3 to 5 days.
- Patients may apply makeup and return to normal activities after treatment.
- Gentle skin care is recommended, along with the use of bland emollients and diligent sun protection.
- Swelling after more aggressive treatments may be managed with a 3-day course of oral steroids.
- Oral anti-inflammatories (nonsteroidal anti-inflammatory drugs [NSAIDs]) and antihistamines may be taken for swelling.
- All topical retinoids and alpha/beta acids should be discontinued for the first week after treatment.
- Diligent sunscreen is mandatory for at least 4 weeks after treatment.

62.5.2 AFR (▶ Fig. 62.4)

- After cleansing face with chlorhexidine and cooling with Zimmer, the open channels are prime for laser assisted drug delivery. For acne scarring and rhytides (atrophic lesions), administer Sculptra©; for hypopigmented scars or lesions, administer bimatoprost; for hypertrophic scars, administer 5-fluorouracil + /– kenalog. Administer medications that can be safely injected into skin or bloodstream.
- Apply brightening serum (such as SkinCeuticals© Discoloration Defense), followed by Alastin© Regenerating Skin Nectar and then Alastin © Recovery Balm.
- Apply TELFA to the treated sites followed by elastic mesh.
- We recommend patients are seen on postoperative day 1, day 3, day 5, day 7, and day 14 to ensure adequate wound healing, detect early signs of infection (presence of pustules, vesicles, increased pain, and inability to re-epithelialize by day 6 postoperatively), and identify early hypertrophic scarring. If any of these signs are present, recommend more frequent follow-up for longer duration.
- Redness and swelling are very common; while swelling may resolve within 1 to 2 weeks, prolonged redness may last up to 3 months.
- Blisters, bleeding, and crusting are common, and patients should be counseled to keep the sites clean and moisturized to prevent infection and scarring (see topical care regimen instructions).
- Oral anti-inflammatories (NSAIDs) and antihistamines may be taken for swelling.
- Pruritus may appear 4 to 7 days post procedure and should be treated with Class 6 or 7 topical steroids.
- Milia formation may be due to use of occlusive topical dressing and should be treated with topical ivermectin.
- All topical retinoids and alpha/beta acids should be discontinued for the first week after treatment.
- Diligent sunscreen is mandatory for at least 8 weeks after treatment.
- Avoidance of smoking will aid in healing. Direct contact with pets should be avoided until re-epithelialized and vinegar soaks are no longer required (usually 7–10 days).
- Prolonged severe erythema greater than 3 weeks should be treated with class 4-6 topical steroid followed by low fluence pulse dye laser.
- In case of hypertrophic scarring, consider low fluence pulse dye laser followed by intralesional 5-fluorouracil and kenalog-10 (9:1).

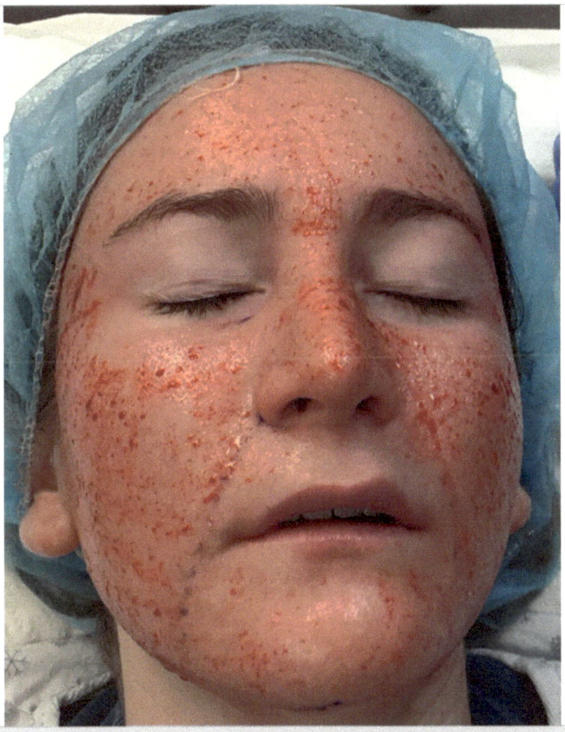

Fig. 62.4 Ablative fractional resurfacing (AFR), immediate post treatment.

62.6 Case Example

A Fitzpatrick Skin Type 2 female presented at the age of 17 for evaluation and treatment of atrophic boxcar and rolling acne scars. She underwent seven NAFR followed by two AFR treatments over 22 months, along with oral and topical therapy to control her residual acne. We noted a considerable (> 75%) improvement in the atrophic lesions (▶ Fig. 62.5).

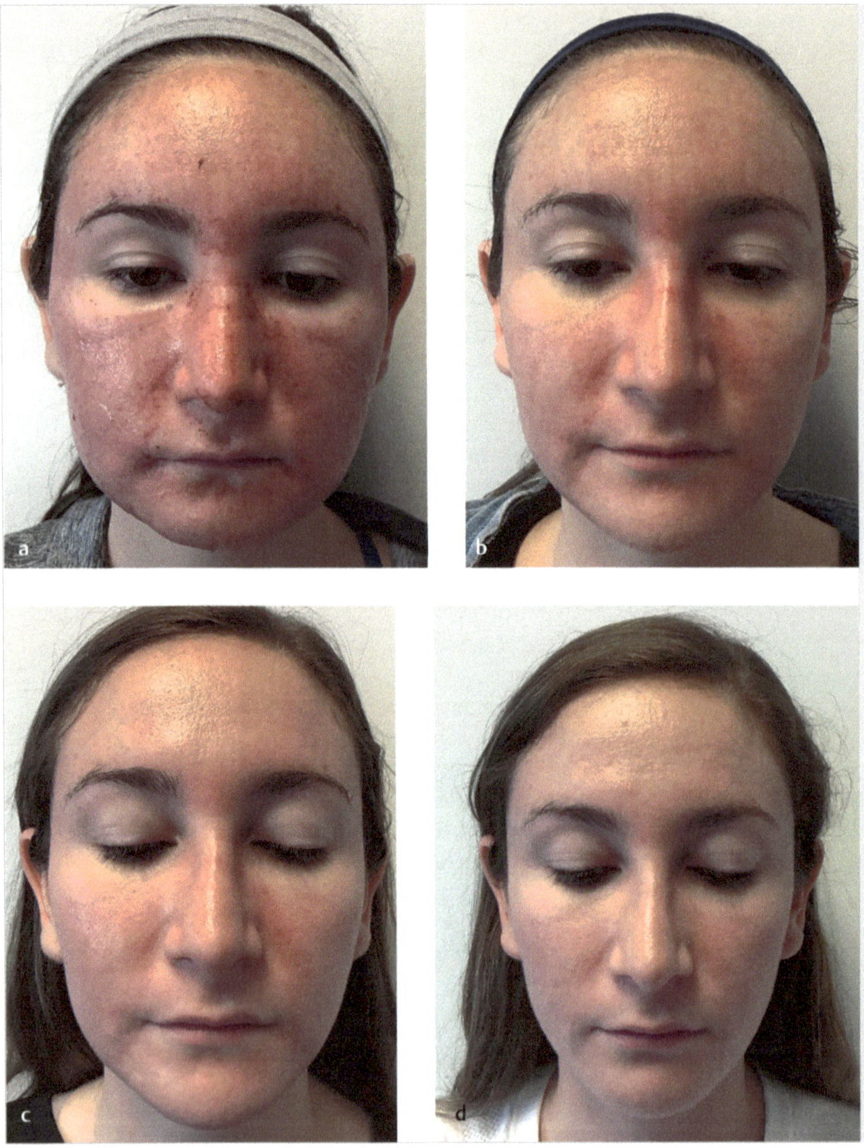

Fig. 62.5 Ablative fractional resurfacing (AFR) **(a)** post-op day 1, **(b)** post-op day 5, **(c)** post-op day 7, and **(d)** post-op day 18.

62.7 Conclusion

NAFR and AFR are the mainstay of facial laser resurfacing. Laser assisted drug delivery can enhance outcomes. Pretreatment topical therapy will effectively prime the skin for laser resurfacing, and post-treatment care is imperative for optimal results. Low density NAFR is favored in darker skin types, but AFR can be used in darker skin types with appropriate settings and prophylactic bleaching regimen.

Further Readings

Alajlan AM, Alsuwaidan SN. Acne scars in ethnic skin treated with both non-ablative fractional 1,550 nm and ablative fractional CO_2 lasers: comparative retrospective analysis with recommended guidelines. Lasers Surg Med. 2011; 43(8):787–791

Geddes ER, Ravanfar P, Friedman PM. Nonablative fractional resurfacing. In: Laser and Light Source Treatments for the Skin. 1st ed. New Delhi, India: Jaypee Brothers Medical Publishers Ltd; 2014

Risner-Rumohr S, Ravanfar P, Friedman PM. Ablative fractional resurfacing. In: Laser and Light Source Treatments for the Skin. 1st ed. New Delhi, India: Jaypee Brothers Medical Publishers Ltd; 2014

Rkein A, Ozog D, Waibel JS. Treatment of atrophic scars with fractionated CO_2 laser facilitating delivery of topically applied poly-L-lactic acid. Dermatol Surg. 2014; 40(6):624–631

Waldman A, Bolotin D, Arndt KA, et al. ASDS Guidelines Task Force: consensus recommendations regarding the safety of lasers, dermabrasion, chemical peels, energy devices, and skin surgery during and after isotretinoin use. Dermatol Surg. 2017; 43(10):1249–1262

63 Microneedling

Tina S. Alster

Abstract

Microneedling has grown in popularity over the past several years for a variety of skin conditions such as scars, striae distensae, rhytides, and photodamage. The advantages of microneedling include its cost-effectiveness, high clinical efficacy, and excellent safety profile with low complication rate. As a result, microneedling is a valuable alternative or complement to more invasive procedures such as laser skin resurfacing and deep chemical peeling. Microneedling can be used as a stand-alone treatment or in combination with other therapies to optimize clinical outcomes.

Keywords: Microneedling, scars, striae distensae, rhytides, photodamage, treatment

Key Points

- The original microneedling devices consisted of evenly distributed needles affixed to a drum-shaped roller.
- Microneedling devices have evolved to include corded and battery-powered pens with disposable tips containing 12 to 36 needles.
- Automated pen devices offer variability of needle depth (0.25 to 3.0 mm) with a single cartridge and are small enough to treat areas difficult to access by a roller device.
- In addition to their enhanced sterility and maneuverability, microneedling pens can more effectively and reliably penetrate into the deeper dermis to produce improved clinical outcomes.
- Microneedling can successfully treat a wide variety of cutaneous conditions, including scars (atrophic, surgical, traumatic), rhytides, striae distensae, prominent pores, and photodamaged skin (actinic keratoses, dyschromia).

63.1 Preoperative Steps

- Assess skin for a treatable condition.
- Avoid areas of inflammation, infection, or recent sun exposure.

63.1.1 Microneedling Setup

- Microneedling device and protective shield.
- Single-use sterile needle tip.
- Gliding gel (hyaluronic acid).
- Ice water in bowl.
- 4″ × 4″ gauze.
- Topical anesthetic.
- Disposable gloves.

63.1.2 Microneedling Key Points

- Conditions treated:
  - Photodamage (actinic keratoses, dyschromia).
  - Prominent pores.
  - Rhytides.
  - Scars (atrophic, surgical, traumatic).
  - Striae distensae.
- Avoid:
  - Active infection or inflammation (e.g., acne, eczema).
  - Recent ultraviolet light exposure or evidence of tan.
- Prep:
  - Mild (nonirritating) cleanser.
  - Topical anesthetic.
  - Antimicrobial solution.
- Technique:
  - Hyaluronic acid gel (or platelet-rich plasma) to facilitate device gliding.
  - Skin traction with perpendicular device tip placement.
  - Cross-hatch microneedling passes.
  - Pinpoint bleeding endpoint.
  - Ice water compression for hemostasis.
- Postcare:
  - Hydrating gel or cream (e.g., hyaluronic acid or hydrocortisone).
  - Mineral sunblock (SPF 30 +).

63.2 Procedural Steps

- Cleanse skin with nonirritating cleanser.
- Apply topical anesthetic cream (30% lidocaine) for 30 to 60 minutes.
- Remove anesthetic with antimicrobial solution (e.g., hypochlorous acid).
- Apply thin layer of hyaluronic acid gel (or platelet-rich plasma) to facilitate gliding action of device (avoid use of excessive gel, which can interfere with the microneedling mechanism).
- Select appropriate needle depth for lesion (deep rhytides and fibrotic scars typically require longer needle lengths of 2.5–3.0 mm, whereas superficial rhytides, shallow scars, and thin skin regions can be treated with shorter 1.0–1.5 mm needles).
- Apply gentle traction of the skin to ensure perpendicular placement of the device tip and to assist smooth, vertical delivery of needles into the dermis (▶ Fig. 63.1).
- Exert minimal pressure to the skin to facilitate gliding action of the device.
- Cross-hatch microneedling passes are made until lesional effacement and/or pinpoint bleeding is evident.
- Apply sterile ice water or saline-soaked gauze to remove excess blood and to achieve hemostasis.

63.3 Postprocedural Care

- Apply soothing balm or hydrating gel/cream (e.g., hyaluronic acid, hydrocortisone).
- Apply mineral (zinc oxide and/or titanium dioxide) sunblock (SPF 30 +).
- Avoid application of substances that are not approved for intradermal use in order to reduce possibility of dermatitis or granuloma formation (microneedle-induced channels remain patent for several hours post-treatment).

63.4 Additional Treatments

- Microneedling can be used in combination with energy-based treatments such as fractionated and pulsed dye lasers, radio frequency, or microfocused ultrasound in order to enhance clinical outcomes.
- Monthly microneedling treatments are advocated until the desired clinical results are achieved.
- Maintenance treatment sessions are often recommended on an annual or semiannual basis in order to enhance cosmetic outcomes.

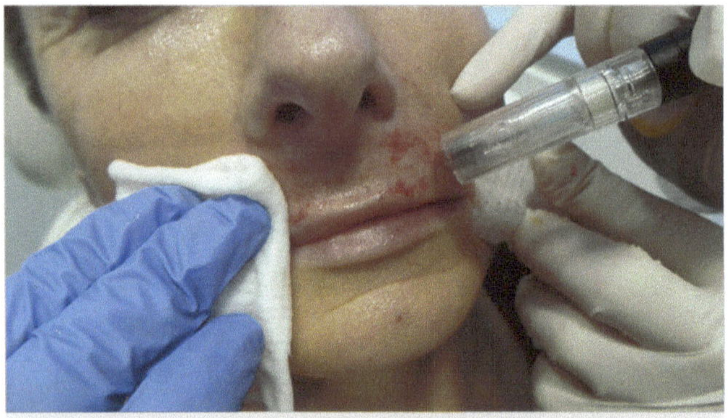

Fig. 63.1 Traction applied during microneedling. (Reproduced with permission from Hausauer AK, Jones DH. PRP and Mikroneedling in Aesthetic Medicine. Thieme; 2019.)

63.5 Case Examples

63.5.1 Case Example 1

Perioral rhytides before and after three microneedling sessions (▶ Fig. 63.2a, b).

63.5.2 Case Example 2

Abdominal surgical scar and striae distensae before and after three microneedling sessions (▶ Fig. 63.3a, b).

63.5.3 Case Example 3

Atrophic scars and enlarged pores on the nose and perinasal creases before and after three microneedling treatments (▶ Fig. 63.4a, b).

63.6 Conclusions

Microneedling is a simple and effective treatment for a variety of cutaneous conditions including dyschromia, photodamage, rhytides, scars, and striae distensae. Its advantages include the ability to treat a wide range of phototypes with rapid post-treatment healing and minimal risk of side effects. Microneedling can be applied as a stand-alone treatment, but can also be integrated into a multimodal approach to enhance skin texture and contour. Monthly treatment sessions are advocated, but standardized protocols (with and without concomitant therapies) have yet to be established to optimize clinical outcomes.

See **Video 63.1**.

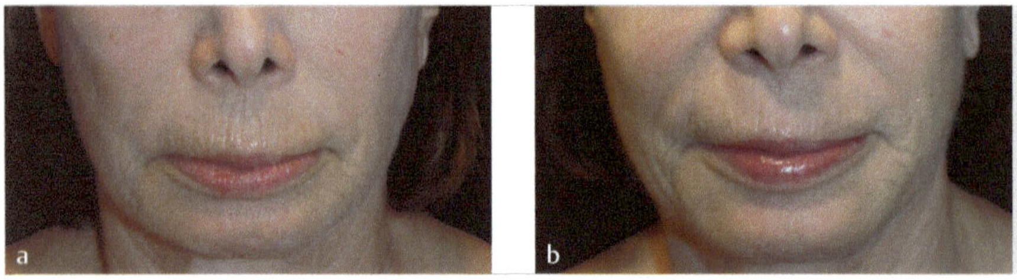

Fig. 63.2 (a, b) Case 1. Perioral rhytides before and after three microneedling sessions.

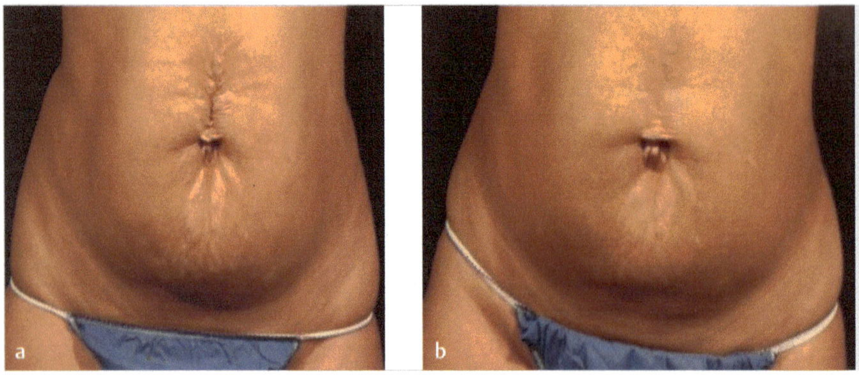

Fig. 63.3 (a, b) Case 2. Abdominal surgical scar and striae distensae before and after three microneedling sessions.

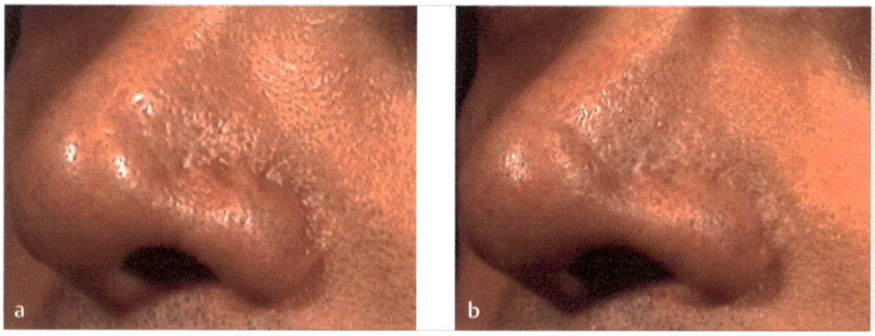

Fig. 63.4 (a, b) Case 3. Atrophic scars and enlarged pores on the nose and perinasal creases before and after three microneedling treatments.

Further Readings

Alster TS, Graham PM. Microneedling: a review and practical guide. Dermatol Surg. 2018; 44(3):397–404

Alster TS, Li MK. Microneedling of scars: a large prospective study with long-term follow-up. Plast Reconstr Surg. 2020; 145(2):358–364

Alster TS, Li MK. Microneedling treatment of striae distensae in light and dark skin with long-term follow-up. Dermatol Surg. 2020; 46(4): 459–464

Pellicane B, Alster TS. Microneedling: clinical applications. In: Hausauer AK, Jones DH, eds. PRP and Microneedling in Aesthetic Medicine. New York: Thieme Medical Publishers Inc.; 2019:69–82

Part X

Breast

X

64 Breast Augmentation

Rafael A. Couto, David Sieber, and William P. Adams Jr.

Abstract

Breast augmentation is not an isolated surgical procedure, but a true process consisting of four steps: (1) patient education and informed consent; (2) tissue-based planning; (3) refined surgical technique/fast-track 24-hour recovery; and (4) defined postoperative care regimen. Following these steps is key to practicing breast augmentation at the highest level, since it optimizes patient outcomes and satisfaction. Details of the process of breast augmentation are discussed and illustrated.

Keywords: Breast augmentation, dual plane, High Five Process, tissue-based planning, 14-point plan

Key Points

- Breast augmentation outcomes are optimized using the process of breast augmentation including: (1) patient education and informed consent, (2) tissue-based planning, (3) refined surgical technique/fast-track 24-hour recovery, and (4) defined postoperative care regimen (▶ Fig. 64.1).
- We advocate performing dual-plane breast augmentation in all patients, except body builders.
- The surgical 14-point plan effectively decreases surgical site infection, capsular contracture, and breast implant-associated anaplastic large cell lymphoma (BIA-ALCL).

64.1 Preoperative Steps

64.1.1 Patient Education and Informed Consent

- This step is critical to an optimal outcome. The surgical team educates the patient about the concepts and goals of the procedure.
- The aim is to create a partnership between the patient and the surgical team for implant selection and postoperative care.

64.1.2 Tissue-Based Planning

- The High Five Process is used to determine preoperatively: Pocket plane, implant size/type, inframammary fold (IMF) position, and incision (▶ Fig. 64.2).
- The soft tissue pinch thickness of the upper and lower poles of the breast is measured (▶ Fig. 64.3a).
- The breast width measurement correlates with the subpectoral implant pocket. It is a linear measurement at the level of the nipple that extends from the medial border to lateral border of the breast (▶ Fig. 64.3b).
- The breast skin stretch is measured by grasping the skin medial to the nipple and pulling anteriorly (▶ Fig. 64.3c).
- The nipple to IMF (N:IMF) distance is measured from the midpoint of the nipple under maximal stretch to the IMF (▶ Fig. 64.3d).
- Three-dimensional imaging is a comprehensive consultation tool. It provides an efficient visual patient education of asymmetries of breast and chest wall, and the final scientifically accurate (98%) visual simulation of the postoperative result.

64.1.3 Breast Markings (▶ Fig. 64.4)

- The patient's midline and IMF are marked.
- The new IMF position is determined based on the established High Five relationships that correlate N:IMF position based on optimal fill volume of the given breast . A simple mnemonic is: the new IMF level can be determined by using the following method: 300 mL implant requires a N:IMF distance of 8.0 cm; for every 10 mL of volumetric change, the N:IMF distance should be adjusted by 0.1 cm. All measurements are always on maximum stretch.

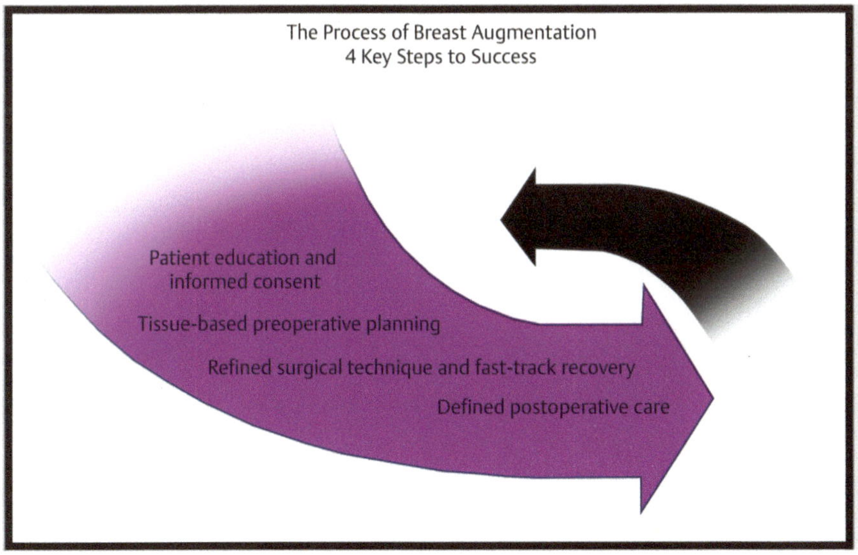

Fig. 64.1 The four key steps for a successful breast augmentation are: (1) patient education and informed consent; (2) tissue-based planning; (3) refine surgical technique; and (4) clear post-operative care regimen. (Reproduced with permission from Adams WP Jr. ed. Breast Augmentation Video Atlas. 2nd ed. New York, NY: Thieme; 2019:2.)

William P Adams, Jr., M.D. Augmentation Mammaplasty Clinical Evaluation for
Patient Preferences, Objectives, Preparation, History, Limitations, Exam, Implant Selection

Size: Pt. Desires: ✖ Natural appearing breast o Unnatural, bulging upper breast
✖ Proportionate to protect tissues o Very large
Approximate Desired Cup «Custom Text 8» Requests specific cc's: ______
o Pt. Chooses Size o Pt. Leaves Size Choice to Dr. Adams
Implant: o Round o Anatomic o Smooth o Textured
o Saline o Silicone o Cohesive o Pt. Leaves Type Choice to Dr. Adams
Pocket Location: ✖ PRP o RM o Dr. Adams to decide
Incision Location: ✖ IM o PA o AX o Incision Choice to Dr. Adams
Pts Initials

Capsular Contracture and Tissue Stretch Factors:
✖ Implant choice may affect risk
✖ Pt. accepts full responsibility for all costs (hospital and anesthesia) for any surgery necessary to treat capsule, tissue stretch deformities and aging implants. Revision surgery may exceed the costs of the original surgery. Pts. Initials______

Patient Has Completed, Read and Signed:
✖ Pt. Educator Consult ✖ Choice Documents
✖ Dr Adams website Pt. Ed. Initials: ______

Discussed/Patient Accepts That:
✖ The larger the implant , the more risks of sensory loss, tissue damage, and increased risk for re-operations
Pts. Initials______

Age «Person_Age»
Height «Custom_Text_12»
Frame: ☐ Sm ☐ Med ☐ Lrg
Torso: o Nl ☐ Wide ☐ Nr
Gravida, Para «Custom_Text_10»
Ages: «Custom_Text_11»

Bra Band Size: 32, 34, 36
Manufacturer: ______
Breast Cup Size (Approx.)
Prior to pregnancy «Custom_Text_6»
Largest with preg «Custom_Text_9»
Current Cup Size «Custom_Text_7»
Desired Cup Size «Custom_Text_8»

Previous Breast Disease:
☐ None
Biopsies: o No o Yes
______

Family Hx. Breast Cancer
☐ No ☐ Yes
Mother Grandmother Aunt
☐ Maternal ☐ Paternal

Previous Mammograms:
☐ No ☐ Yes
Date: «Person_Warning»
Interpretation: ☐ Normal
Other: ______

Pertinent Medical History:
«Custom_List_6»

PSH: «Custom_Memo_1»

Smoker: ☐ No ☐ Yes ____
Allergies: «Person_Allergy_List»

Current Meds, Herbs, Vits:
«Person_Current_Medication_List»

Companion: «Person_Spouse»
Relation: ______

Specific Limitations Discussed with Patient:

✖ Your breasts will never match

✖ You may lose some or all sensation

✖ You may see or feel edges of your implant due to thin tissues

✖ You may require reoperations and additional costs in the future due to implant size requested and tissue stretch characteristics.

✖ We give no guarantee of cup size

✖ Any reoperation may require an inframammary incision

✖ Patient vocalizes under-standing and acceptance of all items checked above. Pt. Initials ______

Breast Masses
☐ None
☐ Size and Location:
______
______

Larger Breast:
☐ Left ☐ Right
Est. Vol. Diff. ____ cc TBD
Nipple Level
Discrepancy ____ cm N/A
IMF Level
Discrepancy ____ cm N/A
Envelope Compliance
☐ Nl ☐ Inc ☐ Dec
☐ Constricted Lower Env.
☐ Short, fixed IMF
☐ Other:
______

☐ **Note Dictated**

Clinical Breast Measurements L/R		Estimating Desired Breast Implant Volume Based on Breast Measurements and Tissue Characteristics High 5 System										
Breast BW		Base Width Parenchyma (cm)	10.5	11.0	11.5	12.0	12.5	13.0	13.5	14.0	14.5	15.0
		Estimated Initial Implant Volume (cc's)	200	250	275	300	300	325	350	375	375	400
SS_{MaxStr}		If SS < 2.0, - 30cc										
		If SS > 3.0, + 30cc										
		If SS > 4.0, + 60cc										
$N:IMF_{MaxSt}$		If N:IMF > 9.5, + 30cc										
Breast Type												
Pt. request												
		Total Estimated Implant Volume										
Estimating the Optimal Level of the Inframammary Fold Relative to the Nipple												
		For each volume indicated	200	250	275	300		325	350	375		400
New IMF		Set new IMF at N:IMF distance (cm.) (measured under maximal stretch)	7.0	7.0	7.5	8		8.25	8.5	9.0		9.5

SNN/N:IMF
R /
L /

R / L

BW /
SS /
AD /
SPP
IPP
PP /

Breast Type:
I/II/III/IV/V

Notes:

Implant Selected: ______ **Volume:** ______ **cc** **BaseD**______**Ht:** ______ **cm.**

1. ST Coverage
SPP>2 SG, DP 1 2 3
SPP<2 RP, DP 1 2 3

4. IMF position ______cm N:IMF
Lower fold N:IMFpost___
_Do not lower fold

5. Incision: ☐ IMF ☐ RT IMF
☐ PA ☐ IT IMF
☐ TA

Top concerns:

Patient Name: **«Person_First_Name» «Person_Last_Name»** **MRN: «Person_ID»**
EDU Date: ____ **Consultation Date:** **«Person_Next_Appt_Date»**

Ref: **«Person_Referral_Source»**

Fig. 64.2 The High Five Process clinical evaluation form. (Reproduced with permission from Adams WP Jr. ed. Breast Augmentation Video Atlas. 2nd ed. New York, NY: Thieme; 2019:26.)

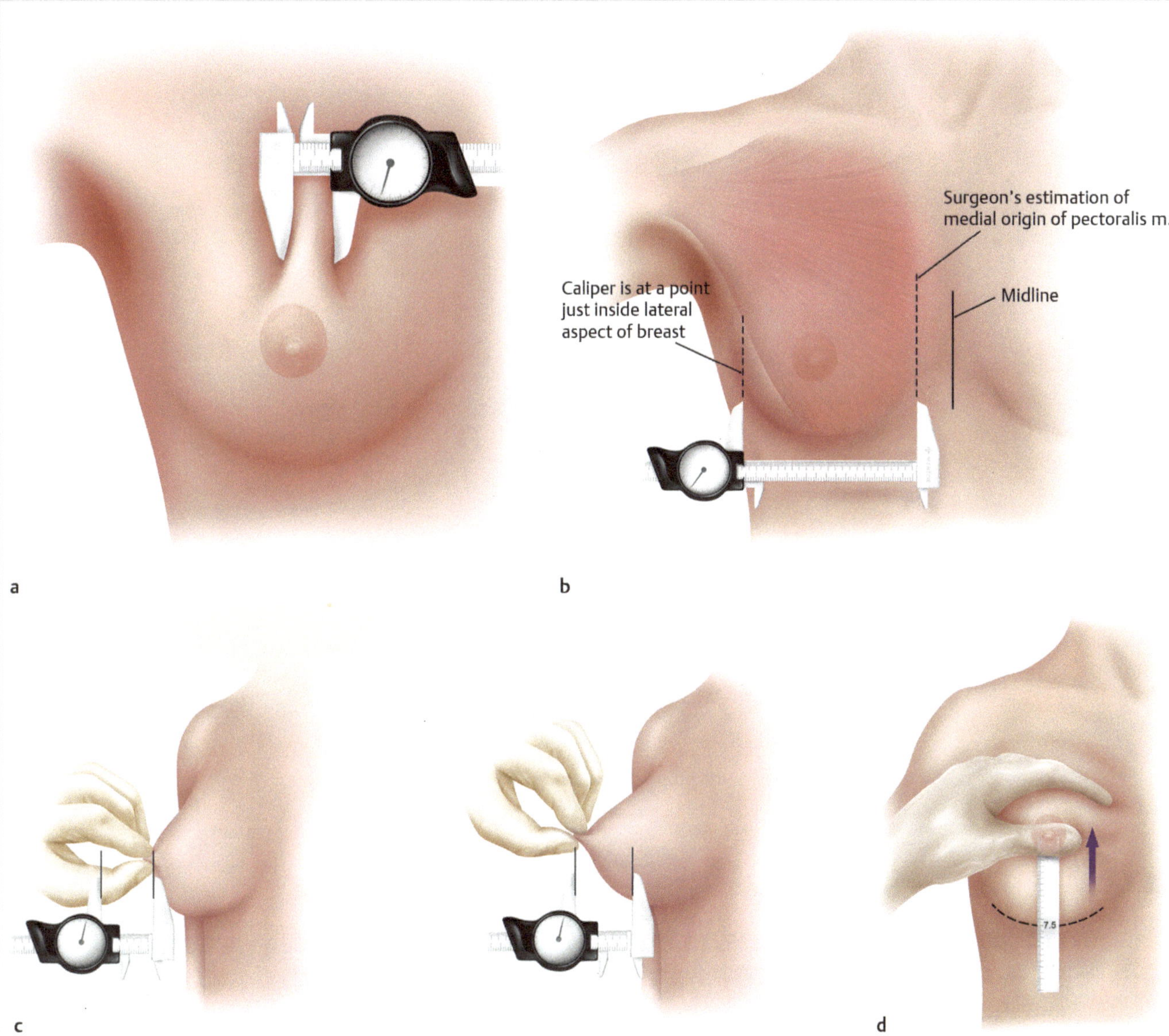

Fig. 64.3 (a–d) The High Five Process measurements: (a) superior pole pinch skin thickness; (b) breast width; (c) anterior skin stretch; and (d) nipple to inframammary fold distance. (Reproduced with permission from Adams WP Jr. ed. Breast Augmentation Video Atlas. 2nd ed. New York, NY: Thieme; 2019:23–25.)

- The incision is marked at the new IMF. The medial extent of the incision is marked on a vertical meridian 1 cm medial to the nipple and it is then extended laterally for 4.5 cm.
- Mark the height and width of the pocket dissection, which are based on the implant dimensions.

64.2 Operative Steps

- The chest is prepped with ChloraPrep™ and draped in sterile fashion and nipple shields are placed.
- Incision is infiltrated with 1% lidocaine with epinephrine (1:100,000) or 0.25% bupivacaine and 1:200,000 epinephrine.
- The breast augmentation is performed following the classic four-part dual-plane dissection (▶ Fig. 64.5).

64.2.1 Skin Incision and Division of Inframammary Fold

- Using a #15 scalpel the skin is incised into the dermis. The remainder of the dissection is performed using electrocautery and under direct visualization as it enables the creation of an atraumatic and bloodless (prospective hemostasis) subpectoral pocket.
- Dissect in a 45-degree angle through the parenchyma down to the pectoralis major muscle.
- Effective and continuous retraction with a double end retractor will facilitate dissection. When the pectoralis major is placed on stretch, it tents anteriorly off the chest wall. This maneuver not only eases the division of the pectoralis major, but also helps its identification from the pectoralis minor below.

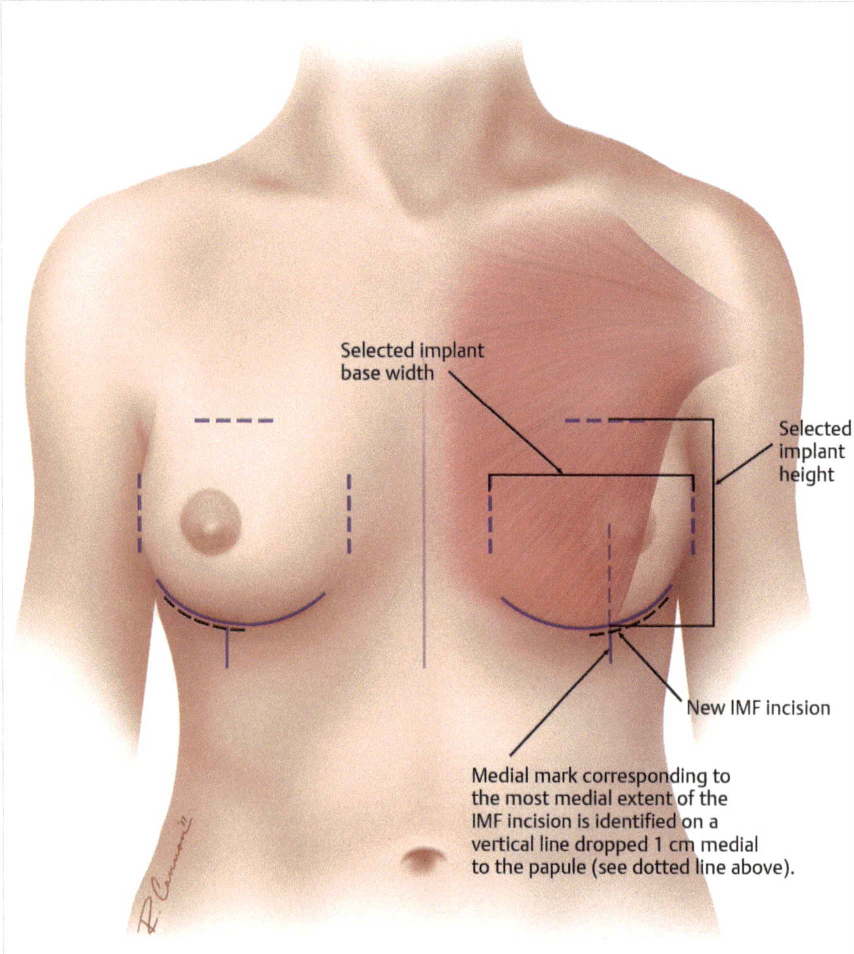

Fig. 64.4 Preoperative breast markings. The breast width and height markings correlate to the subpectoral implant pocket dissection. The dimensions of the subpectoral pocket should be equal to the dimensions of the implant chosen. Other markings include the midline, existing inframammary fold (IMF), and location and length of the new IMF incision. (Reproduced with permission from Adams WP Jr. ed. Breast Augmentation Video Atlas. 2nd ed. New York, NY: Thieme; 2019:81.)

- The pectoralis major is divided parallel and 1 cm above the planned IMF, thus entering the subpectoral space. It is critical to preserve the sternal origins of the muscle. Medial subpectoral pocket dissection is stopped at the medial breast width markings.

64.2.2 Lateral Subpectoral Pocket Dissection

- Sweep your dissection laterally to separate the pectoralis major off the pectoralis minor and serratus anterior. The dissection stops at the lateral breast width markings.

64.2.3 Superior Subpectoral Pocket Dissection

- Switch to a long fiber optic retractor with smoke evacuation capability and dissect the pocket superiorly. The dissection should be limited to the height of the implant, which is guided by the superior breast markings.

64.2.4 Medial Subpectoral Pocket Dissection

- Dissect subpectoral pocket medially and divide any accessory origins of the pectoralis major. Avoid dissecting beyond the medial breast width markings.

64.2.5 Dual-Plane Assessment and Adjustments

- Insert fingers into the subpectoral space and lift the pectoralis major and breast parenchyma to the expected level of expansion. Using your other hand, assess the degree of breast and skin tissue mobility relative to the pectoralis major. Breasts with greater ptosis will require a greater dual-plane adjustment.
- Using the electrocautery, incrementally separate the pectoralis major from the glandular tissue. The goal is to achieve the desired implant–parenchyma interface with the least amount of dissection.

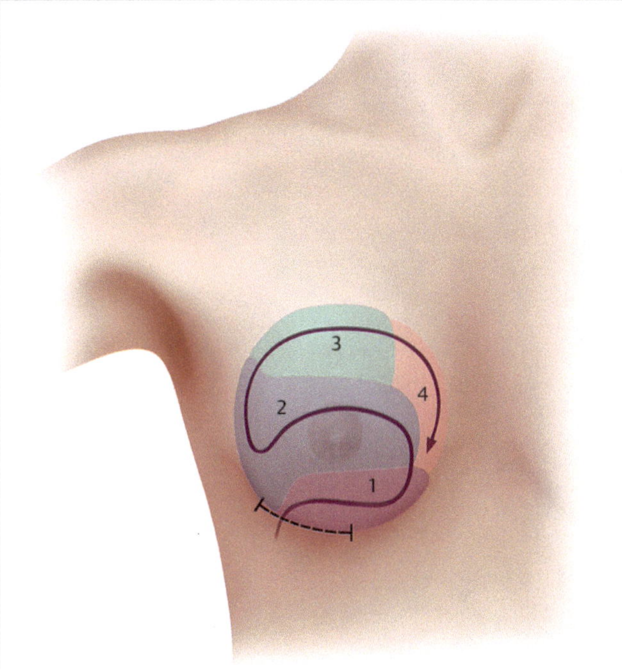

Fig. 64.5 Systematic dissection of a dual-plane breast augmentation involves four steps: (1) division of the inferior pectoralis major origins; (2) lateral pocket definition; (3) superior pocket dissection; and (4) division of medial accessory origins of the pectoralis major. (Reproduced with permission from Adams WP Jr. ed. Breast Augmentation Video Atlas. 2nd ed. New York, NY: Thieme; 2019:87.)

64.2.6 Pocket Preparation and Implant Insertion

- Similar to the process of breast augmentation, which optimizes patient outcomes, the breast pocket irrigation protocol optimizes the results in implant pocket preparation.
- Irrigate pocket with 150 cc of normal saline, followed by 150 cc of betadine-triple solution (i.e., 50 cc of 10% betadine, 500 cc of normal saline, 1 g cefazolin, 80 mg gentamycin).
- Re-prep incisions with small chlorhexidine prep stick, dip/clean retractors into betadine-triple antibiotic solution, and place it inside the breast pocket. After changing gloves, the implants are manually inserted into the breast pocket.
- After implant insertion, the aesthetic shape of the breast is examined and any final adjustments are made.

64.2.7 IMF Fixation and Skin Closure

- IMF fixation is performed in individuals with increased risk of implant malposition such as:
  - Nulliparous/tight envelope.
  - Constricted lower pole breasts.
  - Base width ≤11 cm and tight envelope (skin stretch <2 cm).
  - Surgically lowering IMF.
- IMF fixation technique consists of a three-point suture that secures the superficial fascia above and below the incision to the deep fascia at the level of the IMF. Using a 3–0 polydioxanone (PDS) suture, the IMF is fixated at one to three points. This stitch may produce a temporary mild indentation to the soft tissue.
- The IMF incision closure involves running a 3–0 PDS suture along the superficial fascia, followed by a subdermal 3–0 poliglecaprone (Monocryl) suture, and a running 4–0 Monocryl subcuticular suture.

64.3 Postoperative Care

64.3.1 Wound Care

- A Band-Aid gel strip is left in place for 7 days. Silicone gel scar therapy is initiated and continued for 3 months, followed by scar massages.

64.3.2 Bra

- No "push up" bra for 6 weeks.

64.3.3 Activity

- Upon arrival at home, 2 hour nap, followed by a 20-minute hot shower and light activity.
- Perform instructed arm raise exercises five times every hour while awake for the next 5 days.
- Light activity—shopping, go out to dinner.

64.3.4 Exercise

- Commence aerobic exercises at 2 weeks, nonchest resistance exercises at 4 weeks, and chest/sit-ups at 6 weeks, post surgery.

64.4 Case Example

Preoperative and postoperative photos of a patient following a breast augmentation in anteroposterior, oblique, and lateral views. This patient underwent a dual-plane breast augmentation using smooth round implants (▶ Fig. 64.6a–f).

64.5 Conclusion

The concept of breast augmentation as a process, instead of an isolated procedure, facilitates patient education and perioperative management, thus optimizing satisfaction and outcome. The key to the aesthetics of the breast is controlling the N:IMF distance to breast width ratio.

See **Video 64.1**.

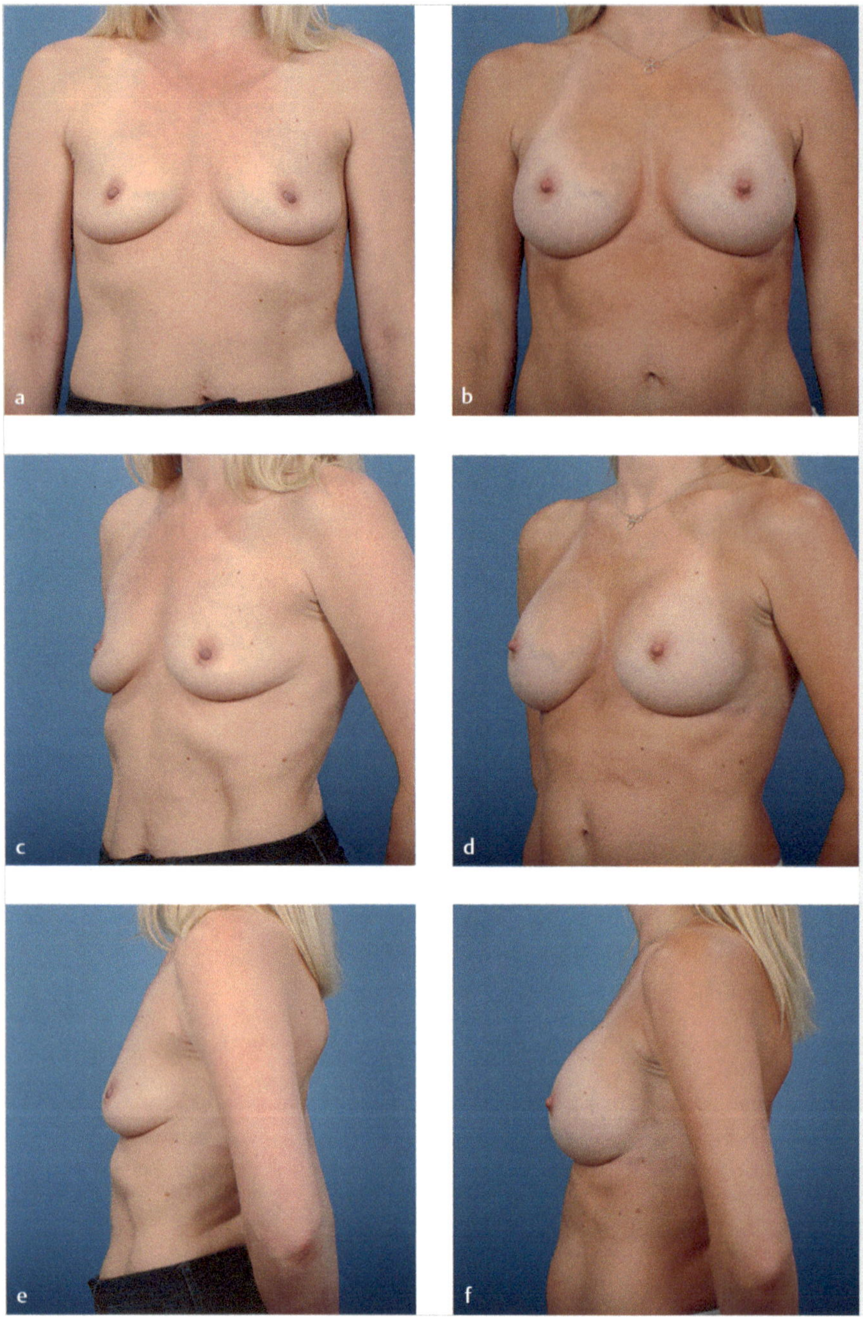

Fig. 64.6 Preoperative and postoperative photos of a patient following a breast augmentation in **(a, b)** anteroposterior, **(c, d)** oblique, and **(e, f)** lateral views. This patient underwent a dual-plane breast augmentation using smooth round implants.

Further Readings

Adams WP Jr, ed. Breast augmentation video atlas. 2nd ed. New York, NY: Thieme; 2019:20–25

Adams WP, Jr. The process of breast augmentation: four sequential steps for optimizing outcomes for patients. Plast Reconstr Surg. 2008; 122(6):1892–1900

Adams WP, Jr, Culbertson EJ, Deva AK, et al. Macrotextured breast implants with defined steps to minimize bacterial contamination around the device: experience in 42,000 implants. Plast Reconstr Surg. 2017; 140(3):427–431

Adams WP, Jr, Rios JL, Smith SJ. Enhancing patient outcomes in aesthetic and reconstructive breast surgery using triple antibiotic breast irrigation: six-year prospective clinical study. Plast Reconstr Surg. 2006; 118(7) Suppl: 46S–52S

Tebbetts JB, Adams WP, Jr. Five critical decisions in breast augmentation using five measurements in 5 minutes: the high five decision support process. Plast Reconstr Surg. 2005; 116(7):2005–2016

65 Subfascial Breast Augmentation

Ryan E. Austin, Frank Lista, and Jamil Ahmad

Abstract

Subfascial breast augmentation is a versatile augmentation mammaplasty technique, wherein a breast implant is placed under the pectoralis major muscle fascia to provide an additional barrier layer between the implant and the breast parenchyma. This technique, similar to subglandular breast augmentation, allows for improvement of breast shape and size in patients with a variety of breast and chest wall morphologies. This chapter will review our surgical technique for performing subfascial breast augmentation in a safe manner with reproducible outcomes.

Keywords: Breast augmentation, implant, subfascial, subglandular

Key Points

- Subfascial breast augmentation is similar to subglandular techniques; instead of placing the implant behind the breast parenchyma, the implant is placed under the pectoralis major muscle (PMM) fascia.
  - Theoretically, this provides an additional barrier layer between the implant and the breast gland to reduce biofilm formation.
- Smooth surface implants can be safely placed in the subfascial or subglandular plane without a significantly increased risk of complications including capsular contracture.

65.1 Preoperative Steps

65.1.1 Patient Selection

- Subfascial breast augmentation is a versatile technique applicable to nearly all patients desiring breast implants.
- Subfascial (and subglandular) breast augmentation is particularly beneficial for patients with certain breast and chest morphologies, including:
  - Patients with a low breast footprint.
    - PMM is present in the upper one-third of the breast footprint only; this provides minimal additional superior pole coverage but increases the risk of implant malposition and animation.
  - Patients with poorly defined breast borders.
    - Subfascial implant placement improves breast border definition without significant implant visibility, palpability, or rippling.
  - Patients with a wide sternum desiring improved medial cleavage.
    - Medial pocket dissection is not limited by sternocostal origin of the PMM.
- Breast base width is measured and a range of possible implant volumes for the patient to select from is determined by maintaining an implant base width within 5 mm of the breast base width and varying the implant projection.
- Smooth, round, optimal shell filled, more cohesive silicone gel implants are routinely used.
- With breast implant technology featuring optimal shell fill and more cohesive silicone gel, we have performed subfascial breast augmentation in patients with ≤2 cm superior pole pinch thickness and achieved excellent aesthetic results.

65.1.2 Preoperative Preparation

- Twice daily for 3 days prior to surgery, patients cleanse the breasts and chest with chlorhexidine gluconate (4%) and apply mupirocin ointment (2%) to the nose, ears, and umbilicus.

65.1.3 Surgical Markings

- The midline of the chest is marked as a vertical line between the sternal notch and the xiphoid process.
- Planned borders for implant pocket dissection are drawn based on the footprint of the breast and base width of the breast implant (▶ Fig. 65.1):
  - Superomedial: The marking is angled to avoid injury to the second and third intercostal perforators during pocket dissection.
  - Medial: The medial extent of the dissection must not pass beyond the medial breast border to avoid implant edge visibility.
  - Superolateral: The marking is extended toward the insertion of the PMM; this helps to recruit skin onto the implant and ablate the zone of adherence inferior to the axillary roll.

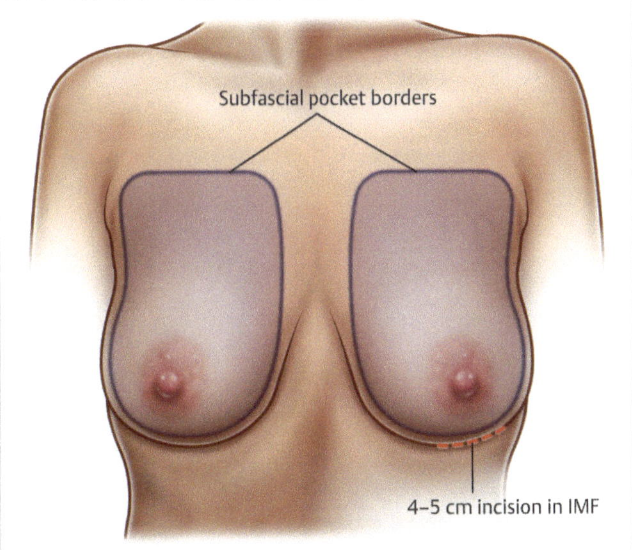

Fig. 65.1 Planned borders for implant pocket dissection are drawn based on the footprint of the breast and base width of the breast implant.

- A 4 to 5 cm incision is planned in the inframammary fold (IMF) for subfascial pocket dissection, starting just lateral to the medial border of the nipple-areolar complex (NAC).
  - All subfascial augmentation is performed through an IMF incision to reduce the risk of bacterial contamination associated with periareolar implant insertion.

65.2 Operative Steps

- Prior to incision, patients receive one dose of intravenous antibiotic:
  - Cefazolin 1 g if patient weighs <80 kg, 2 g if weight is ≥80 kg.
  - Clindamycin 600 mg if there is documented penicillin allergy.
- Chlorhexidine gluconate solution (4%) is used for surgical field preparation.
- A transparent adhesive film dressing (Tegaderm™ transparent film dressing, 3M, St. Paul, MN) is placed over the NAC prior to incision.
  - Helps to prevent ductal bacterial flora from contaminating the surgical field.
- IMF incision and borders of the planned pocket are infiltrated with 20 mL of 1% lidocaine with epinephrine (1:100,000) in the subcutaneous plane to improve hemostasis.
- Incision is carried down sharply into the breast gland using a #15 blade scalpel.
  - Dissection is angled slightly superior toward the inferior origin of the PMM, aided by gentle superior traction with a Miller-Senn retractor.
  - Two layers of dense superficial fascia can be clearly identified and divided prior to reaching the PMM fascia.
    - These fascial layers will later provide strength to incision closure.
- A hand-switching monopolar electrocautery is used to develop the implant pocket with the aid of a lighted breast retractor; care is taken to ensure prospective hemostasis during dissection.
- The implant pocket is developed under the PMM fascia (▸ Fig. 65.2).
- Pocket dissection continues up to the preoperative markings of the breast borders.
  - The superior pocket can be slightly over-dissected to allow for soft tissue redraping over the implant.
  - Avoid over-dissection medially to prevent visibility of the implant edge.
  - We prefer to slightly under-dissect the pocket laterally to maximize medial cleavage and reduce the risk of lateral implant malposition.
- During pocket dissection, a radial cut of the breast capsule is performed at the medial and lateral ends of the incision.
  - It allows for expansion of the lower pole of the breast.
  - Performing this release also aids in retraction and facilitates pocket visualization.
- Ensure symmetry between the pockets and confirm hemostasis before proceeding to implant insertion.
- Each implant pocket is irrigated with three 60 mL syringes of antibiotic solution; the peri-incisional skin is cleansed with the same solution.
  - Antibiotic solution (in 500 cc of saline): Cefazolin 1 g, Gentamycin 80 mg, and 50 cc of 10% Povidone-iodine solution.
    - From this point forward, any instrument inserted into the pocket is cleansed with antibiotic solution prior to insertion.
- "Minimal-Touch" technique of implant insertion:
  - Implant is only handled by the operating surgeon.
  - Prior to accepting the implant onto the sterile field, the surgeon changes into new sterile gloves.
  - The implant is kept sealed in its inner sterile package until ready for insertion.
    - A blunt 18-gauge needle is inserted through the sterile paper packaging and each implant is irrigated with 30 mL of antibiotic solution to reduce electrostatic charge on the implant surface.
  - Implant is transferred from its package to an implant insertion sleeve (Keller Funnel®2, Allergan Inc., Dublin, Ireland) that has been rinsed with antibiotic solution.
  - Deaver retractor is inserted into the pocket to assist with implant insertion.

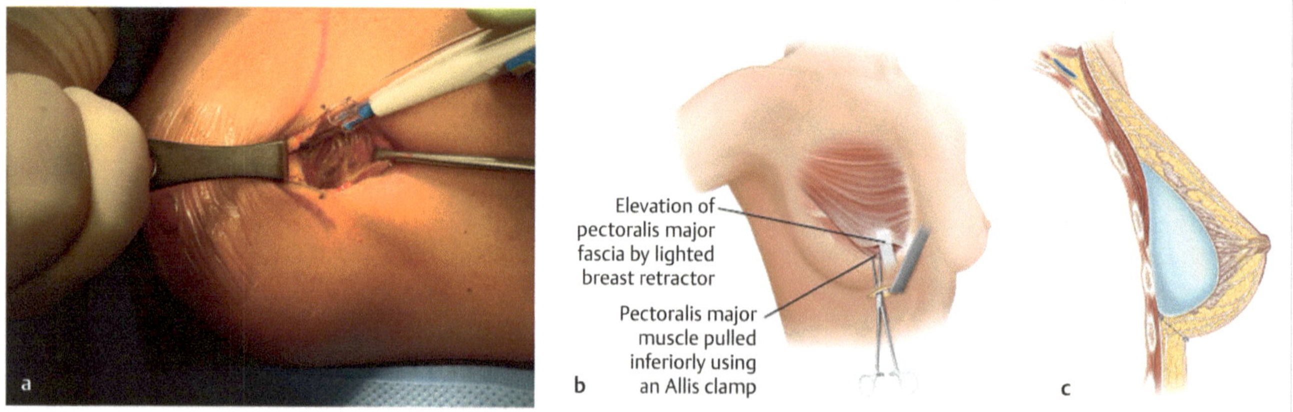

Fig. 65.2 (a–c) A subfascial pocket is created. (Reproduced with permission from Jones GE. Bostwick's Plastic and Reconstructive Breast Surgery. 4th ed. Thieme; 2020.)

 - Tip of the implant insertion sleeve is introduced completely into the pocket before expelling the implant to prevent contact with the skin.
   - Ensure that the implant is inserted with the proper device orientation.
 - Avoid excessive manipulation of the implant and pocket.
   - If manual adjustment is required, the surgeon should cleanse their gloves and instruments in antibiotic solution prior to manipulation.
- An 18-gauge angiocatheter is inserted into the inferolateral aspect of the pocket under direct visualization.
- Incision is closed in multiple layers to ensure a "watertight" closure.
 - A three-point 2–0 Vicryl Plus (Ethicon, Inc., Somerville, NJ) suture is used to repair the superficial layers of the breast capsule to the deep fascia, thus reconstituting the IMF.
   - Two or three sutures are typically required.
 - The superficial breast capsule repair is reinforced using 2–0 Vicryl Plus (Ethicon, Inc., Somerville, NJ) interrupted inverted sutures.
 - Skin edges are reapproximated using a 3–0 Vicryl Plus (Ethicon, Inc., Somerville, NJ) continuous inverted deep dermal suture.
 - Skin edges are reopposed using a 4–0 Monocryl Plus (Ethicon, Inc., Somerville, NJ) continuous intradermal suture.
- Through the angiocatheter, 10 mL of a solution containing local anesthetic (0.25% bupivacaine with 1:100,000 epinephrine) and anti-inflammatory (ketorolac 15 mg) is infiltrated into each breast pocket.
 - This helps to minimize postoperative discomfort, limits postoperative opioid requirements, and expedites recovery.
- Angiocatheter is withdrawn and nipple shields are removed.
- A water-resistant barrier dressing is placed over the incision (Dermabond® Prineo® Skin Closure System, Ethicon Inc, San Lorenzo, PR, USA).

65.3 Postoperative Steps

- All patients are discharged home on the day of the procedure (postoperative day [POD] #0).
- Patients return on POD #1 and are instructed to shower daily, covering the incisions with a nonadherent gauze dressing in their surgical bra.
- Water-resistant barrier dressing removed at 2-week postoperative visit.
 - Patients also instructed to start implant massage for 5 minutes 5-10x per day.
- Patients are instructed to wear a surgical bra at all times for 4 weeks following surgery.
- Avoid strenuous physical activity (including exercise) for 4 weeks following surgery.
- Patients are instructed to lay on their chest for 10 minutes 1-2x per day starting at 1 month postoperatively.
- Silicone bandages are applied to the incisions once all wounds have completely healed for 4 to 6 months postoperatively.

65.4 Case Example

Pre- and postoperative views of a patient 6 months following subfascial breast augmentation in the anteroposterior (AP), oblique, and lateral views. This 36-year-old female had previously undergone a 70 lbs weight loss following bariatric surgery. Breast augmentation was performed using a 385-cc smooth round silicone gel implant (▶ Fig. 65.3a–c).

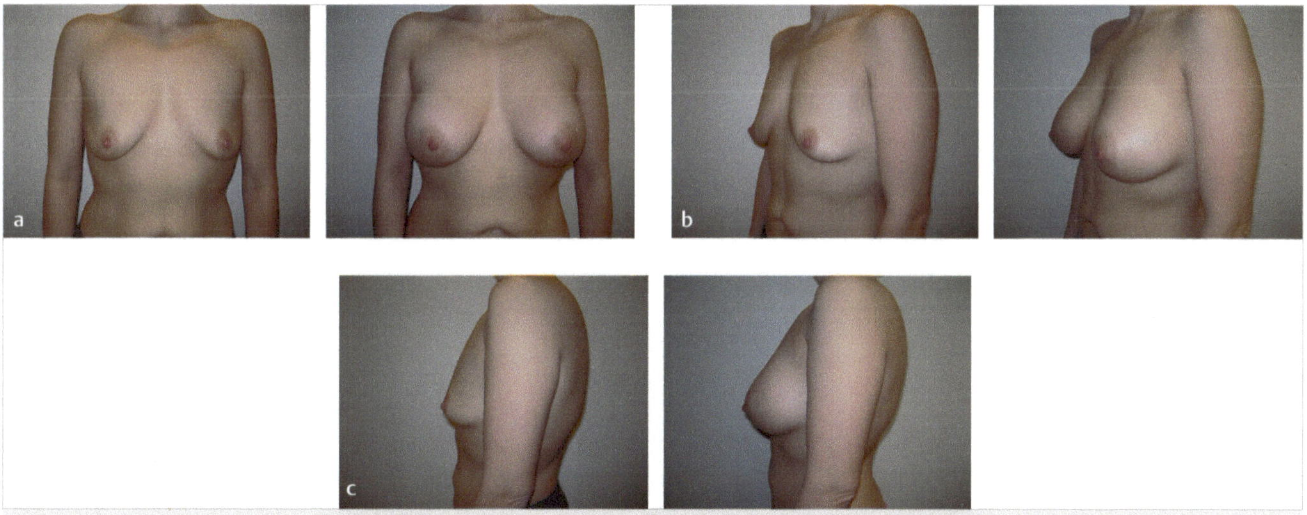

Fig. 65.3 Pre- and postoperative views of a patient 6 months following subfascial breast augmentation in the **(a)** anteroposterior (AP), **(b)** oblique, and **(c)** lateral views. This 36-year-old female had previously undergone a 70 lbs weight loss following bariatric surgery. Breast augmentation was performed using a 385-cc smooth round silicone gel implant.

65.5 Conclusion

Subfascial breast augmentation is a versatile technique applicable to nearly all patients desiring breast implants. Subfascial implant placement is particularly beneficial for patients with a low breast footprint, patients with poorly defined breast borders, and patients with a wide sternum desiring improved medial cleavage. Smooth surface implants can be safely placed in the subfascial or subglandular plane without a significantly increased risk of complications (including capsular contracture). Adherence to surgical techniques intended to minimize bacterial contamination of the breast implant, including a "minimal-touch" technique, is important for reducing the risk of complications in subfascial breast augmentation.

See **Video 65.1**.

Further Readings

Adams WP, Jr, Culbertson EJ, Deva AK, et al. Macrotextured breast implants with defined steps to minimize bacterial contamination around the device: experience in 42,000 implants. Plast Reconstr Surg. 2017; 140(3): 427–431

Lista F, Ahmad J. Evidence-based medicine: augmentation mammaplasty. Plast Reconstr Surg. 2013; 132(6):1684–1696

Lista F, Austin RE, Saheb-Al-Zamani M, Ahmad J. Does implant surface texture affect the risk of capsular contracture in subglandular breast augmentation and breast augmentation-mastopexy? Aesthet Surg J. 2020;40(5): 499–512

Lista F, Tutino R, Khan A, Ahmad J. Subglandular breast augmentation with textured, anatomic, cohesive silicone implants: a review of 440 consecutive patients. Plast Reconstr Surg. 2013; 132(2):295–303

Tebbetts JB, Adams WP. Five critical decisions in breast augmentation using five measurements in 5 minutes: the high five decision support process. Plast Reconstr Surg. 2005; 116(7):2005–2016

66 Vertical Scar Mastopexy with Autoaugmentation Flap

Ryan E. Austin, Jamil Ahmad, and Frank Lista

Abstract
Vertical scar mastopexy is a reliable short-scar breast lift technique, similar to vertical scar breast reduction. However, instead of resecting the excess parenchyma of the inferior pole, we use this tissue to create a centrally based autoaugmentation flap that can increase superior pole volume and projection without the need for a breast implant. This chapter will review our surgical technique for performing vertical scar mastopexy with autoaugmentation flap in a safe manner with reproducible outcomes.

Keywords: Autoaugmentation, breast lift, mastopexy, vertical scar

Key Points

- The technique is similar to vertical scar breast reduction; instead of resecting the tissue in the inferior pole it is used as a centrally based autoaugmentation flap to increase superior pole volume and projection.
- It is ideal for patients with grade 2–3 ptosis desiring an improved aesthetic appearance of the breast, but who do not want to increase breast size and/or decline a breast implant.

66.1 Preoperative Steps

- Vertical scar mastopexy is a versatile procedure that can be adapted to the majority of patients seeking correction of breast ptosis.
  - Patients with significant deflation of the breast and insufficient tissue of the inferior pole are not suitable candidates for this technique.
- We do not perform this procedure on patients with a body mass index (BMI) $\geq$35.0 kg/m^2 or on active smokers due to a significantly higher risk of complications.
- Preoperative mammography is not required prior to vertical scar mastopexy; national or regional screening guidelines for mammography should be followed.
- **Note:** This technique should not be performed in patients with breast implants as the blood supply to the autoaugmentation flap is disrupted during previous placement of the breast implant.

66.1.1 Surgical Markings (▶ Fig. 66.1)

- Mark the midline of the chest and the inframammary fold (IMF).
- Central axis of the breast is marked by drawing a straight line from the midpoint of the clavicle (7–8 cm lateral to midline) through the nipple-areolar complex (NAC).
- Level of the IMF is transposed anteriorly onto the breast and marked; this represents the new location of the superior border of the NAC (point A).
  - Height of the point A marking is transposed to the contralateral breast to avoid asymmetry of the NAC as a result of IMF asymmetry.
  - In comparison to breast reduction where there is unweighting of the breast and the NAC is typically located higher than was marked preoperatively, mastopexy does not involve unweighting of the breast so the NAC typically remains where it is marked.
- Mark a point 5 to 10 cm superior to point A as a reference for autoaugmentation flap inset.
- Inferior extent of the planned skin excision is marked 2 to 4 cm above the IMF (point B).
  - It prevents migration of the vertical scar onto the chest.
- Site for new superior border of the NAC is drawn as a mosque dome starting at point A and extending to points C and D.
  - It is drawn such that when points C and D are brought together, the mosque dome forms a circle.
- Vertical limbs are drawn as curved lines extending from point B to points C and D.
  - Medial and lateral displacement of the breast can assist in approximating these lines.
  - Compared to breast reduction where more breast tissue is removed between the pillars necessitating more skin excision, during mastopexy typically 0 to 100 g of breast tissue is removed from the autoaugmentation flap so less skin can be excised between the pillars.

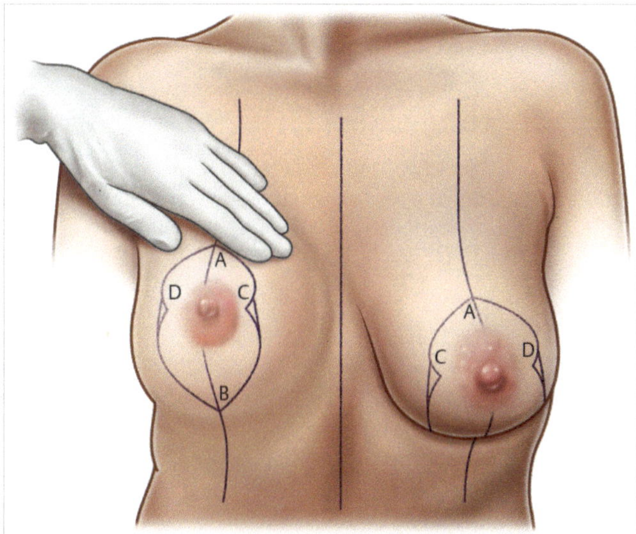

Fig. 66.1 Illustration of the skin markings for vertical scar mastopexy with autoaugmentation flap. ***Point A*** represents the new location of the superior border of the nipple-areolar complex (NAC). ***Point B*** is the inferior extent of the vertical scar, located 2 to 4 cm above the inframammary fold (IMF). ***Points C and D***, the blocking triangles, should create a circle of the mosque-dome pattern when brought together. The tissue of the inferior pole within the marked vertical limbs will become a centrally based autoaugmentation flap.

   - Planned resection can be tested by coning the breast to approximate the planned vertical incisions; it should come together with minimal tension.
   - Inferior extent of the vertical scar should have a "V" shape to minimize dog-ear formation.
   - Blocking triangles at points C and D prevent a "teardrop deformity" of the NAC.
- **Note:** The tissue of the inferior pole within the marked vertical limbs will become a centrally based autoaugmentation flap.

66.2 Operative Steps

See **Video 66.1**.

66.2.1 Infiltration

- Stab incision made at the inferior extent of the planned vertical scar; tumescent solution (1 L of Ringer's Lactate + 1 mL of epinephrine 1:1,000) infiltrated under the planned vertical incisions and throughout the superficial breast parenchyma, as well as the lateral chest and axillary roll if liposuction of these areas is indicated.
   - Avoid infiltration of the inferior pole where the autoaugmentation flap will be created; tumescent fluid distorts the tissues making dissection more difficult and may hydro-dissect the autoaugmentation flap off the pectoralis major muscle (PMM) fascia.
   - Infiltration performed using the simultaneous separation tumescence (SST) technique with a 4 mm exploded-tip cannula and power-assisted liposuction (PAL).
      - Avoid use of SST in the central and deep breast parenchyma as this can disrupt the autoaugmentation flap.
   - Each breast is typically infiltrated with approximately 100 to 200 mL of tumescent solution; more may be infiltrated to the lateral chest and axillary roll if liposuction is required.

66.2.2 Pedicle Selection

- Breast tourniquet applied to maintain tension on the skin.
- New NAC outlined using a circular metal washer (approximately 44 mm diameter) centered over the nipple.
- If any part of the new areola lies superior to an imaginary line drawn between the blocking triangles (points C and D), a superior pedicle is used. If all of the new areola lies inferior to this line, a superomedial pedicle is used (▶ Fig. 66.2a, b).
   - If the NAC is positioned medially, a superolateral pedicle may be required to allow rotation and insetting.
- The selected pedicle is drawn with a 2.5 cm border around the edge of the new areola.
   - For a superomedial pedicle, a 1:2 width-to-length ratio of the pedicle should be maintained to preserve blood supply to the new NAC.

66.2.3 Autoaugmentation Flap

- With the breast tourniquet in place, the planned pedicle and inferior pole autoaugmentation flap are de-epithelialized.
   - It is important to leave the deep dermis intact:
      - Pedicle: Helps to maintain the subdermal vascular supply.
      - Autoaugmentation flap: Dermis acts as a strong tissue layer for suspension of the flap to the PMM fascia in the superior pole.
- The dermoglandular pedicle is developed to a depth of approximately 2.5 cm to protect the neurovascular supply that runs approximately 1 to 1.5 cm deep to the dermis.
   - Beyond this depth, dissection is beveled superiorly and continued down to PMM fascia.
      - This will protect the neurovascular supply and also preserve sufficient tissue on the autoaugmentation flap to maximize superior pole augmentation.
- Medial parenchymal pillar is developed by incising along the medial limb of the vertical pattern straight down to a depth of approximately 2.5 cm.
   - At this depth, it is important to bevel the dissection medially to avoid undermining the base of the autoaugmentation flap.
   - Dissection is carried down to the PMM fascia.
- Lateral limb of the vertical pattern is incised to a depth of approximately 2.5 cm.
   - Similar to the medial pillar, at this depth the incision is beveled laterally to avoid narrowing the base of the

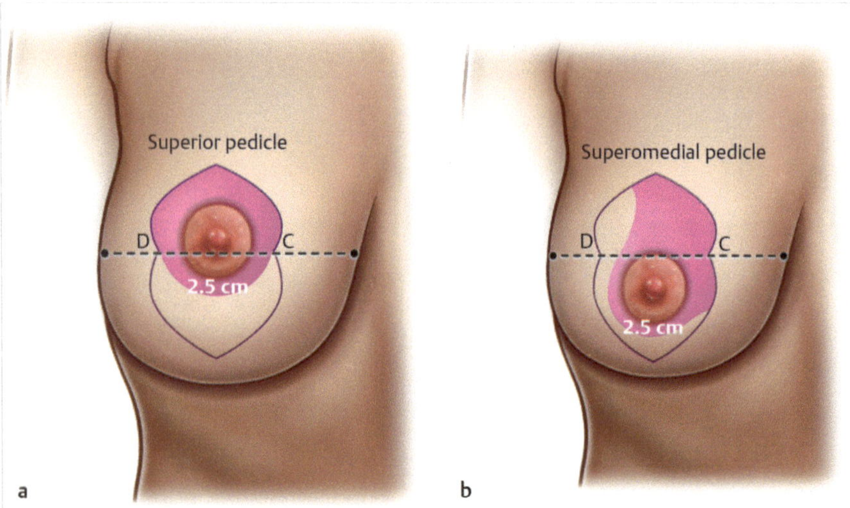

Fig. 66.2 Illustration of dermoglandular pedicle selection. If any part of the new areola lies superior to an imaginary line drawn between the blocking triangles (points C and D), a superior pedicle is used **(a)**. If all of the new areola lies inferior to this line, a superomedial pedicle is used **(b)**. The selected pedicle is drawn with a 2.5 cm border around the edge of the new areola.

autoaugmentation flap; dissection continues down to the PMM fascia.
- **Note:** Be mindful of your surgical assistant; excessive retraction can distort perception of the autoaugmentation flap and result in narrowing of the flap base.
- At the inferior extent of the vertical incision, the skin is thinned to leave tissue on the autoaugmentation flap.
  - Dissection is carried below the IMF to minimize the risk of injury to the centrally based blood supply of the autoaugmentation flap.
- Once the flap has been created, a subglandular pocket is developed in the superior pole almost to the level of the clavicle along the central axis of the breast to allow for flap inset.
  - It is important to leave the PMM fascia intact during dissection, as this fascia will be used to anchor the autoaugmentation flap.
- Autoaugmentation flap is tested to ensure it can be easily mobilized into the superior pole with minimal tension.
  - If tension remains, further release of the medial, lateral, and inferior flap base is required.
- **Note:** If breast size asymmetry is present, parenchyma can be excised from the superficial superior, medial, and lateral surfaces of the autoaugmentation flap on the larger side to reduce breast volume without undermining the flap base.
- Autoaugmentation flap is inset into the superior pole at the level of the third intercostal space using #0 PDS suture (Ethicon Inc., Somerville, NJ).
  - It typically requires two sutures placed through the de-epithelialized dermis at the superomedial and superolateral corners of the autoaugmentation flap.
- In patients with larger autoaugmentation flaps or significant tissue laxity, the parenchyma of the flap may herniate laterally after superior inset.
  - In this case, the lateral dermis of the flap can be sutured to the PMM fascia to maintain central and medial projection.
- It is important to ensure that the autoaugmentation flaps are inset at the same height to improve symmetry between the breasts.

66.2.4 Glandular Reshaping

- Medial and lateral pillars are reapproximated over the autoaugmentation flap using inverted #1 Vicryl sutures (Ethicon, Inc., Somerville, NJ) placed through the breast capsule; two parenchymal pillar sutures are typically required.
  - Inferior pillar suture should be no closer than 4 cm from the inferior end of the incision to prevent creating a standing-cone deformity which predisposes to dog-ear formation.
  - Superior pillar suture should be no closer than 2 cm from the NAC to avoid distortion.
- NAC is rotated into position and inset prior to closure of the vertical incision.
  - NAC is inset with 3-0 Monocryl Plus (Ethicon, Inc., Somerville, NJ) interrupted inverted deep dermal sutures at the 3, 6, 9, and 12 o'clock positions.
    - NAC is closed using a 3-0 Monocryl Plus (Ethicon, Inc., Somerville, NJ) continuous intradermal suture.
- 3-0 Monocryl Plus (Ethicon, Inc., Somerville, NJ) four-point inverted deep dermal box sutures are used to gather the skin of the vertical incision and shorten the length of the vertical scar to approximately 8 to 10 cm.
  - Box sutures are placed starting at the inferior apex of the vertical incision and working toward the NAC; each suture should be placed immediately adjacent to the previous suture to maximize gathering.
  - Box sutures often cause horizontal pleats along the vertical incision; these must be corrected with inverted deep dermal sutures to prevent creating permanent horizontal lines within the vertical scar.
  - Skin within 2 cm of the areola is not gathered to prevent distortion of the areola.
- The remainder of the wound is closed with 3-0 Monocryl Plus (Ethicon, Inc., Somerville, NJ) interrupted inverted deep dermal sutures.
- Skin staples are used along the vertical wound for final closure.
- Breast skin medial and lateral to incision is injected with 10 mL of 0.5% bupivacaine with 1:200,000 epinephrine for postoperative pain relief.
- Incisions are dressed with a paraffin-impregnated antiseptic gauze, dry gauze, and abdominal pads; patient is placed into a postsurgical bra.

66.3 Postoperative Steps

- All patients are discharged home on the day of the procedure (postoperative day [POD] #0).
- Patients return on POD #1; they are instructed to wash their incisions daily with soap and water.
- Skin staples are removed on POD #5/6 and replaced with Steri-Strips (3 M, St. Paul, MN).
- Patients start massage to the lateral chest if liposuction has been performed at 1 week postoperatively and to the breast at 2 weeks postoperatively.
  - Warn patients to be gentle with massage in the superior pole of the breast in the area of the autoaugmentation flap.
- Patients are instructed to wear a postsurgical bra at all times for 4 weeks following surgery.
- Avoid strenuous physical activity (including exercise) for 4 weeks following surgery.
- Silicone bandages are applied to the incisions once all wounds have completely healed in 4 to 6 months postoperatively.

66.4 Case Example

Pre- and postoperative views of a 44-year-old patient 6 months following vertical scar mastopexy with autoaugmentation flap in the (a) anteroposterior (AP), (b) oblique, and (c) lateral views. Mastopexy was performed using a superior dermoglandular pedicle bilaterally, and 49 g of tissue was removed from the right side with 59 g removed from the left side (▶ Fig. 66.3a–c).

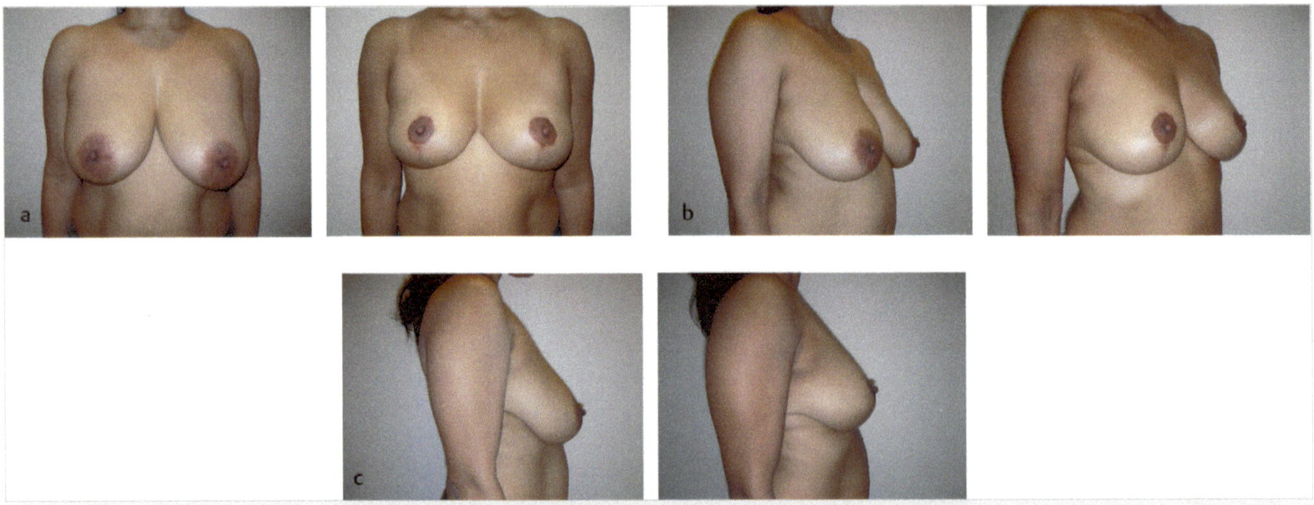

Fig. 66.3 Pre- and postoperative views of a 44-year-old patient 6 months following vertical scar mastopexy with autoaugmentation flap in the **(a)** anteroposterior (AP), **(b)** oblique, and **(c)** lateral views. Mastopexy was performed using a superior dermoglandular pedicle bilaterally, and 49 g of tissue was removed from the right side with 59 g removed from the left side.

66.5 Conclusion

Vertical scar mastopexy with autoaugmentation flap is a reliable breast lift technique for patients looking to achieve improved breast shape, including superior pole volume and projection, without the use of a breast implant. Although care must be taken to avoid undermining the centrally based autoaugmentation flap, it is equally important to maintain adequate tissue on the medial and lateral parenchymal pillars to prevent contour deformities in the lower pole of the breast. Breast size asymmetry can be corrected using this technique. Parenchyma can be excised from the superficial surfaces of the autoaugmentation flap on the larger side to reduce breast volume without undermining the central flap base.

Further Readings

Biggs TM, Graf R, Taneja A. Maintaining shape in mastopexy. Aesthet Surg J. 2003; 23(5):391–392

Graf R, Reis de Araujo LR, Rippel R, Neto LG, Pace DT, Biggs T. Reduction mammaplasty and mastopexy using the vertical scar and thoracic wall flap technique. Aesthetic Plast Surg. 2003; 27(1):6–12

Hammond DC, O'Connor EA. The lower island flap transposition (LIFT) technique for control of the upper pole in circumvertical mastopexy. Plast Reconstr Surg. 2014; 134(4):655–660

Lista F, Austin RE, Singh Y, Ahmad J. Vertical scar reduction mammaplasty. Plast Reconstr Surg. 2015; 136(1):23–25

Rohrich RJ, Thornton JF, Jakubietz RG, Jakubietz MG, Grünert JG. The limited scar mastopexy: current concepts and approaches to correct breast ptosis. Plast Reconstr Surg. 2004; 114(6):1622–1630

67 Inverted-T Mastopexy

Jacob G. Unger and G. Patrick Maxwell

Abstract

Inverted-T mastopexy is a powerful procedure to create lasting and elegant breast shape improvement. This chapter shows a step-by-step approach to reliably create predictable and aesthetic breast contours in mastopexy surgery. You will learn operative techniques, as well as preoperative guidance and postoperative care of these patients. Video is included for a visual guide to help elucidate the particular key steps of this surgery.

Keywords: Mastopexy, breast lift, autoaugmentation, breast fat grafting, inverted-T mastopexy, superior pedicle, breast ptosis repair

Key Points

- Mastopexy can be used to create a better overall breast shape and a more youthful appearance to the breast.
- Mastopexy will improve breast proportions, but will not lead to long-term upper pole fullness.

67.1 Preoperative Steps

67.1.1 History

- Take a detailed family and past medical history, especially in regards to breast cancer.
- Take a detailed past surgical history regarding any previous breast surgeries, which may impact pedicle choice.

67.1.2 Analysis

- Evaluate the breast for overall shape, degree of ptosis, skin quality, breast volume, patient height, sternal length, and breast asymmetries.
- Measure key points of sternal notch to nipple, nipple to inframammary fold (IMF), and base width to determine the best pedicle to utilize.

67.2 Operative Steps

See **Video 67.1**.

67.2.1 Top-Down Approach—Setting the Nipple Height

- Mark the IMF on each side, the lateral mammary folds, the sternal notch, and the midline.
- Mark the new nipple position preoperatively with the patient in the seated position.
- Determine ideal nipple position based on Pitanguy's point, sternal height, patient height, and overall breast volume: Usually between 20 and 23 cm of sternal notch to nipple distance (SN-N).
- Mark 2 cm above ideal nipple position for the upper aspect of the circumvertical portion of the pattern.
- Determine the pedicle to be used. Typically, for < 5 cm of elevation use superior pedicle, for 5 to 10 cm of elevation, utilize superomedial pedicle, and for >10 cm of elevation consider inferior pedicle unless already experienced with superomedial pedicle technique.
- Utilize a 13 cm circumvertical pattern for a 38 mm cookie cutter nipple, and 14 cm pattern for a 42 mm cookie cutter.
- The width of the inferior opening of your circumvertical drawing will be the future width of your vertical pillars, most commonly 4 to 6 cm apart (▶ Fig. 67.1).
- Inscribe nipple with a #15 blade after using cookie cutter around the nipple-areolar complex (NAC).
- Tailor-tack your nipple vertically into position with three staples to the top of your circumvertical drawing. First staple at 12 o'clock, and then 10 o'clock and 2 o'clock (▶ Fig. 67.2).

67.2.2 Setting the Vertical Pillars

- Take the inferior aspect of your circumvertical pattern and bring medial to lateral; this is the coning of the breast step.
- Begin to tailor-tack the skin by imbricating in a straight line from the 6 o'clock position of the nipple marching inferiorly (top-down).
- Keep the medial and lateral pillars on similar stretch. There should be physiologic tension on your staples but they should not be struggling to stay together.

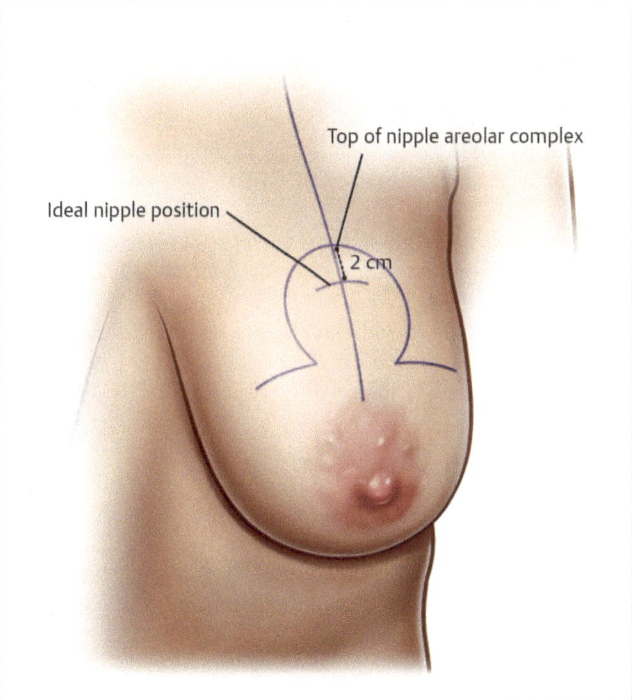

Fig. 67.1 The width of the inferior opening of your circumvertical drawing will be the future width of your vertical pillars, most commonly 4 to 6 cm apart.

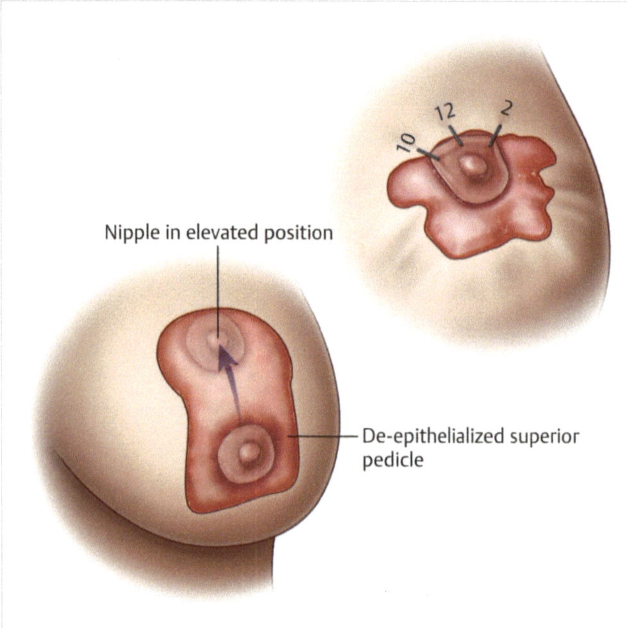

Fig. 67.2 Tailor-tack your nipple vertically into position with three staples to the top of your circumvertical drawing. First staple at 12 o'clock, and then 10 o'clock and 2 o'clock.

- Continue to create this staple line until the nipple–IMF distance is your desired length. This is best measured via cephalic-most staple to fold, which represents infra-areola to fold distance (which is nipple to IMF − 2 cm) (remember final NAC diameter is 38 mm) (▶ Fig. 67.3).

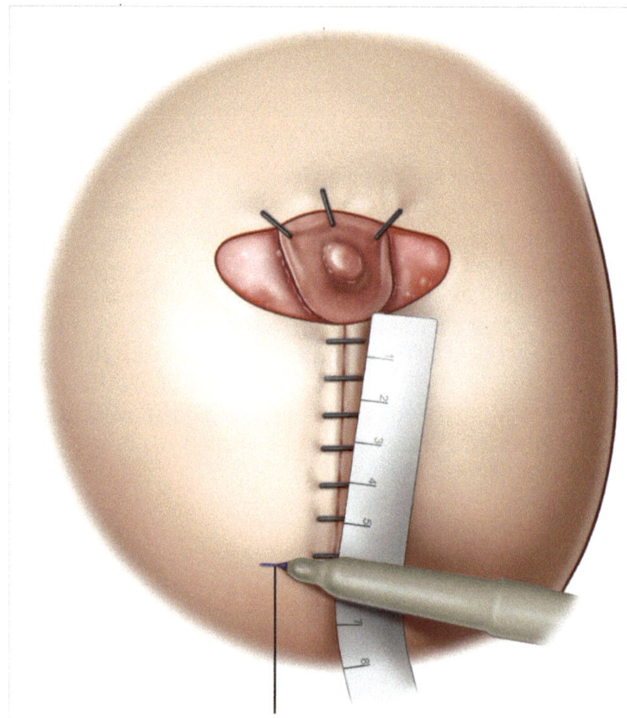

Fig. 67.3 Create a staple line until the nipple–inframammary fold (IMF) distance is your desired length. This is best measured via cephalic-most staple to fold, which represents infra-areola to fold distance (which is nipple to IMF − 2 cm) (remember final nipple-areolar complex [NAC] diameter is 38 mm).

67.2.3 Removing the Vertical Excess

- Once the nipple to inframmary fold (N-IMF) is set by imbricating the transverse excess we can then work on removal of the vertical excess.
- Begin by tacking the inferior extent of the plication and tailor-tacking this point to the IMF with two staples (one on each vertical limb).
- This will set the height of the transverse excision.
- Tailor-tack from the midline medially and laterally from the new level of the desired IMF to the actual IMF.
- Laterally if the resection requires extension lateral to the anterior axillary line, follow the lateral border of the breast cephalically to avoid creating a boxy breast.

67.2.4 Check for Symmetry

- Once tailor-tacking is performed on both sides *sit* the patient *up* to check for symmetry.
- Once you are satisfied with the overall shape and contours, lay the patient back down and use a marking pen to mark all of the tailor-tacked areas. Ensure to mark where your medial and lateral pillars meet along the IMF.
- Take all staples out and use a #10 blade to inscribe the circumvertical, vertical, and transverse incisions.

67.2.5 Excision of Tissue

- De-epithelialize the pedicle within the pattern.
- Remove the lower tissue en bloc below the pedicle down to ensure there is space for pillar re-approximation and to remove the ptotic breast tissue. This maneuver will allow for additional tissue removal from the larger side than the smaller side automatically as the fuller side additional tissue will all rest in the lower pole.
- Release the pedicle and dermis in a gradual fashion, only releasing enough soft tissue to allow for tension-free elevation of the NAC into its new position.
- Obtain meticulous hemostasis prior to closure.

67.2.6 Closure

- First suture is 2–0 PDS on CT-1 Needle 3 Point suture from superficial fascia (SFS) of the base of the vertical pillars to the IMF fascia.
- Then close the fascia of the vertical pillars with 2–0 PDS interrupted sutures.
- Close the medial and lateral flaps from SFS to the IMF.
- Close the deep dermis with 3–0 Monocryl interrupted sutures.
- Inset the nipple with 8 to 10 3–0 Monocryl deep dermals.
- Run 4–0 Monocryl subcuticular suture circumareolar, vertical, and transverse to the incisions.
- Use eight-pointed star Steri-Strips for the NAC, and along the vertical and transverse incisions as well.

67.2.7 Adjunctive Procedures

- For patients desiring slightly more fullness or an improved upper pole contour, consider fat grafting.

- For lower volume, empty breasts, utilizing an autoaugmentation technique by maintaining the inferior tissue and elevating cephalically can help increase breast projection and size modestly.
- Performed via Coleman technique with 16-gauge needle incisions and 17-gauge, 1.5 mm blunt cannulas with 10-cc syringe.
- For patients with very poor soft tissue support and dermal quality, consider dissolving mesh internal support such as GalaFLEX to help prevent lower pole stretch.

67.3 Postoperative Care

- Compressive supportive bra at all times for 6 weeks postoperative.
- Showering OK from 2 day.
- Normal activity allowed next day and walking encouraged.
- No strenuous cardio exercise for 2 to 4 weeks.
- Full release to all exercise at 6 weeks.

67.4 Case Example

This is a 42-year-old G2P2 nonsmoker woman desiring breast lift and improvement in overall breast shape. Her sternal notch to nipple distance was 28 cm and she is 5′4″. She received a superior pedicle approach with inverted-T skin pattern resection, autoaugmentation, and fat grafting to the upper poles of both breasts. Sternal notch to nipple height was set at 21 cm. These pictures are 1 year post-op. She is shown in all views. She also received an abdominoplasty at the time of her mastopexy. No other procedures were performed at the time of her mastopexy (▶ Fig. 67.4a–e).

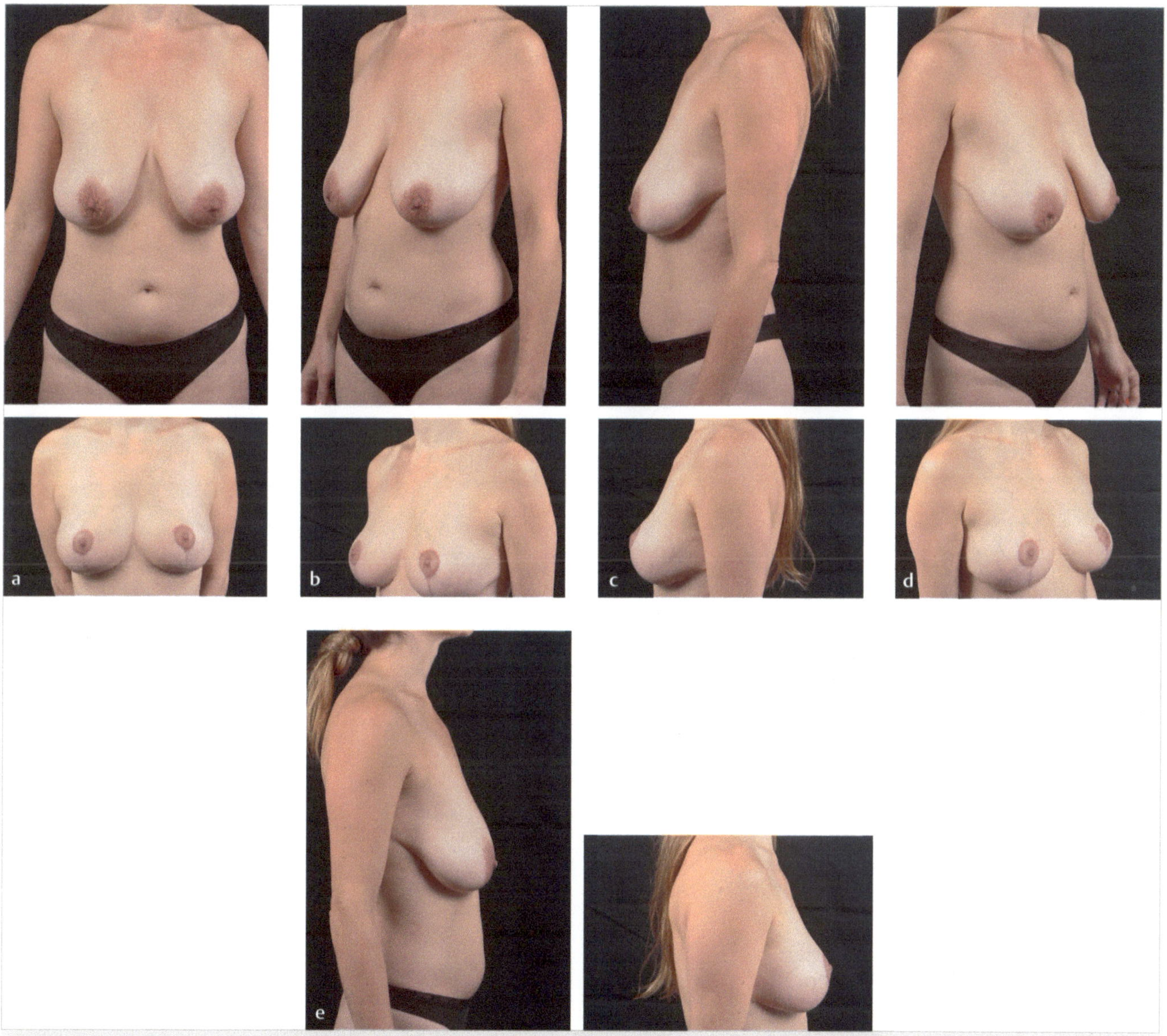

Fig. 67.4 (a–e) This is a 42-year-old G2P2 nonsmoker woman desiring breast lift and improvement in overall breast shape. Her sternal notch to nipple distance was 28 cm and she is 5′4″. She received a superior pedicle approach with inverted-T skin pattern resection, autoaugmentation, and fat grafting to the upper poles of both breasts. Sternal notch to nipple height was set at 21 cm. These pictures are 1 year post-op. She is shown in all views. She also received an abdominoplasty at the time of her mastopexy. No other procedures were performed at the time of her mastopexy.

67.5 Conclusion

Mastopexy can be achieved with a high degree of success and symmetry with tailor-tacking and checking for symmetry. Utilizing an “inverted-T” approach allows direct removal of excess tissue in both the vertical and transverse dimensions. Fat grafting is a helpful adjunct to create more upper pole volume and overall breast volume. There is no reliable way to create lasting upper pole fullness to the same extent an implant can obtain.

Further Readings

Lee MR, Unger JG, Adams WP, Jr. The tissue-based triad: a process approach to augmentation mastopexy. Plast Reconstr Surg. 2014; 134(2):215–225

Sarosiek K, Maxwell GP, Unger JG. Getting the most out of augmentation-mastopexy. Plast Reconstr Surg. 2018; 142(5):742e–759e

Wong C, Vucovich M, Rohrich R. Mastopexy and reduction mammoplasty pedicles and skin resection patterns. Plast Reconstr Surg Glob Open. 2014; 2(8):e202

68 Safe Augmentation Mastopexy

Kyle Sanniec and William P. Adams Jr.

Abstract
Augmentation mastopexy is as challenging as it is popular. It remains a difficult procedure fraught with complications even in experienced hands. The dilemma of tissue reduction (mastopexy) with tissue expansion (augmentation) have led to high revision rates, wound complications, and poor patient satisfaction. This has all led many authors to recommend staging all procedures. However, reliable and reproducible results can be achieved by following a standardized processed approach. This processed approach has led to a highly predictable aesthetic result with a very low reoperation rate. The patient selection, preoperative planning, and intraoperative nuances of this processed approach are presented, with a key toward gearing the surgeon to attaining safe, achievable, and predictable results.

Keywords: Augmentation mastopexy, single-stage augmentation mastopexy, tissue-based triad, process of augmentation mastopexy, staging criteria for augmentation mastopexy, implant mastopexy

Key Points

- The tissue-based triad in augmentation mastopexy allows for a safe and reliable one-stage procedure with high predictability and the lowest peer-reviewed published reoperation rates.
- The control of the nipple to fold length on the breast mound allows for total control of breast shape.
- Following a process-based approach to augmentation mastopexy increases consistency in delivering high-quality results for patients in a procedure that can be fraught with complications.

68.1 Preoperative Steps

68.1.1 Tissue-Based Triad (▶ Fig. 68.1, ▶ Fig. 68.2, and ▶ Fig. 68.3)

- The patients breast base width (BBW), nipple to fold (NIMF) skin stretch (SS), and vertical excess (VE) are measured and used to objectively determine which patients can undergo augmentation versus one- versus two-stage augmentation mastopexy.
  - SS < 4 *and* NIMF < 10 cm can be treated with dual-plane augmentation alone.
  - SS > 4 or NIMF > 10 cm has skin laxity warranting skin excision in addition to implant placement alone.
  - VE is the key measurement in *determining staging*, with VE > 6 cm requiring two-stage augmentation mastopexy.

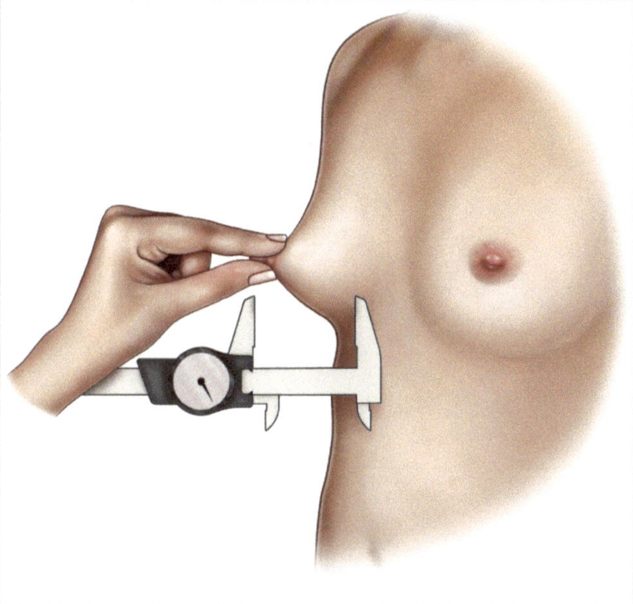

Fig. 68.1 Schematic illustration demonstrating skin stretch measurement.

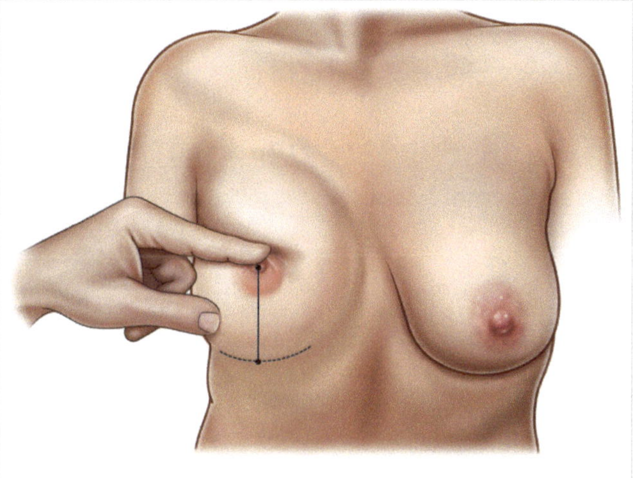

Fig. 68.2 Schematic illustration demonstrating nipple to fold measurement on maximum stretch.

68.1.2 Implant Selection

- The implants are selected with a sufficient height to fill the upper pole only, based upon the patient's breast width less 1 cm, which usually corresponds to 200 to 300 cc implants.
- The amount of breast parenchyma determines the profile of the implant.
  - Minimal breast tissue = moderate profile implant to provide volume that is missing from the breast tissue.

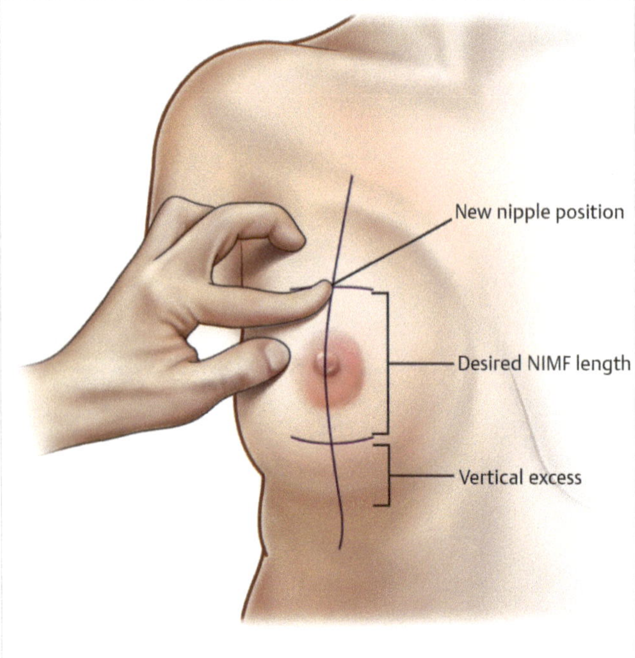

Fig. 68.3 Schematic illustration of vertical excess measurement.

- Adequate breast tissue = low or low plus profile implant to provide upper pole fullness.

68.2 Operative Steps

See **Video 68.1**.

68.2.1 Markings (▶ Fig. 68.4)

- The breast meridian, midline, and inframammary fold (IMF) are marked for reference with the patient in an upright position.
- The nipple is marked by method of Pitanguy with confirmation based on manually raising the nipple to the most aesthetically pleasing place on the breast and then marking this position.
  - The nipple position is then confirmed to be symmetric by ensuring the sternal notch to nipple is equivalent on both sides.
- The ideal NIMF is marked on stretch in an arc from this ideal nipple position. This arc will be the new inferior border of the breast.
  - All points along this arc are equidistant to the new nipple position.
- Everything below this mark is the **VE**, the additional distance between the desired nipple to fold length and the current IMF.
- The technique is called a bottom-up method as the VE determines the length of the IMF incision and the angle of divergence of the vertical limbs by superimposing the distance of the VE medially and laterally from the breast meridian.
- The new fold mark and the existing fold are marked at the point the VE length connects the two horizontal markings.

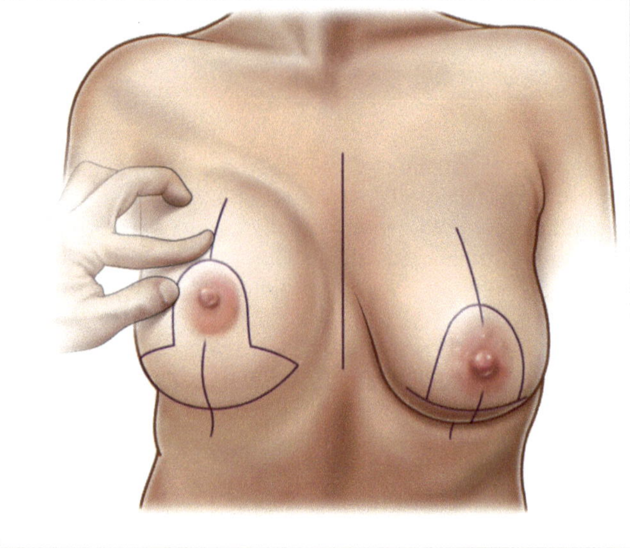

Fig. 68.4 Illustration of preoperative markings.

- The vertical limbs are marked just outside the areola from the ideal nipple position to where the lateral and medial widths of the horizontal incision start.
- A mark demonstrating the width and height of the implant is also marked to ensure the pocket is not over-dissected.

68.2.2 Augmentation

- An IMF incision within the mastopexy markings is created and a four-part dissection performed with prospective hemostasis to create a tight pocket that just fits the dimensions of the implant.
- The pocket is then prepared using the 14-point plan to decrease bacterial load on the implant.
- After the implant is placed, the superficial fascia is closed in two layers with running suture, with the second layer starting lateral to the incision to imbricate and ensure a watertight seal of the implant.

68.2.3 Mastopexy

- The bottom-up technique uses a central mound, and inverted-T incision pattern marking is confirmed to make sure the skin isn't too tight and that the vertical limbs and T point will come together.
- After the vertical and horizontal limbs are incised, the area around the central mound pedicle is de-epithelialized.
- The inferior wedge in the lower pole is removed full thickness as is some parenchyma to remove lower pole bulk on the incision site, with the exception of the Adams dermal flap that is only de-epithelialized. This flap is then used during the closure to cover the implant pocket and to allow dermal tissue under the T point should it break down.
- The skin flaps are raised medially and laterally to right above the superficial fascial system, and only raised enough to

allow the flaps to come together at the T point without much tension.

- The T point is then closed and the Adams dermal flap is pulled cranially under the T point and a three-point suture connecting the dermal flap and lateral and medial limbs is used to offload tension on the T point.
- IMF fixation sutures from the deep fascia to the superficial fascia are performed on the medial and lateral horizontal limb to pull skin and incision down into the fold.
- The vertical incision is stapled close and the ideal nipple position is measured.
  - Skin hooks on the superior and inferior portion of the vertical limb are used to get the skin on full stretch.
  - The ideal position is based off the final breast width with the NIMF approximately BW × 0.7 + 1 cm to get the ideal ratio of nipple to breast mound.
  - Marking the nipple at the end of the procedure allows for better control of optimal nipple position on the breast.

68.3 Postoperative Care

- Steri-Strips remain in place for 7 days and allow for even compression over the areola.
- Scar therapy is started once the Steri-Strips are off.

68.4 Case Example

Preoperative and postoperative images 12 months after single-stage augmentation mastopexy. The patient underwent a dual-plane augmentation with placement of 270-cc implants and then inverted-T central mound mastopexy (▶ Fig. 68.5).

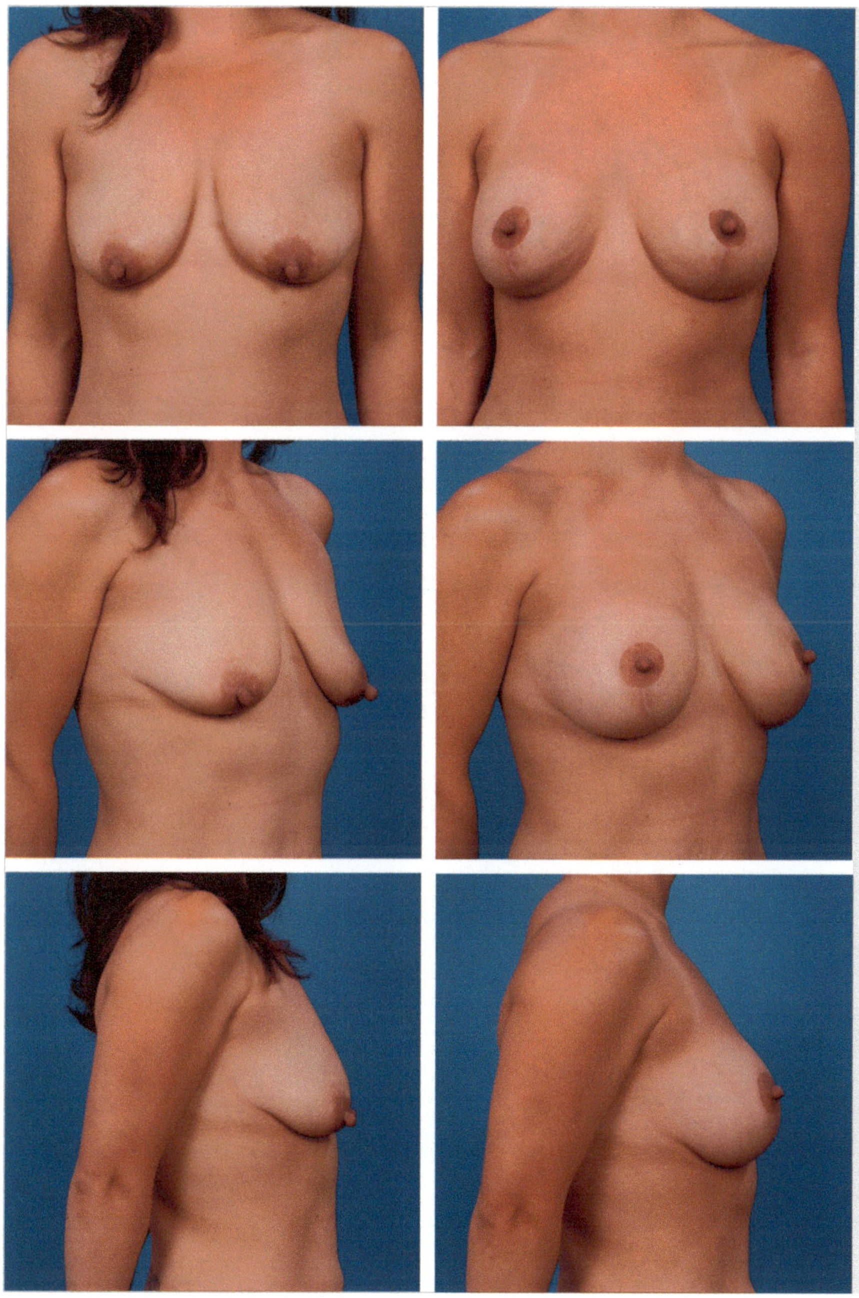

Fig. 68.5 Preoperative and postoperative images 12 months after single-stage augmentation mastopexy. The patient underwent a dual-plane augmentation with placement of 270-cc implants and then inverted-T central mound mastopexy.

68.5 Conclusion

The tissue-based triad provides objective measures to categorize which patients need augmentation versus augmentation mastopexy and whether it is safe to perform them in a one- versus two-stage procedure. Use of a process-based approach allows for a decrease in complications and enhanced outcomes. A systematic approach for augmentation mastopexy allows the surgeon a framework to base decisions and a streamlined process for efficient surgical planning and execution.

Further Readings

Adams WP, Jr, Small KH. The process of breast augmentation with special focus on patient education, patient selection and implant selection. Clin Plast Surg. 2015; 42(4):413–426

Beale EW, Ramanadham S, Harrison B, Rasko Y, Armijo B, Rohrich RJ. Achieving predictability in augmentation mastopexy. Plast Reconstr Surg. 2014; 133(3): 284e–292e

Lee MR, Unger JG, Adams WP, Jr. The tissue-based triad: a process approach to augmentation mastopexy. Plast Reconstr Surg. 2014; 134(2):215–225

Sanniec K, Adams WP, Jr. The tissue-based triad in augmentation mastopexy: single-stage technical refinements. Aesthet Surg J. 2019; 39(12):1331–1341

Tebbetts JB. A process for quantifying aesthetic and functional breast surgery: I. Quantifying optimal nipple position and vertical and horizontal skin excess for mastopexy and breast reduction. Plast Reconstr Surg. 2013; 132 (1):65–73

69 Refining Augmentation Mastopexy

Daniel J. Gould, Nathaniel L. Villanueva, and W. Grant Stevens

Abstract

Augmentation mastopexy has always been viewed as a difficult procedure due to the combination of two seemingly conflicting goals, lifting the breast by removing skin from the envelope while adding volume with an implant to provide superior pole fullness. Arguably, it is common to add volume and correct ptosis in many procedures in plastic surgery and over the last 20 years several groups have demonstrated safety and excellent results in augmentation mastopexy. Given the difficulty of this procedure, secondary mastopexy augmentation is common with a rate of 16.9%, with 5% desiring implant size change and 5% due to poor scaring. The procedure does not stop the aging process—over time patients often require revision and refinement. The purpose of this chapter is to discuss techniques and principles for secondary augmentation mastopexy revision.

Keywords: Breast lift, augmentation mastopexy, secondary augmentation mastopexy

Key Points

- Refinement of augmentation mastopexy is often a difficult procedure—identify common reasons to perform secondary augmentation mastopexy.
- Let patients define success in the preoperative consult.
- Secondary mastopexy augmentation should utilize aggressive lifting of the breast envelope while preserving blood flow to the nipple—avoid complications.
- Implant and breast size are critical factors in downsizing or upsizing.
- Different techniques and materials may help provide long-lasting results.
- Know how to treat complications.

69.1 Preoperative Steps

- Discuss the plan for surgery and have the patient define success.
- Know the blood supply to the breast and nipple (▸ Fig. 69.1a, b) and how previous incisions may have compromised nipple blood supply.
- Identify the sternal notch to nipple distance and plan the amount of nipple translation needed based on the Pitanguy's point (or inframammary fold [IMF]).
- Mark the meridian of the breast and the breast footprint. Move the nipple up toward the meridian.
- Avoid placing the implant too high and the nipple too low—set your implant at the correct height during the augmentation step by designing the correct pocket on table; do not accept implants that "will settle" with time or a bandeau.
- Design the skin excision based on a planned nipple to IMF (N:IMF) distance of 6 to 8 cm.
- Use a pinch test to identify the safe amount of skin that can be excised, both in the vertical and horizontal direction.
- The authors prefer an owl-shaped skin incision to address vertical correction as well as horizontal excess; there are several options (▸ Fig. 69.2).
- Submuscular implants are safest, as they preserve myocutaneous perforators to the breast—avoid subglandular or subfascial augmentation.
- In revision mastopexy augmentation, do not convert a previous subglandular implant to a subpectoral pocket.
- Breast skin flaps should be no less than 1 cm thick; limit skin undermining.
- Implant selection is based on desired goals, breast footprint, and choice of texture versus smooth (all smooth now).
- Internal bra via laser de-epithelialization or through use of GalaFLEX or GalaFORM or other mesh if needed.

69.2 Operative Steps

- Utilize permissive normotension; inject with local anesthesia before prep.
- Plan all skin incisions and make incision around the nipple.
- Make a vertical incision through the breast parenchyma down to the breast implant pocket—preserve a cuff of tissue caudally (at the base) for closure and to avoid a T-junction if possible.
- Preserving blood flow to the nipple is paramount; so after the initial skin incision, steps are taken to protect the vascularity (Hitch Stitch and Goalpost).
- Excise the implant capsule if needed or create a neosubpectoral pocket if needed to recreate a tight implant pocket, in order to account for significant downsizing or other implant malposition (▸ Fig. 69.3a, b).
- Select the new implant and utilize sizers to confirm ideal position.
- Place implant and close deep fascia then tailor-tack again.
- Utilize acellular dermal matrices at this point if needed for improved aesthetic result or to reduce recurrent capsular contracture.
- Commit to the inferior skin incision and recut the proposed nipple location.
- Release and undermine minimally around the future base of the nipple and vertical limbs.
- Approximate vertical pillars deep to cover the dual-plane breast implant, to decrease the horizontal width of the breast and to add support to the mastopexy.
- Place a corset mesh at this point if desired, tabbed or nontabbed, custom shaped or preformed.

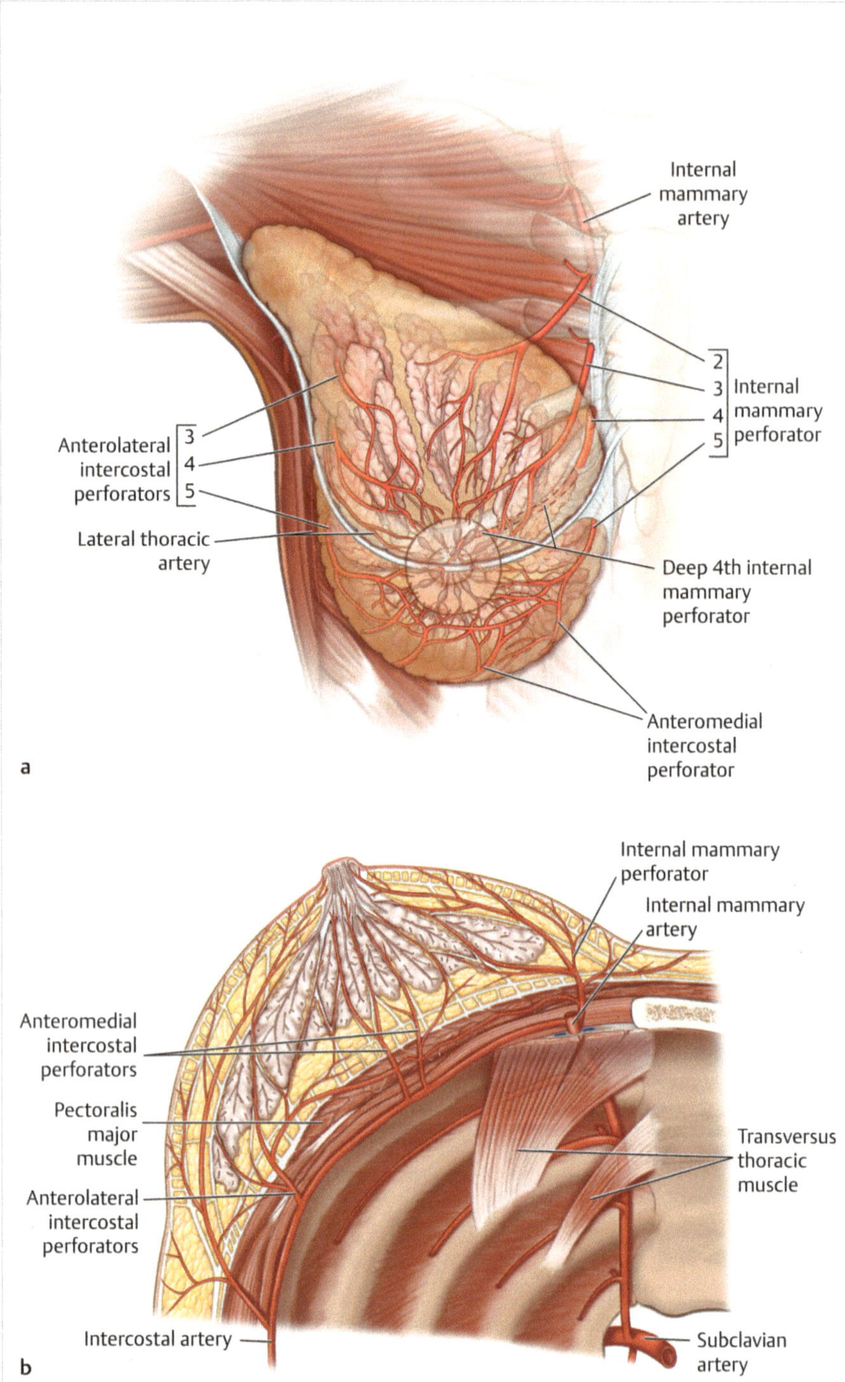

Fig. 69.1 (a, b) Vascular supply of the breast.

- Close all incisions with deep and subcuticular sutures. No drains are needed, and no external or removable sutures are needed typically but this is at the discretion of the surgeon.

69.3 Postoperative Care

- Postoperative monitoring for nipple viability; use nitropaste if needed. See on post-op day 1, and change xeroform. RTC day 3 and then at 1 week.
- Supportive wrap without binders.
- Standard scar management.
- Wait to begin implant massage till postoperative 2 week.

69.4 Case Example

This 43-year-old mother complained of breast asymmetry and right breast capsular contracture. She had undergone right breast subglandular augmentation for breast asymmetry 25 years earlier. She underwent right capsulectomy and

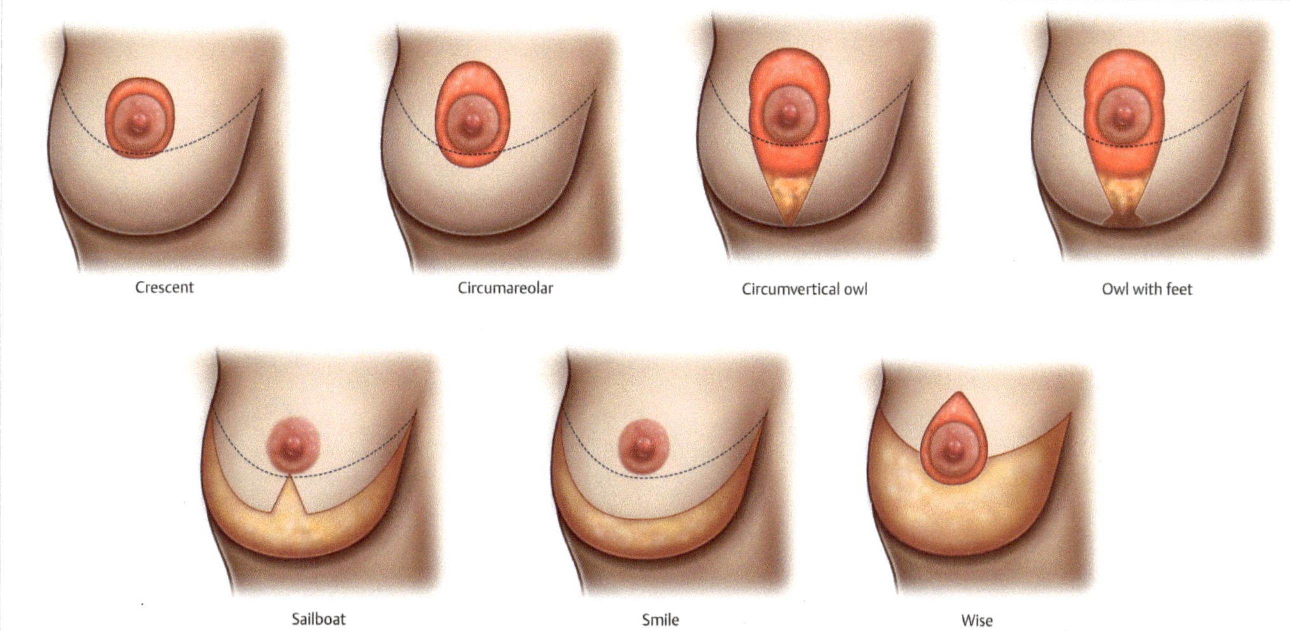

Fig. 69.2 There are many options for revisional incisions—pick the one that allows control of the skin envelope but preserves most blood flow.

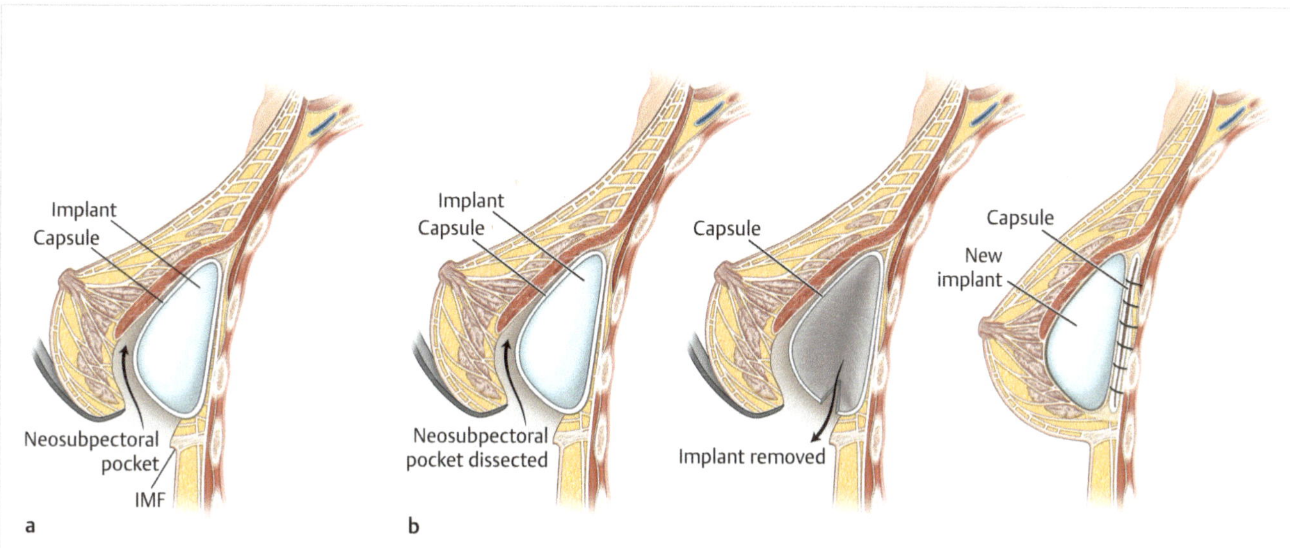

Fig. 69.3 **(a)** The neosubpectoral pocket is created with the implant left in situ to facilitate dissection. **(b)** After the neosubpectoral pocket is dissected, the old implant is removed and the anterior capsule is tacked loosely. The inferior capsule reinforces the inframammary fold.

explantation of a ruptured gel implant. After 2 months, she had one-stage bilateral breast augmentation with 275-cc Moderate Plus Profile Mentor gel implants in a submuscular pocket and bilateral mastopexy with inverted-T scars. She is shown (▶ Fig. 69.4a, c, e) before and (▶ Fig. 69.4b, d, f) 6 months following the secondary augmentation and mastopexy procedure.

69.5 Conclusion

Mastopexy augmentation can be performed safely as a primary or secondary procedure by preserving the blood supply to the nipple. Careful dissection and appropriate implant selection make the biggest impact.

See **Video 69.1**.

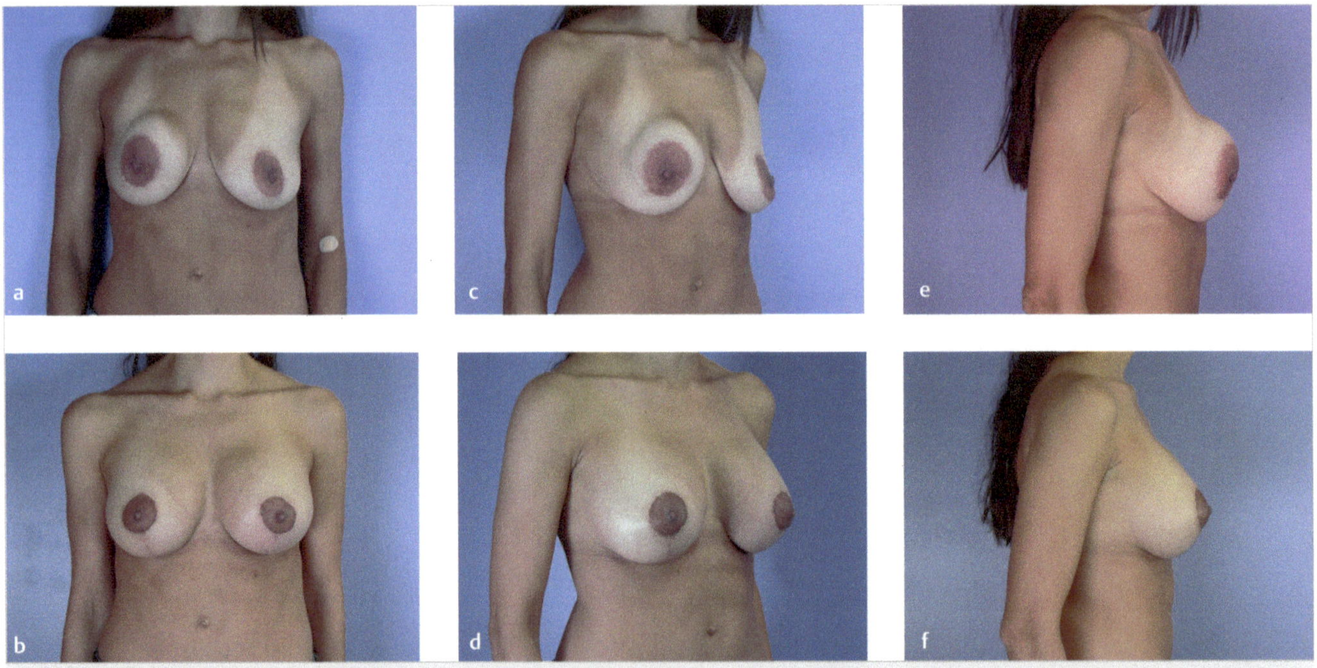

Fig. 69.4 (a–f) This 43-year-old mother complained of breast asymmetry and right breast capsular contracture. She had undergone right breast subglandular augmentation for breast asymmetry 25 years earlier. She underwent right capsulectomy and explantation of a ruptured gel implant. After 2 months she had one-stage bilateral breast augmentation with 275-cc Moderate Plus Profile Mentor gel implants in a submuscular pocket and bilateral mastopexy with inverted-T scars. She is shown **(a, c, e)** before and **(b, d, f)** 6 months following the secondary augmentation and mastopexy procedure.

Further Readings

Georgiade NG, Georgiade GS. Aesthetic surgery of the breast. W.B. Saunders Company; 1990

Messa CA, Messa CA. One-stage augmentation mastopexy: a retrospective ten-year review of 2183 consecutive procedures. Aesthet Surg J. 2019; 39(12):1352–1367

Sanniec K, Adams WP. The tissue-based triad in augmentation mastopexy: single-stage technical refinements. Aesthet Surg J. 2019; 39(12):1331–1341

Spear SL, Pelletiere CV, Menon N. One-stage augmentation combined with mastopexy: aesthetic results and patient satisfaction. Aesthetic Plast Surg. 2004; 28 (5):259–267

Tebbetts JB. Augmentation mastopexy. In: Augmentation Mammaplasty. Amsterdam: Mosby Elsevier; 2010:501–551

70 Augmentation Mastopexy with and without Fat Grafting

Rod J. Rohrich and Dinah Wan

Abstract

Single-stage augmentation mastopexy can be performed in a safe and reliable manner using the Wise pattern, inferior pedicle/central mound technique. By making precise preoperative markings, the surgeon can commit to the mastopexy incisions without the need for tailor-tacking. Implant size is limited to <300 cc to facilitate tension-free closure and optimize long-term results. Autologous fat grafting can be performed in conjunction to further enhance breast contour.

Keywords: Augmentation, mastopexy, augmentation mastopexy, breast implant, fat grafting, fat transfer

Key Points

- Single-stage augmentation mastopexy can be performed in a predictable manner using the Wise pattern, inferior pedicle/central mound technique.
- Implants are used to restore upper pole fullness, rather than volume enlargement.
- Autologous fat grafting may be used in lieu of, or in addition to, implants to further enhance breast contour and cleavage.

70.1 Preoperative Steps

70.1.1 Analysis

- Patients with mild to moderate degree of ptosis (grade 1 to 2) and requiring 4 cm or less of nipple elevation are favorable candidates for single-stage augmentation mastopexy.
- Patients with severe degree of ptosis (grade 3) or requiring greater than 4 to 6 cm of nipple elevation should be assessed for two-stage augmentation mastopexy.
- Obese or massive weight loss patients and prior smokers should be evaluated for two-stage augmentation mastopexy.
- Surgery should not be offered to patients who are actively smoking.
- Implant selection should be limited to low or moderate profile implants no larger than 300 cc.

70.2 Operative Steps

See **Video 70.1**.

70.2.1 Markings

- With the patient in standing position, mark the breast meridians.
- Mark Pitanguy's point by transposing the inframammary fold onto the breast meridian. Confirm the distance from sternal notch to Pitanguy's point is approximately 21 cm bilaterally.
- Mark 8- to 9-cm vertical limbs from Pitanguy's point. Keep the splay angle narrow, just spanning the width of the areola.
- Mark the inframammary fold, curving up 30 degrees laterally at the level of the anterior axillary fold.
- While gently lifting the breast, draw a straight line medially and laterally from the vertical limbs to the inframammary fold.

70.2.2 Isolate Inferior Pedicle/Central Mound

- Incise around the areola using a 42-mm cookie cutter.
- Make all Wise pattern incisions.
- De-epithelialize the inferior pedicle, maintaining a wide base.
- Preserve a superior bridge of de-epithelialized tissue above the areola.

70.2.3 Elevate Skin Flaps

- Excise medial and lateral wedges of breast as needed for symmetry.
- Elevate 2-cm thick medial and lateral breast skin flaps (▶ Fig. 70.1). Limit dissection above the level of the areola.
- Undermine skin flaps for 4 to 5 cm, or just enough to gain mobility for closure.

70.2.4 Create Subpectoral Pocket

- Dissect lateral to the inferior pedicle parenchyma to identify the inferolateral border of the pectoralis major muscle.

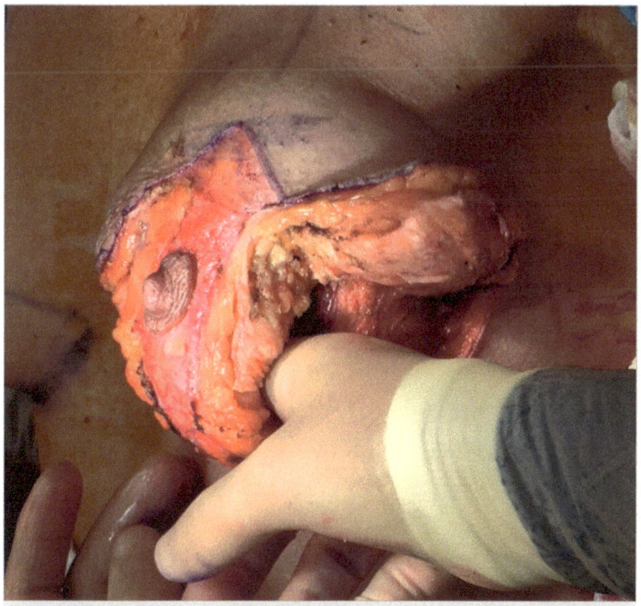

Fig. 70.1 Undermining of thick lateral breast skin flap with preservation of inferior pedicle/central mound and a superior bridge of de-epithelialized tissue.

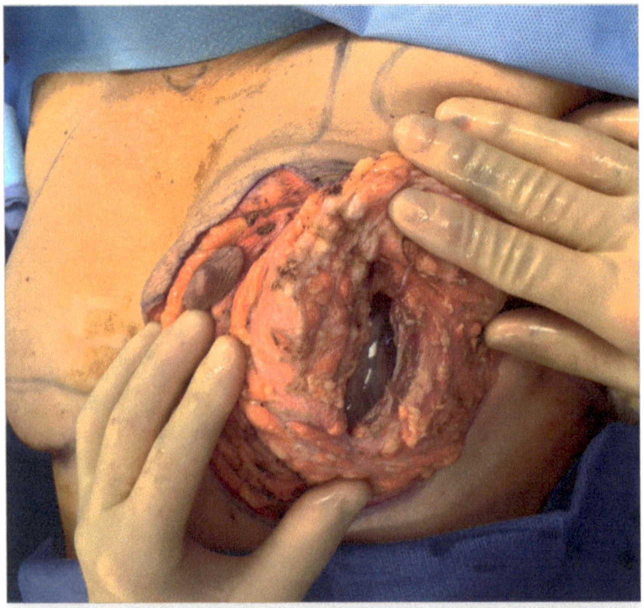

Fig. 70.2 Implant placement in the subpectoral pocket via a split incision in the lateral two-thirds of the pectoralis major muscle. The lateral pectoralis muscle serves as a lateral support sling for the implant pocket.

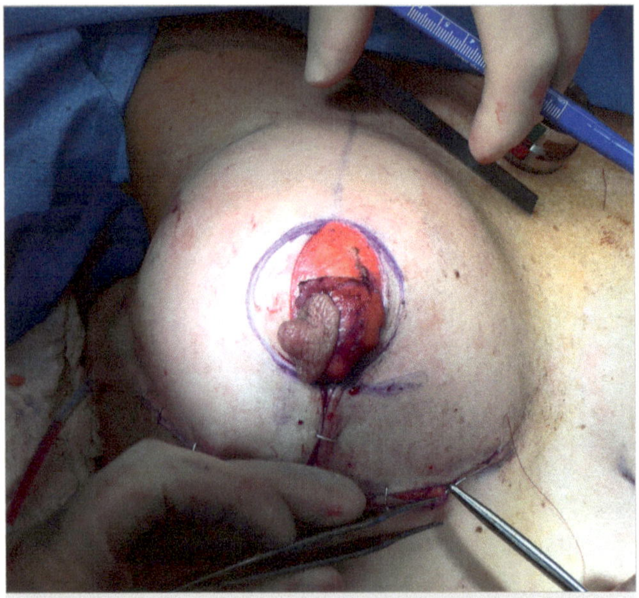

Fig. 70.3 The lower border of the areolar inset is marked 4 to 5 cm above the inframammary incision.

- Split the pectoralis major muscle at the lateral two-thirds along the direction of the muscle fibers (▶ Fig. 70.2).
- Elevate the subpectoral pocket from lateral to medial.
- Release the inferior attachments of the pectoralis major to create a dual-plane pocket.

70.2.5 Place Sizer/Implant

- Obtain hemostasis.
- Irrigate the subpectoral pocket with saline and then with triple-antibiotic solution.
- Place sizer/implant and tailor-tack breast to assess closure. If needed, downsize the implant (<300 cc) or release skin flaps further to obtain a tension-free closure.
- Place a 15-French drain in the subpectoral pocket, exiting the lateral inframammary fold.

70.2.6 Closure and Areolar Inset

- Tailor-tack the closed breast.
- Mark the inferior border of the areola at a distance of 4 to 5 cm from the inframammary fold to account for lower pole stretch over time (▶ Fig. 70.3).
- Inset the areola with a 38- to 40-mm cookie cutter.
- Complete closure of the horizontal and vertical incisions in a layered fashion.

70.2.7 Fat Grafting (if indicated)

- Infiltrate the medial thighs or abdomen with 200 to 300 cc of 0.25% lidocaine with epinephrine.
- Use a 3- to 3.5-mm liposuction cannula to harvest fat into an "in-line" collection canister. Drain off unwanted crystalloid.
- Load fat into 60-cc syringes attached to 14-gauge Coleman cannula for injection.
- Inject via multiple entry sites along the inframammary fold. Use a fanning pattern and keep the cannula moving at all times.
- Direct most of fat injection in the superomedial pole to improve cleavage. Avoid injection around the areola or in the central mound/inferior pedicle.
- A total of 100 to 200 cc of fat is injected in the subcutaneous space of each breast (and not directly into the breast tissue).

70.3 Postoperative Care

- Drains are removed after output is less than 30 cc over a 24-hour period (usually in 2–5 days).
- A supportive bra should be worn after surgery. Patients may transition to underwire bra after 6 weeks.
- Scar therapy is initiated at 2 to 3 weeks.
- Strenuous activity and exercise are avoided until 3 weeks after surgery.
- Smoking cessation must be continued.

70.4 Case Example

A 36-year-old female underwent single-stage augmentation mastopexy using 175 cc of moderate profile silicone gel implants. Preoperative and postoperative photos at 3 months are shown (▶ Fig. 70.4a–c and ▶ Fig. 70.5a–c).

70.5 Conclusion

Precise preoperative markings using 8- to 9-cm vertical limbs and a broad pedicle base allow the surgeon to commit to mastopexy incisions without tailor-tacking in single-stage augmentation mastopexy. Use of small subpectoral implants (<300 cc)

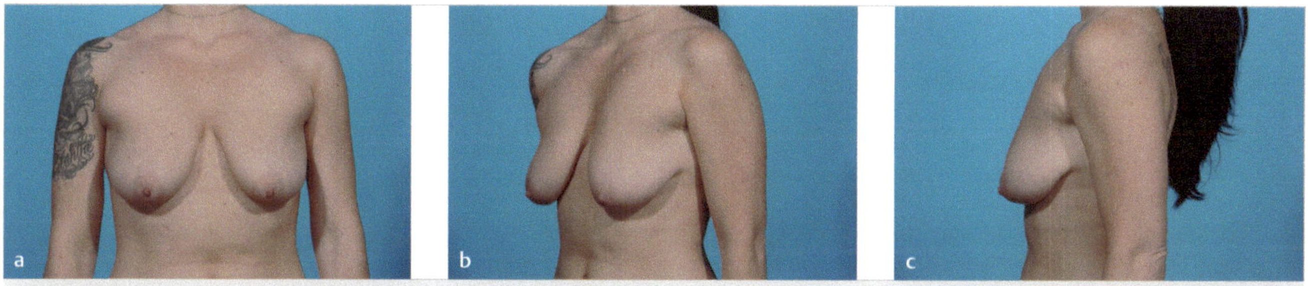

Fig. 70.4 Preoperative photos of single-stage augmentation mastopexy using 175 cc of moderate profile silicone gel implants: **(a)** frontal, **(b)** oblique, and **(c)** lateral views.

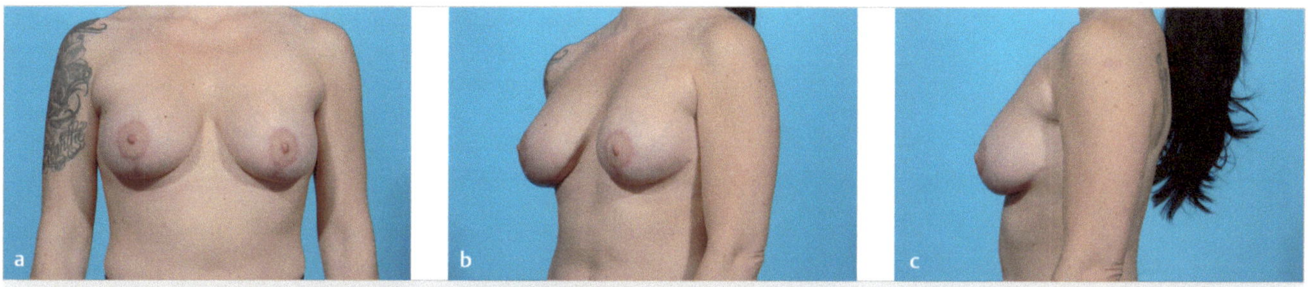

Fig. 70.5 Postoperative photos 3 months after single-stage augmentation mastopexy using 175 cc of moderate profile silicone gel implants: **(a)** frontal, **(b)** oblique, and **(c)** lateral views.

is key to achieving tension-free closure and consistent long-term results. By limiting skin flap undermining and periareolar dissection to only the amount needed to redrape the skin envelope, blood supply is maximized to the skin flaps and nipples. Autologous fat grafting can be performed with mastopexy to enhance breast contour and cleavage.

Acknowledgments

The authors would like to express special appreciation to Erez Dayan, MD and Amy Xue, MD for their assistance with the video.

Further Readings

Beale EW, Ramanadham S, Harrison B, Rasko Y, Armijo B, Rohrich RJ. Achieving predictability in augmentation mastopexy. Plast Reconstr Surg. 2014; 133(3): 284e–292e

Del Vecchio D, Rohrich RJ. A classification of clinical fat grafting: different problems, different solutions. Plast Reconstr Surg. 2012; 130(3):511–522

Kerfant N, Henry AS, Hu W, Marchac A, Auclair E. Subfascial primary breast augmentation with fat grafting: a review of 156 cases. Plast Reconstr Surg. 2017; 139(5): 1080e–1085e

Khavanin N, Jordan SW, Rambachan A, Kim JY. A systematic review of single-stage augmentation-mastopexy. Plast Reconstr Surg. 2014; 134(5):922–931

Rohrich RJ, Parker TH, III. Aesthetic management of the breast after explantation: evaluation and mastopexy options. Plast Reconstr Surg. 2007; 120(1):312–315

71 Vertical Scar Breast Reduction

Ryan E. Austin, Jamil Ahmad, and Frank Lista

Abstract
Vertical scar breast reduction is a reliable technique for short-scar reduction mammaplasty which aims to improve symptomatic mammary hypertrophy and enhance the long-term shape of the breasts while minimizing visible scarring on the breast. This chapter will review our surgical technique for performing vertical scar breast reduction in a safe manner with reproducible outcomes.

Keywords: Breast reduction, liposuction, reduction mammaplasty, short scar, vertical scar

Key Points

- Vertical scar breast reduction aims to improve symptomatic mammary hypertrophy while enhancing the long-term shape of the breasts with minimal scarring.
- Postoperative breast size will likely remain larger by using a vertical scar technique. Patients with significant mammary hypertrophy desiring a small postoperative breast size may not be ideal candidates for this procedure.
- It is commonly combined with liposuction of the lateral chest and axillary roll to improve chest contour and aesthetic outcome of the breast reduction.

71.1 Preoperative Steps

71.1.1 Patient Selection

- Vertical scar breast reduction is a versatile procedure that can be adapted to the majority of patients seeking reduction mammaplasty.
  - Patients with severe mammary hypertrophy desiring a very small postoperative breast size are not suitable candidates for this technique.
- Symptomatic mammary hypertrophy can significantly impact patient's quality of life. Patients presenting with two or more of the following symptoms typically show the greatest improvement from breast reduction:
  - Upper back pain.
  - Neck pain.
  - Shoulder pain.
  - Arm pain.
  - Upper extremity numbness.
  - Skin rashes.
  - Bra strap grooving.
- We do not perform this procedure on patients with a body mass index (BMI) ≥35.0 kg/m^2 or on active smokers due to a significantly higher risk of complications.
- Preoperative mammography is not required prior to vertical scar breast reduction; national or regional screening guidelines for mammography should be followed.

71.1.2 Surgical Markings (▶ Fig. 71.1)

- Mark the midline of the chest and the inframammary fold (IMF).
- Central axis of the breast is marked by drawing a straight line from the midpoint of the clavicle (7–8 cm lateral to midline) through the nipple-areolar complex (NAC).
- Level of the IMF is transposed anteriorly onto the breast and marked; this represents the new location of the superior border of the NAC (point A).
  - Height of the point A marking is transposed to the contralateral breast to avoid asymmetry of the NAC as a result of IMF asymmetry.
  - If breast size asymmetry is present (≥100 g), point A on the larger side should be marked 1 to 2 cm lower than the smaller side to account for differential unweighting of the breasts.
- Inferior extent of the planned skin excision is marked 2 to 4 cm above the IMF (point B).
  - This helps prevent migration of the vertical scar onto the chest.
  - The larger the reduction the more superior elevation of the IMF that will occur, so a greater distance should be left between the IMF and point B.
- Site for the new NAC is drawn as a mosque dome starting at point A and extending to points C and D.
  - It is drawn so that when points C and D are brought together, the mosque dome forms a circle.
- Vertical limbs are drawn as curved lines extending from point B to points C and D.

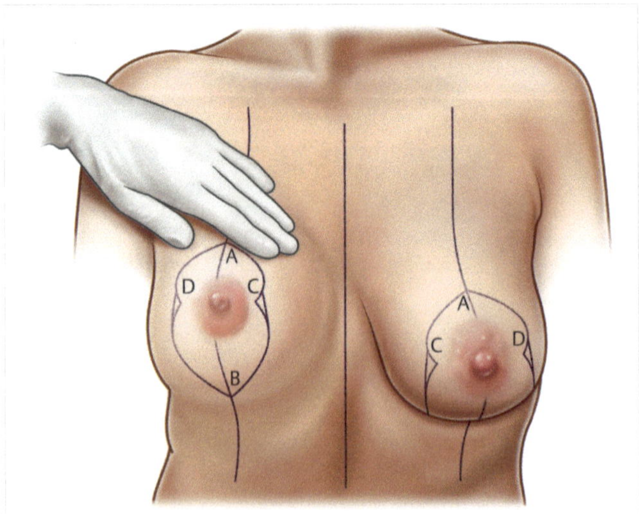

Fig. 71.1 Illustration of the skin markings for vertical scar mastopexy with autoaugmentation flap. ***Point A*** represents the new location of the superior border of the nipple-areolar complex (NAC). ***Point B*** is the inferior extent of the vertical scar, located 2 to 4 cm above the inframammary fold (IMF). ***Points C and D***, the blocking triangles, should create a circle of the mosque-dome pattern when brought together.

- Medial and lateral displacement of the breast can assist in approximating these lines.
- Inferior extent of the vertical scar should have a "V" shape to minimize dog-ear formation.
- Blocking triangles at points C and D prevent a "teardrop deformity" of the NAC.
- Areas for liposuction of the lateral chest and axillary roll are marked.

71.2 Operative Steps

See **Video 71.1**.

71.2.1 Infiltration

- Stab incision made just superior to point B within planned resection margins; tumescent solution (1 L of Ringer's Lactate + 1 mL of epinephrine 1:1,000) infiltrated under the planned vertical incisions and throughout the breast parenchyma, lateral chest, and axillary roll.
  - Infiltration performed using the simultaneous separation tumescence (SST) technique with a 4-mm exploded-tip cannula and power-assisted liposuction (PAL).
  - Each breast is typically infiltrated with approximately 500 mL of tumescent solution.

71.2.2 Pedicle Selection

- Breast tourniquet is applied to maintain tension on the skin.
- New NAC is outlined using a circular metal washer (approximately 44 mm diameter) centered over the nipple.
- If any part of the new areola lies superior to an imaginary line drawn between the blocking triangles (points C and D), a superior pedicle is used. If all of the new areola lies inferior to this line, a superomedial pedicle is used (▶ Fig. 71.2).
  - If the NAC is positioned medially, a superolateral pedicle may be required to allow for rotation and insetting.
- The selected pedicle is drawn with a 2.5 cm border around the edge of the new areola.
  - For a superomedial pedicle, a 1:2 width-to-length ratio of the pedicle should be maintained to preserve blood supply to the new NAC.

71.2.3 Glandular Resection

- Planned pedicle is de-epithelialized with the breast tourniquet in place.
  - It is important to leave the deep dermis intact to minimize injury to the subdermal vascular supply.
- Excision is performed en bloc using #20 blade scalpel, following the preoperative skin markings.
- Dermoglandular pedicle is raised maintaining a flap thickness of at least 2.5 cm.
  - Perforator vessels to the superior and superomedial pedicles are approximately 1 to 1.5 cm deep to the dermis; raising a 2.5 cm thick pedicle will protect the neurovascular supply while allowing for maximum parenchymal volume reduction.
- Medial parenchymal pillar is developed by incising along the medial limb of the vertical pattern straight down to a level just above pectoralis fascia.

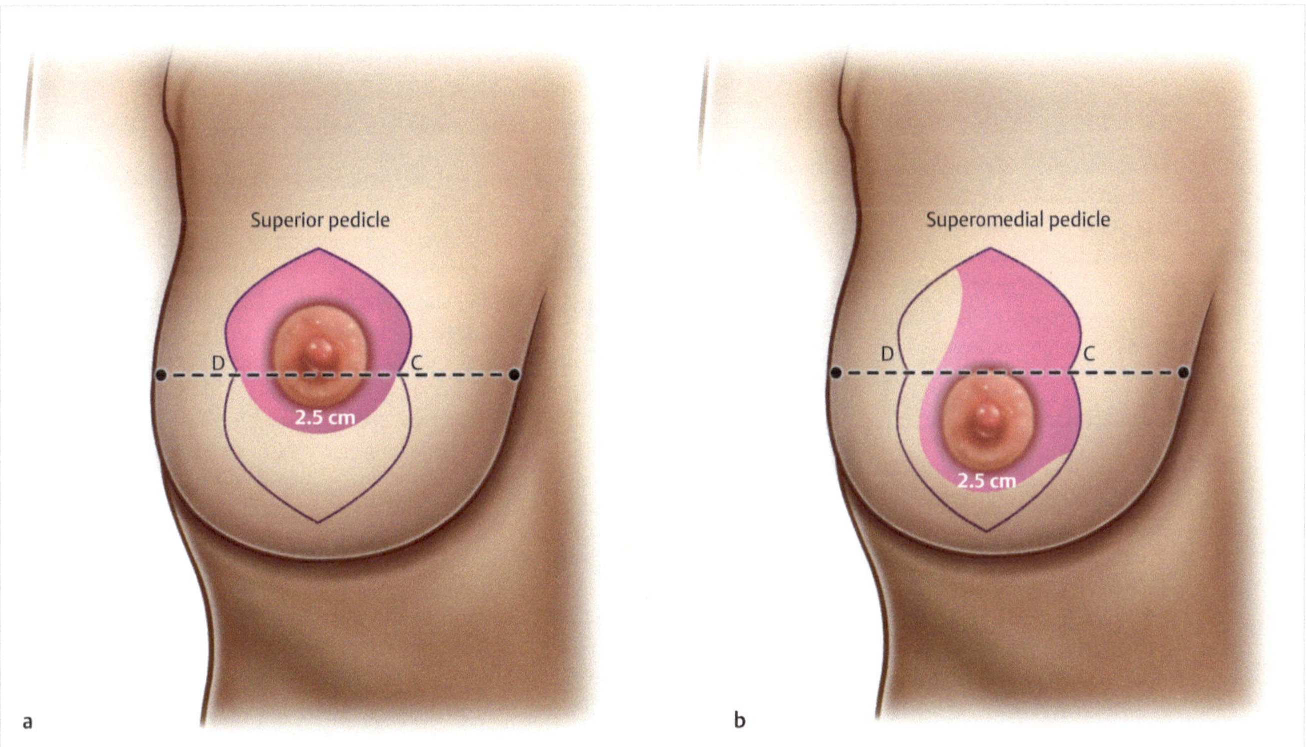

Fig. 71.2 Illustration of dermoglandular pedicle selection. If any part of the new areola lies superior to an imaginary line drawn between the blocking triangles (points C and D), a superior pedicle is used **(a)**. If all of the new areola lies inferior to this line, a superomedial pedicle is used **(b)**. The selected pedicle is drawn with a 2.5 cm border around the edge of the new areola.

   - This maintains medial breast fullness and a better breast aesthetic.
- Lateral limb of the vertical pattern is incised to a depth of 2.5 cm. The lateral parenchymal pillar is developed by maintaining this 2.5 cm flap thickness as dissection is carried toward the lateral breast border.
   - Reduction volume can be adjusted by leaving a greater thickness to the lateral pillar; lateral pillar should never be less than 2.5 cm in thickness to prevent contour and shape abnormalities.
- Tissue to be resected is elevated off the pectoralis fascia from inferior to superior.
   - Once freed from the pectoralis fascia, inferiorly directed retraction on the resection specimen allows for more extensive parenchymal excision from the superior and superolateral poles.
      - This is a useful technique when trying to maximize reduction volume.
- Resection is completed by connecting the medial, lateral, and superior glandular incisions.
- Tissue between the inferior extent of the vertical incision and IMF is thinned to minimize dog-ear formation.
   - A layer of fat should be left on the pectoralis fascia to prevent skin tethering.
- Once excision is complete, the medial, superior, and lateral skin flaps should feel smooth in contour with even tissue thickness.

71.2.4 Liposuction

- Liposuction is performed using a 4-mm, three-hole blunt cannula on PAL according to the separation, aspiration, and fat equalization (SAFE) liposuction technique.
- Liposuction of the lateral chest wall and axillary roll is performed through the vertical incision following glandular resection.
   - Avoid direct liposuction of the medial and lateral pillars; these are required for later glandular reshaping.
   - Avoid overaggressive liposuction of the transition between the lateral breast and the anterolateral chest.
      - Lateral chest wall skin is advanced onto the lateral breast during closure; aggressive liposuction may create contour deformities of the lateral breast.

71.2.5 Glandular Reshaping

- Medial and lateral pillars are reapproximated using inverted #1 Vicryl sutures (Ethicon, Inc., Somerville, NJ) placed through the breast capsule; two parenchymal pillar sutures are typically required.
   - Inferior pillar suture should be no closer than 4 cm from the inferior end of the incision to prevent creating a standing-cone deformity which predisposes to dog-ear formation.
   - Superior pillar suture should be no closer than 2 cm from the NAC to avoid distortion.
- NAC is rotated into position and inset prior to closure of the vertical incision:
   - NAC is inset with 3-0 Monocryl Plus (Ethicon, Inc., Somerville, NJ) interrupted inverted deep dermal sutures at the 3, 6, 9, and 12 o'clock positions.
   - NAC is closed using a 3-0 Monocryl Plus (Ethicon, Inc., Somerville, NJ) continuous intradermal suture.
- 3-0 Monocryl Plus (Ethicon, Inc., Somerville, NJ) four-point inverted deep dermal box sutures are used to gather the skin of the vertical incision and shorten the length of the vertical scar to approximately 8 to 10 cm.
   - Box sutures are placed starting at the inferior apex of the vertical incision and working toward the NAC; each suture should be placed immediately adjacent to the previous suture to maximize gathering.
   - Box sutures often cause horizontal pleats along the vertical incision; these must be corrected with inverted deep dermal sutures to prevent creating permanent horizontal lines within the vertical scar.
   - Skin within 2 cm of the areola is not gathered to prevent distortion of the areola.
- The remainder of the wound is closed with 3-0 Monocryl Plus (Ethicon, Inc., Somerville, NJ) interrupted inverted deep dermal sutures.
- Skin staples are used along the vertical wound for final closure.
- Breast skin medial and lateral to incision is injected with 10 mL of 0.5% bupivacaine with 1:200,000 epinephrine for postoperative pain relief.
- Incisions are dressed with a paraffin-impregnated antiseptic gauze, dry gauze, and abdominal pads; patient is placed into a postsurgical bra.

71.3 Postoperative Steps

- All patients are discharged home on the day of the procedure (postoperative day [POD] #0).
- Patients return on POD #1; they are instructed to wash their incisions daily with soap and water.
- Skin staples are removed on POD #5/6 and replaced with Steri-Strips (3M, St. Paul, MN).
- Patients start massage to liposuction sites and breast at 1 week postoperatively.
- Patients are instructed to wear a postsurgical bra at all times for 4 weeks following surgery.
- Avoid strenuous physical activity (including exercise) for 4 weeks following surgery.
- Silicone bandages are applied to the incisions once all wounds have completely healed for 4 to 6 months postoperatively.

71.4 Case Example

Pre- and postoperative views of a 51-year-old patient 6 months following vertical scar breast reduction in the (a) anteroposterior (AP), (b) oblique, and (c) lateral views. Breast reduction was performed using a superior dermoglandular pedicle bilaterally. On the right side, 415 g of tissue was resected along with 400 cc of liposuction from the lateral chest wall. On the left side, 340 g

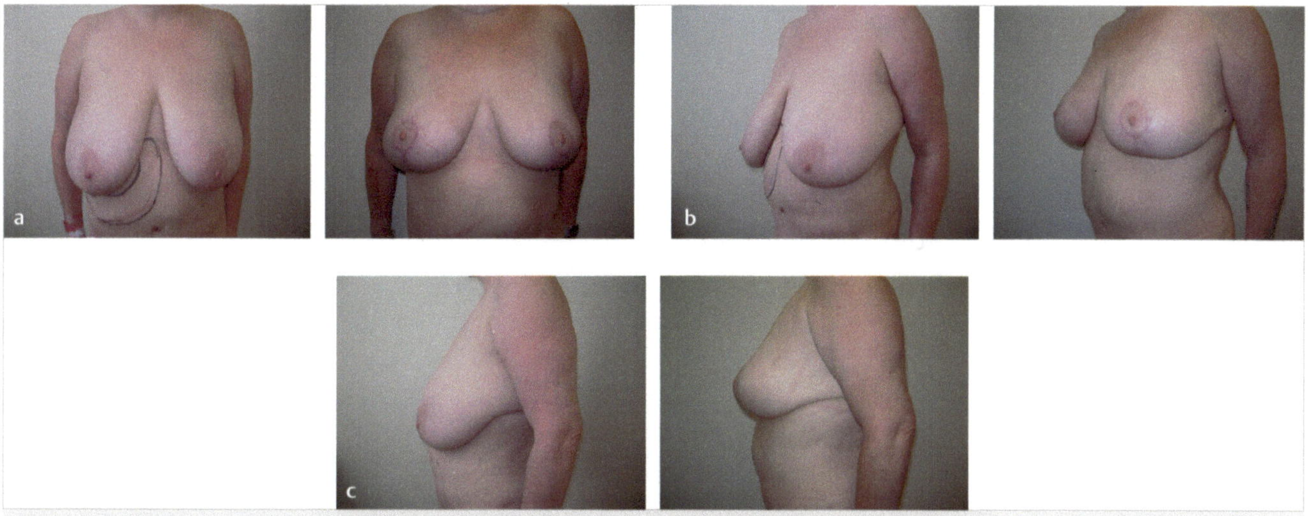

Fig. 71.3 Pre- and postoperative views of a 51-year-old patient 6 months following vertical scar breast reduction in the **(a)** anteroposterior (AP), **(b)** oblique, and **(c)** lateral views. Breast reduction was performed using a superior dermoglandular pedicle bilaterally. On the right side, 415 g of tissue was resected along with 400 cc of liposuction from the lateral chest wall. On the left side, 340 g of tissue was resected along with 400 cc of liposuction from the lateral chest wall.

of tissue was resected along with 400 cc of liposuction from the lateral chest wall (▸ Fig. 71.3a–c).

71.5 Conclusion

Vertical scar breast reduction is a reliable technique that can be adapted to the majority of patients seeking reduction mammaplasty. Final position of the NAC is higher (about 1.0 cm) than predicted by the preoperative markings, as unweighting the inferior pole of the breast reduces traction on the dermoglandular pedicle. This is particularly important in cases of size asymmetry with differential resection volumes. It is important to keep the inferior extent of the planned vertical scar 2 to 4 cm above the IMF to prevent migration of the vertical scar onto the chest wall skin. Liposuction of the lateral chest wall and axillary roll is an important adjunctive procedure to improve chest contour and the aesthetic outcome of the vertical scar breast reduction.

Further Readings

Ahmad J, Lista F. Vertical scar reduction mammaplasty: the fate of nipple-areola complex position and inferior pole length. Plast Reconstr Surg. 2008; 121(4): 1084–1091

Ahmad J, McIsaac SM, Lista F. Does knowledge of the initial technique affect outcomes after repeated breast reduction? Plast Reconstr Surg. 2012; 129(1):11–18

Austin RE, Lista F, Ahmad J. Management of recurrent or persistent macromastia. Clin Plast Surg. 2016; 43(2):383–393

Lista F, Austin RE, Singh Y, Ahmad J. Vertical scar reduction mammaplasty. Plast Reconstr Surg. 2015; 136(1):23–25

Lista F, Ahmad J. Vertical scar reduction mammaplasty: a 15-year experience including a review of 250 consecutive cases. Plast Reconstr Surg. 2006; 117(7):2152–2165, discussion 2166–2169

72 Wise Pattern Breast Reduction

Francesco M. Egro and Kenneth C. Shestak

Abstract

Wise pattern breast reduction is an optimal technique to improve the functional and aesthetic impairment caused by moderate to severe macromastia. This technique allows repositioning of the nipple-areolar complex, removal of excess parenchyma, and skin redraping to fit the new breast shape and size. This book chapter reviews the preoperative, intraoperative, and postoperative steps to obtain optimal aesthetic results in patient undergoing a Wise pattern breast reduction to treat macromastia.

Keywords: Breast reduction, reduction mammaplasty, reduction mammoplasty, Wise, inverted-T, inferior pedicle, breast contour, breast aesthetics, macromastia

Key Points

- Wise pattern breast reduction is an optimal technique to improve the functional and aesthetic impairment caused by moderate to severe macromastia.
- This technique allows repositioning of the nipple-areolar complex (NAC), removal of excess parenchyma, and skin redraping to fit the new breast shape and size.
- Breast reduction requires careful patient selection, planning, and surgical delivery for optimal aesthetic results.

72.1 Preoperative Steps

72.1.1 Analysis

- The first step is to understand the patient's expectations and assess whether they can be met.
- A thorough history should focus on personal or family history of breast cancer, prior breast surgery, and current and desired breast size.
- A detailed examination includes assessment of breast symmetry, "footprint," size, shape, degree of ptosis, skin quality and elasticity, presence of axillary tissue, inframammary fold (IMF) level, and NAC size and shape.

72.1.2 Markings

- In the standing position, the breasts are marked including midline, breast meridian, midline, IMF, Pitanguy's point, and new nipple position.
- An inverted "V" is drawn from the nipple position with the limbs measuring approximately 9 cm with the degree of divergence based on the amount of resection planned.
- The outline of the new areola (4 cm diameter) is drawn with the upper aspect of the areola marked 2 cm above Pitanguy's point.
- The mid breast meridian is transposed to the lower chest area marking the mid portion of the inframammary incision (outlined 2 cm above the IMF).
- Medial and lateral limbs are extended to join the inframammary incision markings. Markings of the Wise pattern are shown in ▶ Fig. 72.1.
- A 7-cm pyramidal pedicle is marked.

72.2 Operative Steps

A description of the key operative steps are shown in **Video 72.1.**

72.2.1 NAC and Pedicle Delineation

- Inject 1:1 mixture of 0.5% bupivacaine and 1.0% xylocaine with 1/100,000 of epinephrine into the deep dermis and superficial subcutaneous adipose layer of each breast (not into parenchyma) for superficial vasoconstriction and extended immediate postoperative analgesia. Approximately 10 cc is placed on each side.
- The new NAC is marked using a 42-mm cookie cutter.

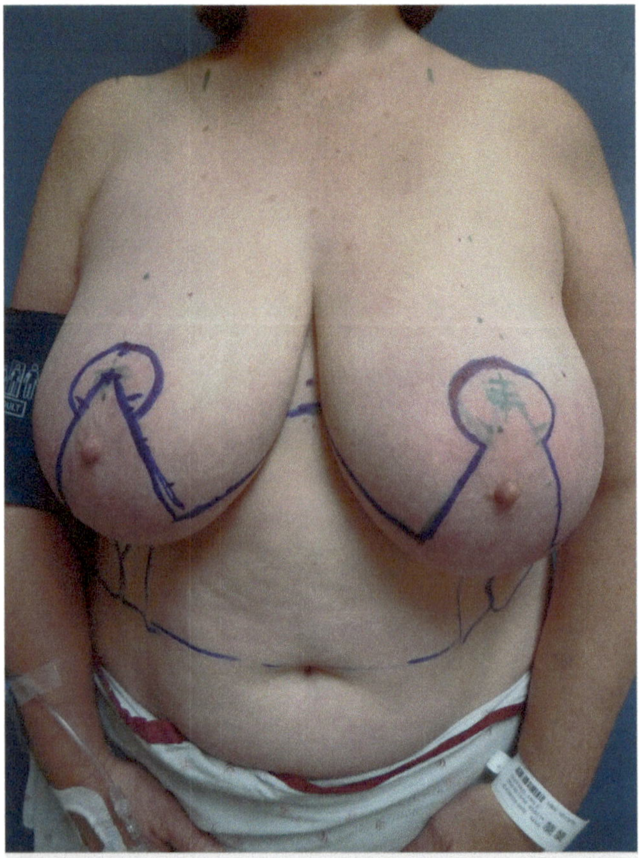

Fig. 72.1 Preoperative marking of a Wise pattern breast reduction.

- Incisions are made along the markings to delineate the NAC and the pedicle.
- The pedicle and NAC are de-epithelialized using a #10 scalpel.

72.2.2 Medial Dissection

- Dissection is started medial to the pedicle by performing a beveling dissection to preserve perforators from the internal mammary system (▶ Fig. 72.2).
- The dissection is then initiated at the level of the junction of the deep subcutaneous tissue anterior breast fascia to raise a flap approximately 1 cm in thickness and is deepened through the breast capsule 2 cm from the medial edge of the pedicle.
- The inferior dissection of the medial triangle is made by beveling cephalad. The dissection is deepened through the superficial fascia system 2 cm above the incision to preserve the IMF.
- The medial triangle is then resected.

72.2.3 Lateral Dissection

- Lateral dissection is similar to the medial dissection.
- Dissection is performed lateral to the pedicle in a beveling fashion to create a pyramidal pedicle to preserve perforators from the lateral thoracic system.
- As the dissection proceeds toward the mid-axillary area of the breast from the lateral edge of the de-epithelialized pedicle, the resection is brought in line with the incised de-epithelialized area. The dissection is deepened down to fascia overlying the serratus anterior muscle.
- The dissection is then advanced in the lateral direction to elevate the lateral limb of the Wise pattern to create a draping flap of at least 2 cm in thickness. Care must be taken not to over-resect the flap and should be thicker closer to chest wall.
- The lateral triangle is then excised by performing a dissection from superior to inferior toward the inframammary incision.
- The inferior dissection of the lateral triangle is again beveled cephalad, coming through the superficial fascial system 2 cm above the incision to preserve the IMF.
- Extra tissue along the lateral chest wall can be elevated and excised to enhance the lateral contour.
- The lateral tissue segment is resected at the level of the muscle fascia. Care is taken not to penetrate the fascia overlying the serratus anterior fascia to preserve the nerve supply, which enters the breast laterally.
- Graphic of the inferior pedicle and resected breast tissue is shown in ▶ Fig. 72.3.

72.2.4 Superior Dissection

- Dissection is then done superior to the pedicle by incising above the NAC and beveling in a cephalad direction down to the prepectoralis major fascia up to the second intercostal space.

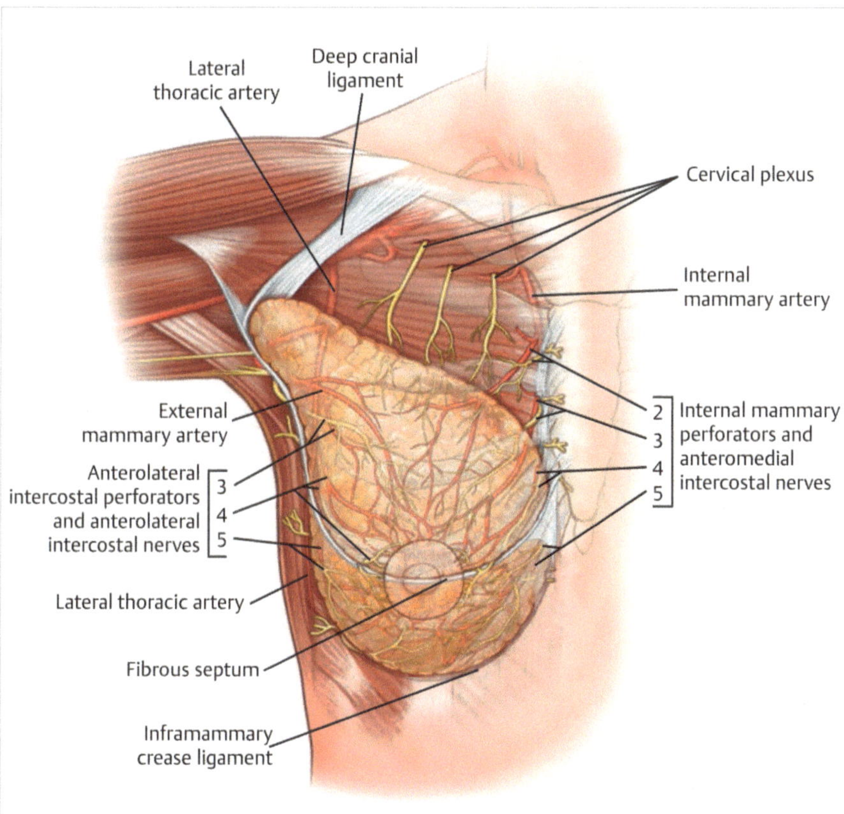

Fig. 72.2 Vascular anatomy of the breast highlighting the internal mammary perforators. (Reproduced with permission from Nahai F. The Art of Aesthetic Surgery. 2nd ed. Thieme; 2011.)

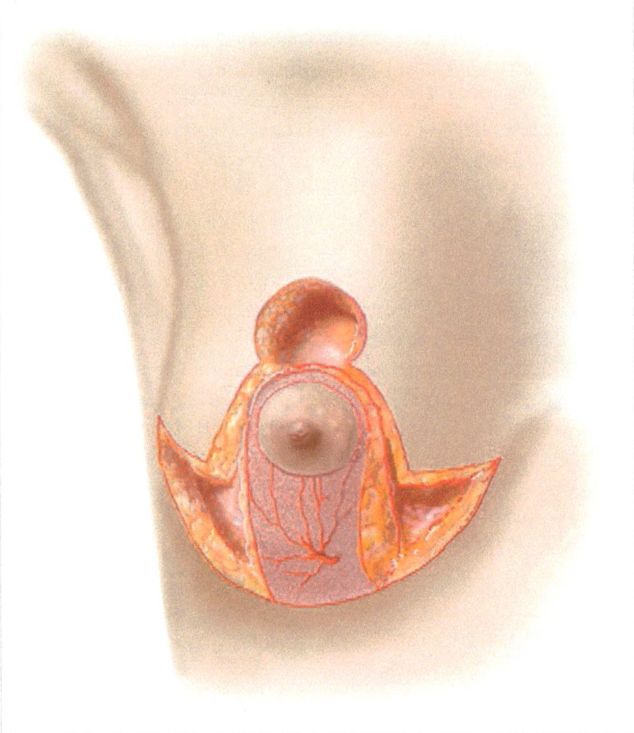

Fig. 72.3 Resected Wise pattern showing the inferior pedicle and resected breast tissue. (Reproduced with permission from Nahai F. The Art of Aesthetic Surgery. 2nd ed. Thieme; 2011.)

- The tissue to be resected is then mobilized by elevating flaps superiorly at a thickness of approximately 1.5 cm. This is done progressing toward the second intercostal space and deepening the dissection as the surgeon moves closer to chest wall to join the dissection already done on the pectoralis fascia.
- The wounds are temporarily closed by placing a tri-point Prolene suture followed by temporary staple closure of the skin wounds.

72.2.5 Contralateral Breast Reduction

- The same process described in steps 1 to 4 are conducted.

72.2.6 Refinements

- Assessment for symmetry, projection, fullness, lateral breast contour, and NAC size and shape is performed.
- Any adjustments can be conducted.
- Additional lateral trimming of the pedicle can be carried out and is frequently necessary. This is can be done on direct vision, beveling away from the pedicle to preserve contributions from the lateral thoracic system.
- The medial skin flap can be thinned with Bovie cautery or scissors.
- Care is taken to leave fullness medially as the medial segment is stapled closed.
- If the pedicle is significantly long, i.e., the distance from the areola at the 6 o'clock position to the IMF is 12 cm or greater, the surgeon can shorten the pedicle with a transverse imbrication of the dermis approximately 3 to 4 cm above the IMF with the imbricated tissue being 3 to 4 cm in height with a running suture of coated 3–0 polyglycolic acid. This increases projection of the pedicle by "pushing" the breast parenchyma posteriorly.
- In patients with significantly compromised skin and breast tissue elasticity, additional skin at the superior edge of the pedicle can be de-epithelialized and sutured to the pectoralis muscle fascia at the level of the third rib using two or three 2–0 coated polyglycolic acid sutures as a means of suspension that can help maintain the breast shape during the first 6 to 8 weeks of healing.

72.2.7 Closure and Dressings

- Once satisfied with the result, closure is carried out with 3–0 Monocryl interrupted deep dermal sutures and 4–0 Monocryl subcuticular suture.
- Apply 0.25 inch paper tape to the incisions.
- Fluffed gauze is applied over the breasts and held in place with a surgical brasserie.

72.2.8 Pearls

- Preserve IMF by beveling dissection cephalad.
- IMF preservation improves breast shape.
- Do not undermine pedicle.
- Shape pedicle in pyramidal fashion.

72.3 Postoperative Care

- Patients are encouraged to wear the surgical or sport brasserie for the first 4 weeks. It is important to avoid brasseries with underwire.
- Patient can shower after 48 hours but incisions should be tapped dry afterwards.
- Trauma or pressure to breasts should be avoided.
- Exercise should be avoided for the first week followed by gentle reintroduction over the course of the following 3 weeks.
- Analgesia is prescribed as needed.
- If a Prolene suture has been placed at the "T" point, it is removed in 7 to 10 days.
- Patients are usually seen 3 days, 1 week, 2 weeks, 5 weeks, and 3 months postoperatively.

72.4 Case Example

Pre- and postoperative photos of a 48-year-old female with macromastia who underwent inferior pedicle Wise pattern breast reduction (▶ Fig. 72.4a, b).

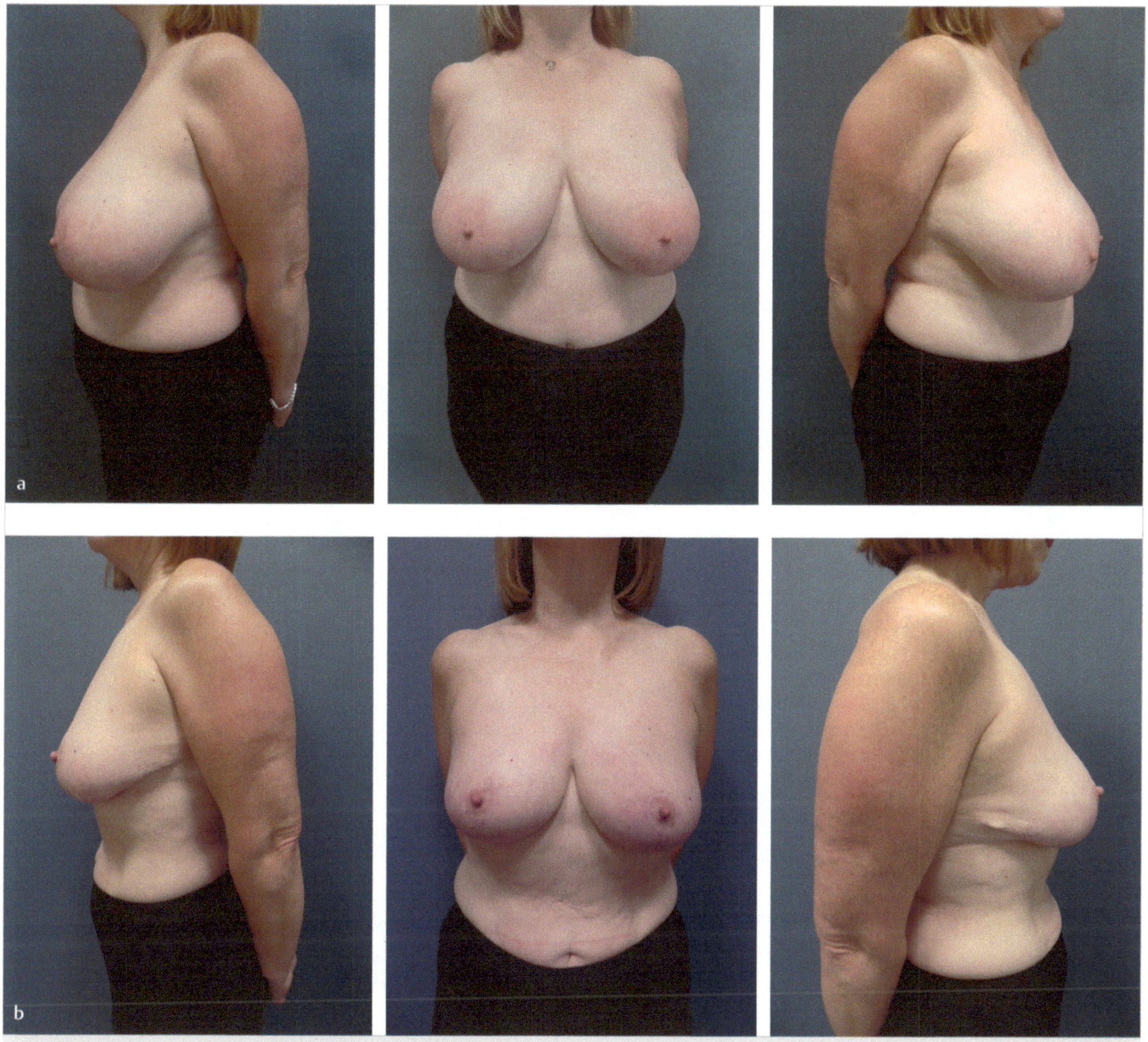

Fig. 72.4 **(a)** Pre- and **(b)** postoperative photos of a 48-year-old female with macromastia who underwent inferior pedicle Wise pattern breast reduction.

72.5 Conclusion

Wise pattern breast reduction is an optimal technique to improve the functional and aesthetic impairment caused by moderate to severe macromastia. Wise pattern breast reduction grants great flexibility in the repositioning of the NAC, parenchymal resection, and amount of skin resection. Breast reduction requires careful patient selection, planning, and surgical delivery for optimal aesthetic results.

Further Readings

Hall-Findlay EJ, Shestak KC. Breast reduction. Plast Reconstr Surg. 2015; 136(4):531e–544e

Nahai F. The art of aesthetic surgery. 2nd ed. Thieme; 2011

Shestak KC, Davidson EH. Assessing risk and avoiding complications in breast reduction. Clin Plast Surg. 2016; 43(2):323–331

van Deventer PV, Graewe FR. The blood supply of the breast revisited. Plast Reconstr Surg. 2016; 137(5):1388–1397

Wise RJ. A preliminary report on a method of planning the mammaplasty. Plast Reconstr Surg (1946). 1956; 17(5):367–375

73 Tuberous/Constricted Breasts

Rafael A. Couto and William P. Adams Jr.

Abstract

Similar to traditional patients, tuberous/constricted breasts follow the four-part breast augmentation process: (1) patient education and informed consent; (2) tissue-based planning; (3) refined surgical technique/fast-track 24-hour recovery, and (4) defined postoperative care regimen; however, the tuberous/constricted breast has distinctive anatomical abnormalities that need to be restored at the time of the augmentation. Herein, we focus in the clinical decision and specific techniques pertaining to the correction of these deformities.

Keywords: Breast augmentation, dual plane, constricted, High Five Process, tissue-based planning, tuberous, 14-point plan

Key Points

- The process of breast augmentation consists of four essential parts: (1) patient education and informed consent, (2) tissue-based planning, (3) refined surgical technique, and (4) clear postoperative care regimen. Integration of these four steps optimizes patient outcomes.
- The constricted breast requires specific maneuvers to correct the deformity including:
  - Using an implant that is wider than the breast width.
  - Lowering the inframammary fold (IMF).
  - Releasing the horizontal constricting fascia/bands in the lower pole of the breast.
  - Using an implant with enhanced gel cohesion and a lower distribution of fill in the breast.
  - Correcting pseudoherniation of the areola.
- Patients with mild to moderate lower pole constriction are candidates for one-stage procedure, whereas individuals with severe IMF constriction may need a two-stage approach.

73.1 Preoperative Steps

73.1.1 Patient Education and Informed Consent

- The more the patient knows, the better the outcome, as well as the satisfaction. During the education and consent phase, key concepts and goals are addressed and reviewed with the patient.
- For further details, see *Chapter 64 Breast Augmentation*.

73.1.2 Tissue-Based Planning

- The High Five Process and its corresponding measurements are used for tissue-based planning. Since the breast width is narrower by definition in the constricted breast, the surgeon uses the desired breast width to calculate the optimal fill volume. For further details, see *Chapter 64 Breast Augmentation*.
- A unique planning technique for tuberous/constricted breasts is anterior distraction at the IMF. This maneuver is used to determine the degree of lower pole breast constriction. A patient who has a distractible IMF (mild constriction) is a candidate for a one-stage procedure; whereas, a patient with a fixed IMF (moderate–severe constriction) will need a two-stage approach: tissue expansions, followed by implant placement (▶ Fig. 73.1).
- In order to maximize lower pole fullness, we prefer to use either anatomical or round implants with high cohesivity. When using anatomical or round implants, it is important to use an implant that is shorter in height in order to shift the distribution of fill in the lower pole of the breast.
- Three-dimensional imaging is a useful tool in these particular cases. It facilitates the surgeon to accurately demonstrate to the patient: (1) a visual simulation of the breasts postoperatively, and (2) an objective assessment of the breast or chest wall.

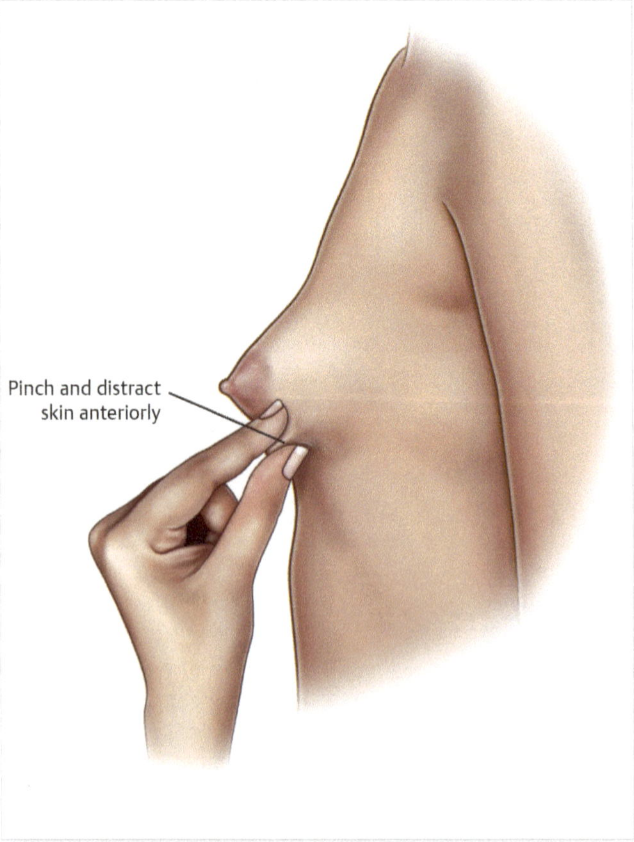

Fig. 73.1 Anterior distraction of inframammary fold (IMF) tests the degree of lower breast pole constriction. The skin overlying the IMF is pinched and distracted anteriorly. Patients with a mobile IMF (mild constriction) may be candidate for a one-stage procedure, while a patient whose IMF is fixed (moderate–severe constriction) will need a two-stage approach: tissue expansion, followed by implant placement.

73.1.3 Marking the Breasts

- The markings utilized for a tuberous/constricted breast augmentation are the same as used for a traditional breast augmentation. See *Chapter 64 Breast Augmentation*, for a detailed description of the markings.
- If the patient requires nipple-areolar complex (NAC) reduction and/or repositioning, a periareolar mastopexy is planned. The appropriate nipple position is first determined by using Pitanguy's point, and then confirmed with a nipple drop technique. In other words, the nipple is raised superiorly to a level that is aesthetically pleasing, and then it is released and marked where the nipple was located. The top of the marking is planned as the nipple, not the superior border of the areola. Symmetry of both nipples is confirmed with sternal notch to nipple measurements. Often times the nipple level is adequate but the periareolar technique is utilized to improve the areolar fullness. Therefore, patients may not require a periareolar technique if the pseudoherniation is mild.
- After determining the new nipple position, the amount of excess skin is estimated and then a periareolar oval shape is marked around the NAC. It is important to keep the periareolar procedure relatively conservative. The flattening that occurs with periareolar procedures is usually a shaping benefit in the constricted breast that is unique to that deformity.
- Planning the new IMF location is done as follows:
  - The implant volume and new IMF location is determined by applying the estimated new breast width to the High Five Process.
  - Because these patients have horizontal and vertical skin envelope deficiency, their breast width and N:IMF distance must be increased.
  - *It is important to note that constricted/tuberous breasts are the exception to the tissue-based planning rule: the implant will be wider than the current breast width.*
  - In order to maintain a proper N:IMF distance to breast width ratio, the IMF needs to be lowered. The new IMF location is determined by applying the selected implant volume to the High Five Process.

73.2 Operative Steps

- Our preference is to use the IMF approach in the tuberous/constricted breast.

73.2.1 Subpectoral Pocket Dissection

- The breast augmentation follows the classic four-part dual-plane dissection under direct vision, precisely, with prospective hemostasis. For a detail description of this part of the procedure, see *Chapter 64 Breast Augmentation*.
- When using anatomical implants, the height of your subpectoral pocket dissection will control the rotation of your implant. Therefore, it is crucial to make a precise pocket, and limit the superior dissection to the height of the implant.

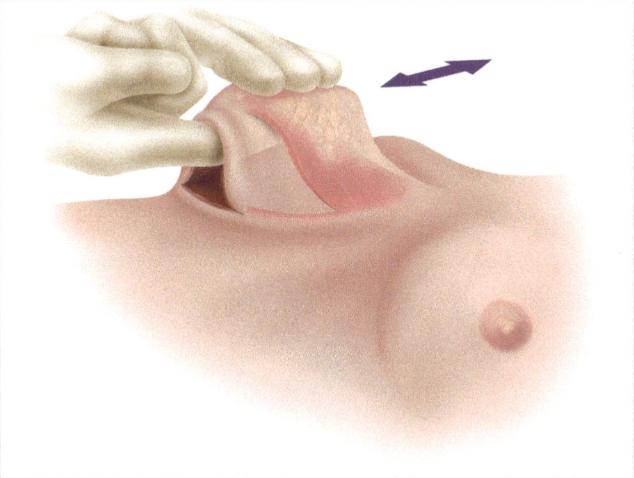

Fig. 73.2 Dual-plane assessment. Using the nondominant hand, the overlying breast parenchyma is palpated bimanually, and the degree of expansion of this parenchyma and vertical laxity are assessed. (Reproduced with permission from Adams WP Jr, ed. Breast Augmentation Video Atlas. 2nd ed. New York, NY: Thieme; 2019:74.)

73.2.2 Dual-Plane Assessment and Adjustment

- Once the subpectoral pocket dissection is completed, the dual plane is assessed and adjusted. Insert fingers into the subpectoral space and lift the pectoralis major and breast parenchyma to the expected level of expansion (▶ Fig. 73.2). Using your other hand, assess the degree of breast and skin tissue mobility relative to the pectoralis major.
- Using the electrocautery, gradually dissect the pectoralis major off the breast tissue. A dual plane II or III is recommended for constricted lower pole breasts as this maximize implant–parenchyma interface, and thus expand the lower breast pole (▶ Fig. 73.3). Avoid releasing the muscle beyond the superior border of the areola, as its cranial displacement can result in poor implant coverage and breast animation deformity.

73.2.3 Breast Parenchyma Scoring

- After achieving the desired dual plane, horizontal constricting bands are divided with radial "scores" to maximize expansion and efface the previous IMF.

73.2.4 Pocket Preparation and Implant Insertion

- The 14-point plan is followed as per routine. Irrigate pocket with 150 cc of normal saline, followed by 150 cc of betadine-triple antibiotic solution (i.e., 50 cc of 10% betadine, 500 cc of normal saline, 1 g cefazolin, 80 mg gentamycin).
- Re-prep incisions with chlorhexidine prep stick, dip/clean retractors into betadine-triple antibiotic solution, and place it inside the breast pocket.

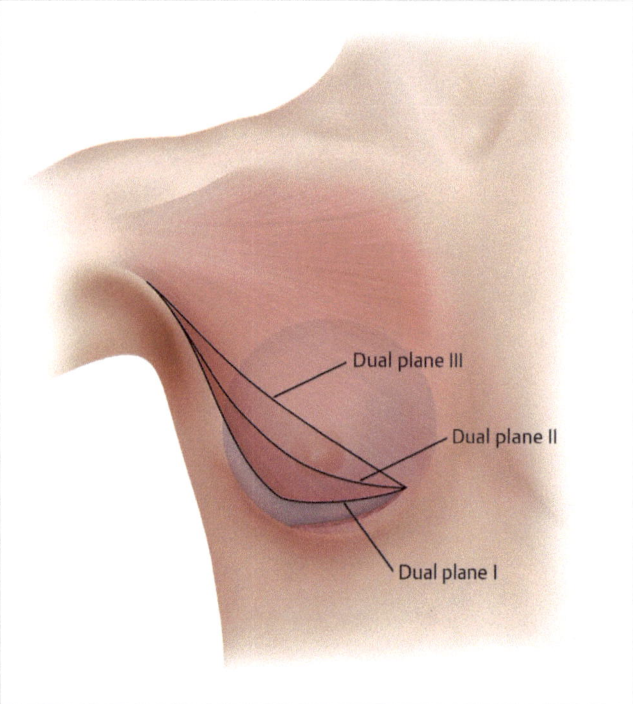

Fig. 73.3 Types of dual planes. The pectoralis major muscle is divided along the inframammary fold in all dual-plane types. The difference between each of them lies in the amount of subglandular dissection that is performed. Type I: No subglandular dissection. Type II: Subglandular dissection to the inferior border of the areola. Type III: Subglandular dissection to the superior border of the areola. (Reproduced with permission from Adams WP Jr, ed. Breast Augmentation Video Atlas. 2nd ed. New York, NY: Thieme; 2019:71.)

- After changing gloves, the implants are manually inserted into the breast pocket using aseptic techniques. If using anatomical implants, ensure that it was placed in the correct orientation.
- The aesthetic shape of the breast is evaluated and any final adjustments are made.

73.2.5 IMF Fixation and Skin Closure

- Tuberous/constricted breasts have an increased risk of implant malposition; thus, IMF fixation is always performed in this patient population.
- IMF fixation technique consists of a three-point suture that secures the superficial fascia above and below the incision to the deep fascia of the IMF. Using a 3–0 polydioxanone (PDS) suture, the IMF is fixated at one to three points. This stitch may produce a temporary mild indentation to the soft tissue (▶ Fig. 73.4).
- The IMF incision closure involves running a 3–0 PDS suture along the superficial fascia, followed by a subdermal 3–0 poliglecaprone (Monocryl) suture, and a running 4–0 Monocryl subcuticular suture.

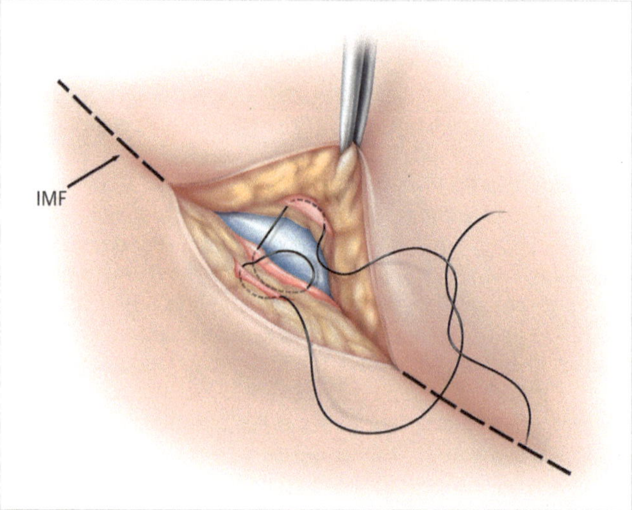

Fig. 73.4 The inframammary fold (IMF) is fixated by securing the superficial fascia above and below the incision to the deep fascia with a 3–0 polydioxanone (PDS) suture. (Reproduced with permission from Adams WP Jr, ed. Breast Augmentation Video Atlas. 2nd ed. New York, NY: Thieme; 2019:104.)

73.2.6 Management of Nipple-Areolar Complex (NAC)

- When correction of NAC is required, a periareolar mastopexy is performed. If a two-stage procedure is been pursued, NAC deformities and breast ptosis are addressed during the second stage.
- The NAC is marked with a 38-mm cookie cutter. The inner and the outer periareolar markings are incised, and then excess skin within these two incisions is de-epithelized.
- To facilitate nipple repositioning and skin approximation, the dermis around the perimeter of the defect can be divided and the surrounding soft tissue cautiously undermined.
- NAC closure involves deep dermal stitches with 3–0 Monocryl suture, followed by a 4–0 Monocryl subcuticular stitch.

73.3 Postoperative Care

- A detailed postoperative care regimen is essential for both a 24-hour fast-track recovery and optimal outcome.
- See *Chapter 64 Breast Augmentation*, for a detailed description of the postoperative management.

73.4 Case Example

Preoperative and postoperative photos of a patient with constricted breasts following a breast augmentation in anteroposterior, oblique, and lateral views. This patient underwent a dual plane III breast augmentation using anatomical implants (▶ Fig. 73.5a–f).

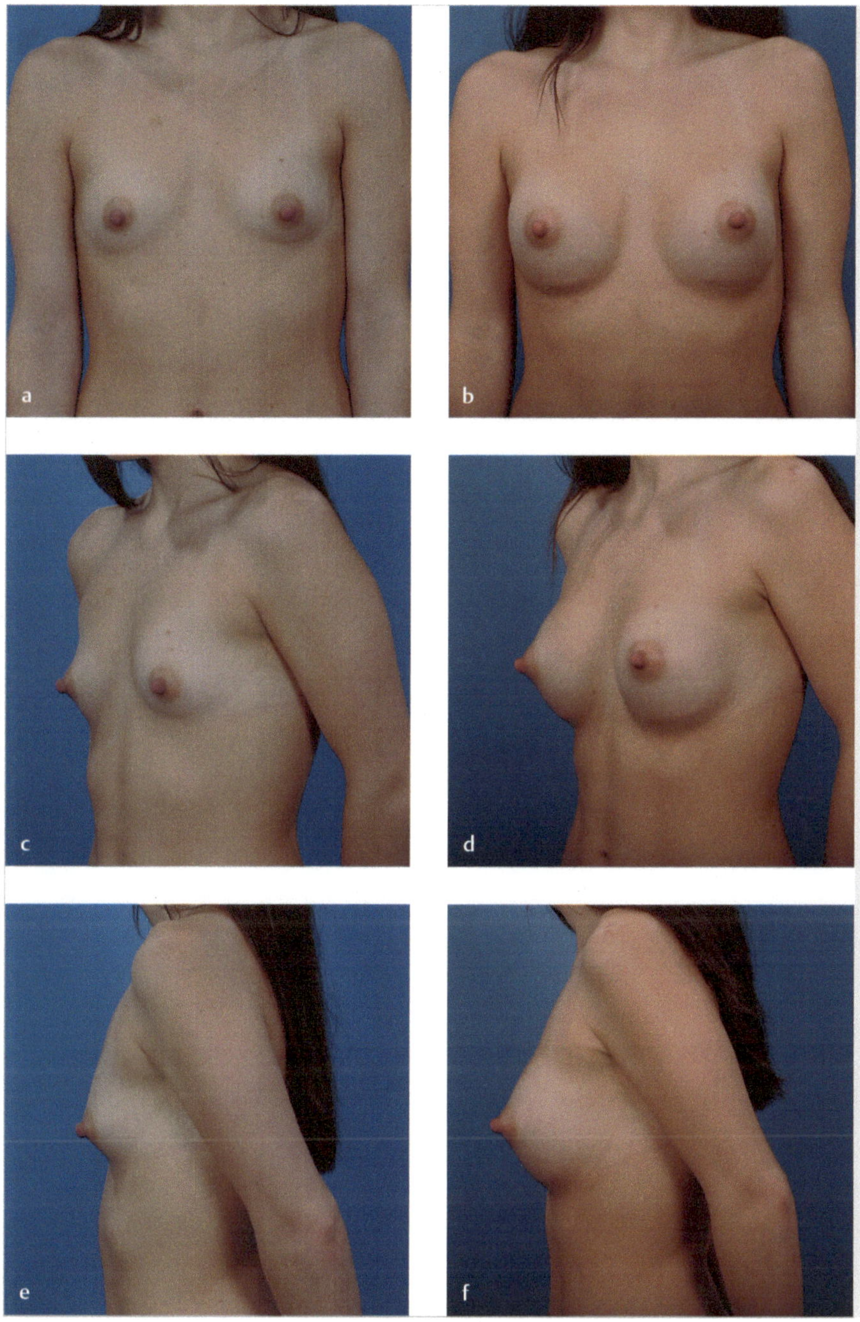

Fig. 73.5 Preoperative and postoperative photos of a patient with constricted breasts following a breast augmentation in **(a, b)** anteroposterior, **(c, d)** oblique, and **(e, f)** lateral views. This patient underwent a dual plane III breast augmentation using anatomical implants.

73.5 Conclusions

The concept of breast augmentation as a process, instead of an isolated procedure, facilitates patient education and perioperative management, thus optimizing satisfaction and outcome. The key to the aesthetics of the breast is controlling the N:IMF distance to breast width ratio. The success of this procedure relies on the preoperative planning and maximizing lower breast pole expansion. The latter is achieved through effective implant selection, dual-plane pocket dissection, and glandular scoring.

See **Video 73.1**.

Further Readings

Adams WP Jr, ed. Breast augmentation video atlas. 2nd ed. New York, NY: Thieme; 2019:20–25

Adams WP, Jr. The process of breast augmentation: four sequential steps for optimizing outcomes for patients. Plast Reconstr Surg. 2008; 122(6):1892–1900

Adams WP, Jr, Afrooz PN, Stuzin JM. Tissue-based planning and technique for breast augmentation with anatomical implants. Plast Reconstr Surg. 2019; 143(6):1634–1636

Hammond D. Tuberous breast deformity. In: Hammond D, ed. Atlas of Aesthetic Breast Surgery. London, UK: Elsevier; 2009:183–194

Kolker AR, Collins MS. Tuberous breast deformity: classification and treatment strategy for improving consistency in aesthetic correction. Plast Reconstr Surg. 2015; 135(1):73–86

Part XI

Body Contouring

XI

74 SAFE Liposuction

Jeffrey R. Claiborne, Kristy L. Hamilton, and Simeon Wall Jr.

Abstract

SAFELipo differs from traditional liposuction and was developed to overcome its shortcomings. Whereas traditional liposuction is strictly a reductive procedure, SAFELipo is a comprehensive body contouring technique for fat, skin, and the fasciocutaneous network. SAFELipo allows the surgeon to expand the resistance differential between tissue planes, whether the goal is to remove more fat, release fibrous scar, redistribute residual fat, or add more fat to the area using expansion vibration lipofilling (EVL). This technique allows for dramatic and thorough liposuction without increasing the risk of contour deformities or damage to the skin and blood supply. It is more than a reductive or additive procedure because it removes, redistributes, blends, and adds fat as needed. It releases and equalizes disparities in skin distribution, simultaneously providing for areas of skin retraction much wider than traditional liposuction treatment areas. SAFELipo also treats deep and superficial tissues without disrupting vascular and stromal networks.

Keywords: SAFELipo, liposuction, body contouring, expansion vibration lipofilling, separation, aspiration, equalization

Key Points

- Heat generated by radiofrequency, ultrasound, and laser liposuction causes ischemia, cell death, and inflammation—all detriments to creating a smooth, natural result.
- The three-step process of SAFELipo (separation, aspiration, and fat equalization) allows greater control, precision, and safety in fat manipulation.
- SAFELipo separation widens the resistance differential which gives the surgeon greater control and precision in manipulating the adipose tissue.
- Fat equalization emulsifies some of the remaining fat, eliminates thicker and thinner areas of fat, and leaves this liquified fat as a smooth layer of local fat grafts to prevent adherence and fill in any imperfections.
- SAFELipo and expansion vibration lipofilling (EVL) are ideal for treating contour deformities, with the majority of time spent in the separation, equalization, and expansion phases for correction of irregularities.

74.1 Preoperative Steps

- Poor skin quality (striae, atrophic type cellulite/dimpling, laxity) can compromise the result and needs to be noted and discussed with the patient.
- Delineate and discuss the fat distribution pattern: intra-abdominal versus extra-abdominal fat and apple versus pear shape.
- Evaluate the muscular framework and define the patients' goals to discern their expectations (lean/thin versus big/broad).
- Carefully examine for any hernias—failure to recognize a fascial defect can lead to a catastrophic visceral injury.
- Skeletal asymmetries (scoliosis, leg-length discrepancies, pelvic tilt, and chest wall deformities) need to be documented and discussed with the patient.
- Patients with a body mass index (BMI) of over 30 typically have a large amount of visceral fat, and it is more difficult to create a rewarding postoperative result. They also have a higher perioperative complication rate.
- Zones of adherence or tethering within the treatment area do not need to be avoided, but rather they need to be clearly marked out preoperatively, as these areas need additional time spent in the separation and equalization phases.
- Carefully plan intraoperative patient positioning, and discuss with the surgical team. For circumferential trunk SAFELipo only, we prefer a 360-degree prep and use a supine–lateral–lateral sequence. For SAFELipo with safe subcutaneous buttock augmentation (SSBA), we use all four positions adding prone to the supine–lateral–lateral sequence.

74.2 Operative Steps

See **Video 74.1**.

74.2.1 Positioning

- Carefully plan intraoperative patient positioning, and discuss with the surgical team.
- We prefer a single whole-body prep so that the patient can be moved frequently into any position intraoperatively rather than struggling from fixed positions.
- For circumferential trunk SAFELipo, we use a supine–lateral–lateral sequence.
- Although the epigastric–thoracic transition area can be treated from the supine position, it is safer and easier from the lateral decubitus position because the adipose tissue falls away from the fascia.
- Treating targeted areas from multiple hidden access sites and patient positions increases cross-hatching and reduces the likelihood of contour irregularities.

74.2.2 Infiltration

- Good infiltration with simultaneous separation and tumescence (SST) provides for wide dispersion and immediate vasoconstriction with initial fat separation, ultimately reducing vascular injury and improving surgeon awareness and control of cannula position by eliminating flexibility misguidance and increasing working space.
- For primary liposuction cases, we recommend an infusion-to-aspiration ratio of 1:1 or 1.5:1.
- In a repeat liposuction procedure (or in patients with highly fibrotic-tethered tissues), additional volume expansion of the target zone is even more vital to being able to precisely

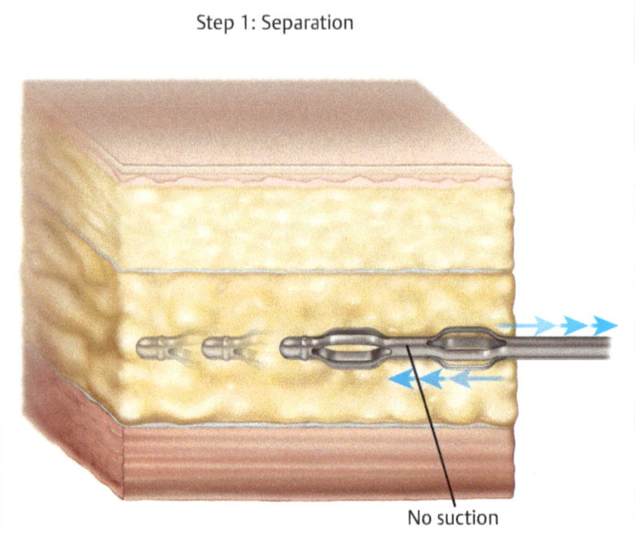

Fig. 74.1 Cross section of adipose tissue, before separation. (Reproduced with permission from Steinbrech DS. Male Aesthetic Plastic Surgery. Thieme; 2020.)

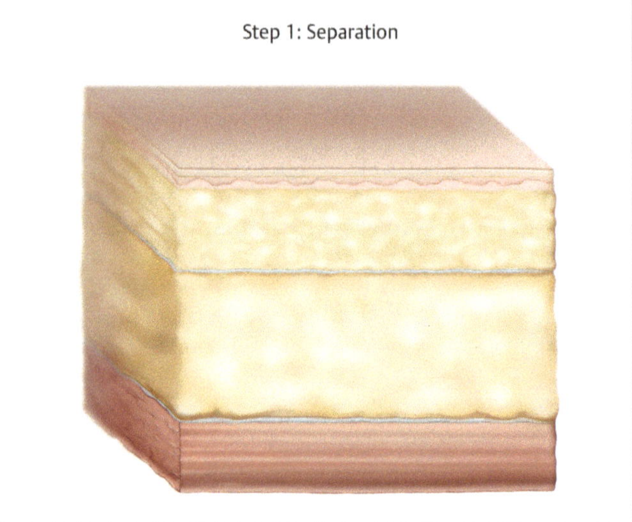

Fig. 74.2 Cross section of adipose tissue, after separation. (Reproduced with permission from Steinbrech DS. Male Aesthetic Plastic Surgery. Thieme; 2020.)

traverse the tissue planes, and a tumescent approach with a ratio of 2:1 or even 3:1 utilizing SST is frequently required.
- Assuming patients have no cardiac, pulmonary, or renal medical history, it is not uncommon to use 6 to 10 L of infiltration when planning to aspirate 3 to 7 L of fat.

74.2.3 Separation

- Separation (including infiltration with SST) accounts for 40% of the total procedural time in primary SAFELipo (▶ Fig. 74.1 and ▶ Fig. 74.2).
- Separation is the process of widening the resistance differential between the target fat and surrounding structures using rapid oscillations of a 4 to 5 mm angled exploded-tip cannula through the adipose tissue to mechanically emulsify the solid fat architecture into a more liquid environment.
- We recommend power-assisted liposuction (PAL) for separation to maximize the oscillations and efficacy of the wings on the exploded-tip cannulas and to minimize effort during liposuction.
- In repeat liposuction cases, the separation step is more critical because the adipose layer can be scarred; scarring narrows the resistance differential between target fat and other, unintended structures, and makes it more difficult for the surgeon to precisely treat this layer.
- The endpoint of the separation step is the loss of resistance with cannula passage, indicating a very wide resistance differential and adequately emulsified fat.

74.2.4 Aspiration

- A 4-mm angled long-port double Mercedes tip cannula is used to aspirate the emulsified, low-resistance fat (▶ Fig. 74.3 and ▶ Fig. 74.4).

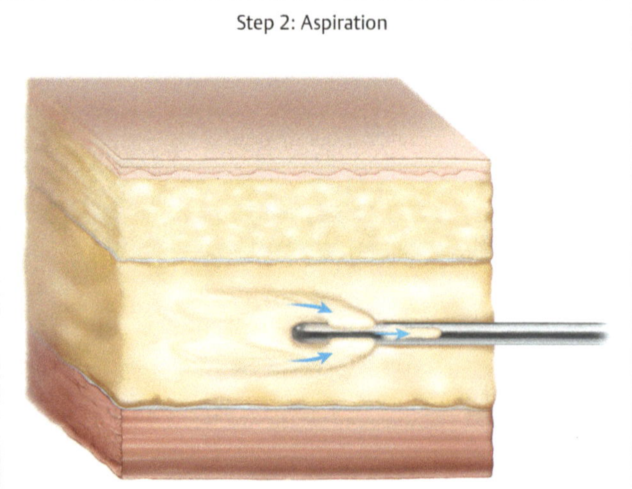

Fig. 74.3 Cross section of adipose tissue, before aspiration. (Reproduced with permission from Steinbrech DS. Male Aesthetic Plastic Surgery. Thieme; 2020.)

- The aspiration step accounts for approximately 40% of the treatment time.
- The liquified fatty layer has a very distinct low-resistance tactile feel, allowing the surgeon greater control and precision.

74.2.5 Equalization

- The final step of SAFELipo is equalization which constitutes 20% of the treatment time.
- This step employs an exploded-tip cannula without suction to rake across the fatty hills and valleys to smooth any inconsistencies in fat thickness (▶ Fig. 74.5 and ▶ Fig. 74.6).

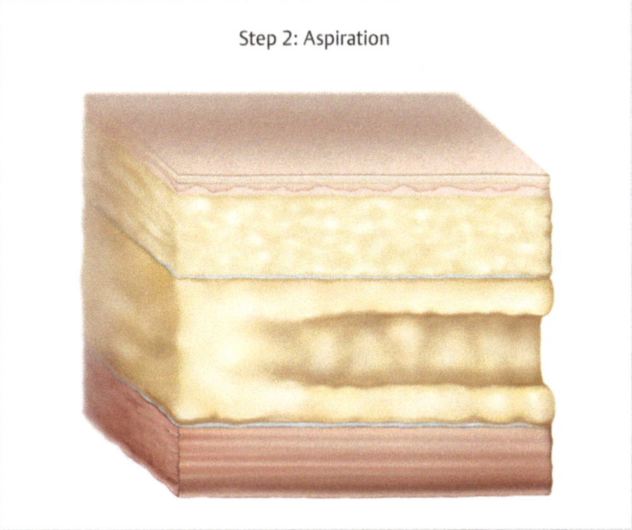

Fig. 74.4 Cross section of adipose tissue, after aspiration.

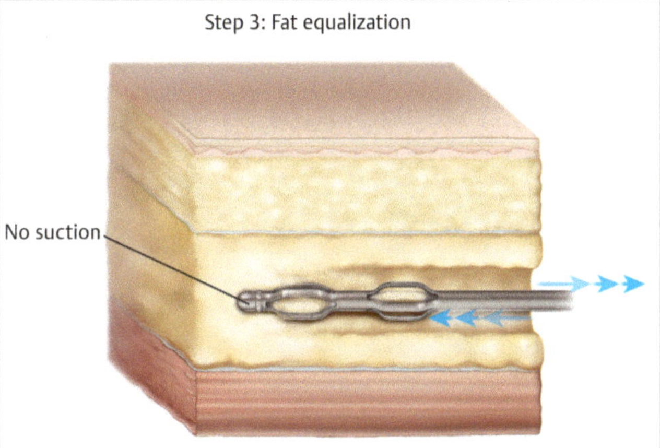

Fig. 74.5 Cross section of adipose tissue, before equalization. (Reproduced with permission from Steinbrech DS. Male Aesthetic Plastic Surgery. Thieme; 2020.)

- Fat equalization emulsifies some of the remaining fat, and this liquified fat graft blanket will fill in any grooves and help prevent adherence of the skin.
- Equalization ensures a consistent tissue thickness and smoothness to the postoperative result even in thinner patients, whereas other forms of liposuction are highly associated with contour deformities when the remaining layer of fat is left thin.
- The endpoint of equalization is a smooth rolling pinch test: The skin is gently pinched and rolled between the fingers to compare smoothness and thickness throughout the treatment area.

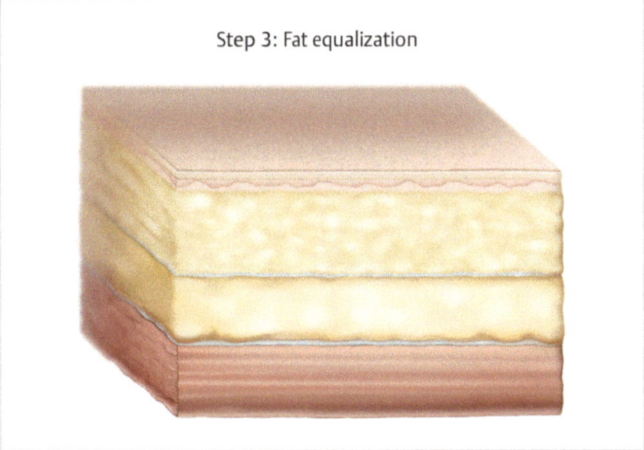

Fig. 74.6 Cross section of adipose tissue, after equalization. (Reproduced with permission from Steinbrech DS. Male Aesthetic Plastic Surgery. Thieme; 2020.)

74.3 Postoperative Care

- For treatment areas that had more than 2 L removed and areas with poor skin elasticity, incisions are left open to drain excess fluid (alternatively, a closed suction drain can be placed).
- Patients are placed into a compression garment plus 0.5- to 1-inch Reston foam (3 M corporation) to control swelling and skin redraping.
- Massage is started at 2 weeks postoperatively on all treated areas.
- Patient wears the compression 24/7 for the first 2 weeks, and then during the day for weeks 3 and 4.
- Foam can usually be discontinued after 4 weeks, and patients transition into a Spanx-type garment for another 2 to 8 weeks to control swelling during the day and especially during activity.
- At 3 to 4 weeks postoperative, patients can begin to increase their activity, but they need to monitor their swelling and adjust their garment and activity accordingly.
- Patients need to monitor their skin for the development of creases which most commonly occurs from constricting clothing, and these areas should promptly be treated with foam compression.

74.4 Case Examples

(▶ Fig. 74.7, ▶ Fig. 74.8, ▶ Fig. 74.9, ▶ Fig. 74.10, ▶ Fig. 74.11, ▶ Fig. 74.12, ▶ Fig. 74.13, ▶ Fig. 74.14, ▶ Fig. 74.15, ▶ Fig. 74.16, ▶ Fig. 74.17, ▶ Fig. 74.18, ▶ Fig. 74.19, and ▶ Fig. 74.20).

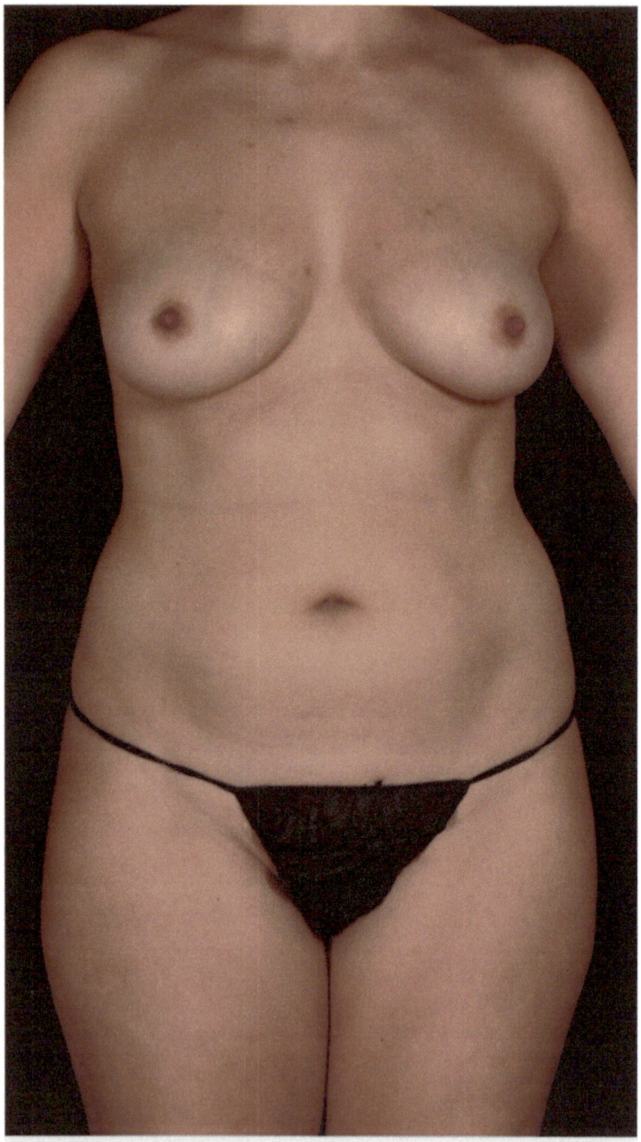

Fig. 74.7 Case example, before.

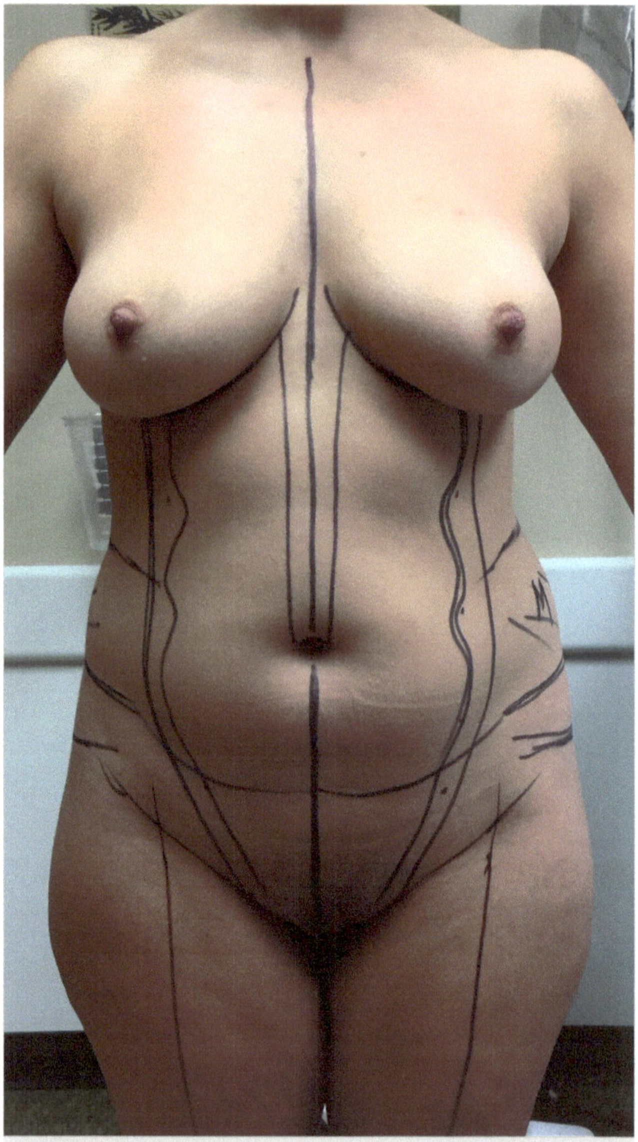

Fig. 74.8 Case example, markings.

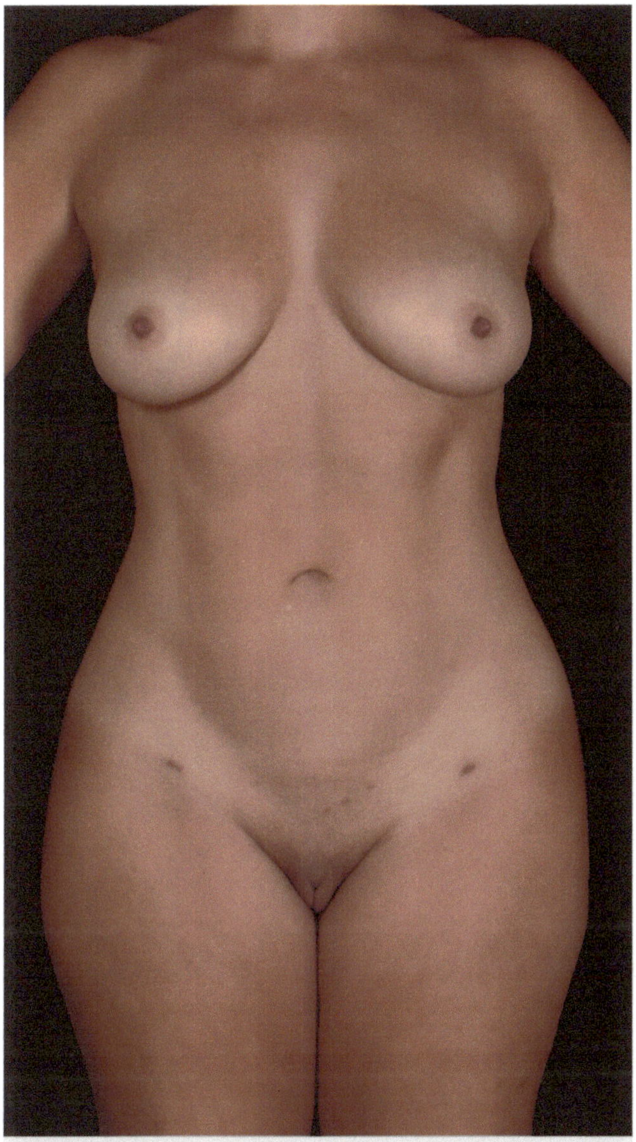

Fig. 74.9 Case example, after.

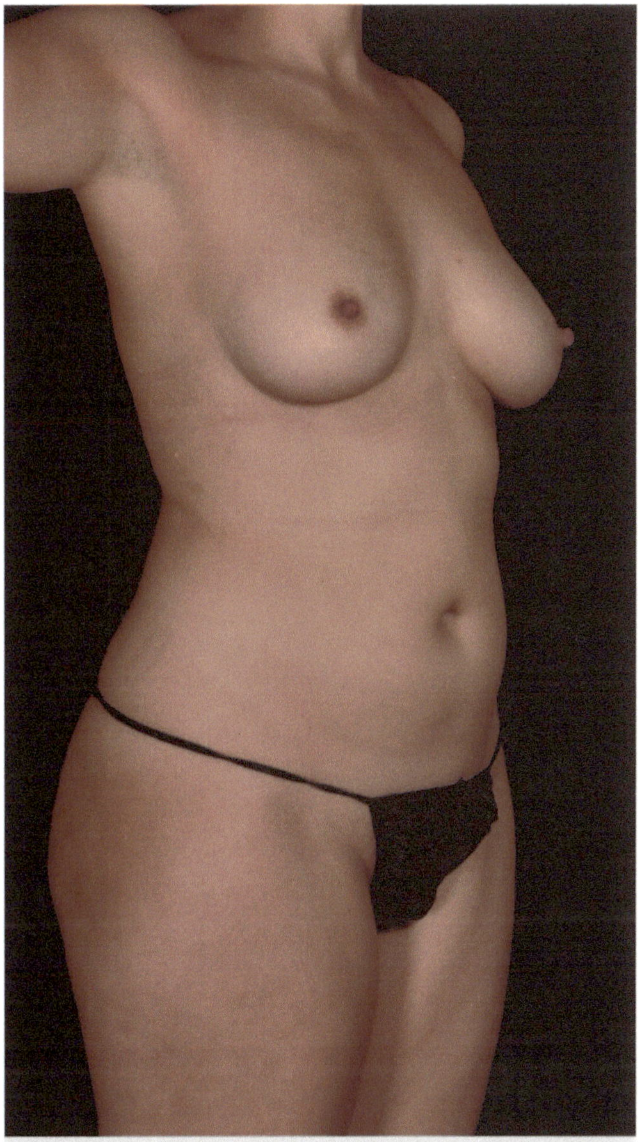

Fig. 74.10 Case example, before.

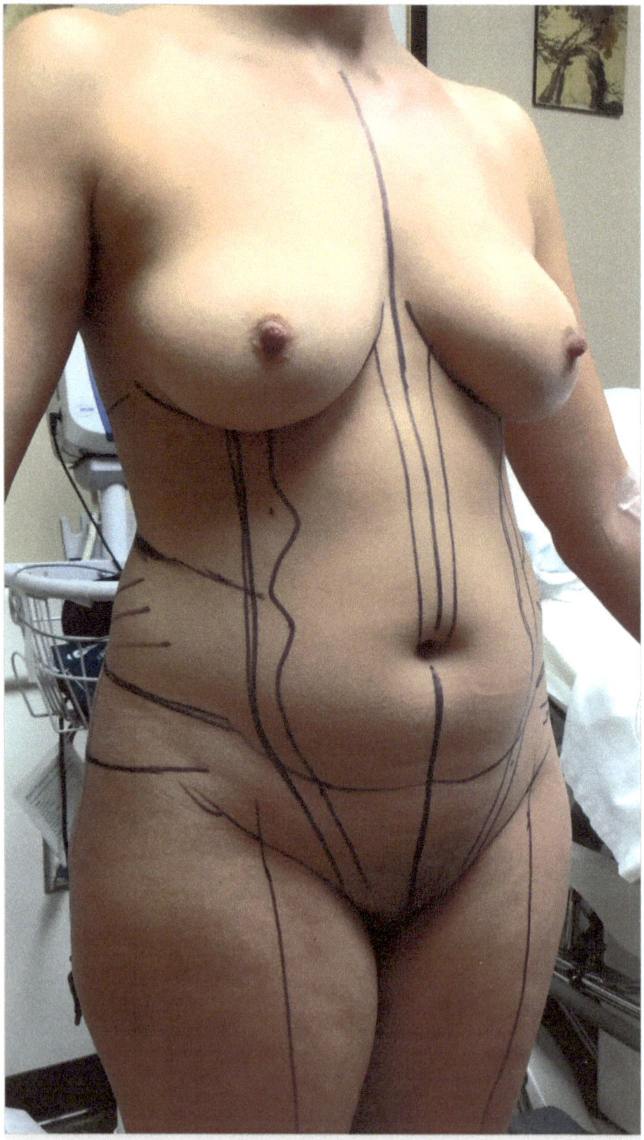

Fig. 74.11 Case example, markings.

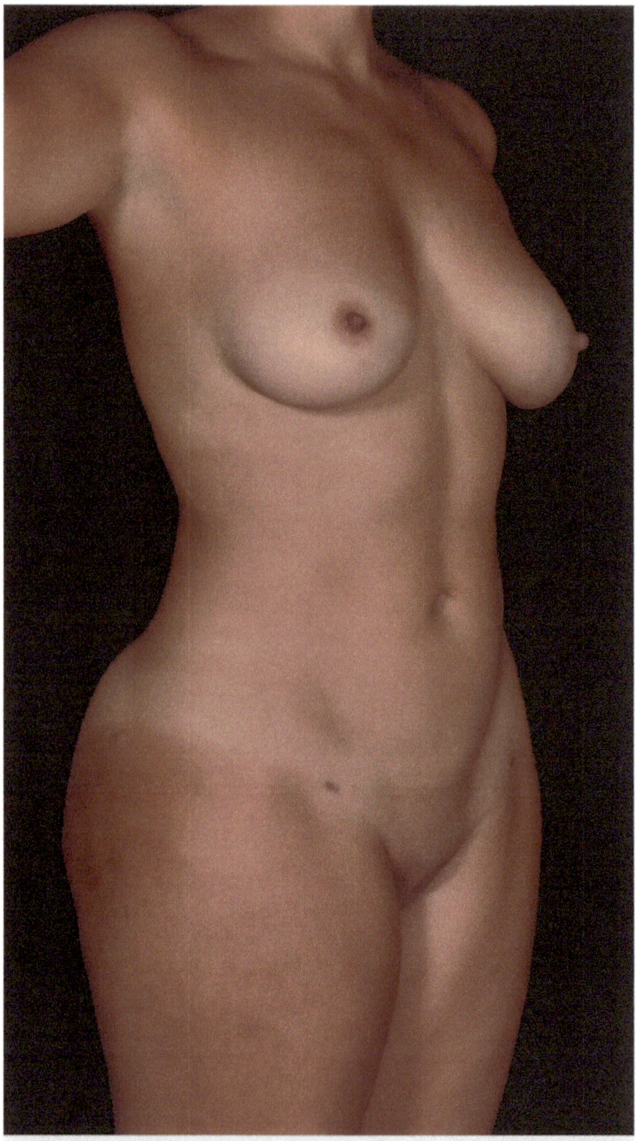

Fig. 74.12 Case example, after.

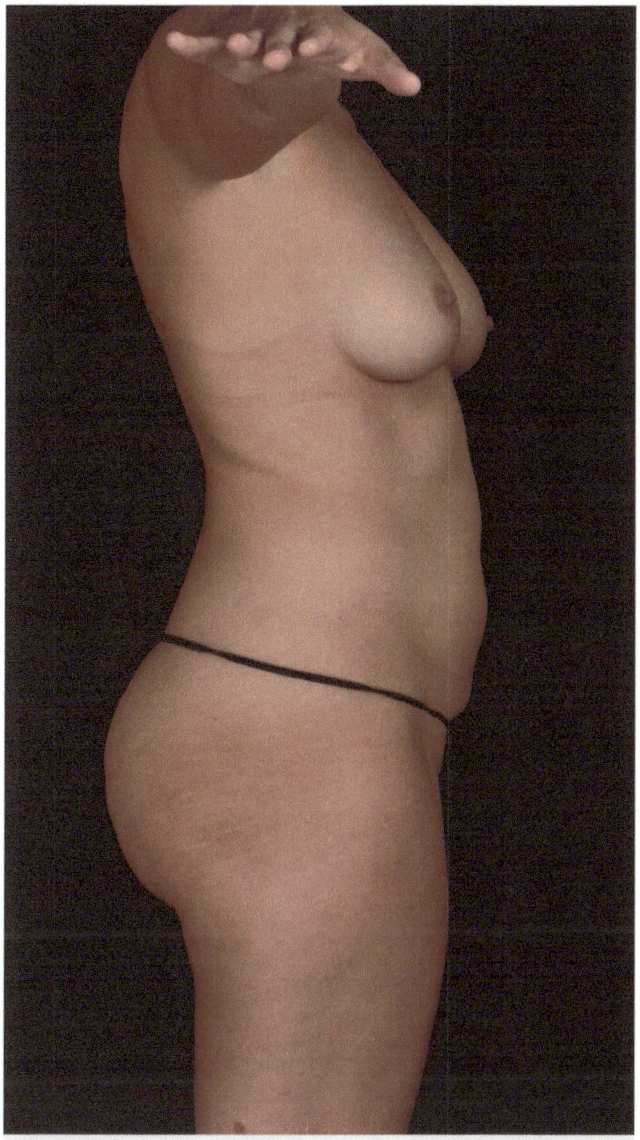

Fig. 74.13 Case example, before.

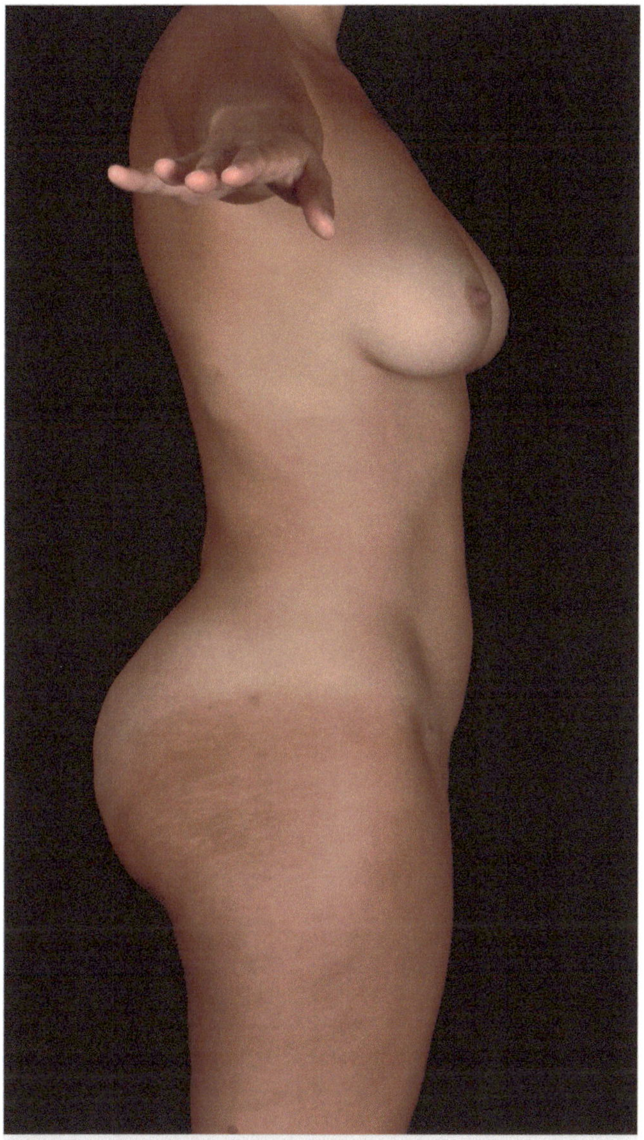

Fig. 74.14 Case example, after.

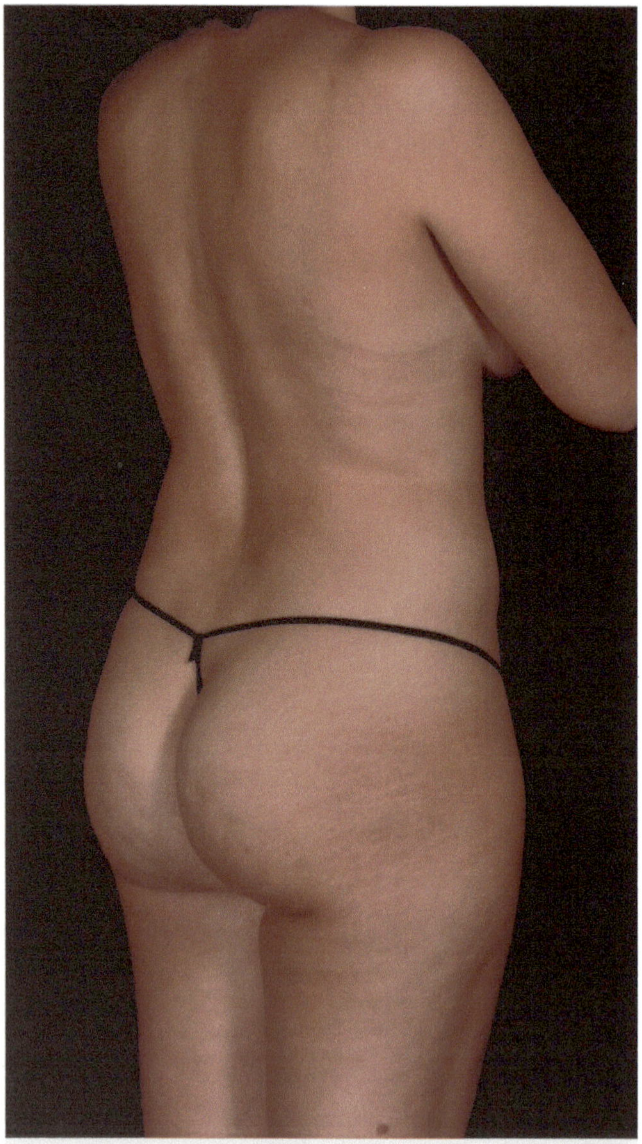

Fig. 74.15 Case example, before.

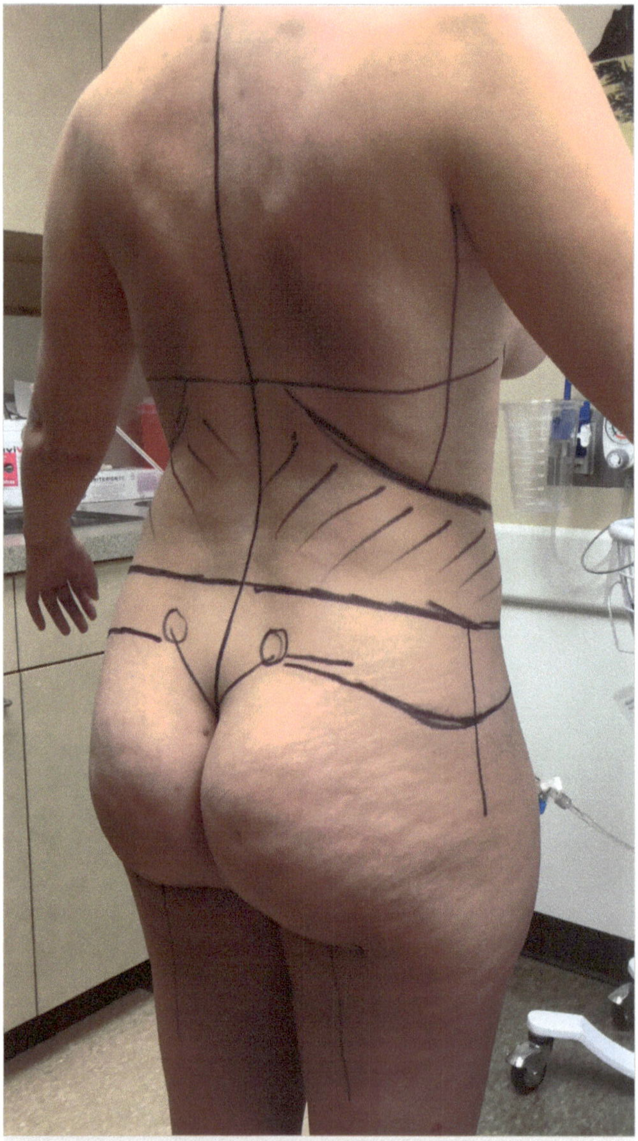

Fig. 74.16 Case example, markings.

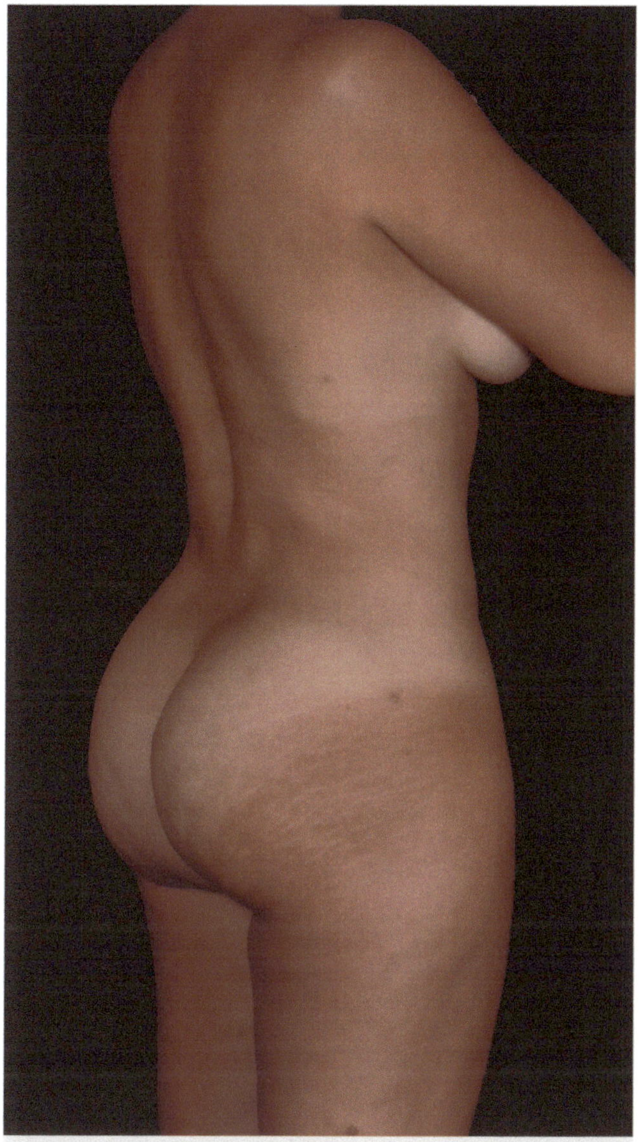

Fig. 74.17 Case example, 1 year after.

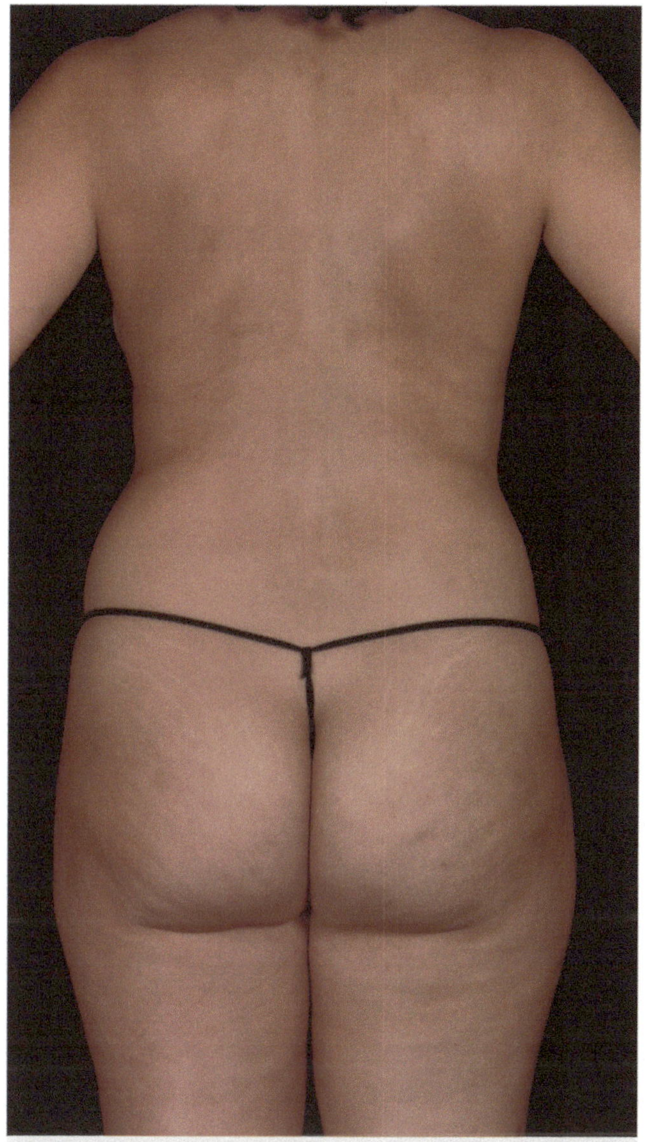

Fig. 74.18 Case example, before.

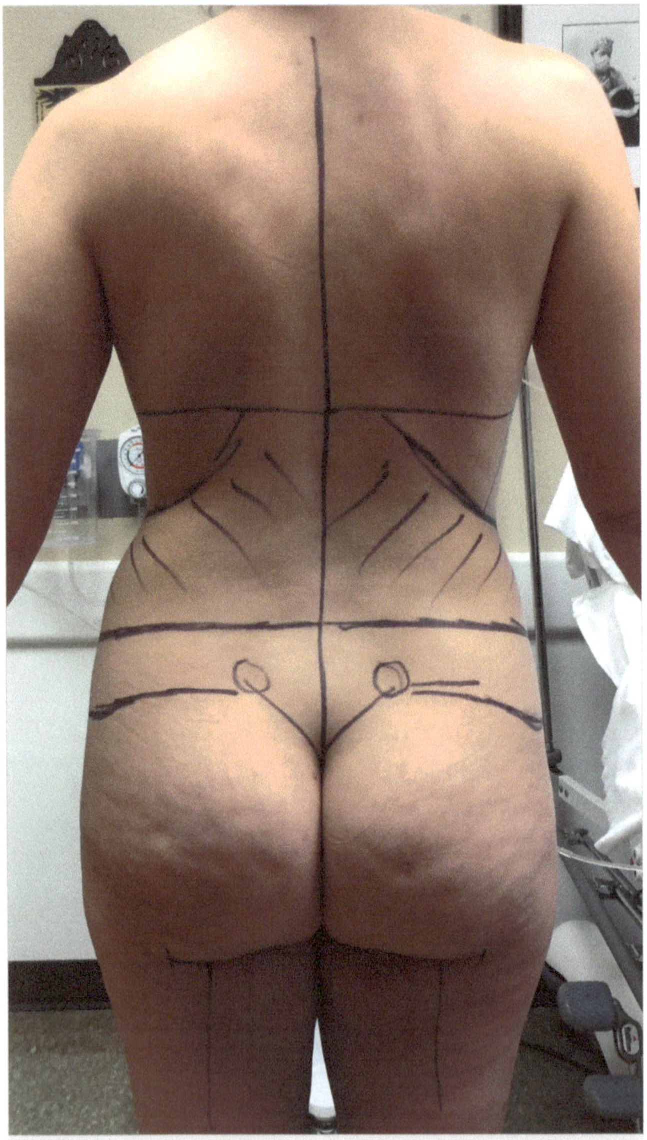

Fig. 74.19 Case example, markings.

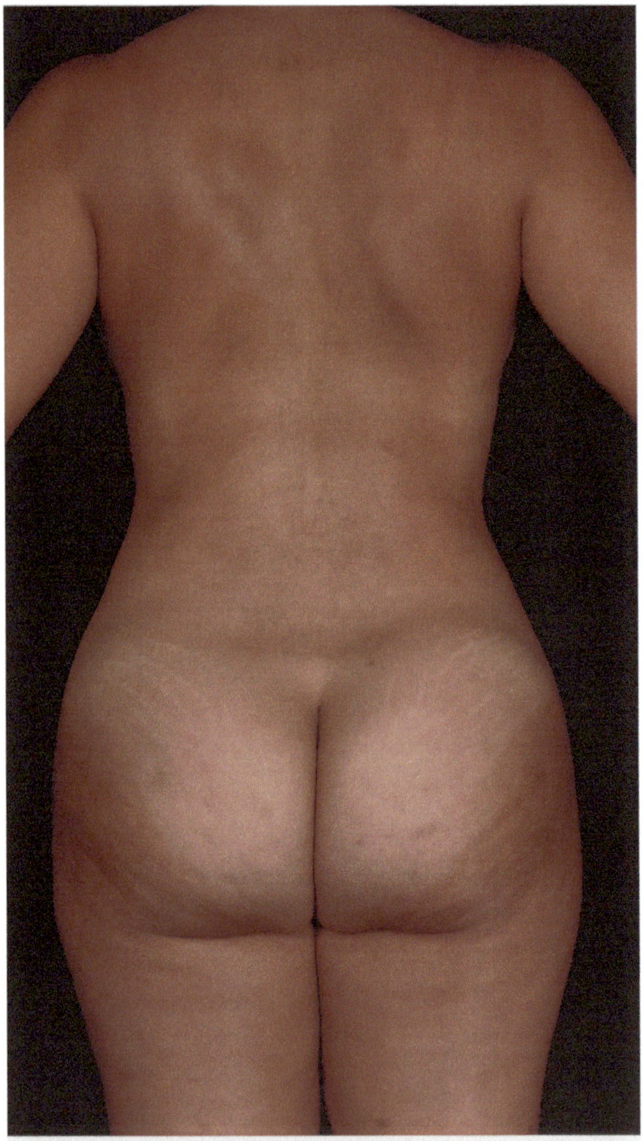

Fig. 74.20 Case example, 1 year after.

74.5 Conclusion

The stepwise approach of SAFELipo allows dramatic fat removal, even in thinner patients, without the associated risks of contour deformities. SAFElipo is more than a reductive procedure—it removes, redistributes, blends, and adds fat as needed to ensure a consistently smooth and natural appearance. Haphazard postoperative protocols and poor compliance can ruin a well-executed operation.

Further Readings

Wall S, Jr. SAFE circumferential liposuction with abdominoplasty. Clin Plast Surg. 2010; 37(3):485–501

Wall SH, Jr, Lee MR. Separation, aspiration, and fat equalization: SAFE liposuction concepts for comprehensive body contouring. Plast Reconstr Surg. 2016; 138(6): 1192–1201

Farkas JP, Stephan PJ, Kenkel JM. Liposuction: basic technique and safety considerations. The Art of Aesthetic Surgery. 2nd ed. St. Louis: Quality Medical Publishing; 2011

Del Vecchio D, Wall S, Jr. Expansion vibration lipofilling: a new technique in large-volume fat transplantation. Plast Reconstr Surg. 2018; 141(5):639e–649e

Wall SH, Jr, Claiborne JR. Discussion: a report of 736 high-definition lipoabdominoplasties performed in conjunction with circumferential VASER liposuction. Plast Reconstr Surg. 2018; 142(3):676–678

75 High-Definition Abdominal Liposculpture with BodyBanking

Ira L. Savetsky and Douglas S. Steinbrech

Abstract

Abdominal contour techniques including selective fat reduction with or without silicone have been limited in terms of inability to achieve muscular appearance in patients with very little muscular bulk in the rectus abdominis. Here we present our technique for achieving superior results in abdominal contouring using selective lipo-contouring with fat grafting.

Keywords: High definition, liposculpture, abdominal etching, fat grafting, abs

Key Points

- Patients are interested in a fitter, more sculpted look with great definition to the musculature.
- Results are maximized using a combination of selective lipo-contouring with measured structural fat grafting.

75.1 Preoperative Panning

75.1.1 Analysis

- The procedure begins with a thorough preoperative analysis to identify areas of lipodystrophy along with desired muscular enhancements and shadowing.
- These areas are carefully marked preoperatively with the patient standing prior to any sedative administration (▶ Fig. 75.1).

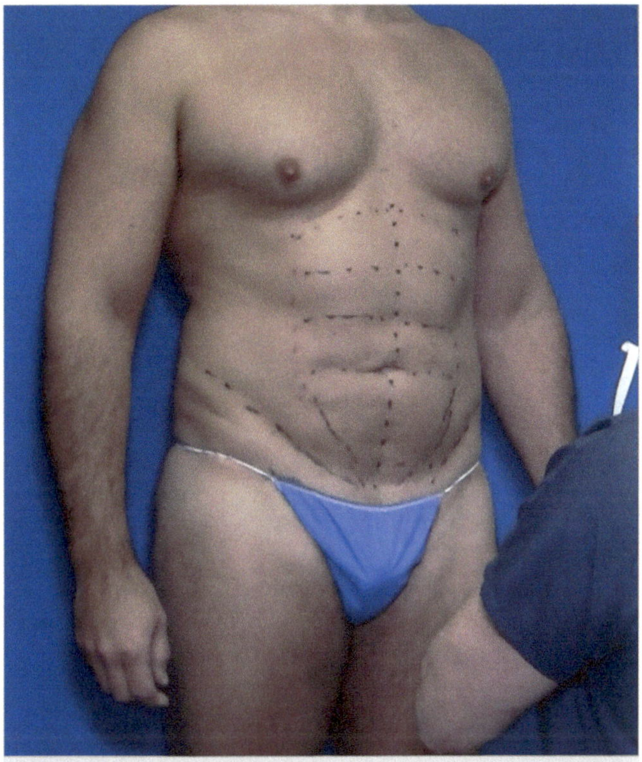

Fig. 75.1 Preoperative markings.

75.2 Operative Steps

See **Video 75.1**.

75.2.1 Access Incisions and Fat Harvest

- Three stab incisions are made in the underwear line to suction the central and lateral inscription as well as for V-flaring of the lower abdominal area.
- Four "hidden" umbilical incisions are made for upper and lower midline contouring.
- Two incisions are made under the nipples for the upper transcription.
- One incision is made laterally for second and third transverse inscription, and one is made in the upper gluteal crease for all posterior lower back and posterior flank.
- The tumescent solution (0.9% saline with lidocaine 0.1% and epinephrine 1:1,100,000) is given 10 minutes to take effect.
- The lipectomy is then carried out using power-assisted liposuction (Power Assisted Liposuction System, MicroAire, Charlottesville, VA) or standard traditional suction lipectomy from the abdominal wall and the linea alba, lateral vertical margin, serratus, and obliques to allow visibility of the rectus sheath and inscription of the rectus abdominis as well as the lower portion of the external oblique (▶ Fig. 75.2).
- The patient is then rotated using a team approach to a prone position and liposuction of the flanks is carried out after tumescent infiltration.

75.2.2 Fat Preparation and BodyBanking

- Average volumes removed from each surgical site to obtain fat and highlight contour are as follows: lower abdomen, 272 cc; muscular inscriptions, 136 cc; lateral anterior abdomen, 313 cc; bilateral flanks, 537 cc; and upper back, 228 cc.
- The fat is drained using a metal strainer and then placed into 20-cc syringes for reinjection.
- The fat is transplanted with a 1.2 Tulip fat grafting cannula (Tulip Medical Products, San Diego, CA) after dermal access of the skin with an 18-gauge needle.
- Average volumes of fat placed into each area are as follows: lower "six-pack," 42 cc each; middle "six-pack," 58 cc each; upper "six-pack," 55 cc each; and serratus muscle, 31 cc each.

75.2.3 Tissue Molding

- By placing the tip of the Penrose drain through a liposuction cannula, Penrose drains are placed through all liposuction sites, both anteriorly and posteriorly.

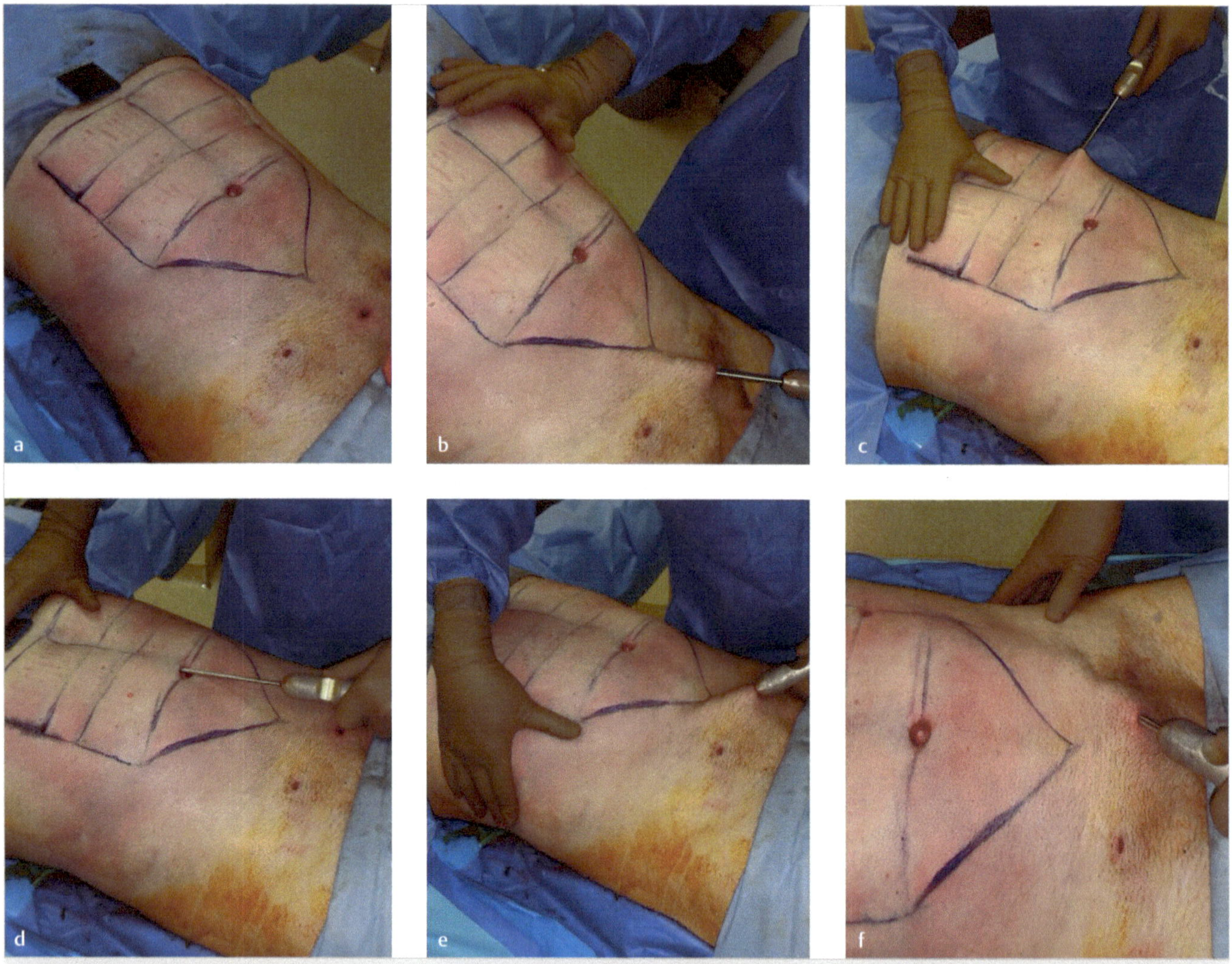

Fig. 75.2 Intraoperative technique of abdominal sculpting demonstrated on a 28-year-old man. **(a)** Tumescence, **(b)** lower abdominal suctioning, **(c)** sculpting of inscriptions, **(d)** midline sculpting, and **(e, f)** contouring of lower abdomen.

- Areas of lipofilling are then molded and preserved using foam tape, foam panels, and compression dressings.
- Foam tape along areas of depression also supports the elevation of adjacent areas that were fat grafted so fat is maintained in the desired locations (▶ Fig. 75.3).

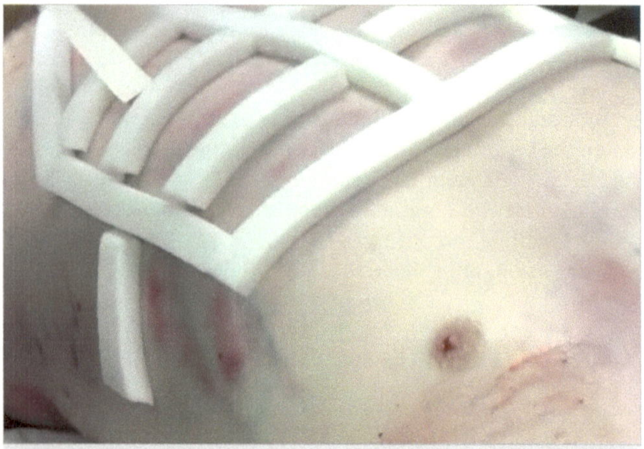

Fig. 75.3 Foam placement.

75.3 Postoperative Care

- Compression garments and foam are removed on the third postoperative day.
- Posterior Penrose drains are removed after 10 days while anterior drains are repositioned and pulled out partially at this time.
- Anterior Penrose drains are fully removed after another 10 days.

75.4 Case Example

Preoperative views of a 28-year-old man seeking improvement in definition of "six-pack." Postoperative result at 1 year after abdominal contouring (▶ Fig. 75.4a–f).

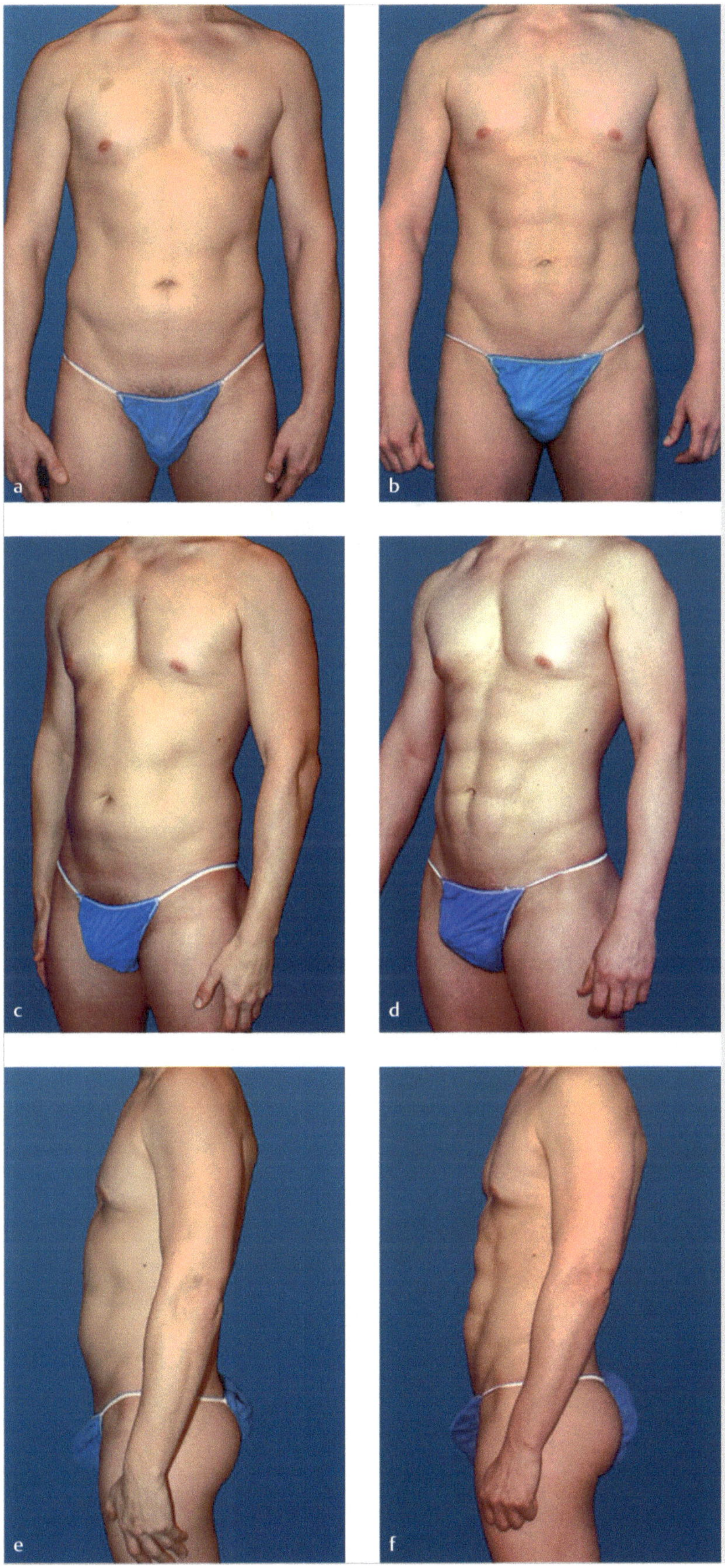

Fig. 75.4 **(a, c, e)** Preoperative views of a 28-year-old man seeking improvement in definition of "six-pack." **(b, d, f)** Postoperative result at 1 year after abdominal contouring.

75.5 Conclusion

Body contouring is a growing field with various techniques and tools available to the plastic surgeon. When used as a primary modality, liposuction may impart significant changes in both volume and contour. Liposuction alone can be limited by rebound fat deposition in undesirable locations, such as in the intra-abdominal cavity and buccal fat pad, among others. Selective liposuction is combined with measured structural fat grafting to combat the effects of rebound fat deposition while achieving synergistic elevations and depression in surgically addressed areas to refine contour.

Further Readings

Almutairi K, Gusenoff JA, Rubin JP. Body contouring. Plast Reconstr Surg. 2016; 137 (3):586e–602e

Chia CT, Neinstein RM, Theodorou SJ. Evidence-based medicine: liposuction. Plast Reconstr Surg. 2017; 139(1):267e–274e

Matarasso A, Levine SM. Evidence-based medicine: liposuction. Plast Reconstr Surg. 2013; 132(6):1697–1705

Steinbrech DR. Male aesthetic plastic surgery. London, England: Thieme; 2019

Steinbrech DS, Sinno S. Utilizing the power of fat grafting to obtain a naturally-appearing muscular "6-pack" abdomen. Aesthet Surg J. 2016; 36(9):1085–1088

76 High-Definition Liposculpture

Alfredo E. Hoyos and Mauricio E. Perez

Abstract

In recent decades, women and men have been constantly looking for an athletic and fit body. Although CrossFit and gym routines are very important for general health, some individuals struggle to get their desired outcomes and do need some help in achieving and keeping them. High-definition (HD) liposculpture was created and then improved through time and expertise to introduce new concepts regarding body contour surgery.

Since the first description of the tumescent technique, many updates and improvements have been done by introducing new technologies and concepts in body contouring. Nowadays, HD liposculpture is not only based on cutting-edge devices for liposuction and fat grafting, but also constantly evolving with evidence-based safety performance. In the following paragraphs we will describe the key points and also warnings that we need to take into account while performing HD liposculpture. Patient inclusion criteria and postoperative care compromise are significant information that need to be addressed before surgery. Some critical basic concepts include: artistic anatomy, lights and shadows, negative and dynamic zones, fat grafting, and stem cell autografts. Finally, the main premises to avoid complications and how to manage them (if they occur) are also reviewed in this chapter. We feel so honored to share our knowledge and expertise with our readers and hope to build on their strategies and techniques while performing body contour surgery.

Keywords: Liposuction, high-definition liposculpture, dynamic definition, ultrasound assisted liposculpture, VASER, fat grafting, stem cells

Key Points

- High-definition (HD) liposculpture is based on the individual's underlying structural anatomy.
- Markings are critical to ensure the correct zones to enhance (lights) and define (shadows) for an optimal result.
- Negative and dynamic zones are determined by the muscles and spaces between them for specific definition.
- HD liposculpture encompasses the whole-body contour, including arms, chest, abdomen, torso, buttocks, thighs, and calves, rather than independent zones.

76.1 Preoperative Steps

76.1.1 Patient Criteria

- General good health.
- Body mass index (BMI) <32 kg/m^2.
- American Heart Association guidelines for low risk patients (ASA < III).
- Nonsmokers or who have quit smoking.
- Patients with comorbidities need attending physician assessment to be cleared for surgery.
- Review the records of any previous procedures or surgeries performed.

76.1.2 Markings

- Optimal markings are essential to recognize deep, superficial, and smooth zones for definition.
- Create your own color code to understand operative procedures on each marked zone.
- Anatomical landmarks and some fat pads should be marked in black (▸ Fig. 76.1).
- Blue can be used in more obese individuals where deep thorough liposuction must be done (▸ Fig. 76.2).
- Red could delineate dynamic and adhesion zones (▸ Fig. 76.2).
- Green markings are used for negative spaces and transition zones where smooth liposuction must be done (▸ Fig. 76.3a).
- Purple could be used for enhancing (light) zones where fat grafting should be considered (▸ Fig. 76.3b).

Warning: Take special consideration of some "forbidden" (adhesion) zones for liposuction (can be marked with another color) if you do not have enough expertise (e.g., trochanteric depression, popliteal zone, lumbar depressions, inner arm and thigh, chest, Cooper's ligament of the breast, inguinal ligament) (▸ Fig. 76.2).

76.2 Operative Steps

See **Video 76.1**.

76.2.1 Stealth Incisions

- Incisions should be placed over hidden skin creases or maybe over the underwear's line, as scaring can leave horrible marks (▸ Fig. 76.4).
- The less the incisions the less the risk of complications.
- Gentle flap and incision manipulation helps in the healing process.

76.2.2 Liposuction

Classic Three-Step Process

- Infiltration:
  - Tumescent solution (1,000 cc Ringer's lactate + 20 cc of 1:100,000 epinephrine in addition to lidocaine 1%) infiltration is done in the superficial and deep layers.
  - Allowing for epinephrine and solution to distribute uniformly within 20 minutes before starting emulsification.
- Emulsification:
  - HD liposculpture is assisted by a third-generation ultrasound device.
  - Vibration amplification of sound energy at resonance (VASER) mode is preferred over the superficial layer with

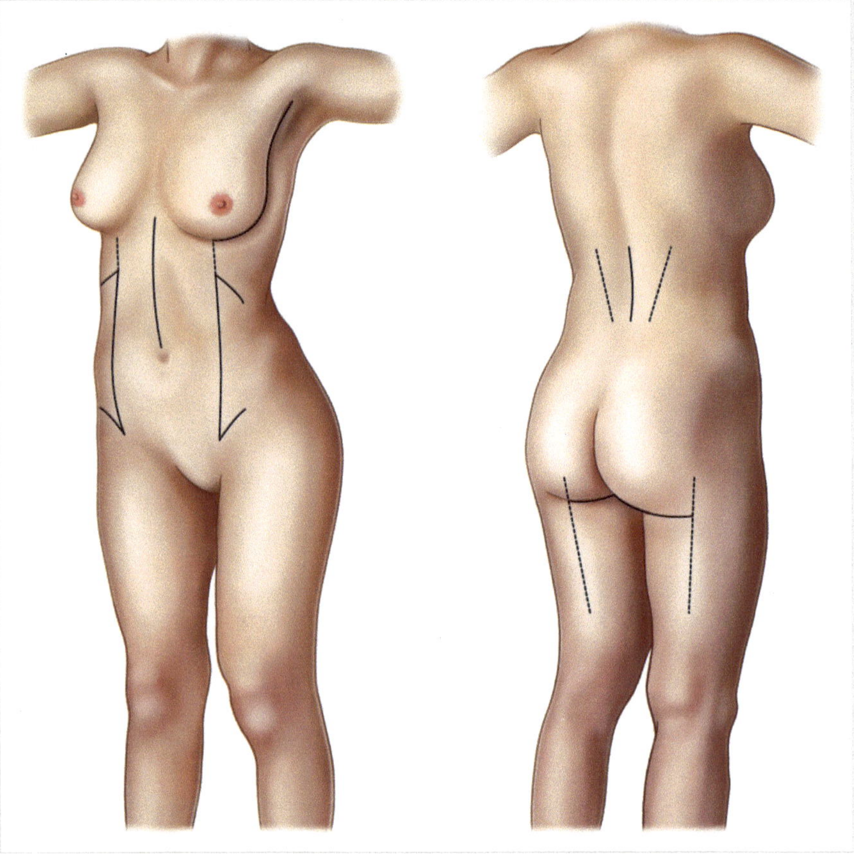

Fig. 76.1 General landmarks are preferably marked with black. Muscle insertions and underlying disposition are marked as a guide.

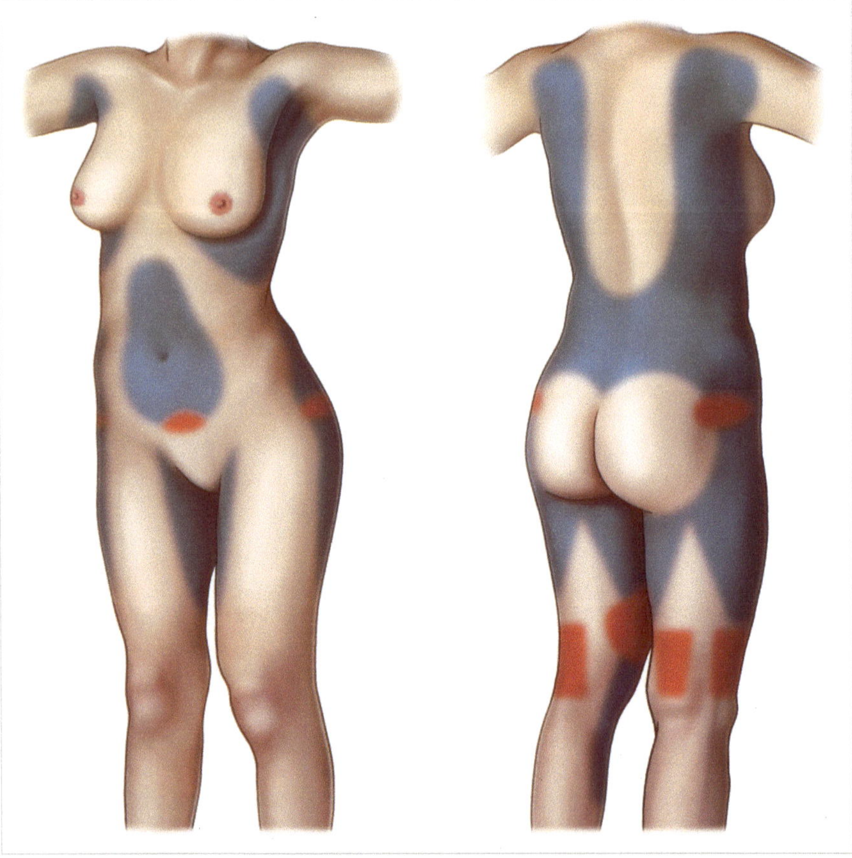

Fig. 76.2 Liposuction on adhesion zones (*red*) need to be avoided, otherwise contour defects and abnormal skin retraction might develop. Deep liposuction should be performed in areas with abundant fat pad deposition (*blue*).

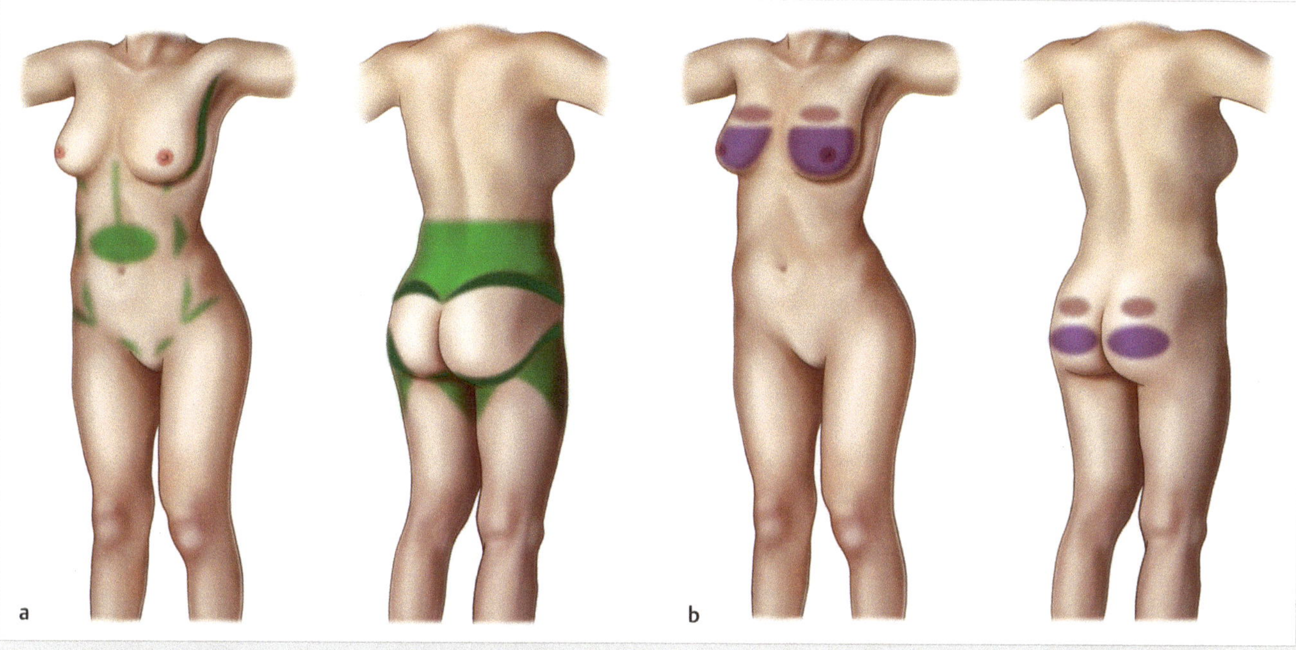

Fig. 76.3 (a, b) Preoperative markings and code of color. Artistic anatomical landmarks and specific negative zones are drawn first **(a)**. Triangles are helpful to delineate areas for smooth definition. Transition zones **(a, b)** are marked later to not only guide superficial and deep liposuction but also define zones for fat grafting **(b)**.

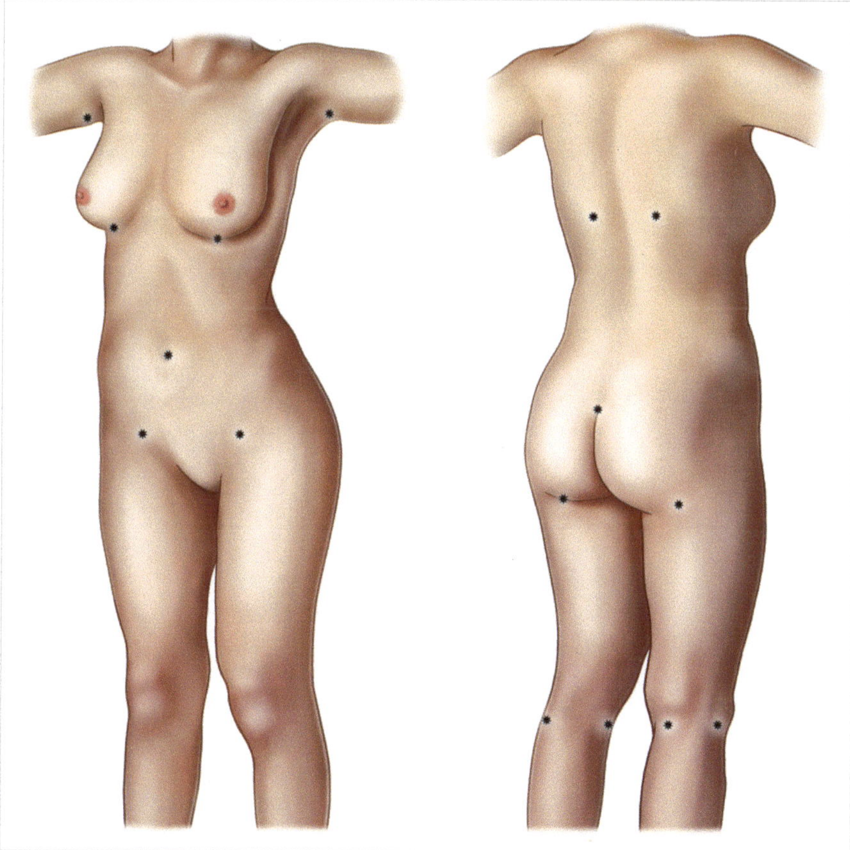

Fig. 76.4 Stealth incisions are covered by underwear or hidden by normal skin folds in order to avoid undesired scarring and visual marks of surgery. This will also masquerade natural results in high-definition liposculpture.

80 to 90% power, depending on fibrosis and/or tissue structure. Continue with gentle movements until no resistance is achieved.
  - Both superficial and deep layers must be emulsified. Deep layer is emulsified in continuous mode.

Warning: Ultrasound probe movements should be continuous and without torquing. This as well as placing wet towels under the ports will prevent burns from happening.

- Liposuction:
  - Once ports are removed, liposuction takes place.
  - Power X and Microaire systems can be used to facilitate aspiration.
  - The amount of fat removal and the cannula diameter will depend on preoperative markings. For convexities (lights), less fat removal should be performed and small (3 mm) curved cannulas are useful. For negative spaces and concavities (shadows), thorough liposuction should be done with thick (3.7–4 mm) and straight cannulas.
  - Controlled deformities are created in the superficial layer by removing almost all fat pad with 3.0-mm cannulas. Smooth areas of transition between muscles is done in women, while sharp ends are preferred in men.
  - Pinch test should be performed in the superficial layer to compare and, if needed, perform additional liposuction to improve definition.

Warning: The deep layer is carved to define group muscles and gross anatomy, while the superficial layer is the artist's keystone, where specific definition is made.

  - Dynamic zones resemble the change of the underlying muscle during contraction versus resting position. Some muscles drastically change its appearance and need to be carefully marked to avoid the unnatural facade of liposculpture surgery. This topic is discussed in depth in *Chapter 77 Male High-Definition Liposculpture*.

76.2.3 Fat Grafting

- Ultrasound assisted lipoaspiration through Power X and Microaire technologies have proven to be useful in fat graft harvesting by controlling negative pressure (<10 mmHg).
- The inner thigh and lower abdomen are rich in stem cells. So they are preferred zones for harvesting.
- Fat graft processing is done by decantation and ultracentrifugation.
- Fat grafting is reserved for volume-lacking areas or zones with desired projection improvement. Most common zones in HD liposculpture are: biceps, deltoids, pectorals, breasts, buttocks, thighs, and calves (▶ Fig. 76.3b).
- Graft is placed in multiple layers with a 3-mm cannula moving in a retrograde fashion.
- Microaire + peristaltic pump device (expansion vibration lipofilling [EVL]) can delicately place the graft between the subcutaneous layer in buttocks fat grafting.

Warning: For safety considerations, the buttocks must be grafted only in the subcutaneous layer. Deltoids and pectorals can be grafted in the intramuscular layer to improve graft survival.

- Once the procedure is concluded. Some stealth incisions are closed primarily with absorbable monofilament subdermal continuous suture.
- Incisions over the inguinal zone and the intergluteal crease are left open and a drain is placed to avoid seroma formation by allowing extra fluid drainage. If needed, other incisions could also be left open.
- Absorbable pads are placed over incisions, then the patient is dressed with foam vests and compression garments.

76.3 Postoperative Care

The adherence to postoperative therapies and recommendations is crucial to achieve the desired results in body sculpting surgery (▶ Fig. 76.5a–h). Patients are subject to the following postoperative care in order to avoid most common complications:

- Patient's head is placed at 30 to 45 degrees in recovery.
- Overnight vigilance is considered for high volume extraction (>6000 mL) or according to any medical condition.
- Discharge is made approximately 6 hours after surgery.
- Daily drainage must be performed by a technician or a nurse for 8 to 10 days postoperatively.
- Compression garments must be used from 4 to 8 weeks, while foams must be used at least 2 to 4 weeks after the procedure.
- Assisted ambulation is mandatory to improve lung and surgical trauma fast recovery.
- Exercise and sexual activity should be avoided for 3 to 4 weeks.
- Cosmetic Active Recovery (CARE) system is a therapeutic method planned to reduce swelling, bruising, pain, and improve healing. It is sometimes used before surgery to prepare the tissue for intervention.

76.4 Complications

Although very uncommon, surgeons and their staff must be aware of any insidious sign of complications:

- Seroma.
- Infection.
- Burns.
- Contour irregularities or asymmetry.
- Abnormal skin retraction.
- Bleeding (excessive bruising or hematoma).
- Others: Pulmonary edema, thromboembolism, fat embolism, perforation, necrosis, lidocaine toxicity.

76.5 Case Example

HD lipoplasty performed on a 38-year-old female patient. Note the localized fat pads and the abdominal contour's absence of

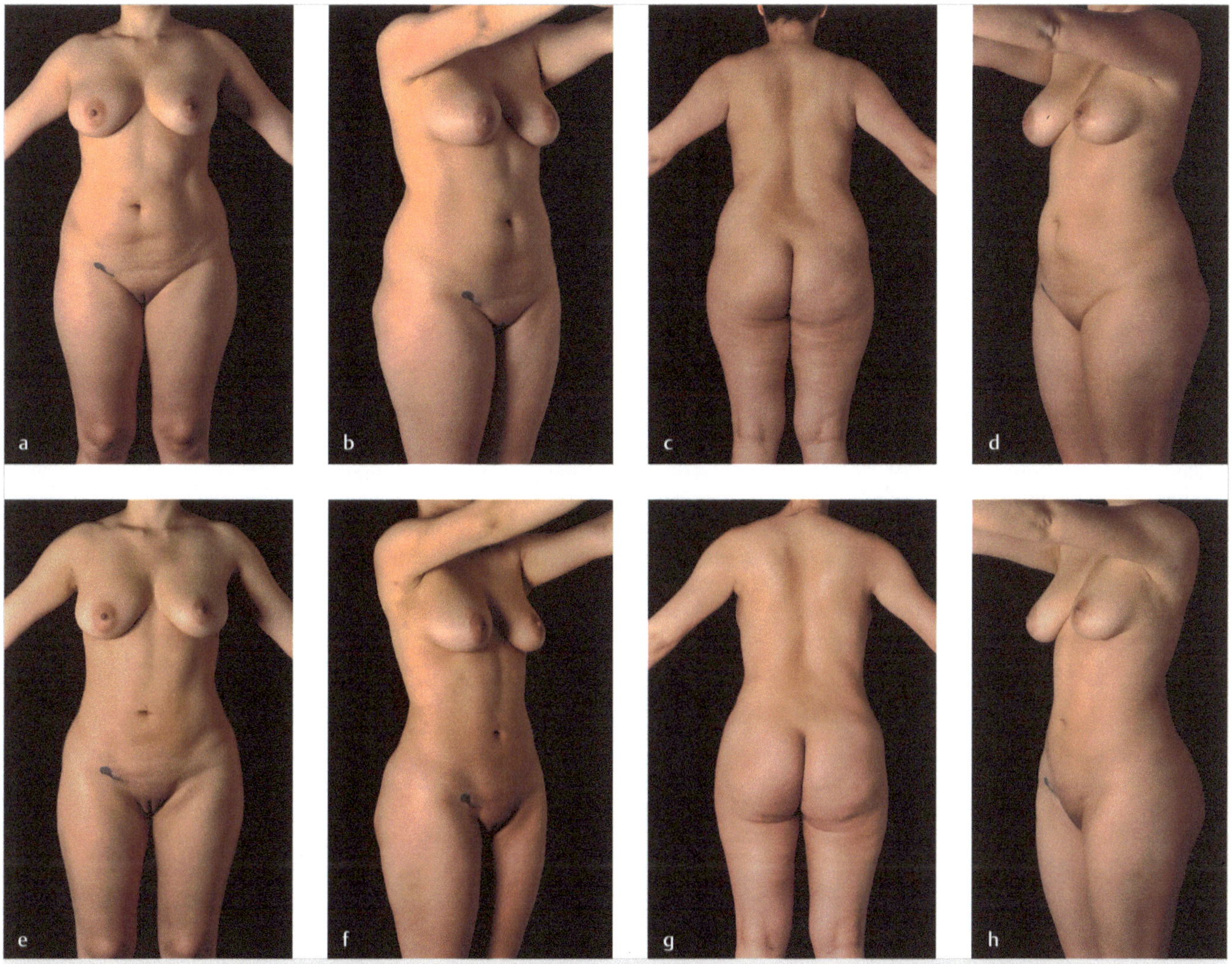

Fig. 76.5 (a–h) High-definition lipoplasty performed on a 38-year-old female patient. Note the localized fat pads and the abdominal contour's absence of definition in the preoperative pictures **(a–d)** compared to the new athletic and slim appearance in the postoperative pictures **(e–h)**. Buttocks are now bigger and rounder than before, with a new defined abdomen and torso.

definition in the preoperative pictures (▶ Fig. 76.5a–d) compared to the new athletic and slim appearance in the postoperative pictures (▶ Fig. 76.5e–h). Buttocks are now bigger and rounder than before, with a new defined abdomen and torso.

76.6 Conclusion

A slim and natural body contour for women and muscular and athletic for men can be achieved by means of HD liposculpture. Artistic anatomy and adequate preoperative markings are essential to get desired outcomes in the lipoplasty technique (▶ Fig. 76.5a–h). New technologies and concepts have been introduced to HD liposculpture in order to improve the natural appearance of the body contour. Fat grafting in addition to superficial and deep lipoplasty are the basic procedures in HD liposculpture. Postoperative care is the basic principle to avoid complications as well as to guarantee long-lasting results.

Further Readings

Del Vecchio D, Wall S, Jr. Expansion vibration lipofilling: a new technique in large-volume fat transplantation. Plast Reconstr Surg. 2018; 141(5):639e–649e

Hoyos AE, Millard JA. VASER-assisted high-definition liposculpture. Aesthet Surg J. 2007; 27(6):594–604

Hoyos AE, Prendergast PM. High definition body sculpting: art and advanced lipoplasty techniques. 1st ed. Berlin, Heidelberg: Springer; 2014

Rohrich RJ, Beran SJ, Kenkel JM. Ultrasound-assisted liposuction. 1st ed. St Louis, USA: Thieme Medical Publishers, Inc.; 1998

Toledo LS. Gluteal augmentation with fat grafting: the Brazilian buttock technique: 30 years' experience. Clin Plast Surg. 2015; 42(2):253–261

77 Male High-Definition Liposculpture

Alfredo E. Hoyos and Mauricio E. Perez

Abstract

Male patients have increasingly become more interested in body contour surgeries, since new technologies and devices have improved outcomes and are now suitable for many of them. The chest, abdomen, and buttocks are the main concern our patients ask about at our office. High definition (HD) lipoplasty is assisted by ultimate generation ultrasound devices and has important differences between male and female procedures, mainly regarding multiple muscle enhancing areas through fat grafting and enhanced muscle definition. The male body shape resemble power and strength throughout history in different cultures around the world, so our main purpose in male HD liposculpture is to restore and define the underlying anatomy to make the body muscular and athletic again. Basic important clues to pursue this goal are: the markings phase, the specific zones for superficial versus deep liposuction, and selective fat grafting. Critical concepts also need to be mastered to understand the principles that rule HD liposculpture. These include artistic anatomy, lights and shadows, negative and dynamic zones, and stem cell fat grafting. Although many safety considerations have been stablished to perform HD lipoplasty, some complications might occur, most of them related to inappropriate postoperative care. Finally, insomuch as many patients have reported above expectations results, immense expertise and good training are needed to achieve the desired results.

Keywords: Male liposculpture, high-definition lipoplasty, male dynamic definition, ultrasound assisted liposculpture, VASER, fat grafting, stem cells

Key Points

- Athletic appearance with pectoral and buttocks enhancement, six-pack sharpness, and deltoid prominence are main concerns that male patients request for at our office.
- Male high-definition (HD) liposculpture has clear differences compared to the female procedure. Buttocks and pectorals usually need volume augmentation.
- As muscular enhancement is crucial for the male figure, dynamic concepts become very important to reach exceptional outcomes.
- Multilayer fat grafting enriched with stem cells is almost always used to enhance some areas lacking projection or volume.

77.1 Preoperative Analysis

77.1.1 Patient Criteria

- General good health.
- Low preoperative risk assessment (ASA < III) according to American Heart Association (AHA) guidelines.
- Body mass index <32 kg/m^2.
- Preferably without previous liposculpture procedures or without severe fibrosis nor biopolymer injections.
- Nonsmokers or who have quit.
- Patients with comorbidities need attending physician's assessment to be cleared for surgery.

77.1.2 Markings

- They are the initial step to understand and plan this kind of procedure.
- Start with the anatomical landmarks (▶ Fig. 77.1): muscles, bony prominences, limits, etc.
- Then, mark the negative spaces as triangles and transition zones for smooth definition (▶ Fig. 77.2a).
- After that, fat grafting zones are drawn in different muscles to improve projection and volume (▶ Fig. 77.2b).

Warning: Remember to use a color code for your own markings. This will help you to differentiate structures and the intraoperative process.

- Some adhesion zones in the male (prohibited in the female) need to be considerably defined as they will enhance the masculine appearance. These comprise the trochanteric depression, paravertebral, and pectoral triangles (▶ Fig. 77.2a).
- In the obese patient, ultrasound may be useful to delimit some additional anatomical features.

77.2 Operative Steps

See **Video 77.1**.

77.2.1 Stealth Incisions

- Incisions should be placed over hidden skin creases or maybe over the underwear's line, as scaring can leave horrible marks (▶ Fig. 77.3).
- As the male patient needs an athletic definition, additional incisions are sometimes needed.
- Gentle flap and incision manipulation helps the healing process.

77.2.2 Liposuction

Classic three-step process is followed.

Infiltration

- Infiltration starts from the deep and then the superficial layers with tumescent solution (1,000 cc Ringer's lactate + 20 cc of 1:100,000 epinephrine in addition to lidocaine 1%) in a 2:1 ratio.
- Allow for epinephrine and solution to distribute uniformly within 20 minutes before starting emulsification.

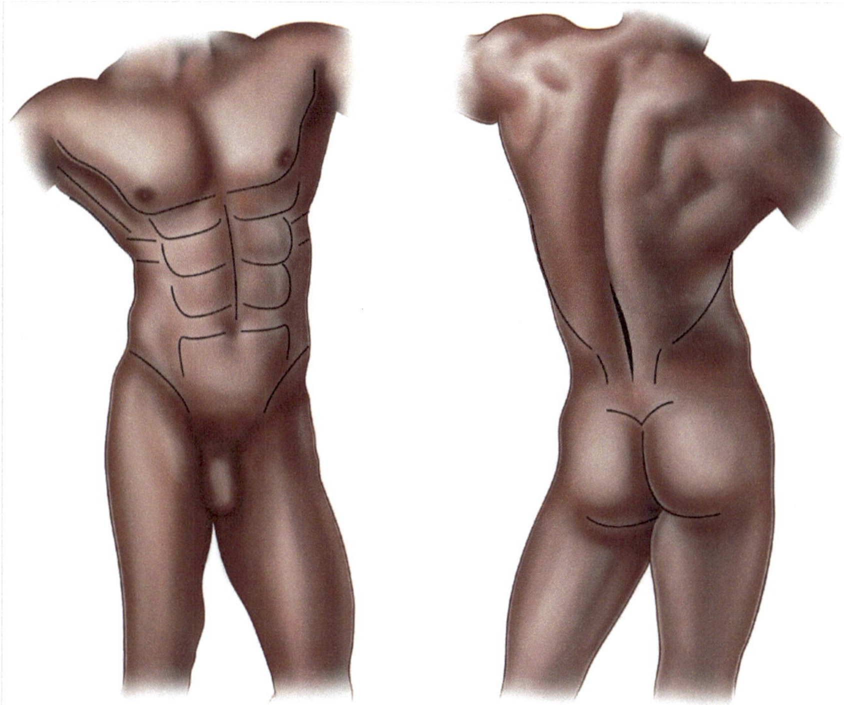

Fig. 77.1 Gross anatomical landmarks: Muscular limits and disposition for subsequent definition.

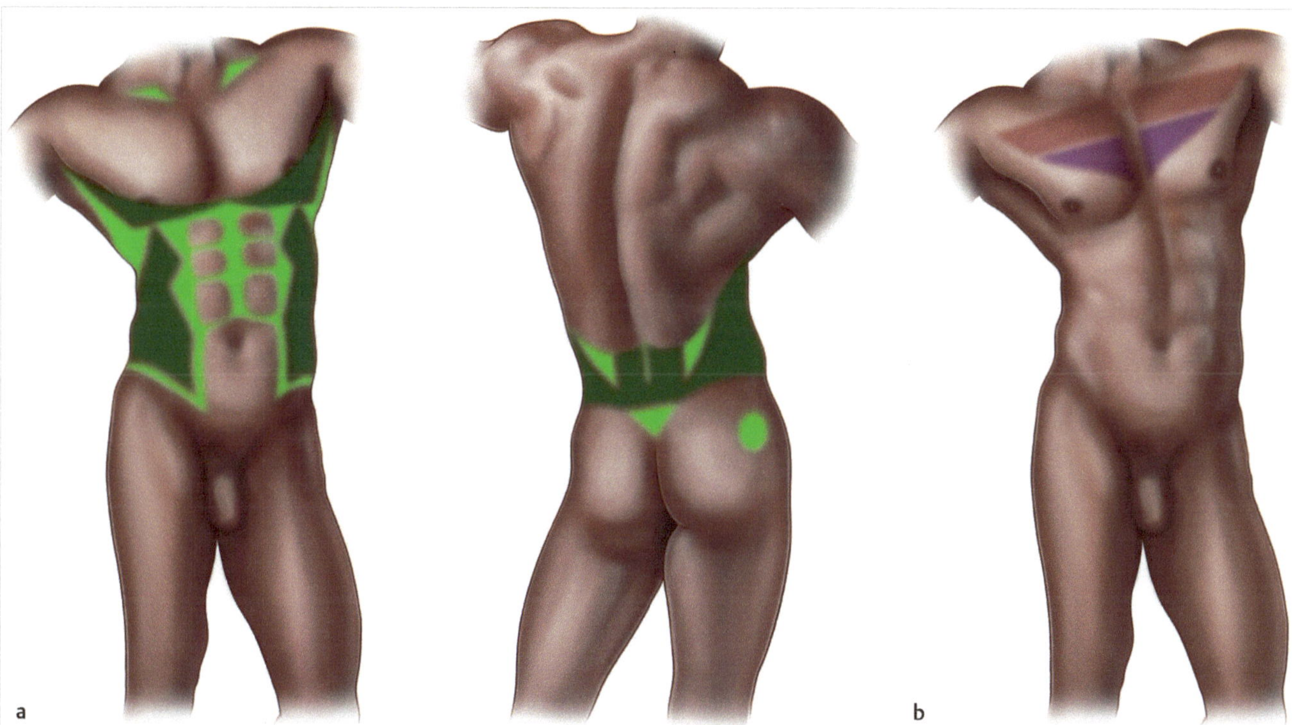

Fig. 77.2 Specific markings (code of color): Negative spaces and transition zones **(a)** are marked in *green* while fat grafting zones **(b)** are drawn with *red and purple*. Note that some adhesion zones **(a)**—prohibited in the female lipoplasty—need to be treated to exalt the muscular appearance.

Emulsification

- We use third-generation ultrasound device to assist liposuction.
- Vibration amplification of sound energy at resonance (VASER) mode is used for the superficial layer with 80 to 90% power, depending on fibrosis and/or tissue resistance.
- Deep layer is emulsified in continuous mode.
- Continue with gentle movements until the probe moves freely.

Warning: Ultrasound probe movements should be continuous and without torquing. This as well as placing wet towels under the ports will prevent burns from happening.

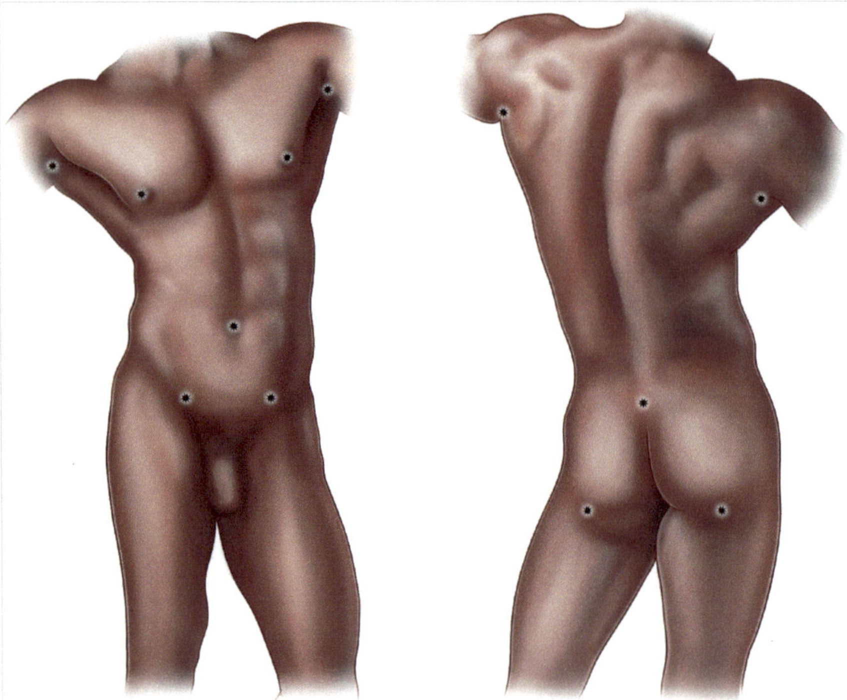

Fig. 77.3 Stealth incisions are usually hidden by normal skin creases (or the underwear line). Male high-definition (HD) liposculpture occasionally need additional incisions over the abdomen to increase the "six-pack" definition.

Liposuction

- Once ports are removed, liposuction takes place.
- Power X and Microaire systems can be used to ease aspiration.
- The amount of fat removal and the cannula diameter will depend on preoperative markings:
  - For convexities (lights), less fat removal should be performed and small (3 mm) curved cannulas are useful.
  - For negative spaces and concavities (shadows), thorough liposuction should be done with thick (3.7–4 mm) and straight cannulas.
- Start liposuction in the deep layer. Once the subcutaneous flap is 1 cm thick, superficial framing can be achieved.
- Sharp ends and close transition zones are preferred in the male patient to build on muscular definition.
- Pinch test and thorough liposuction should be done in the superficial layer to improve athletic definition (▶ Fig. 77.4).
- Thorough definition must be performed on *dynamic zones,* which will resemble the change of the underlying muscle during contraction versus resting position (▶ Fig. 77.5). Comparatively, smooth definition must be achieved on negative spaces surrounding them.

Warning: Dynamic zones in the male include: pectorals (▶ Fig. 77.5a), deltoids, triceps (▶ Fig. 77.5b), serratus, rectus abdominis, latissimus dorsi, quadriceps, and gastrocnemius.

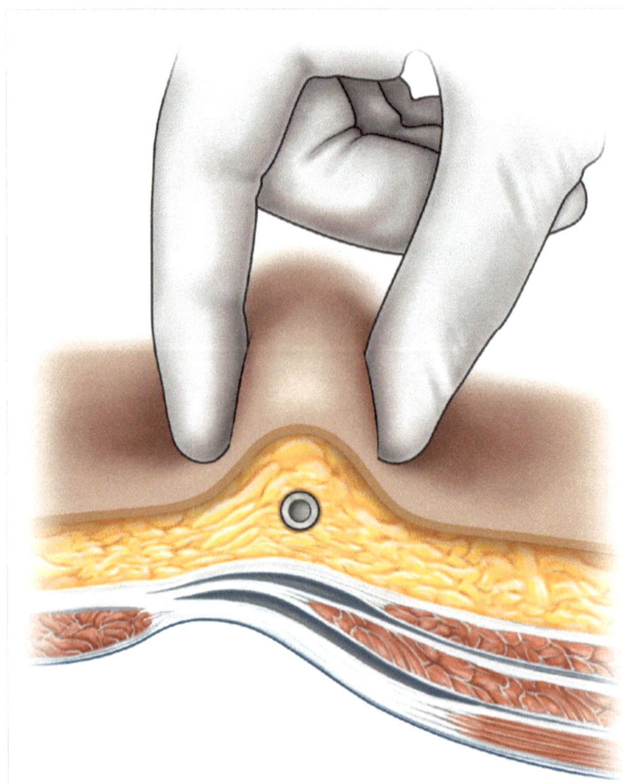

Fig. 77.4 Pinch maneuver in order to perform superficial framing. This allows us to reduce the skin flap thickness, which in turn will ease the postoperative adherence to the muscular surface, resulting in better definition.

77.2.3 Fat Grafting

- Ultrasound assisted lipoaspiration through Power X and Microaire technologies have proven to be useful in fat graft harvesting by controlling negative pressure (<10 mmHg).

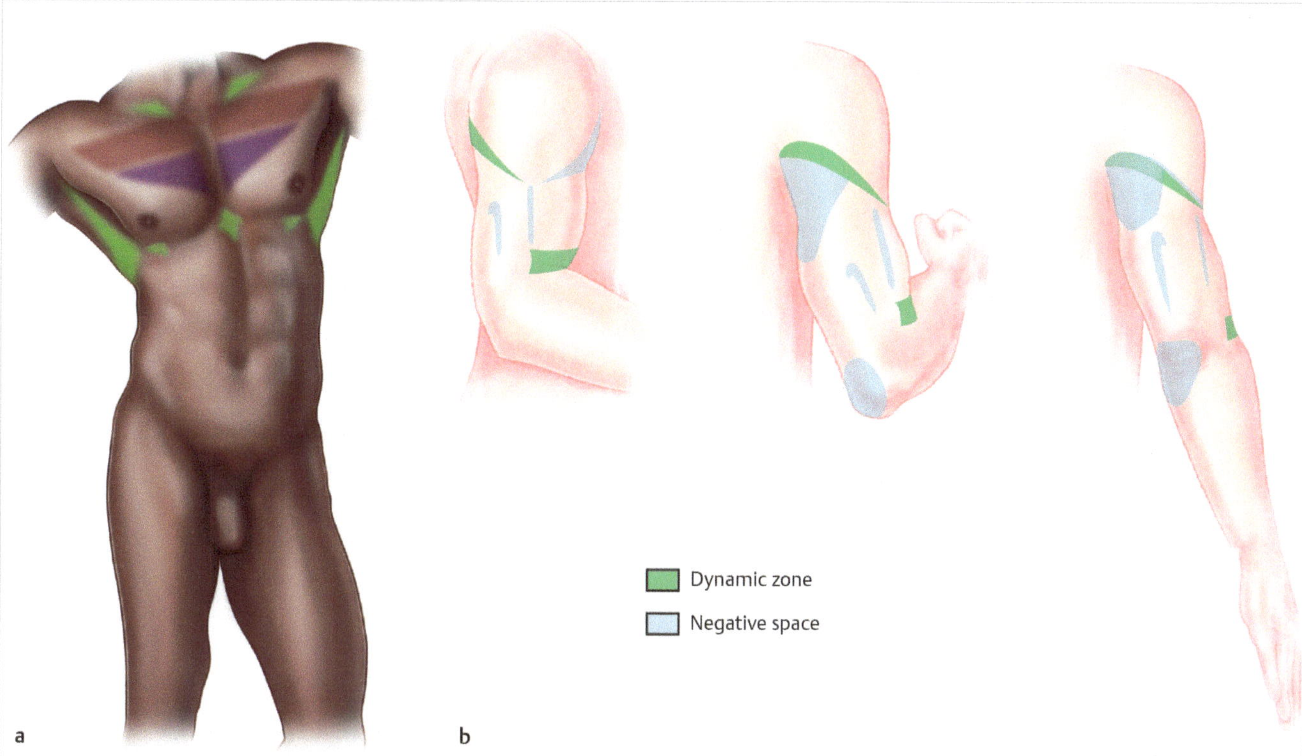

Fig. 77.5 Pectoral etching **(a)** and arm definition **(b)** pictures. Triangles are helpful to delineate areas for smooth definition surrounding keen muscular edges **(a)**. Dynamic zones **(a, b)** are marked later to not only guide superficial and deep liposuction but also define negative zones and muscles for fat grafting (deltoid, pectorals).

- The inner thigh and lower abdomen are rich in stem cells. Fat graft processing is done by decantation and ultracentrifugation.
- Fat grafting is reserved for volume-lacking areas or zones with desired projection improvement. Most common zones in male HD liposculpture are: Biceps, deltoids, pectorals (▸ Fig. 77.5a and ▸ Fig. 77.6a), buttocks (▸ Fig. 77.6b), thighs, and calves.
- Microaire + peristaltic pump device (expansion vibration lipofilling [EVL]) can delicately place the graft between the subcutaneous layer in buttocks fat grafting.

Warning: The buttocks must be grafted only in the subcutaneous layer due to safety considerations. Deltoids and pectorals can be grafted in the intramuscular layer to improve graft survival.

- Once the procedure is concluded, most incisions are closed with absorbable monofilament subdermal continuous suture.
- Incisions over the inguinal zone and the intergluteal crease are left open and a drain is placed to avoid seroma formation by allowing extra fluid drainage. If needed, other incisions could also be left open.
- Absorbable pads are placed over incisions; then the patient is dressed with foam vests and compression garments.

77.3 Postoperative Care

- Patient's head is placed at 30 to 45 degrees in recovery.
- Overnight vigilance is considered for high volume extraction (>6000 mL) or any other medical condition.
- Discharge is made approximately 6 hours after surgery.
- Adherence to postoperative therapies and recommendations must be given and precisely followed by the patient to ensure optimum results (▸ Fig. 77.7a–h).
- Daily drainage must be performed by a technician or nurse for 8 to 10 days after surgery.
- Compression garments must be worn for 6 to 8 weeks. Foams are mandatory for at least 4 weeks after the procedure.
- Progressive assisted ambulation is recommended to improve lung and surgical trauma recovery.
- Exercise and sexual activity should be avoided for 3 to 4 weeks.
- Cosmetic Active Recovery (CARE) system is a therapeutic method planned to reduce swelling, bruising, pain, and

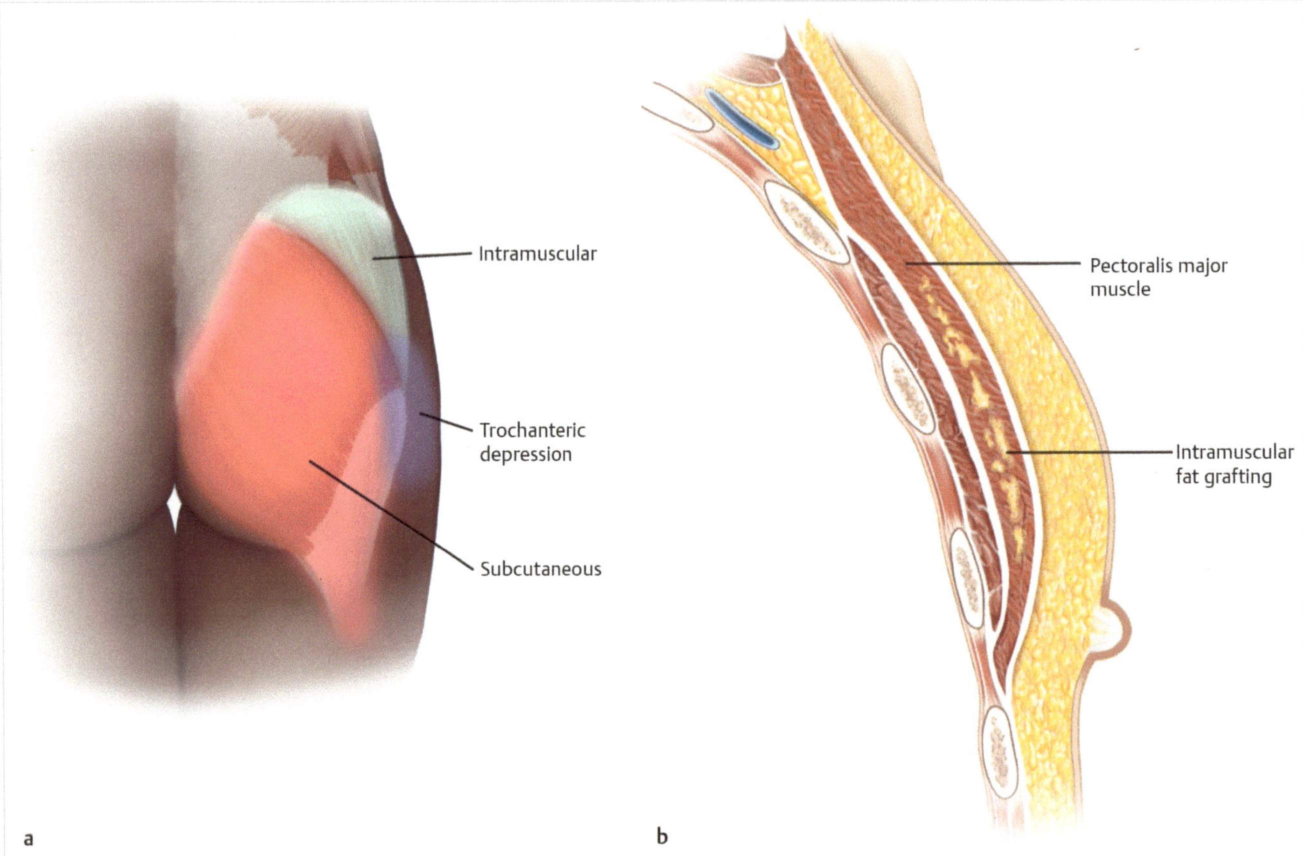

Fig. 77.6 Fat grafting: Subcutaneous approach is preferred on the gluteal area **(a)** to reduce the risk of migration. Gluteus medius could be grafted in a multilayer fashion as it is performed on the pectoralis muscle **(b)** and other muscles (deltoid, biceps, calves).

improve healing. Lymphatic drainage, radiofrequency, and ultrasound are used to stimulate recovery.

77.4 Complications

- Seroma.
- Infection.
- Bleeding (excessive bruising or hematoma).
- Contour irregularities or asymmetry.
- Abnormal or aberrant skin retraction.
- Burns.
- Others: Pulmonary edema, thromboembolism, fat embolism, perforation, necrosis, lidocaine toxicity.

77.5 Case Example

HD lipoplasty performed on a 34-year-old male patient. Lack of chest projection and definition is observed in the preoperative pictures (▶ Fig. 77.7a–d) in addition to deficient upper limb muscularity. The new chest enhancement and athletic appearance of the arm as well as abdomen muscular definition can be perceived in the postoperative pictures (▶ Fig. 77.7e–h).

77.6 Conclusion

Muscular and athletic body appearance in the male patient can be achieved through HD lipoplasty. Accurate markings as well as dynamic, negative, and transition zones are determinant concepts that need to be mastered in order to perform an exceptional male HD liposculpture. Male liposculpture needs sharp definition and muscular enhancement to accomplish the goal of a masculine appearance. Volume and projection augmentation can be performed by selective multilayer fat grafting in some major muscles. HD liposculpture in the male patient is a safe and reproducible procedure. Specific knowledge of the artistic anatomy and basic HD principles in addition to a significant learning curve are required to achieve optimal results.

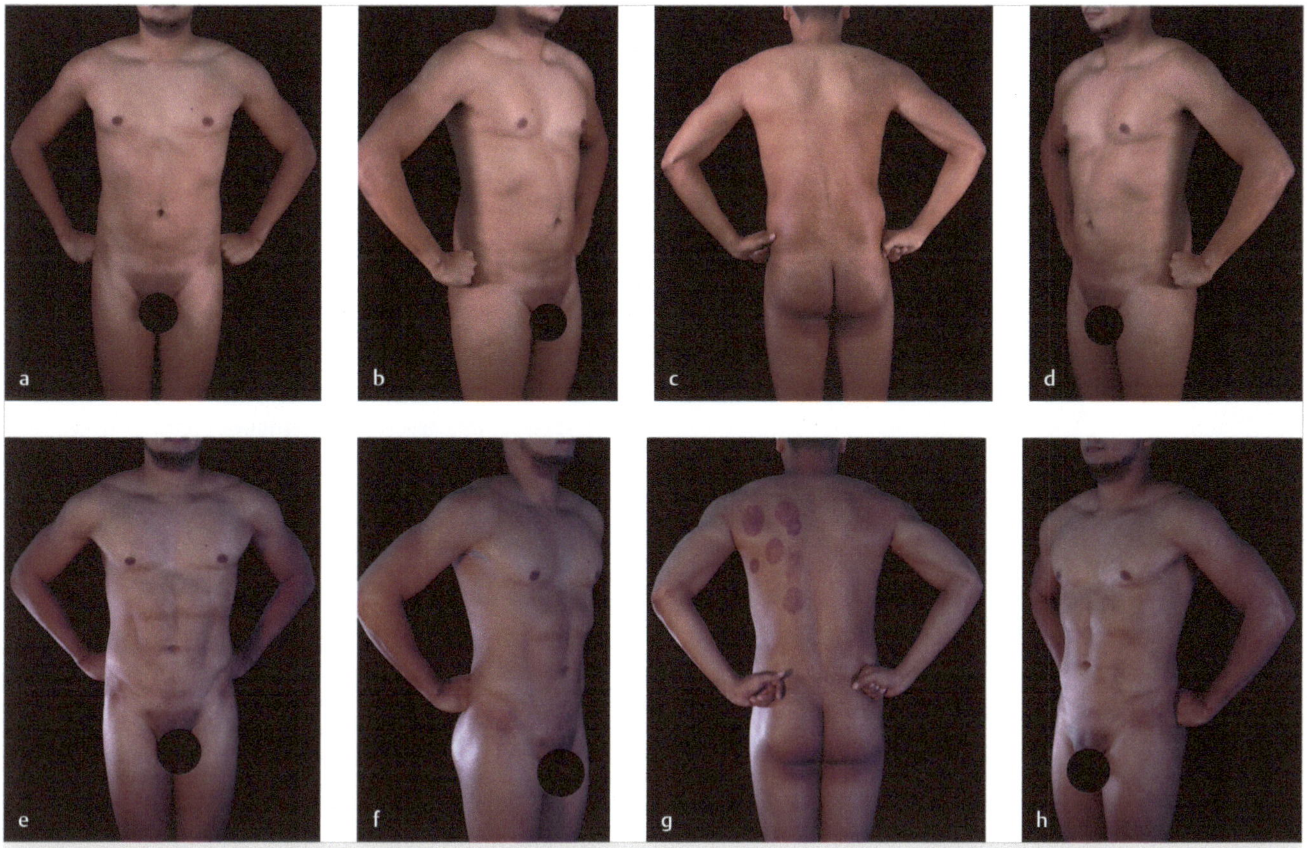

Fig. 77.7 (a–h) High-definition (HD) lipoplasty performed on a 34-year-old male patient. Lack of chest projection and definition is observed in the preoperative pictures **(a–d)** in addition to deficient upper limb muscularity. The new chest enhancement and athletic appearance of the arm as well as abdomen muscular definition can be perceived in the postoperative pictures **(e–h).**

Further Readings

Del Vecchio DA, Villanueva NL, Mohan R, et al. Clinical implications of gluteal fat graft migration: a dynamic anatomical study. Plast Reconstr Surg. 2018; 142(5):1180–1192

Hoyos AE, Millard JA. VASER-assisted high-definition liposculpture. Aesthet Surg J. 2007; 27(6):594–604

Hoyos AE, Prendergast PM. High definition body sculpting: art and advanced lipoplasty techniques. 1st ed. Berlin, Heidelberg: Springer; 2014

Hoyos A, Perez M. Dynamic-definition male pectoral reshaping and enhancement in slim, athletic, obese, and gynecomastic patients through selective fat removal and grafting. Aesthetic Plast Surg. 2012; 36(5):1066–1077

Rohrich RJ, Beran SJ, Kenkel JM. Ultrasound-assisted liposuction. 1st ed. St Louis, USA: Thieme Medical Publishers, Inc.; 1998

78 Gynecomastia Excision with BodyBanking

Ira L. Savetsky and Douglas S. Steinbrech

Abstract

Chest contour techniques including selective fat and glandular tissue reduction have been limited in terms of inability to achieve muscular appearance in patients with very little muscular bulk in the pectoralis major musculature. Here we present our technique for achieving superior results in chest contouring using selective lipo-contouring with fat grafting.

Keywords: Gynecomastia, male breasts, pseudogynecomastia, liposuction, fat grafting

Key Points

- Gynecomastia is typically idiopathic; however, physiologic and pathological causes must be ruled out.
- Minimize inferior areolar incisions, obliterate the inframammary fold, and perform near-complete excision of breast glandular tissue.
- Goal is a flat chest contour with accentuation of the underlying pectoral major muscle.
- Results are maximized using a combination of suction lipectomy, direct excision, along with measured structural fat grafting.

78.1 Preoperative Steps

78.1.1 Analysis

- The procedure begins with a thorough preoperative analysis to identify areas of glandular and/or fatty tissue along with desired muscular enhancements and shadowing.
- These areas are carefully marked preoperatively with the patient standing prior to any sedative administration.

78.2 Operative Steps

See **Video 78.1**.

78.2.1 Direct Excision, Access Incisions, and Suction Lipectomy

- Along the inferior areolae, 3-mm stab incisions are made.
- The tumescent solution (0.9% saline with lidocaine 0.1% and epinephrine 1:1,100,000) is infiltrated and given 10 minutes to take effect.
- The lipectomy is then carried out using power-assisted liposuction (Power Assisted Liposuction System, MicroAire, Charlottesville, VA).
- Incisions are made with a #15 blade and deepened with electrocautery, and then near-complete excision of glandular tissue is removed en bloc (▶ Fig. 78.1).
- To avoid a contour depression or "dish saucer deformity," 2 to 3 mm of subareolar tissue is left behind in very athletic patients while 5 mm of subareolar tissue is left behind in slightly overweight patients.
- Wide undermining of the inframammary is performed sharply from the inferior areolar incisions to allow excess skin to obliterate the fold and allow the skin to redrape and contract.

78.2.2 Fat Harvest, Preparation, and BodyBanking

- The areas for fat harvest are determined preoperatively depending on patient's desires and areas of lipodystrophy.
- Stab incisions are made in an inconspicuous area.
- The tumescent solution (0.9% saline with lidocaine 0.1% and epinephrine 1:1,100,000) is infiltrated and given 10 minutes to take effect.
- The lipectomy is then carried out using power-assisted liposuction (Power Assisted Liposuction System, MicroAire, Charlottesville, VA) or standard traditional suction lipectomy (▶ Fig. 78.2).
- The fat is drained using a metal strainer and then placed into 20-cc syringes for reinjection.
- The fat is transplanted with a 1.2 Tulip fat grafting cannula (Tulip Medical Products, San Diego, CA) after dermal access of the skin with an 18-gauge needle to the superior chest to accentuate the underlying pectoral major muscle (▶ Fig. 78.3).

78.2.3 Tissue Molding

- By placing the tip of the Penrose drain through a liposuction cannula, Penrose drains are placed through all liposuction sites.
- Areas of lipofilling are then molded and preserved using foam tape, foam panels, and compression dressings.
- Foam tape along areas of depression also supports the elevation of adjacent areas that were fat grafted so that fat is maintained in the desired locations.

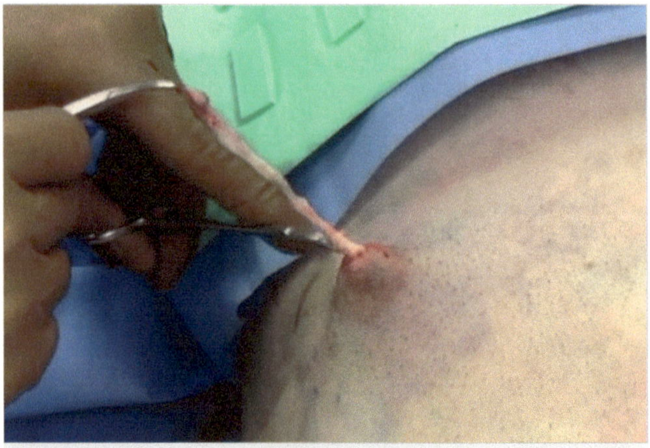

Fig. 78.1 En bloc excision of glandular tissue.

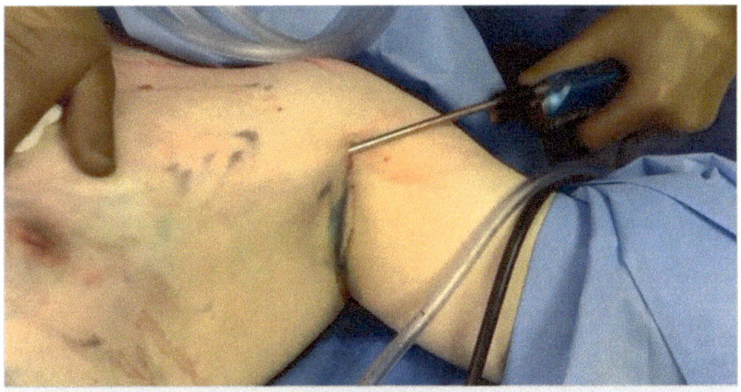

Fig. 78.2 Lipectomy using power-assisted liposuction.

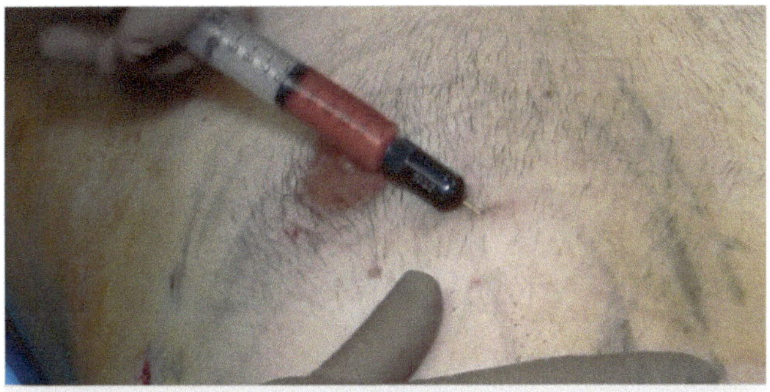

Fig. 78.3 Fat grafting with a 1.2 Tulip fat grafting cannula.

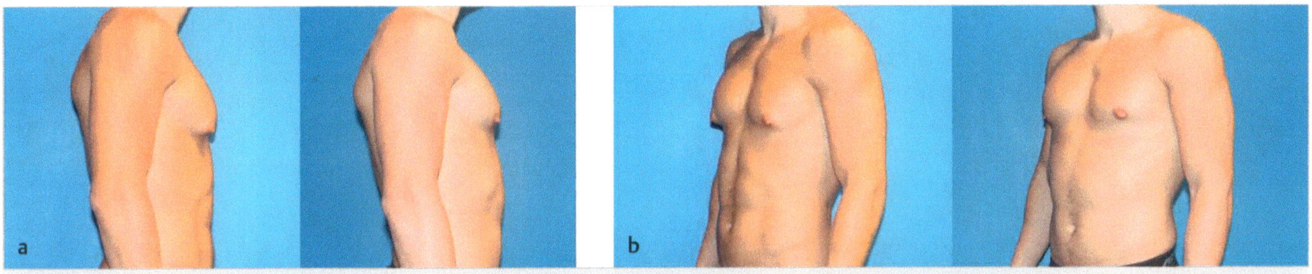

Fig. 78.4 (a, b) Pre- and postoperative lateral and oblique views of a male patient after undergoing gynecomastia excision with autologous fat transfer to the chest.

78.3 Postoperative Management

- Compression garments and foam are removed on the third postoperative day.
- Penrose drains are repositioned and pulled out partially after 10 days.
- Penrose drains are fully removed after another 10 days.

78.4 Case Example

Pre- and postoperative lateral and oblique views of a male patient after undergoing gynecomastia excision with autologous fat transfer to the chest (▶ Fig. 78.4a, b).

78.5 Conclusion

Body contouring is a growing field with various techniques and tools available to the plastic surgeon. When used as a primary modality, liposuction may impart significant changes in both volume and contour. Liposuction alone can be limited by rebound fat deposition in undesirable locations, such as in the intra-abdominal cavity and buccal fat pad, among others. Selective liposuction is combined with measured structural fat grafting to combat the effects of rebound fat deposition while achieving synergistic elevations and depression in surgically addressed areas to refine contour.

Further Readings

Blau M, Hazani R, Hekmat D. Anatomy of the gynecomastia tissue and its clinical significance. Plast Reconstr Surg Glob Open. 2016; 4(8):e854

Blau M, Hazani R. Correction of gynecomastia in body builders and patients with good physique. Plast Reconstr Surg. 2015; 135(2):425–432

Khouri RK, Jr, Khouri RK. Current clinical applications of fat grafting. Plast Reconstr Surg. 2017; 140(3):466e–486e

Lista F, Ahmad J. Power-assisted liposuction and the pull-through technique for the treatment of gynecomastia. Plast Reconstr Surg. 2008; 121(3):740–747

Steinbrech DR. Male aesthetic plastic surgery. London, England: Thieme; 2019

79 Mommy Makeover Finesse

Matthew Schulman

Abstract

In current society, there is an increasing demand for more product, delivered quickly and efficiently. Today's plastic surgery demand is no different. Patients desire a total body improvement in a single operation. Modern surgical techniques, together with advanced anesthetic technology, make it possible to perform combined procedures safely. The term "mommy makeover" is used to refer to a single operation composed of multiple procedures that addresses different areas of the body simultaneously. This is generally used to reverse the common changes associated with pregnancies, but is also used to improve changes associated with aging and weight fluctuations. This most commonly used procedures include abdominoplasty, liposuction, and cosmetic breast surgery, but will vary from patient to patient. This chapter will discuss what most commonly constitutes a "mommy makeover"—how to choose appropriate patients and procedure combinations, how to modify your techniques when combining procedures, and how to perform combined surgeries efficiently, thereby minimizing operative time and reducing surgical risk.

Keywords: Mommy makeover, combination, abdominoplasty, breast, liposuction, pregnancy

Key Points

- "Mommy makeover" refers to a combination of procedures, performed during a single operation, to reverse commons signs of aging and pregnancies.
- Advances in surgical and anesthesia techniques have enabled us to do combination surgery more safely.
- The specific combinations are unique and customized to each patient.
- Proper combination surgery requires that the surgeon consider each procedure individually and also how each relates to and affects the other.

79.1 Defining a "Mommy Makeover"

- Single operation consisting of multiple procedures, each designed to address specific areas of the body.
- Most commonly used when referring to surgery to reverse effects of pregnancy.
- The term is a misnomer, and patients need not be mothers or have had prior pregnancies.
- Also used to refer to combined surgery to correct changes from normal aging process, congenital abnormalities, or fluctuations in weight.

79.2 Most Common Procedures

- Breast procedures:
  - Augmentation mammoplasty, mastopexy, augmentation, mastopexy, reduction mammoplasty.
- Abdominal procedures:
  - Abdominoplasty, extended abdominoplasty, mini abdominoplasty.
- Liposuction.
- Buttock augmentation.
- May include virtually any procedure since each operation is customized for individual patients.
- Circumferential approach will offer the most dramatic improvement.
- Most commonly involves procedures for the breast and body, although facial procedures are not excluded.

79.3 Preoperative Considerations

79.3.1 Patient Selection

- Surgeries tend to be longer so patient selection is critical.
- Healthy patients with appropriate medical clearance.
- Complete blood count (CBC), prothrombin time (PT)/partial thromboplastin time (PTT), basic metabolic panel, electrocardiogram (ECG), chest X-ray (CXR) (if over 50 years old), physical examination, and written medical clearance by primary medical doctor or any relevant specialists.
- Hemoglobin >12.5 g/dL.
- Optimization of any pre-existing medical issues.
- Nicotine cessation for a minimum of 4 weeks prior to and 8 weeks after surgery.
- Patients with realistic expectations who understand that combination procedures require longer recovery periods and higher revision rates.
- No immediate plans for pregnancy.
- Minimum of 9 months post-partum.

79.3.2 Selecting Procedure Combinations

- Combination should be selected to maximize patient improvement and minimize operative time, while understanding how combinations affect healing and results.
- Anticipated postoperative pain and required time off from work or away from family responsibilities are a consideration and should be discussed with patients.
- It is best to address the areas that bother the patient the most, knowing that it is not always possible to safely address all the areas in a single operation.
- Anterior-only combinations—abdominoplasty, breast surgery, and anterior/lateral liposuction:
  - Allows for ease in operative positioning and more rapid operative time.

- Positioning during recovery period will be supine.
- May not offer maximal improvement since posterior defects are not addressed.

- Addition of posterior procedures—posterior liposuction, skin removal, and buttock contouring:
  - Will require position changes in the operating room with additional operative time.
  - Positioning during recovery period will be supine or lateral since prone positioning can adversely affect results of abdominoplasty or breast surgery.
  - Increased risk of dependent seroma formation after posterior liposuction and placement of posterior drain may be indicated.
  - When buttock contouring with fat grafting is performed, there will be increased risk of fat resorption from pressure of supine positioning during recovery.

79.3.3 Surgical Markings

- Surgical markings are made as per usual, with some specific considerations.
- When combining breast surgery with an abdominoplasty, you must consider the inferior stretch on the inframammary fold (IMF) (▶ Fig. 79.1).
  - Breast markings must be adjusted to account for inferior IMF displacement and should be made while the abdomen skin is "on-stretch."
  - Failure to anticipate IMF displacement will result in visible scars on the superior abdominal wall that would normally be concealed within the IMF.
  - IMF displacement will alter the nipple to IMF distances which is important during breast lift and reduction procedures.

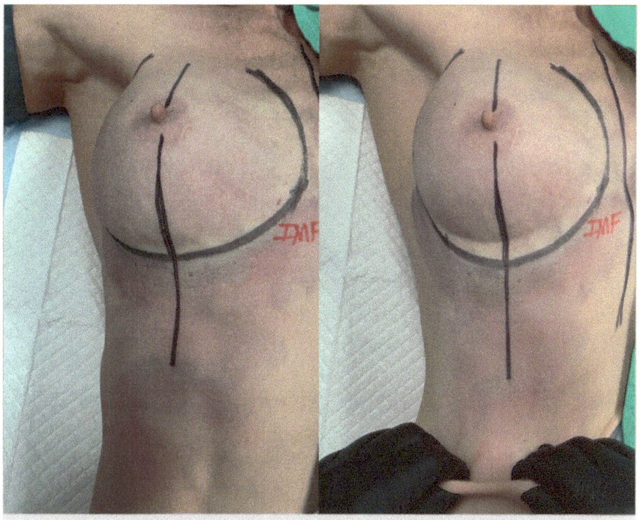

Fig. 79.1 Demonstration of anticipated breast scar migration during a simultaneous breast and abdominal surgery. On the left, you will see how the marker remains within the inframammary fold (IMF). On the right, you will see where that "incision" will be after abdominal skin retraction of an abdominoplasty. The placement of the IMF incision should account for the anticipated migration.

79.4 Operative Steps

See **Video 79.1**.

79.4.1 In Presurgical Holding Area

- Preoperative hydration with 1,000 cc of normal saline or lactated Ringers.
- Intravenous antibiotics 20 minutes prior to incision.
- Further reviews about the risks, alternatives, and benefits of planned procedure.

79.4.2 Sequence of Procedures

- Order will depend on the specific procedures being performed.
- Sterility of procedure and necessary patient positioning will determine sequence.
- When possible, placement of breast implants as the first procedure minimizes risk of contamination.
- When using a circumferential approach, patient cannot be placed prone after completion of an abdominoplasty or complex breast procedure:
  - Start prone and perform the posterior procedures.
  - Turn patient supine and then perform anterior procedures, starting with breast procedures.
  - Liposuction of the anterior torso is performed last and this will allow most accurate shaping since the other procedures have already been completed.
  - Additional fat grafting to the hips can be performed, if necessary, from this anterior approach.

Specific Sequencing Example: Breast Procedure (Lift, Lift with Implants, Implants), Tummy Tuck, and Brazilian Butt Lift

- Prone position.
- Liposuction of the posterior torso with fat grafting to the buttock and hips.
- Turn supine.
- Breast lift and implants.
- Abdominoplasty.
- Liposuction of the flanks, bra line, and any other anterior areas.
- Additional fat grafting to hips from and anterior approach (if necessary).

79.4.3 Patient Positioning

- Position changes increases patient risk:
  - Increased operative time.
  - Increased exposure and hypothermia.
  - Anesthetic concerns—airway, blood pressure, and oxygenation.
- Two position approach:
  - Anterior and posterior.
  - No lateral positioning.
- No more than two positions to avoid unnecessary operative time and increased risk associated with moving the patient:
  - Avoid anterior → posterior → anterior.
- Appropriate airway control and patient cushioning.

79.5 Minimizing Operative Time

- Operative and anesthesia time can almost always be reduced by being more efficient with aspects not related to the actual operating.

79.5.1 Staff Communication

- Keep good communication with your surgical team about the next steps in your operation.
- Give accurate time updates about how long between steps so that they can be prepared.
- When you are finishing a specific procedure, your team should be preparing for the next procedure to avoid unnecessary delays.

79.5.2 Efficiency in Patient Repositioning

- Significant delays can be avoided with an efficient patient reposition.
- Efficiency of the repositioning is critical and this should be practiced, much like a NASCAR pit crew practices a tire change.
- You should be timing the reposition for self-audit and improvement:
  - The process should take as little as 30 seconds in skinny patients and no more than 60 seconds in heavier patients.
  - This takes a consistent surgical team and practice so it is much easier to perfect in an in-office setting.
- The repositioning can be done rapidly and safely with four team members (▶ Fig. 79.2a–d).

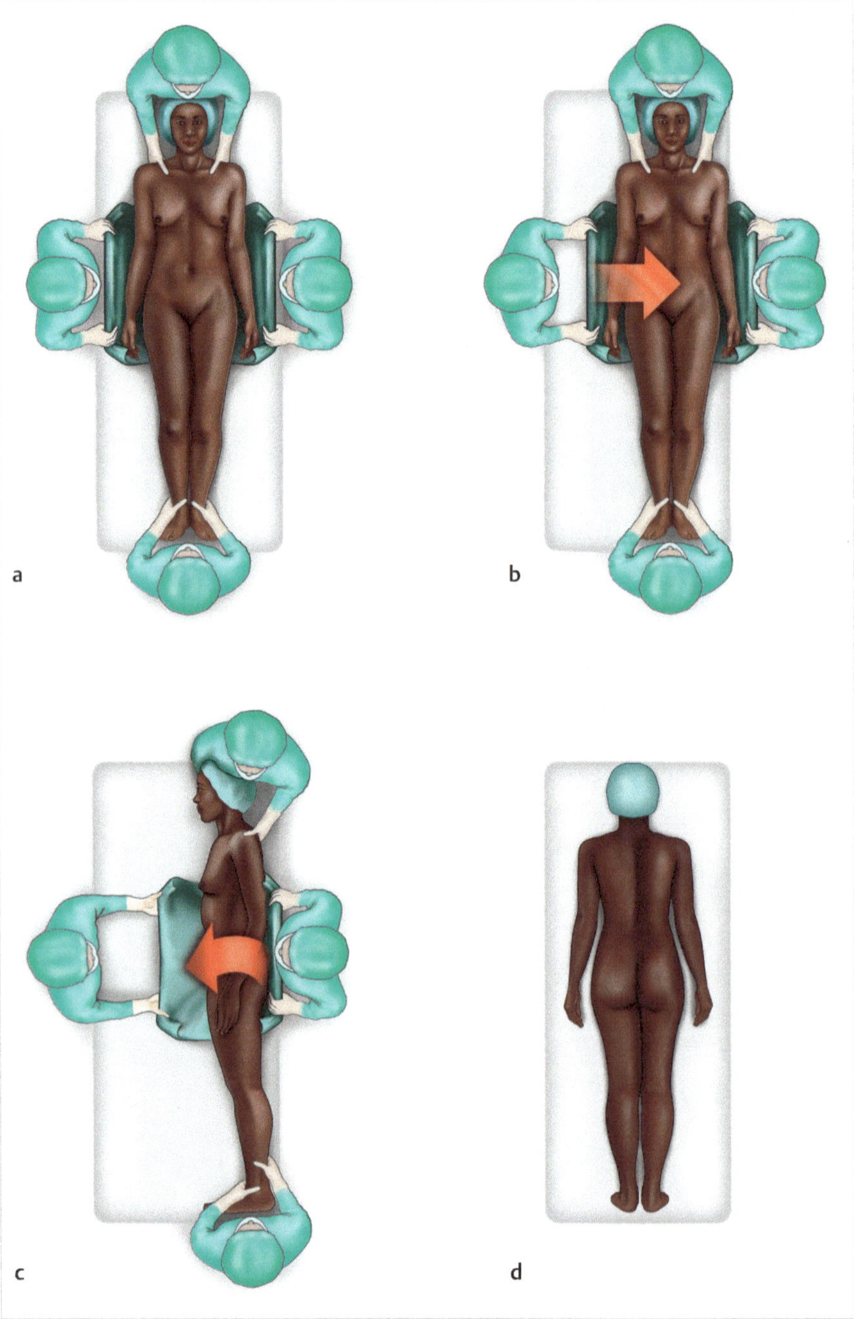

Fig. 79.2 (a–d) Schematic demonstration of an efficient "on-table flip", or repositioning a supine patient to the prone position using four team members and three maneuvers ("slide", "turn", "flip"). **(a)** Positioning of team member at the head, feet, and both sides. **(b)** The "slide": A prepositioned draw sheet is used to move the patient laterally to edge of bed. **(c)** The "turn": The patient is turned on her side in a lateral decubitus position. **(d)** The "flip": The patient is then tipped to the prone position with the primary team member "catching." At this point, the arms can be positioned and side rolls and/or chest rolls can be placed.

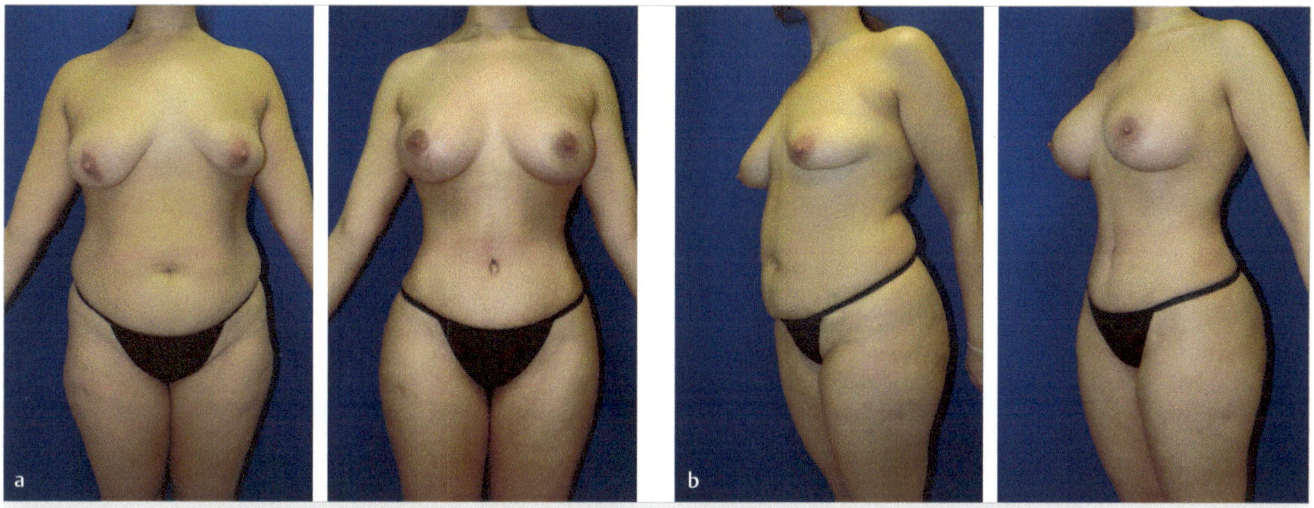

Fig. 79.3 Follow-up of a "mommy makeover" at 16 months in **(a)** anteroposterior (AP) and **(b)** oblique views. The combined procedure consisted of a breast augmentation with circumareolar lift and correction of volume asymmetry with differential implant volumes, full abdominoplasty, and circumferential liposuction with fat grafting to the hips and buttock. The patient was most concerned about achieving a smooth body contour and 1,400 cc of fat was grafted into the lateral buttock and "hip dips."

  - Anesthesia monitoring the head and airway.
  - Surgeon on one side.
  - Assistant on other side.
  - Assistant at the feet.
- A draw sheet should already be in position before the patient is put to sleep.
- There are three maneuvers: "slide," "turn," and "flip."

79.6 Postoperative Care

- The postoperative care will depend on the specific procedures.
- The procedure with the most postoperative restrictions will take precedent and is usually the abdominoplasty.
- Overall recovery will be longer after a mommy makeover and postoperative edema is more significant, particularly when the surgery is circumferential.
- As with any surgery, you must stress patience and realistic expectations.

79.7 Consistency of Results

- Mommy makeover is simply a combination of procedures that you are already proficient in.
- The key to consistent results is the preoperative decision-making and operative planning.
- A circumferential approach will always produce better cosmetic results and should be discussed with your patients.
- Safety is always most important and procedures, including a circumferential approach, should be avoided if it will likely extend total anesthetic time by greater than 6 hours or otherwise increase perioperative risks.
- A staged approach always remains the safest option and has the advantage of allowing small revisions on surgeries done previously.
- When in doubt, stage!

79.8 Case Example

Anteroposterior (AP) and oblique views of 16 months follow-up of a "mommy makeover.". The combined procedure consisted of a breast augmentation with circumareolar lift and correction of volume asymmetry with differential implant volumes, full abdominoplasty, and circumferential liposuction with fat grafting to the hips and buttock. The patient was most concerned about achieving a smooth body contour and 1,400 cc of fat was grafted into the lateral buttock and "hip dips" (▶ Fig. 79.3a, b).

79.9 Conclusion

Current surgical and anesthetic techniques now allow us to safely combine multiple procedures in a single operation. This allows us to dramatically improve the body and reverse common signs of aging, weight fluctuations, and pregnancies in a single operation. People are getting busier and busier, so there is an increasing desire to minimize the number of surgical procedures they will need to undergo. Patients are more likely to choose a combined mommy makeover, with increased cost and longer recovery, than select multiple smaller procedures done separately.

Further Readings

Hardy KL, Davis KE, Constantine RS, et al. The impact of operative time on complications after plastic surgery: a multivariate regression analysis of 1753 cases. Aesthet Surg J. 2014; 34(4):614–622

Hoyos A, Perez ME, Guarin DE, Montenegro A. A report of 736 high-definition lipoabdominoplasties performed in conjunction with circumferential VASER liposuction. Plast Reconstr Surg. 2018; 142(3):662–675

Matarasso A, Smith DM. Combined breast surgery and abdominoplasty: strategies for success. Plast Reconstr Surg. 2015; 135(5):849e–860e

Matarasso A, Smith DM. Strategies for aesthetic reshaping of the postpartum patient. Plast Reconstr Surg. 2015; 136(2):245–257

Rinker B, Veneracion M, Walsh CP. The effect of breastfeeding on breast aesthetics. Aesthet Surg J. 2008; 28(5):534–537

80 Brachioplasty

Rod J. Rohrich and Paul D. Durand

Abstract

With a growing massive weight loss population, upper arm contouring continues to rise in popularity. Refinements in technique, such as modification of skin excision patterns and the adjunct use of liposuction, have allowed for safe and reproducible results. Patient selection remains of utmost importance in selecting the best approach for upper arm contouring. In this chapter, a clinical algorithm is presented that can be used to select the best surgical method based on careful aesthetic analysis of the upper arm. This is followed by detailed descriptions of the operative steps involved in each type of procedure.

Keywords: Brachioplasty, limited-incision brachioplasty, extended brachioplasty, upper arm contouring, body contouring

Key Points

- With a growing massive weight loss population, upper arm contouring continues to rise in popularity.
- Refinements in technique, such as modification of skin excision patterns and the adjunct use of liposuction, have allowed for safe and reproducible results.
- Patient selection is of utmost importance in selecting the best approach for upper arm contouring.

80.1 Preoperative Steps

- Proper preoperative analysis is key in determining the best method for upper arm contouring for each patient.
- A pinch test can be used to determine excess fat; it will usually account for more than 1.5 cm of additional tissue thickness that should be factored into the resection.
- Skin laxity is a separate issue that can be present alone or in combination with excess fat; it can be measured by pinching excess skin between fingers and measuring the *length* of excess skin.
- Redundant tissue has to be evaluated in at all locations of the upper arm: proximal, middle, and distal aspects.
- A classification system can serve to stratify patients and narrow down what technique would be effective for each (▶ Table 80.1).

80.2 Operative Steps

See **Video 80.1**.

80.2.1 Liposuction Alone

- Access incision are made along radial aspect of distal humerus and proximally along posterior aspect of the arm.
- Areas of liposuction are infiltrated using a superwet technique with a solution of 1 L of lactated Ringer's solution, 30 cc of 1% lidocaine, and one ampule of 1:1000 epinephrine.
- Excess fat is removed from intermediate and superficial with ultrasound-assisted liposuction (UAL) or suction-assisted liposuction (SAL) alone.
- Superior to the brachial groove the authors use SAL exclusively, whereas inferiorly better skin retraction has been noted if SAL is combined with UAL.

80.2.2 Limited-Incision Brachioplasty

- Ideal in patients with proximal skin laxity and limited fat excess.

Markings

- With the arm in repose, the anterior and posterior limits of the axillary incision are marked in the axillary skin crease; limiting the incision between these points ensures that the scar will be hidden within the axilla.
- The arm is then abducted to 90 degrees and the two points are connected in the axillary fold.
- The amount of skin excision is marked in a semi-elliptical fashion; it usually measures 3 to 5 cm in vertical distance at the most central point.
- With the arm in the abducted position, areas of liposuction are then marked, with the bicipital groove as the most anterior point for liposuction.

Table 80.1 Classification system for the brachioplasty patient

Skin laxity		Location of redundant skin	Treatment
Type I	No	No skin laxity	UAL/SAL
Type II			
A	Yes	Minimal medial lower arm laxity	Lib-Medial brachioplasty
B	Yes	Moderate medial lower arm laxity	Extended medial brachioplasty
Type III			
A	Yes	Entire lower arm	Inferior or medial brachioplasty
B	Yes	Entire lower arm and lateral chest wall	Extended inferior brachioplasty

Abbreviations: SAL, suction-assisted liposuction; UAL, ultrasound-assisted liposuction.

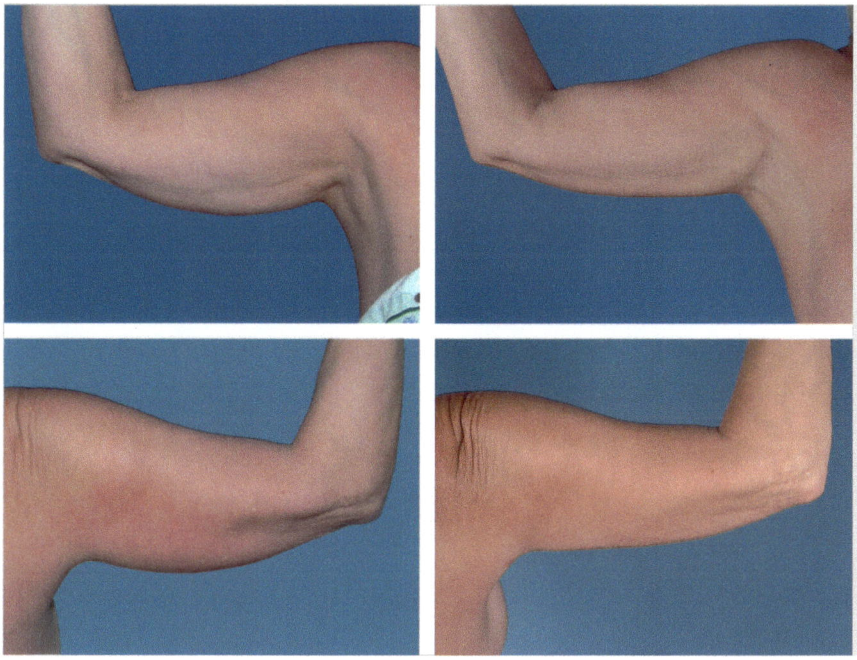

Fig. 80.1 This 54-year-old female desired improvement at her arms. She had a medial arm lift. The left photo is before surgery, the right photo is 18 months after surgery.

Liposuction

- Areas of liposuction are infiltrated using a superwet technique with a solution of 1 L of lactated Ringer's solution, 30 cc of 1% lidocaine, and one ampule of 1:1000 epinephrine.
- Using a 3.7-mm cannula, liposuction of the middle fat layer is performed radially.
- Approximately 100 to 300 cc of lipoaspirate are usually retrieved depending on the degree of lipodystrophy.

Skin Excision

- After the liposuction is complete, incision is made in the previously marked medial axillary skin fold.
- It is important for excision to be very superficial in subcutaneous plane in order to maximize lymphatic and nerve preservation. Posteriorly, where the fat layer is more robust, a deeper plane can be excised to aid in final incision contour.
- After meticulous hemostasis, very minimal undermining of the distal incision and medial incision can be performed.
- Excess undermining would be detrimental and cause untoward scar migration.

Closure

- Closure is then approximated with staples, carefully advancing any excess centrally and avoiding dog-ear formation.
- Layered closure is performed with 3–0 Vicryl interrupted sutures deep in subcutaneous tissue followed by 4–0 Vicryl sutures in the deep dermis. A 5–0 polydioxanone running subcuticular suture is then used as a final layer followed by application of Dermabond glue.

Case Example

This 54-year-old female desired improvement at her arms. She had a medial arm lift.

The left photo is before surgery, the right photo is 18 months after surgery (▶ Fig. 80.1).

80.2.3 Extended Brachioplasty

Markings

- Markings are made with the patient in the upright position with the arms abducted 90 degrees.
- First draw a line from the medial epicondyle to the midaxillary line as a reference point.
- Then draw the ideal position of the resultant scar slightly posterior along the posterior midline.
- If the deformity extends onto lateral chest, the planned scar should be drawn following on the lateral chest wall. If needed, scar can be tapered toward the inframammary fold.
- Some authors advocate drawing a notch in the axillary apex to prevent webbing of the scar across the axilla.
- A gentle skin pinch can be used to calculate the planned excision with adequate tapering at the ends to prevent any deformities.
- Areas of additional liposuction alone are also delineated at this time in the lateral chest wall, axilla, and/or elbow.
- Liposuction access points are marked in the mid-arm (area to be resected), elbow (away for the ulnar nerve), and lateral chest wall.

Liposuction

- Areas of liposuction are infiltrated using a superwet technique with a solution of 1 L of lactated Ringer's solution, 30 cc of 1% lidocaine, and one ampule of 1:1000 epinephrine.
- UAL is set at 50% and performed in a superficial plane away from ulnar nerve located close to the elbow.
- SAL with a 4.6-mm cannula is focused in the superficial layer only in the area that is planned to be excised.

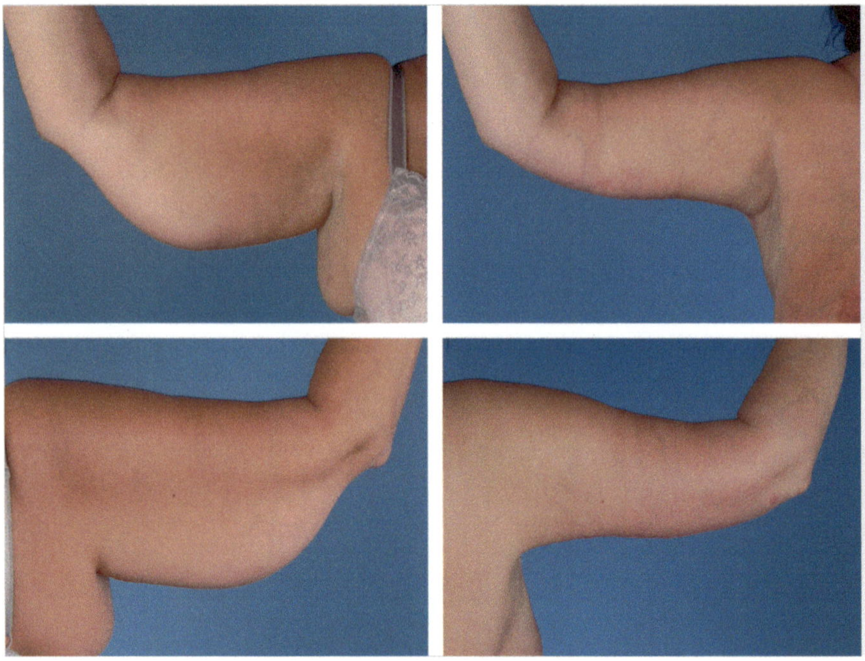

Fig. 80.2 This 47-year-old female desired improvement at her arms after losing weight. She had an extended arm lift. The left photo is before surgery, the right photo is 11 months after surgery.

- SAL can be extended almost circumferentially but should primarily focus on area marked for excision, where liposuction should be more aggressive.

Skin Excision

- After aggressive liposuction of area that is planned for excision, markings are re-checked with pinch test.
- Incisions are made down to superficial fascia and a Kocher clamp is used to grasp the tissue proximally.
- The tissue is then gently removed with continuous traction and countertraction from proximal to distal, decreasing damage to vessels, nerves, and lymphatics as compared to sharp tissue dissection.
- Excellent hemostasis is performed.

Closure

- Closure is then approximated with staples, carefully advancing any excess centrally and avoiding dog-ear formation.
- Layered closure is performed with 3–0 Vicryl interrupted sutures deep in subcutaneous tissue followed by 4–0 Vicryl sutures in the deep dermis. A 5–0 polydioxanone running subcuticular suture is then used as a final layer followed by application of tissue adhesive glue.

Case Example

This 47-year-old female desired improvement at her arms after losing weight. She had an extended arm lift. The left photo is before surgery, the right photo is 11 months after surgery (▶ Fig. 80.2).

80.3 Postoperative Care

- Patient is dressed in a long arm compression garment with Topifoam in place.
- Arm elevation is recommended at 90 degrees for 3 weeks.
- Topifoam is removed on second postoperative day and patient is allowed to shower.
- Compression garment is kept in place 24/7 for 3 weeks except for showering.
- Patient can resume all activities of daily living after 1 week.

80.4 Conclusion

An array of techniques is available for successful upper arm contouring. Proper patient selection is key in determining which procedure can be used for each particular patient. In the massive weight loss patient with significant skin excess, skin excision remains the gold standard.

Further Readings

Appelt EA, Janis JE, Rohrich RJ. An algorithmic approach to upper arm contouring. Plast Reconstr Surg. 2006; 118(1):237–246

Hurwitz D, Brachioplasty. Clin Plast Surg. 2014; 41(4):745–751

Knotts CD, Kortesis BG, Hunstad JP. Avulsion brachioplasty: technique overview and 5-year experience. Plast Reconstr Surg. 2014; 133(2):283–288

Nguyen AT, Rohrich RJ. Liposuction-assisted posterior brachioplasty: technical refinements in upper arm contouring. Plast Reconstr Surg. 2010; 126(4): 1365–1369

Shermak MA. Aesthetic refinements in body contouring in the massive weight loss patient: Part 2. Arms. Plast Reconstr Surg. 2014; 134(5):726e–735e

Trussler AP, Rohrich RJ. Limited incision medial brachioplasty: technical refinements in upper arm contouring. Plast Reconstr Surg. 2008; 121(1):305–307

81 Medial Thighplasty

Rod J. Rohrich, Erez Dayan, and Joshua M. Cohen

Abstract

Liposuction-assisted medial thighplasty is a safe, efficient, and reproducible procedure that should follow a four-step algorithm: (1) L-shaped anterior markings, (2) superwet infiltration, (3) circumferential combined superficial ultrasound-assisted/suction-assisted liposuction, and (4) predesigned and patterned skin excision and layered closure. It simplifies the markings and resection, and the procedure preserves the lymphatics and nerves, minimizes blood loss, and maintains the saphenous vein system to prevent skin loss and wound breakdown. It produces reliable and predictable results, with optimal outcomes. This technique offers another refinement in the evolution of medial thigh contouring.

Keywords: Medial thigh lift, thighplasty, body contouring

Key Points

- Traditional medial thigh lift has been associated with postoperative problems such as inferior wound migration, scar widening, lateral traction deformities of the vulva, and early recurrence of ptosis. Possible surgical damage to the lymphatic vessels increases the risk of seroma and recovery can be painful due to the sensitivity of the area.
- A modified approach to the medial thigh lift presented in this chapter avoids many of the complications associated with traditional thigh lift while allowing for predictable aesthetic outcomes.

81.1 Preoperative Steps

- The patient is marked to create an inverted L-shaped incision, which leads to a predesigned and patterned skin excision. The patient is marked first in the standing position with the legs slightly apart. The final desired location of the incision is along the medial thigh from the lower aspect of the knee to the crease.
- Using a skin pinch method, the medial thigh skin is assessed for redundancy and mobility by transposing in both the anterior and posterior directions to meet the previously drawn line. This demonstrates the amount of skin to be removed. This maneuver leads to an ellipse pattern skin excision that tapers at the medial knee. The width of the ellipse is based on the skin pinch and typically ranges between 10 and 15 cm (▶ Fig. 81.1).
- The anterior, proximal incision is drawn such that a gentle curve is achieved in an inverted L-shaped anterior marking. The superior and inferior end of the incision ends up conical.

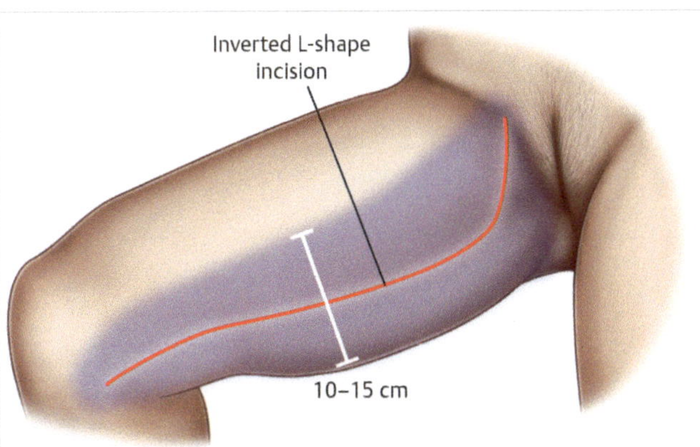

Fig. 81.1 Preoperative markings for excision (*blue*) and final scar location (*red*).

81.2 Operative Steps (▶ Fig. 81.2)

- Liposuction access points are distal to the groin crease within the region to be resected, midthigh, and just proximal to the medial knee.
- The thigh is infiltrated using a superwet technique circumferentially. The preferred solution is 1 L of lactated Ringer's solution, 30 cc of 1% lidocaine, and one ampule of 1:1000 epinephrine.
- Circumferential combined suction-assisted and/or ultrasound-assisted liposuction using 3.5 to 4.0 mm cannulas is performed circumferentially except in the area to be excised. The saphenous vein system is avoided by maintaining a superficial plane of liposuction in the area to be excised. This is key to avoid skin breakdown and infection. The undermined tissue is

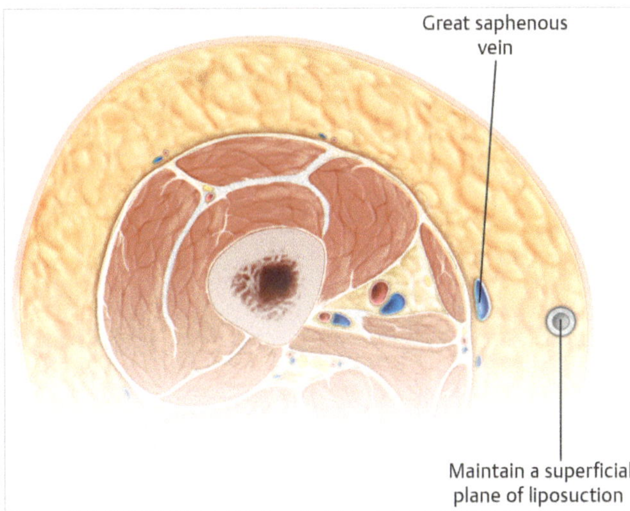

Fig. 81.2 Anatomy of the medial thigh. The saphenous vein system is avoided by maintaining a superficial plane of liposuction in the area to be excised, which is key to avoid skin breakdown and infection.

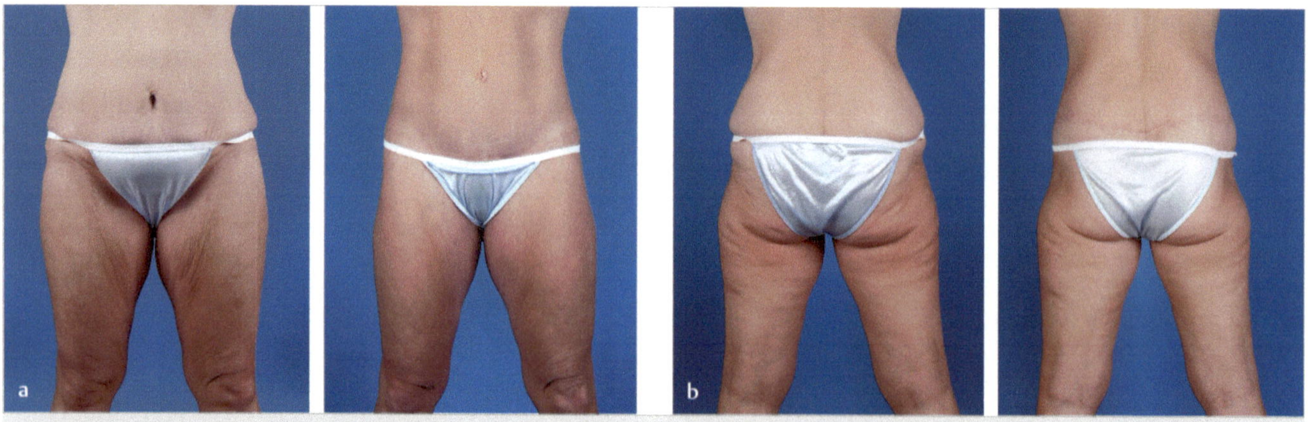

Fig. 81.3 (a, b) This 38-year-old female desired body contouring procedures after losing 100 lbs status post gastric bypass. The photo on the right is a medial thigh lift staged 6 months after a circumferential body lift.

re-checked via a pinch test to verify excisional marks and avoid over-resection of skin.

- The predesigned and patterned skin excision is performed followed by a layered closure with postoperative compression.
- Hemostasis is checked and a 19 French Blake drain is placed, exiting at the inferior-most aspect of the incision. Wound margins are then tailor-tacked with staples and any excess tissue is trimmed. The staples from the distal- and proximal-most ends of the incision are removed incrementally, and a two-layer closure is performed. Staples are maintained in the middle of the incision, at the area of most tension. These are removed once the patient returns to the office.

81.3 Postoperative Care

- The surgical staples are removed on postoperative 5 day.
- The usual post-op course involves some edema and ecchymosis. This typically resolves in 3 to 4 weeks and is aided by the use of a compression garment. There is no need for an elaborate dressing as the incision areas are sealed with Dermabond.
- Most patients return to work after 2 weeks.

81.4 Case Example

This 38-year-old female desired body contouring procedures after losing 100 lbs status post gastric bypass. The photo on the right is a medial thigh lift staged 6 months after a circumferential body lift (▶ Fig. 81.3a, b).

81.5 Conclusion

Historic complications of medial thigh lift surgery can be avoided by limiting injury to the saphenous vein system and surrounding lymphatics of the medial thigh. This is accomplished by superficial liposuction and removal of excess tissue while preserving these structures.

See **Video 81.1**.

Further Readings

Armijo BS, et al. Four-step medial thighplasty: refined and reproducible. Plast Reconstr Surg. 2013::e717–e-725

Mathes DW, Kenkel JM. Current concepts in medial thighplasty. Clin Plast Surg. 2008; 35(1):151–163

Mathes DW. Current techniques in medial thighplasty. In: Shiffman MA, DiGiuseppe A, eds. Body Contouring, Part 7. Berlin: Springer; 2010:815–826

Schultz RC, Feinberg LA. Medial thigh lift. Ann Plast Surg. 1979; 2(5):404–410

82 Postbariatric Body Contouring: Brachioplasty

Francesco M. Egro and J. Peter Rubin

Abstract

Massive weight loss patients may develop significant body deformities including severe arm ptosis due to significant volume loss with extensive skin laxity. Contouring of postbariatric patients usually requires the arm, axilla, and lateral chest wall to be addressed together as a combined aesthetic unit. Brachioplasty involves a trade-off of arm shape for scar. This book chapter reviews the preoperative, intraoperative, and postoperative treatment of severe arm ptosis.

Keywords: Brachioplasty, arm contouring, body contouring, bariatric surgery, postbariatric, massive weight loss

Key Points

- Contouring of postbariatric patients usually requires the arm, axilla, and lateral chest wall to be addressed together as a combined aesthetic unit.
- Brachioplasty involves a trade-off of arm shape for scar.

82.1 Preoperative Steps

82.1.1 Analysis

- The first step is to understand the patient's expectations and assess whether they can be met.
- A thorough history should focus on weight loss, nutritional status, bariatric surgery, personal or family history of venous thromboembolic event, and smoking status. The ideal candidate should have a stable weight, preferably with a body mass index (BMI) under 30 for at least 3 months.
- A detailed examination of the whole body should be performed to determine the timing and stages of the body contouring procedures. It is important to note the distribution and extent of skin laxity and adiposity in the arm, axillary region, and lateral chest wall.
- To obtain adequate results, postbariatric patients usually need the arm, axilla, and lateral chest wall addressed together as a combined aesthetic unit.

82.1.2 Markings

- The patient is marked in the standing or sitting position with the arms abducted 90 degrees and the elbows bent at 90 degrees (▶ Fig. 82.1).
- The bicipital groove is marked to the level of the elbow (point C) and it represents the final position of the incision.
- The anterior axillary line is marked along the chest.
- The margins of the superior incision line are marked by placing caudal traction on the arm, with the proximal end (point A) set high in the dome of the axilla.
- A pinch test is performed to determine point A'.
- Points A' and B are then connected to determine the posterior extent of axillary skin resection.
- A pinch test is performed to determine the inferior line of resection.
- Vertical hashmarks are drawn for alignment.

82.2 Operative Steps

See **Video 82.1**.

82.2.1 Positioning and Prepping

- The shoulder, lateral chest wall, and arm are prepped in a sterile fashion with betadine.
- The distal arm is wrapped in a sterile towel to allow full mobility during surgery. Intravenous access and monitoring devices can be attached on the forearm or the lower extremity.

82.2.2 Superior and Anterior Axillary Line Incision, and Flap Elevation

- The superior and anterior axillary line markings are incised.
- Dissection begins in the middle third of the incision pattern, superficial to the brachial fascia leaving a thin layer of fat on the deep fascia.
- Then dissection becomes more superficial distally to avoid the medial antebrachial cutaneous nerve.
- An even flap is elevated to the estimated inferior marking line (▶ Fig. 82.2).

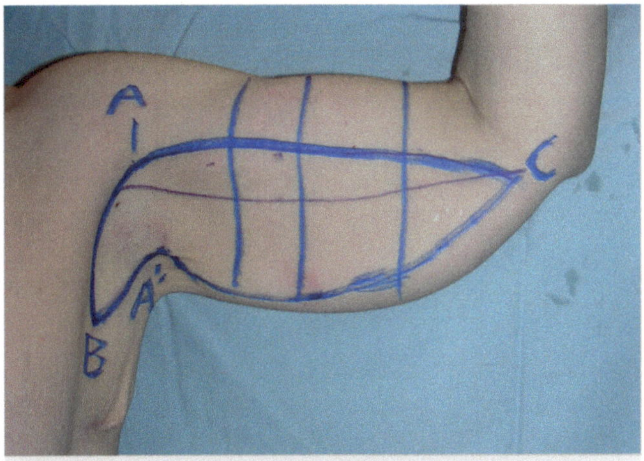

Fig. 82.1 Brachioplasty preoperative markings. (Reproduced with permission from Strauch B, Herman CK. Encyclopedia of Body Sculpting after Massive Weight Loss. Thieme, 2010.)

82.2.3 Axillary Tissue and Arm Excess Tissue Resection

- The superior incision line is transposed beneath the flap using heavy forceps to decide how much tissue can be excised inferiorly (▶ Fig. 82.3). This technique is used at the three vertical hashmarks previously drawn.
- The flap is vertically incised to the transposed points of the inferior incision line and these skin landmarks are kept approximated using towel clips (▶ Fig. 82.4).
- After checking point A' and the lateral chest wall markings again, the excess axillary tissue is excised.
- The flap superficial fascial system is suspended from point A' to the clavipectoral fascia in the axillary dome with permanent 0-braided nylon sutures.
- The definitive inferior incision line is drawn by joining horizontally the transposed points between the towel clips (▶ Fig. 82.5).
- The excess arm tissue is excised.

82.2.4 Closure and Dressings

- A 15F round closed suction drain is placed along the arm with the end exiting 3 to 4 cm proximal to the distal extent of the chest wall incision.

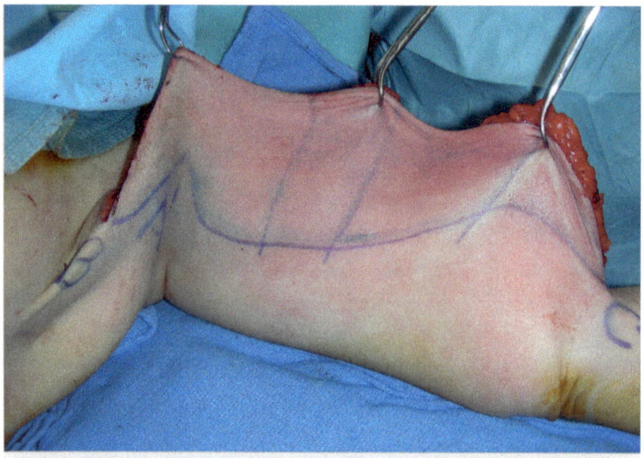

Fig. 82.2 Superior and anterior axillary line incision, and flap elevation. (Reproduced with permission from Strauch B, Herman CK. Encyclopedia of Body Sculpting after Massive Weight Loss. Thieme, 2010.)

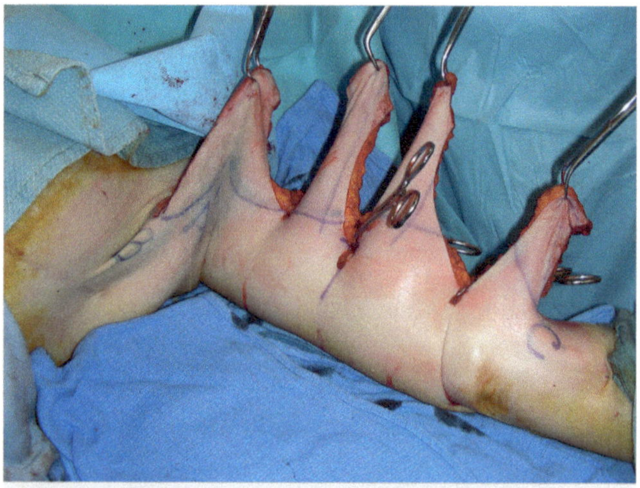

Fig. 82.4 Vertical incision of flap to the transposed points of the inferior incision line. (Reproduced with permission from Strauch B, Herman CK. Encyclopedia of Body Sculpting after Massive Weight Loss. Thieme, 2010.)

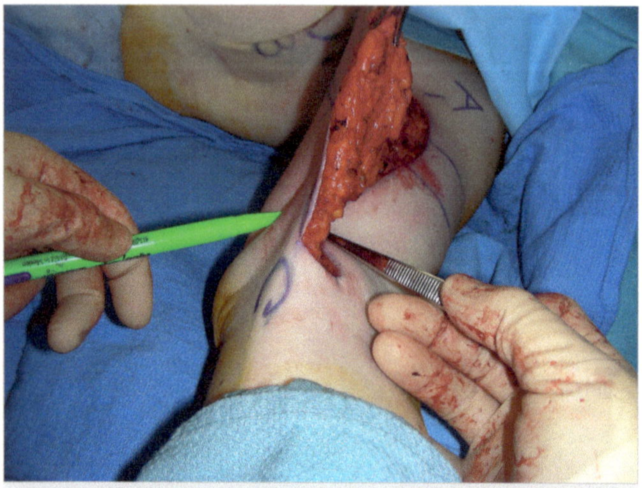

Fig. 82.3 Superior incision line transposition. (Reproduced with permission from Strauch B, Herman CK. Encyclopedia of Body Sculpting after Massive Weight Loss. Thieme, 2010.)

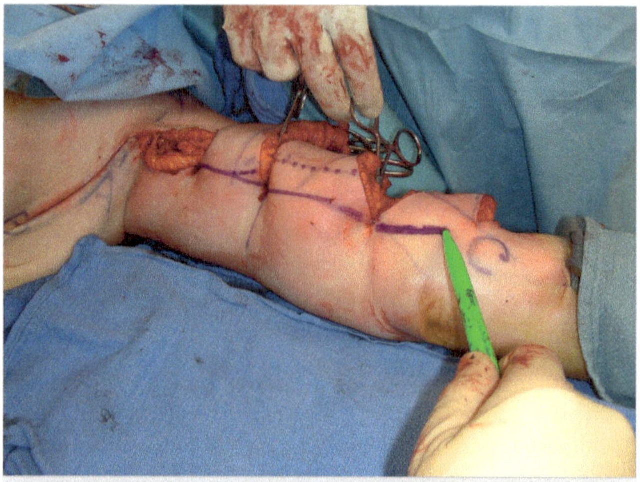

Fig. 82.5 Superficial fascial system suspension to clavipectoral fascia and definitive inferior incision line marking. (Reproduced with permission from Strauch B, Herman CK. Encyclopedia of Body Sculpting after Massive Weight Loss. Thieme, 2010.)

- The skin is temporarily closed with staples (▶ Fig. 82.6).
- A layered closure is performed. The superficial fascial system is closed with interrupted 2–0 Vicryl sutures, followed by 3–0 Biosyn interrupted deep-dermal sutures and 3–0 V-Loc running subcuticular suture.

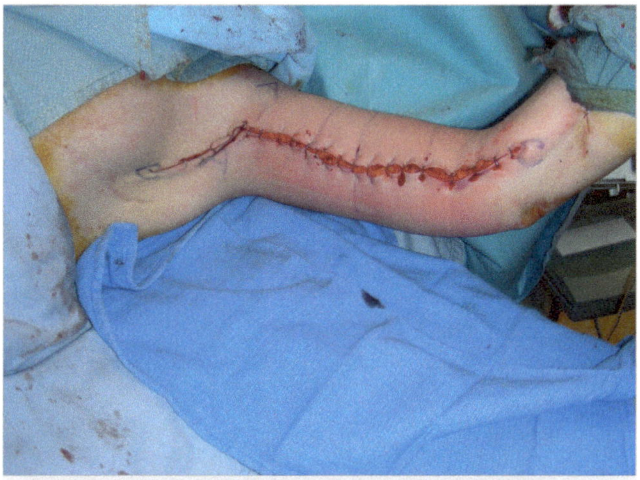

Fig. 82.6 Temporary skin closure with staples. (Reproduced with permission from Strauch B, Herman CK. Encyclopedia of Body Sculpting after Massive Weight Loss. Thieme, 2010.)

- The incision is covered with Kerlix gauze and 6-inch FlexMaster ACE bandage from hand to shoulder.

82.3 Postoperative Care

- Patients should keep the ACE bandage in place until the first follow-up visit. At that point the patient can either wear ACE bandage or a support stocking to be worn for several more weeks.
- Patient should sleep in a "lounge chair position" for a few days.
- Patient can sponge bath after 24 hours and may shower after first follow-up appointment, but incisions should be tapped dry afterwards.
- Trauma or pressure to breasts should be avoided.
- Rest for 2 weeks with intermittent walks. Arms should not be extended above shoulder level for 2 weeks followed by gentle reintroduction afterwards.
- Analgesia is prescribed as needed.
- Drain will remain in place until daily output is less than 30 cc.
- Patients are usually seen 1 week, 2 weeks, 5 weeks, and 3 months postoperatively.

82.4 Case Example

A 53-year-old woman following a 131 lbs weight loss underwent brachioplasty. Preoperative views and markings (▶ Fig. 82.7a–c), postoperative view at 3 months (▶ Fig. 82.7d), postoperative view at 6 months (▶ Fig. 82.7e), postoperative view at 14 months

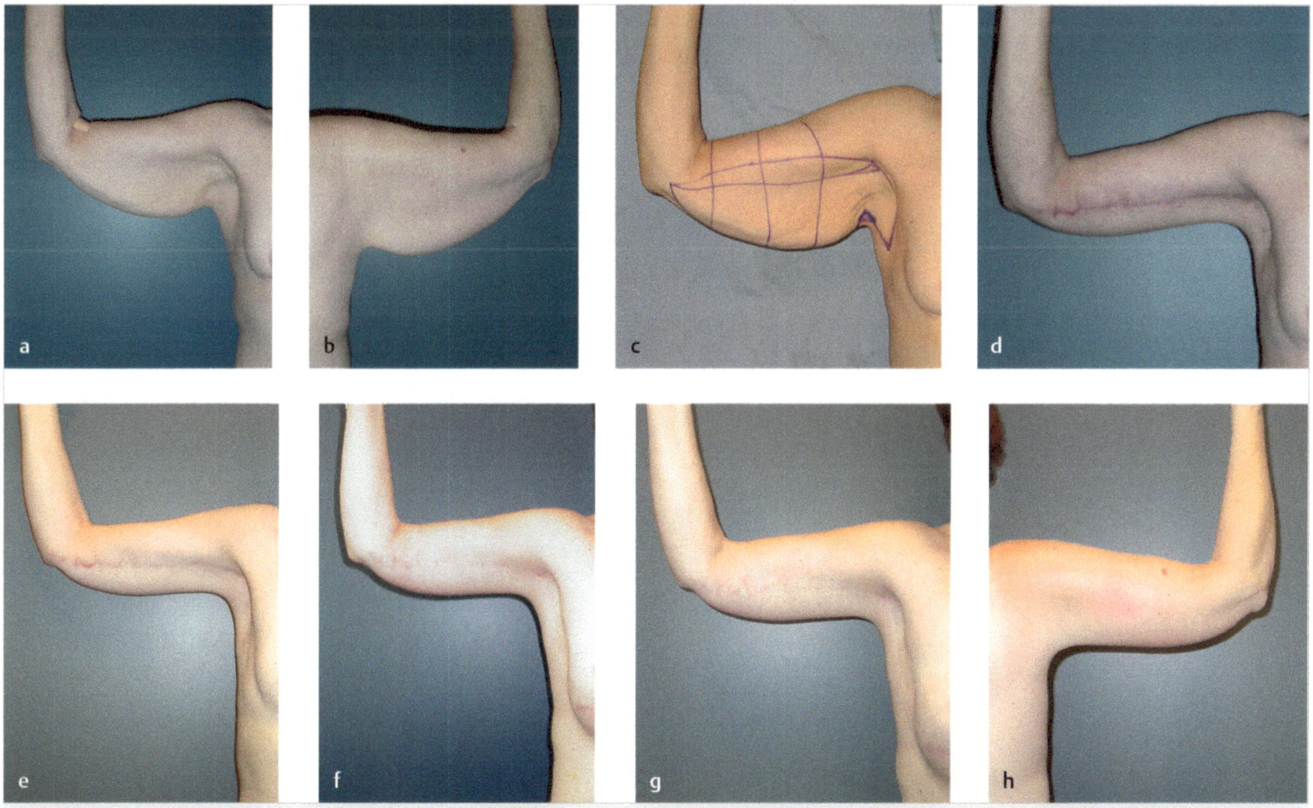

Fig. 82.7 A 53-year-old woman following a 131 lbs weight loss underwent brachioplasty. **(a–c)** Preoperative views and markings. **(d)** Postoperative view at 3 months. **(e)** Postoperative view at 6 months. **(f)** Postoperative view at 14 months. **(g, h)** Postoperative view at 19 months. (Reproduced with permission from Strauch B, Herman CK. Encyclopedia of Body Sculpting after Massive Weight Loss. Thieme, 2010.)

(▶ Fig. 82.7f), and postoperative view at 19 months (▶ Fig. 82.7g, h) are shown.

82.5 Conclusion

Brachioplasty is a powerful operation in massive weight loss patients. It involves a trade-off of arm shape for scar. Contouring of postbariatric patients usually requires the arm, axilla, and lateral chest wall to be addressed together as a combined aesthetic unit.

Further Readings

Gusenoff JA, Coon D, Rubin JP. Brachioplasty and concomitant procedures after massive weight loss: a statistical analysis from a prospective registry. Plast Reconstr Surg. 2008; 122(2):595–603

Lockwood T. Brachioplasty with superficial fascial system suspension. Plast Reconstr Surg. 1995; 96(4):912–920

Knotts CD, Kortesis BG, Hunstad JP. Avulsion brachioplasty: technique overview and 5-year experience. Plast Reconstr Surg. 2014; 133(2):283–288

Strauch B, Herman CK. Encyclopedia of body sculpting after massive weight loss. Thieme; 2010

83 Postbariatric Body Contouring: Lower Body Lift

Jonathan P. Brower and Jeffrey A. Gusenoff

Abstract

The lower body lift is an excellent option to treat stigmata of massive weight loss in the buttocks, primarily skin excess and volume loss. The procedure can be performed with or without autoaugmentation to address volume deficit and contour irregularities. The lower body lift is often combined with other procedures, including medial thigh lift or abdominoplasty. It is essential to optimize nutritional status and manage expectations preoperatively to achieve patient safety and satisfaction. Markings are essential to ensure appropriate shape, symmetry, and tension. Suction-assisted lipectomy is a useful adjunct to improve contour and provide discontinuous undermining to assist in closure. Patients are generally admitted to the hospital for 1 to 2 nights to ensure adequate nursing care and facilitate early ambulation to combat venous thromboembolism.

Keywords: Lower body lift, massive weight loss, body contouring, buttock reshaping, gluteal autoaugmentation, saddlebag deformity

Key Points

- The lower body lift provides circumferential contouring of the trunk, buttock, and thigh regions particularly problematic in the massive weight loss (MWL) patient.
- The lower body lift is "lower" than a belt lipectomy and aims to restore normal shape of the buttocks and saddlebag regions. The belt lipectomy is based higher and improves the lower back or love handles without much benefit to the lower buttocks or outer thigh.
- The lower body lift can be performed with or without gluteal autoaugmentation, and can be combined with an abdominoplasty or inner thighplasty.

83.1 Preoperative Steps

83.1.1 Preoperative Evaluation

Optimizing Surgical Candidacy

- A weight loss history is essential for appropriate patient selection. A body mass index (BMI) less than 30 kg/m^2 is optimal.
  - A higher BMI before bariatric surgery and at the time of evaluation for body contouring after MWL are associated with higher complication rates.
  - Patients may need to achieve further weight loss to be an appropriate candidate.
- Patients should be at least 1 year out from their bariatric procedure and have stable weight for 3 months.
- Medical history is focused on evaluating cardiopulmonary and metabolic comorbidities, including coronary artery disease, obstructive sleep apnea, and diabetes mellitus. Any history of thrombotic events should be further investigated.
- Medications with antiplatelet activity, including some herbal remedies and supplements, are discontinued 2 weeks before surgery.
- All nicotine exposure must be discontinued 4 weeks prior to surgery.
- Physical examination should include noting of all surgical scars and hernias.
- Nutritional deficiencies are common among patients who have had bariatric surgery.
  - Goal protein intake is 70 to 100 g/day. Serum albumin and prealbumin should be measured as history alone is not adequate to rule out protein malnutrition.
  - Common micronutrient deficiencies in bariatric patients include iron, calcium, B_{12}, folate, and thiamine.
- A psychiatric history is an important part of the initial evaluation.
  - Mood and personality disorders are prevalent in obese patients and typically do not resolve with weight loss.
- Expectations are carefully managed, emphasizing that excess skin will be traded for a long scar.
  - The goal is to achieve improvement in body contour, not perfection.
- The social support system is evaluated, including living situation and availability of family and friends to assist the patient postoperatively.
- Preoperative medical evaluation includes labs (complete blood count, electrolytes, renal function, coagulation studies, and blood type and screen).
- An electrocardiogram (EKG) is obtained for patients over age 40.
- The patient is evaluated by the primary care physician, any necessary specialists, and/or anesthesia to provide medical clearance and guidance for perioperative medical management.

Anatomic Analysis of the Buttock

- Note overall shape of the buttocks and degree of adiposity and deflation.
- Assess contour of skin over lower back, flanks, buttocks, and thighs, including indentations and folds.
- Lifting of the buttocks can simulate the flattening effect if no autoaugmentation is planned.

83.1.2 Markings

- With the patient in the standing position, the sinusoidal point of the hip is identified just lateral to the posterior superior iliac spine. A pinch test is performed in the midline to

determine the central extent of a gullwing-shaped upper incision line. This point may be above the gluteal cleft in a patient with significant deflation.
- The lower incision is determined by pinch test.
- Hatch marks are drawn to guide tissue reapproximation every 6 cm. Four reference bars are typically drawn out to the midaxillary line.
- If gluteal augmentation is planned, a paddle of tissue is marked out to the third reference line. The designed dermoadipofascial flaps will be liberated and rotated caudally to provide desired augmentation.
- The lateral extent of the incision is transitioned to a planned abdominoplasty incision about the hip or into an inner thighplasty.

83.2 Operative Steps

- Prophylactic doses of heparin and antibiotics are initiated preoperatively. Antibiotics are re-dosed intraoperatively as appropriate.
- Pneumatic compression boots are applied.
- A Foley catheter is placed and then the patient is intubated on the stretcher and turned prone onto the operating table. Appropriate padding and attention to eye pressure is critical. The bed is lightly jackknifed to simulate tension if a concomitant abdominoplasty is planned.
- Tumescent solution is infiltrated over the areas to be addressed with liposuction (i.e., lateral thighs). All incision lines are injected with dilute epinephrine solution (1:100,000).
- If gluteal autoaugmentation is not planned, the upper incision is made and dissection is carried inferiorly along the gluteal fascia to the level of the planned lower incision. The inferior extent can be committed to in a serial fashion to avoid over-resection.
- If gluteal autoaugmentation is planned, the upper incision is made and the intended flaps are de-epithelialized. The surgeon must commit to an upper and lower incision; therefore, checking the planned excision with towel clamps prior to proceeding is advised.
- Pockets are created inferiorly above the gluteal fascia such that the dissected dermoadipofascial flaps can be rotated into them:
  - The flaps themselves are not undermined to avoid any injury to blood supply, thereby avoiding future fat necrosis.
- The flaps are rotated into the pockets and secured with 2–0 braided absorbable horizontal mattress sutures being sure to take bites that help round and shape the buttocks.
- Liposuction of the lateral saddlebags proceeds as necessary.
- The lateral hip tissue beyond the autoaugmentation flaps is excised. Arm board on the lower part of the bed can be used to help abduct the legs and improve the amount of tissue to be excised laterally.
- Hemostasis is obtained and drains are placed.
- The incision is closed in layers and with glue and the patient is turned supine to complete the abdominoplasty or thighplasty portion of the procedure anteriorly.

83.3 Postoperative Care

- No garment is typically used. If an abdominoplasty is also performed, a standard abdominal binder is used.
- Patients are admitted to the hospital for 1 to 2 nights depending on the amount of surgery performed.
- Compression stockings and pneumatic compression boots remain functional for the duration of hospitalization, along with chemoprophylaxis.
- An incentive spirometer is provided and patients are coached to achieve adequate pulmonary toilet.
- Ambulation is encouraged as soon as possible.
- Patients should avoid bending over for 3 weeks to avoid splitting the incision.
- Drains are removed when less than 30 mL over 24 hours.

83.4 Case Example

This is a 40-year-old female with a history of 137 lbs weight loss from diet and exercise. Preoperative photos, operative markings for lower body lift with autoaugmentation, and 14-month follow-up are shown (▶ Fig. 83.1a–c).

83.5 Conclusion

When combined with abdominoplasty, the lower body lift provides circumferential contouring of the torso, lower buttock, and outer thighs. The procedure may include autoaugmentation, which serves to improve buttock shape and projection, but increases the risk of wound healing complications.

See **Video 83.1**.

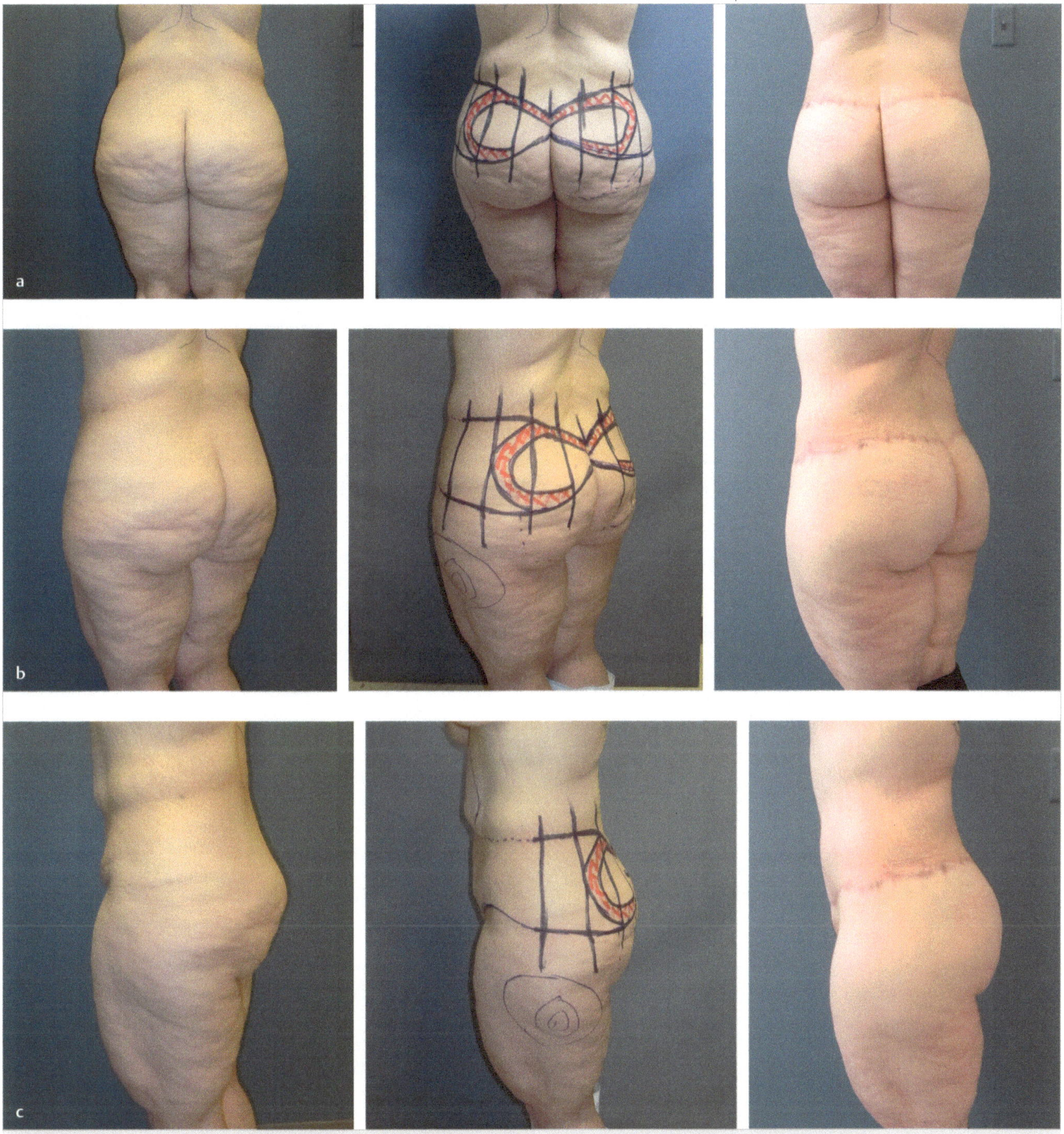

Fig. 83.1 (a–c) This is a 40-year-old female with a history of 137 lbs weight loss from diet and exercise. Preoperative photos, operative markings for lower body lift with autoaugmentation, and 14-month follow-up are shown.

Further Readings

Dreifuss SE, Beidas OE, Rubin JP, Gusenoff JA. Characterizing the saddlebag deformity after lower body lift. Aesthet Surg J. 2018; 38(10):1115–1123

Kitzinger HB, Cakl T, Wenger R, Hacker S, Aszmann OC, Karle B. Prospective study on complications following a lower body lift after massive weight loss. J Plast Reconstr Aesthet Surg. 2013; 66(2):231–238

Richter DF, Stoff A. Circumferential body contouring: the lower body lift. Clin Plast Surg. 2014; 41(4):775–788

Srivastava U, Rubin JP, Gusenoff JA. Lower body lift after massive weight loss: autoaugmentation versus no augmentation. Plast Reconstr Surg. 2015; 135 (3):762–772

84 Postbariatric Body Contouring: Vertical Thigh Lift

Joseph P. Hunstad and Vasileios Vasilakis

Abstract

The vertical thigh lift addresses the medial and circumferential thigh lipodystrophy and skin laxity following massive weight loss. It can be combined with circumferential liposuction and incorporates the relatively atraumatic avulsion of the planned resection area in order to preserve the lymphatic and neurovascular structures. This enhances healing and reduces common complications such as seroma and lymphocele formation. The scar is well hidden in the medial aspect of the thighs. Complications are typically incisional and managed with minor revision and wound care. The outcome is predictable, circumferential tightening.

Keywords: Vertical thigh lift, avulsion thighplasty, liposuction, massive weight loss, body contouring, excess adiposity, skin atrophy, skin laxity

Key Points

- Vertical thigh lift is the optimal technique to treat medial and circumferential thigh lipodystrophy, as well as skin laxity following massive weight loss.
- Avulsion of the planned resection area (avulsion thighplasty) allows for maximal preservation of branching vessels, cutaneous nerves, and lymphatics that run superficial to the deep muscle fascial system in the medial thigh.
- Preservation of the lymphatic and neurovascular structures enhances healing, and reduces seroma, lymphedema, and in particular lymphocele, a recognized complication of this operation.
- Thorough, complete liposuction of the planned resection area accomplishes relatively atraumatic removal of skin and fat.
- Vertical thigh lift can be performed as a second-stage procedure preceded by circumferential liposuction, or safely executed in combination with circumferential liposuction.

84.1 Preoperative Steps

- Counsel patients about the high risk of minor wound complications and potential need for scar revision.
- Determine the extent of the scar depending on the deformity and patient preference.
- Perform standard preoperative laboratory analysis.
- Assess nutritional status in the massive weight loss patients.
- The need for coagulation tests is assessed on a case-by-case basis depending on the medical history.
- No smoking for 6 weeks preoperatively and 4 weeks postoperatively.

84.2 Operative Steps

See **Video 84.1.**

84.2.1 Markings

- First, the ideal position of the vertical marking corresponding to the proposed final medial thigh incision is drawn from the pubic area to the knee, with the marking on each side being mirror image of the other.
- Proximally, the marking originates at the origin of the gracilis muscle in the pubic area and extends distally as a straight line to the inferior aspect of the deformity near the medial condyle of the femur.
- In patients with significant soft tissue laxity, the incision could be extended proximally into the inguinal crease or distally beyond the knee, where the linear scar is broken up at the knee area to avoid contracture.
- In order to estimate the planned soft tissue resection, bimanual strong skin pinch of the redundant tissue is performed on both sides of the proposed vertical incision, and the estimated resection area is marked accordingly.
- Realignment markings to ensure accurate closure are placed (▸ Fig. 84.1).

84.2.2 Intraoperative Details

- Preoperative antibiotics are administered, sequential compression devices are applied, and general anesthesia is induced; venous thromboembolism chemical prophylaxis is administered only if warranted based on the preoperative work-up.
- The patient is supine, with the legs supported in the "frog leg" position.

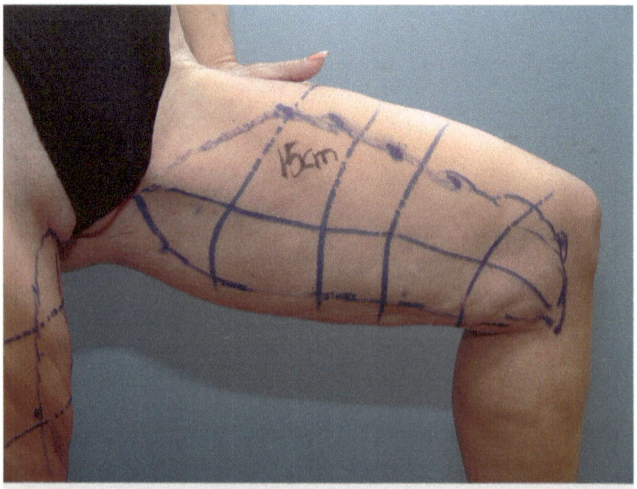

Fig. 84.1 Vertical thigh lift markings.

- Realignment markings are tattooed outside the resection pattern with methylene blue to prevent wash-off during the procedure.
- Tumescent solution is infiltrated only throughout the area of the planned resection.
- If circumferential liposuction is to be performed, the patient is repositioned prone to perform liposuction of the entire posterior thigh, then turned supine to complete the circumferential liposuction and vertical thigh lift.
- Aggressive, complete liposuction of the area to be resected is performed using a 4-mm basket cannula until complete thinning of the soft tissue is achieved as indicated by a sharp step-off in the edges of this area (dished-out deformity).
- Complete removal of fat from the area to be resected is key in order to perform the avulsion thighplasty with maximal preservation of the branching vessels, cutaneous nerves, and lymphatics; the pinch test should reveal virtual complete absence of subcutaneous fat.
- Prior to the incision, the markings are assessed once more using staples to ensure desired thigh shape with a tight and smooth contour under appropriate tension.
- Once the markings are finalized, circumferential incisions through the dermis are made and the avulsion is performed using a Kocher clamp from proximal to distal while applying strong counter-pressure, removing skin only.
- Upon completion, the aforementioned superficial structures are seen intact in the wound and hemostasis is achieved using electrocautery.
- The skin edges are stapled together to approximate the tissues prior to the onset of significant swelling.
- Drains are reserved only for cases when significant circumferential liposuction is performed in combination with the vertical thigh lift, with the entry site being in the groin area.
- Closure is performed in two layers using interrupted 3–0 poliglecaprone (Monocryl) sutures in the superficial fascial system/deep dermis followed by a 4–0 running subcuticular poliglecaprone (Monocryl) suture.
- Securing interrupted 4–0 polypropylene sutures are placed at 2 cm intervals and removed as swelling subsides.
- Tape is applied to the incision, split every 3 cm to allow for postoperative swelling.
- Use 4-inch wraps from the base of the toes up to the knees, and 6-inch wraps over absorbent gauze to cover the incisions from the knee to the groin.

84.3 Postoperative Care

- Sequential compression devices remain until discharge.
- Early ambulation is encouraged, starting in the first postoperative evening.
- Prolonged periods of standing or sitting for the first few weeks are avoided.
- When not ambulating, the feet should be elevated at a lever higher than the heart.
- Dressings are changed as needed and the incision is assessed usually on postoperative day 1, and no later than postoperative day 4.
- Close follow-up allows early diagnosis and wound care in case of dehiscence or other incisional complications.
- Topical scar treatment commences as early as 2 to 3 weeks postoperatively in the absence of complications.

84.4 Case Example

Pre- and postoperative photos of a patient 13 months following a vertical avulsion thigh lift (**a**) anteroposterior (AP) (**b, c**) oblique, and (**d**) posterior views (▶ Fig. 84.2a–d).

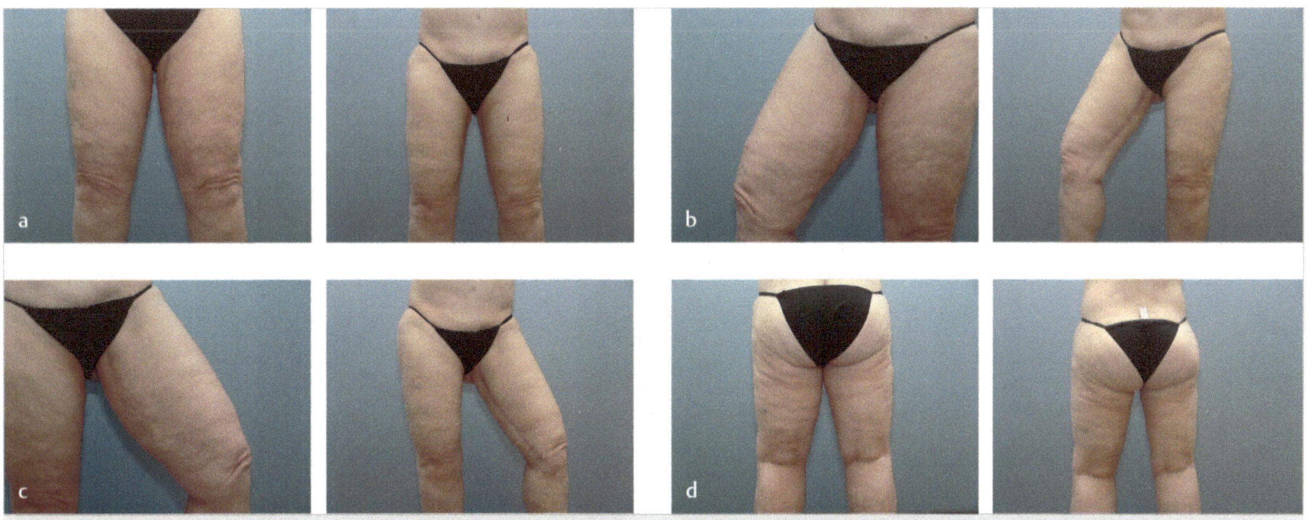

Fig. 84.2 Pre- and postoperative photos of a patient 13 months following a vertical avulsion thigh lift (**a**) anteroposterior (AP), (**b, c**) oblique, and (**d**) posterior views.

84.5 Conclusion

Vertical thigh lift, with or without circumferential liposuction, provides predictable circumferential tightening following massive weight loss. The key steps to its successful execution are the frequent intraoperative verification of the markings in order to achieve balance between tight contour and appropriate tension, and complete liposuction of the proposed resection tissue to allow for atraumatic preserving avulsion. Avulsion thighplasty achieves the separation of tissue and preservation of superficial structures in order to reduce postoperative complications such as seroma, lymphocele, and lymphedema.

Further Readings

Bertheuil N, Chaput B, Berger-Müller S, et al. Liposuction preserves the morphological integrity of the microvascular network: flow cytometry and confocal microscopy evidence in a controlled study. Aesthet Surg J. 2016; 36(5):609–618

Hunstad JP, Repta R. Lower body lift and thighplasty. In: Thorne CH, Chung KC, Gosain AK, et al, eds. Grabb and Smith's Plastic Surgery. Philadelphia, PA: Lippincott Williams & Wilkins; 2014:696–706

Hunstad JP, Kortesis BG, Knotts CD. Avulsion thighplasty: technique overview and 6-year experience. Plast Reconstr Surg. 2016; 137(1):84–87

Knotts CD, Kortesis BG, Hunstad JP. Avulsion brachioplasty: technique overview and 5-year experience. Plast Reconstr Surg. 2014; 133(2):283–288

85 Postbariatric Body Contouring: Upper Back Contouring—The Bra-Line Back Lift

Joseph P. Hunstad and Matthew H. Isakson

Abstract

The bra-line back lift is a powerful technique that addresses the entirety of the complex back deformity following massive weight loss. The zones of adherence in the back result in horizontal and vertical laxity, particularly after massive weight loss, which is not treated by a traditional lower body lift or other techniques. The bra-line back lift allows the surgeon to address this deformity with a horizontal scar that is well tolerated and easily concealed in a brasserie or swimsuit top. Complications are rare and can usually be managed with minor revision and wound care. The procedural learning curve is gentle, yielding consistent and predictable results with high patient satisfaction.

Keywords: Back lift, torsoplasty, trunkplasty, bra-line back lift, upper body lift, transverse upper body lift

Key Points

- The bra-line back lift is a powerful technique that allows the surgeon to address the entirety of the complex back deformity, including excess adiposity and skin laxity.
- Zones of adherence in the upper back result in horizontal and vertical laxity that are not addressed by a traditional lower body lift.
- The bra-line back lift allows the surgeon to address this common upper back deformity with a scar that is well tolerated and easily concealed in a bra or swimsuit top.
- Morbidity has proven to be minimal. Complications are rare and can usually be managed by minor wound care or revision under local anesthetic.
- The procedural learning curve is gentle, yielding consistent and predictable results with high patient satisfaction.

85.1 Preoperative Steps

85.1.1 Counseling

- A comprehensive discussion regarding body contouring and goals is held with the patient. Photographs are reviewed with patients to ensure expectations are appropriate, and they understand incision placement, risks, and complications.
- Routine labs including complete blood counts, comprehensive metabolic panels, and coagulation profiles are drawn and reviewed.
- Discontinue nonsteroidal anti-inflammatory medications and herbal supplements 2 weeks before surgery. Smoking abstinence should be reviewed with patients; active nicotine abuse is a relative contraindication.

85.1.2 Analysis and Marking

- Patients with concerns of upper back tissue excess are evaluated for skin quality, striae, subcutaneous adiposity, and excess or hanging skin.
- Redundant tissue is firmly grasped with bimanual palpation to demonstrate the final outcome in terms of tissue resection. Patients are encouraged to bring their most revealing top or bra the day of surgery to individualize scar placement.
- Patients are marked in a standing position with their arms at their sides.
- Bimanual palpation is used to strongly gather redundant skin and adiposity such that it centers on the final incision line. The resection pattern is strongly tapered into the inframammary fold at the level of the anterior axillary line to prevent a dog-ear.
- Precise realignment of tissues is important to the ultimate outcome, and closure is facilitated by vertical realignment marks placed preoperatively (▶ Fig. 85.1).

85.2 Operative Steps

- A penetrating towel clamp is used to the confirm preoperative markings and assess tension at multiple points. Difficulty in closing the clamp signifies excessive tension and adjustment of these lines is common.
- Realignment markings are tattooed with methylene blue as "permanent" skin markers rarely provide markings that last the entirety of a case.
- Dissection proceeds, without beveling or undermining, straight down to the loose areolar plane above the muscle fascia. The tissue directly superficial to muscle fascia is

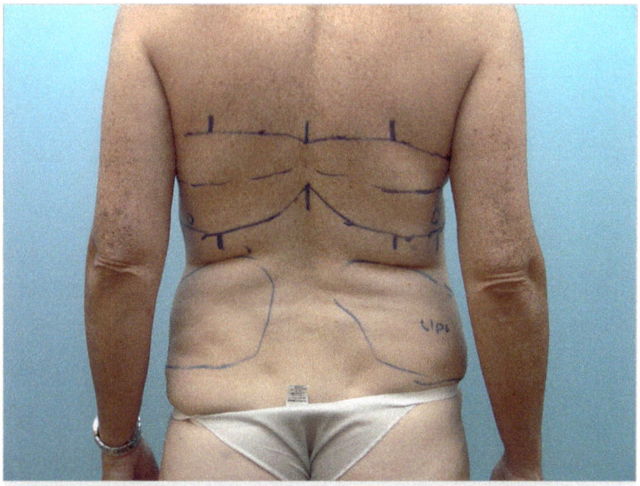

Fig. 85.1 Bra-line back lift preoperative markings.

preserved to help with pain control and to provide an anchor for space-obliterating sutures.

- Accurate bites of the superficial fascial system (SFS) are of vital importance to the closure. Tension is maximal on the SFS and immaculate closure will prevent scar migration or widening. The SFS may seem to retract in relation to the overlying dermis when the towel clamps are placed.
- Based on tension, either a 0 or number 1 polyglactin (Vicryl, Ethicon Inc, Somerville, NJ) suture is used. The closure begins laterally and progresses toward the spine. This suture is a three-point, space-obliterating suture, eliminating the need for drains.
- Towel clamps or staples can be progressively used at selective points of higher tension closure in order to ensure that good opposition is secured.
- The deep dermis is closed with a 2–0 polyglactin (Vicryl) suture in a buried fashion. The final layer is finished with an intracuticular running 4–0 poliglecaprone suture (Monocryl, Ethicon Inc, Somerville, NJ).
- Should this procedure be combined with a mastopexy, breast reduction, or reverse abdominoplasty, a temporary V-Y closure can be performed anterolaterally as far as the table permits.
- The suture line is then treated with paper tape; it is important to split the tapes every 3 cm to allow for swelling and to avoid shearing forces. If tape is not split, the skin will shear resulting in blistering and postinflammatory hyperpigmentation.

85.3 Postoperative Care

- Patients are encouraged to shower on postoperative day 1 if comfortable. Paper tape is left in place for a shower and patients are instructed to pat dry.
- Patients are routinely seen on postoperative day 1, though depending on their availability they can be seen within the first four postoperative days.
- Patients are reminded to keep their arms adducted while shampooing their hair.
- Range of motion is gradually increased based on patient comfort, with full range of motion achieved within 6 weeks.
- If abducting arms becomes painful or creates undue tension, patients are advised to scale back their activity.
- Skin tapes are changed weekly in clinic and removed after 2 to 3 postoperative weeks.
- Scar therapy is begun at 3 weeks postoperatively, consisting of silicone cream application two times daily.

85.4 Case Example

Pre- and postoperative photos of a patient undergoing bra-line back lift (▶ Fig. 85.2, ▶ Fig. 85.3, ▶ Fig. 85.4, ▶ Fig. 85.5, and ▶ Fig. 85.6).

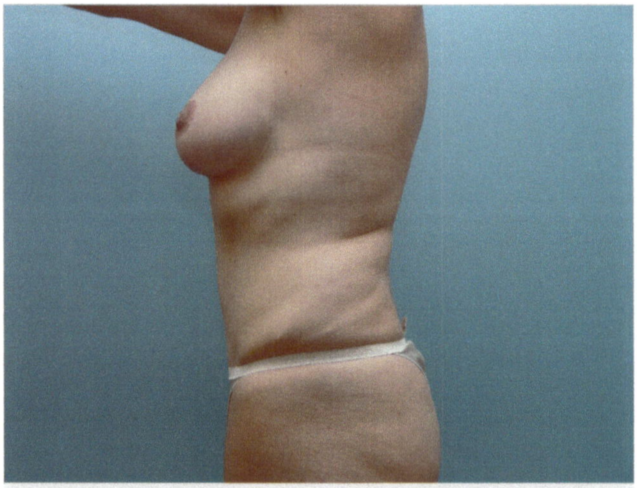

Fig. 85.3 Preoperative appearance of bra-line back lift, lateral view.

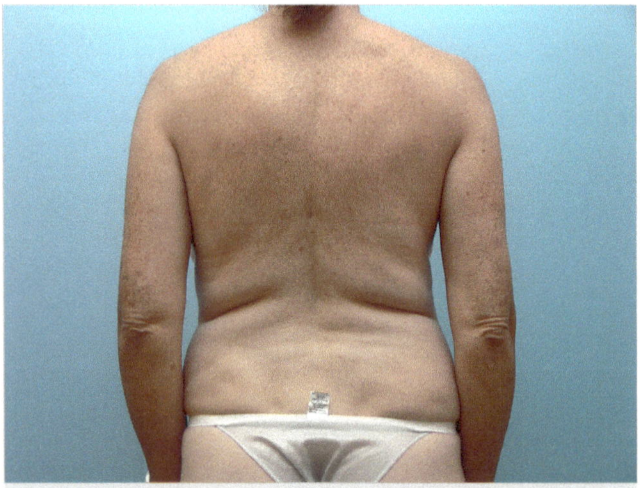

Fig. 85.2 Preoperative appearance of bra-line back lift, anteroposterior view.

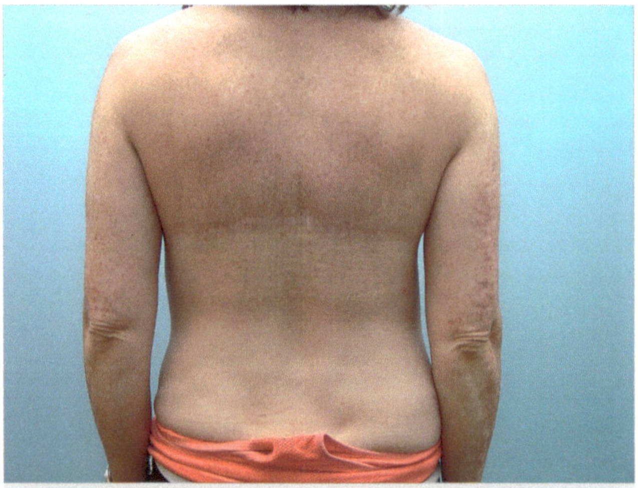

Fig. 85.4 Bra-line back lift postoperative appearance, anteroposterior view.

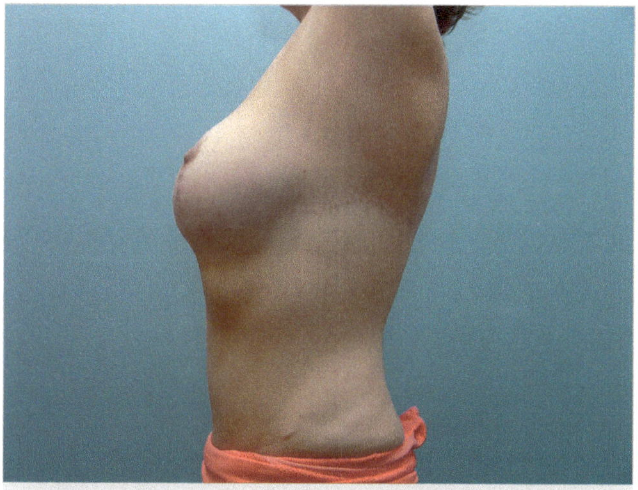

Fig. 85.5 Bra-line back lift postoperative appearance, lateral view.

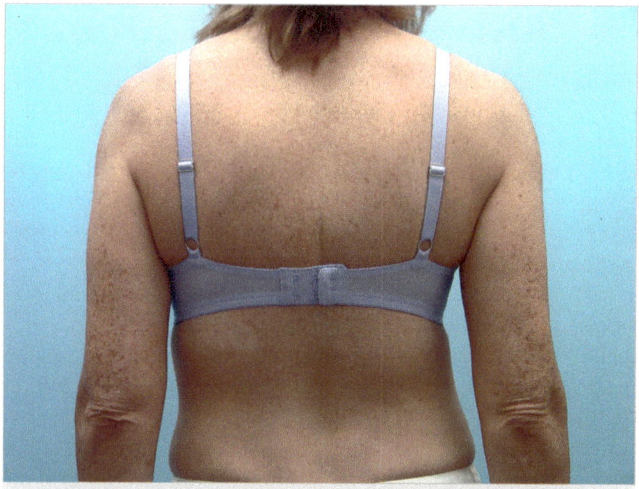

Fig. 85.6 Bra-line back lift postoperative appearance; note how scar is hidden by undergarments.

85.5 Conclusion

The transverse upper body lift that the authors refer to as the *bra-line back lift* is a powerful tool that delivers consistent and safe results. It has proven useful for both normal and massive weight loss patients who have experienced weight fluctuations and subsequent laxity. The procedure allows a rapid recovery, and the final scar is concealed beneath the bra or swim suit line. Complications are rare and can usually be managed by minor wound care or revision under local anesthetic. Morbidity associated with this procedure is minimal. Mastering this technique has a gentle learning curve and serves as a useful tool in the armamentarium of body contouring. Overall patient satisfaction has been universally high.

See **Video 85.1**.

Further Readings

Hunstad J, Chen C, Abbed T. Bra-line back lift. Clin Plast Surg. 2019; 46(1):77–84

Hunstad JP, Knotts CD. Transverse upper body lift. In: Rubin JP, ed. Body Contouring and Liposuction. Philadelphia, PA: Elsevier; 2013:159–165

Hunstad JP, Urbaniak RM. Bra-line back lift. In: Strauch B, Herman CK, eds. Encyclopedia of Body Sculpting After Massive Weight Loss. New York, NY: Thieme; 2011:230–239

Shermak MA. Management of back rolls. Aesthet Surg J. 2008; 28(3):348–356

Soliman S, Rotemberg SC, Pace D, et al. Upper body lift. Clin Plast Surg. 2008; 35(1): 107–114, discussion 121

86 Buttock Augmentation: S-Curve®

Nathaniel L. Villanueva and Ashkan Ghavami

Abstract

The S-Curve® procedure is an effective and powerful way to enhance patients' silhouette. Patient selection and preoperative planning are critical in achieving excellent outcomes. Execution of the procedure requires an understanding of gluteal aesthetics and anatomy. During the procedure selective release of ligamentous anatomy allows for intraoperative expansion and shaping of the buttock. The fat transfer should only be in the subcutaneous space to improve the safety of the procedure. Postoperatively, patients should be educated on key recommendations to improve graft survival and optimal trunk contour. Overall, this procedure provides an aesthetically pleasing S-shaped silhouette by narrowing the waist and augmenting the buttocks.

Keywords: Buttock augmentation, S-curve, gluteal augmentation, fat transfer, Brazilian butt lift

Key Points

- Patient selection and management of expectations are important in achieving safe, good outcomes and patient satisfaction.
- Preoperative planning and markings with a thorough understanding of the patient's anatomy are critical to obtaining an aesthetically pleasing S-curve silhouette (▶ Fig. 86.1).
- Precise contouring of the waist and thighs with suction-assisted lipectomy are as important as the fat transfer to the buttocks in order to achieve ideal silhouette and transitions from back and thighs to buttocks.
- Buttock fat transfer should be performed with small aliquots in the subcutaneous space **only** with continuous motion.
- Overcorrection should be avoided because increased pressure may decrease graft survival and may create unwanted future buttock ptosis.

86.1 Preoperative Steps

86.1.1 Patient Selection

- Ideal patients will have sufficient donor fat for gluteal fat transfer.
- Thinner patients can also achieve dramatic results with modest trunk liposuction and fat transfer to select zones in the gluteal region.
- Patients with insufficient donor fat can be instructed to gain weight with a diet targeted to increase fat lobule volume.
- Patients with personal or family history of hematologic disorders (deep venous thrombosis, pulmonary emboli, bleeding diathesis, etc.) may be contraindicated for the procedure but should be evaluated by hematologist prior to proceeding.

86.1.2 Understand the Patient's Anatomy

- Knowing subcutaneous, neurovascular, muscular, and ligamentous anatomy is key to getting optimal results.
- There are four general trunk and buttock shapes: A frame (desirable), V frame, H frame, and round (▶ Fig. 86.2).

86.1.3 Markings

- Marking is done in standing position.
- Liposuction zones adjacent to buttock should be delineated with the augmentation zones in mind.
- Areas requiring release and grafting should be identified.

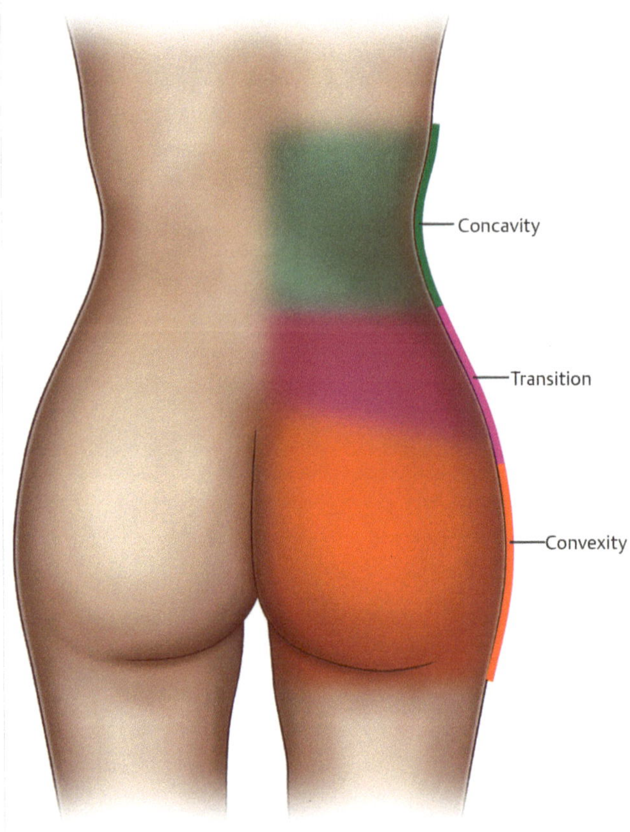

Fig. 86.1 The S-Curve®. The aesthetically pleasing S-curve silhouette is composed of superior concavity, a transition zone, and a convexity in the gluteal region.

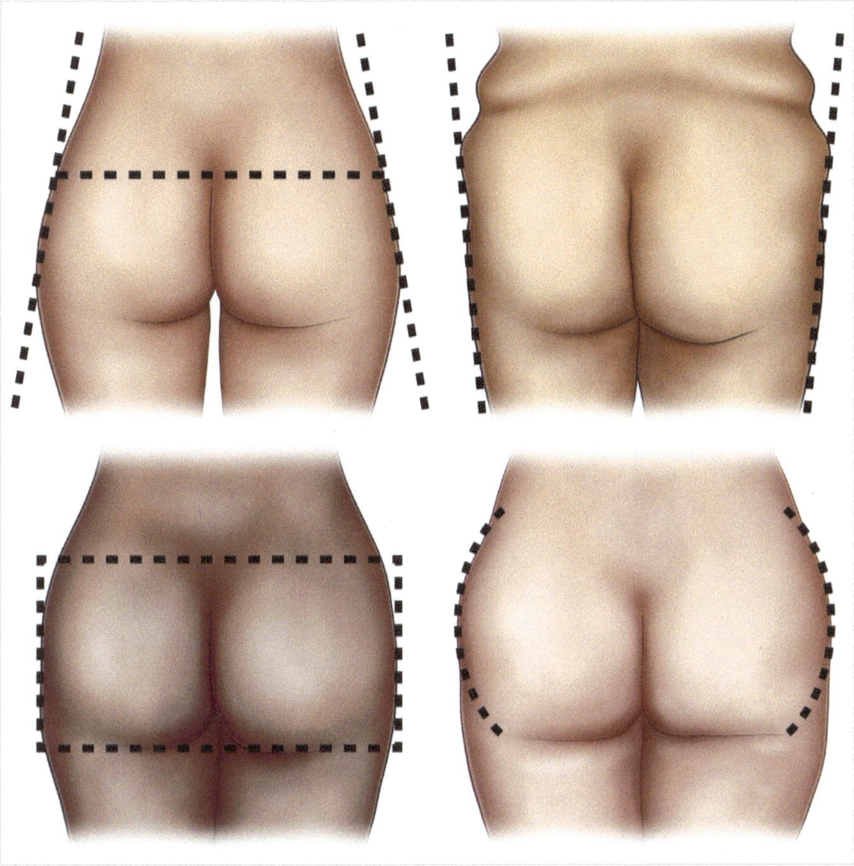

Fig. 86.2 Buttock shapes. There are four general trunk and buttock shapes: A frame (top left), V frame (top right), H or square frame (bottom left), and round frame (bottom right).

86.2 Operative Steps

See **Video 86.1**.

86.2.1 Liposuction

- Power-assisted aspiration of donor fat and contouring with 4 to 5 mm cannulas with the surgeon's preferred wetting solution (our preference is superwet, 1:1 wetting solution to lipoaspirate).
- Prerelease and postrelease are highly effective in separating fat to be aspirated and providing an even layer of tissue after lipectomy.
- Use multiple access sites allowing crisscrossing passes.
- Aggressive liposuction of the flanks, lower back, and sacral area is critical for improving the projection of upper pole of the buttock and generating the S-curve silhouette.

86.2.2 Fat Preparation

- The goal is to separate viable fat from the aqueous component of the lipoaspirate in a sterile fashion.
- Allow the fat to separate from the aqueous component in the liposuction cannister, and decant fluid and blood.
- The fat is then strained through a commercial straining without touching the fat, which helps remove oil, blood, and fibrous tissue especially in secondary liposuction.
- Mix 300 mg of clindamycin solution in each strained batch.
- Transfer fat to 60 mL Toomey syringes and prepare for injection.

86.2.3 Buttock Fat Transfer

- The patient is placed in prone jack knife position at 30 to 45 degrees.
- The preliminary release and first stage fat grafting allows for some intraoperative expansion.
- Fat acquired in supine position is injected prior to liposuctioning in prone position which allows time for wetting solution epinephrine to achieve full efficacy.
- Inject small aliquots of fat using continuous motion only in the subcutaneous space.
- Multiple passes are required to ensure graft take and a homogenous distribution.
- Resistance should be felt during every pass and overcorrection is not recommended.
- During all stages of buttock fat grafting, selectively release the osseocutaneous and fasciocutaneous ligaments to prevent

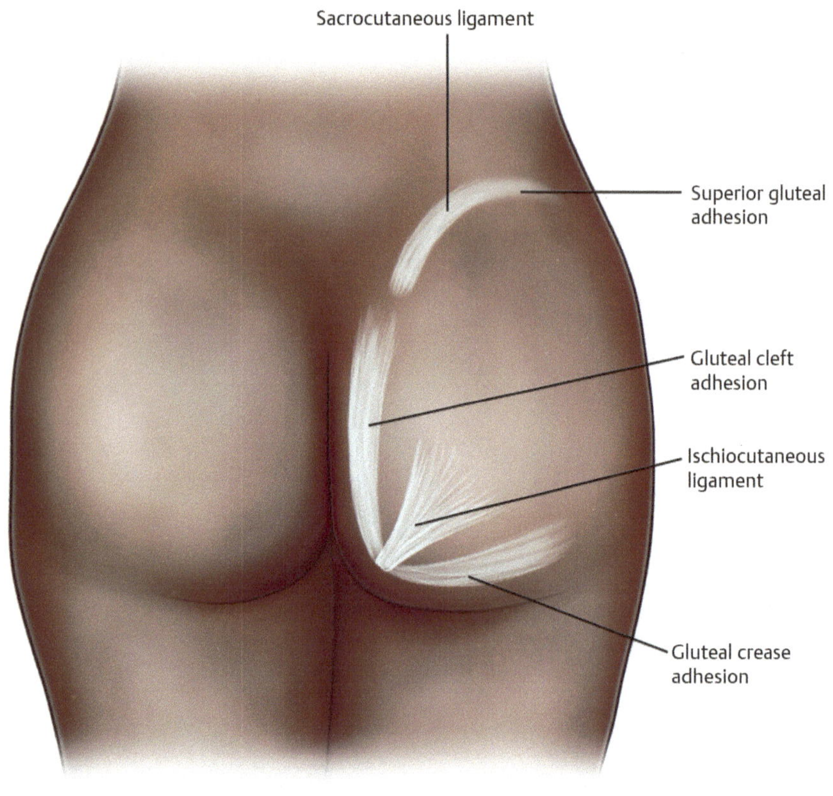

Fig. 86.3 The osseocutaneous and fasciocutaneous ligaments of the buttock. Selective release of the ligaments allows for expansion of the fat grafted regions, but complete disruption should be avoided.

cannula misguidance and improve irregularities transmitted to the skin which cause dimpling (▶ Fig. 86.3).
- Access incisions are closed in layers.

86.3 Postoperative Care

- Antibiotic prophylaxis is given for 5 days.
- Immediate ambulation following surgery with meticulous hygiene.
- Compression of the liposuction sites with foam pads is important for seroma avoidance and adherence of skin to superficial fascio/muscular framework (removed after 7 to 10 days).
- The garment is worn for up to 2 months.
- Avoid sitting or lying on the buttock for 2 to 8 weeks.

86.4 Case Example

This is a 28-year-old female with an A-shaped silhouette who underwent the S-Curve® procedure as described with a total of approximately 600 cc of fat transferred to each buttock. The patient is satisfied with her improved contour which has been maintained at 3 years postoperatively (▶ Fig. 86.4).

86.5 Conclusion

S-curve gluteal augmentation has the ability to significantly improve and transform patients' silhouette and waist to hip ratios. The procedure can be performed safely and has a low complication profile when using proper technique and adhering to recommended injection guidelines.

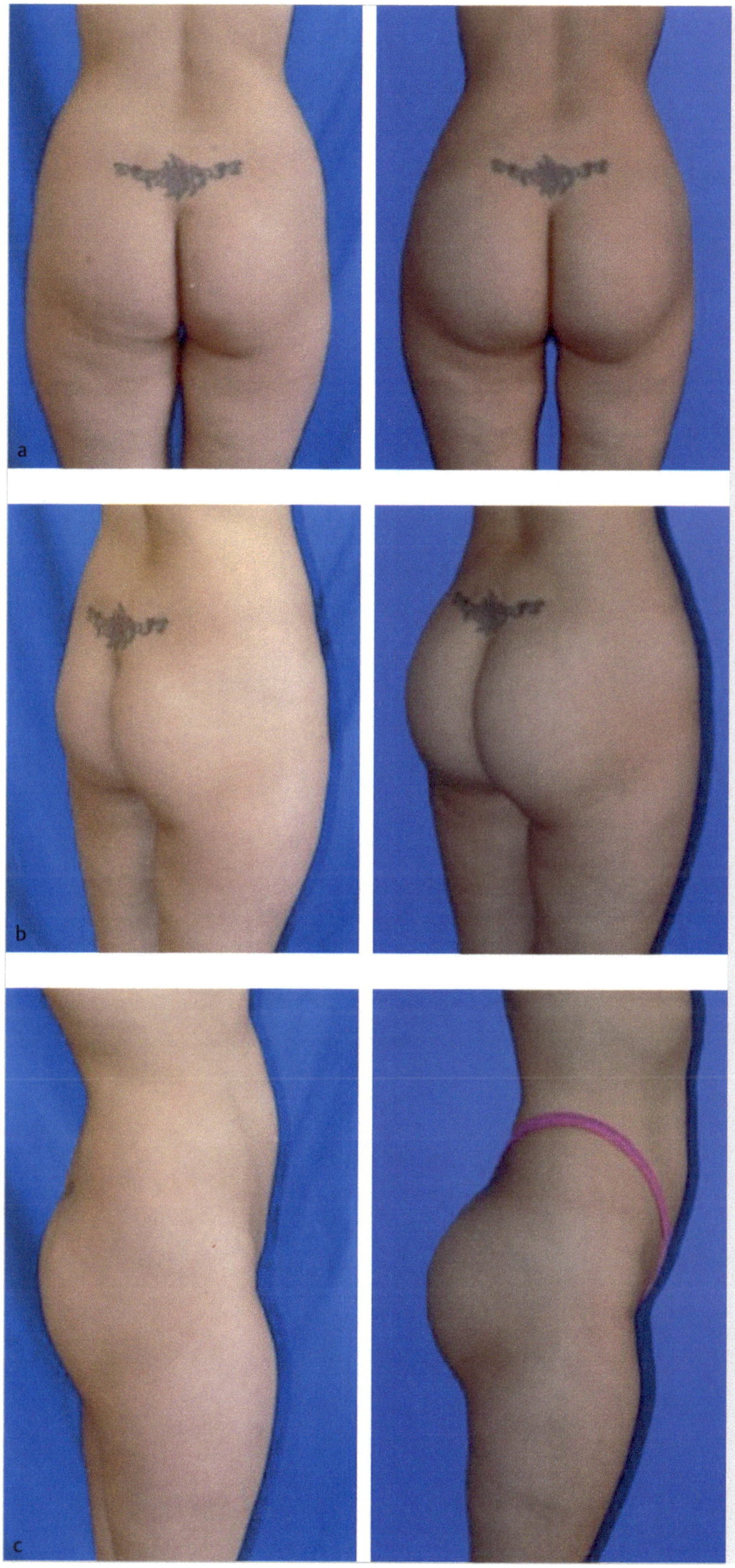

Fig. 86.4 (a–c) Case example. Preoperative photos (left), 3-year postoperative photos (right).

Further Readings

Ghavami A, Cohen MN, Thaller SR. Gluteal augmentation. Unfavorable Result Plast Surg Avoid Treat. 2018:499–516

Ghavami A, Villanueva NL. Gluteal augmentation and contouring with autologous fat transfer: Part I. Clin Plast Surg. 2018; 45(2):249–259

Ghavami A, Villanueva NL, Amirlak B. Gluteal ligamentous anatomy and its implication in safe buttock augmentation. Plast Reconstr Surg. 2018; 142(2):363–371

Nahai F, Ghavami A. The art of aesthetic surgery: principles and techniques. 3rd ed. Thieme;.

Wall S, Jr, Delvecchio D, Teitelbaum S, et al. Subcutaneous migration: a dynamic anatomical study of gluteal fat grafting. Plast Reconstr Surg. 2019; 143(5): 1343–1351

87 Safe Subcutaneous Buttock Augmentation

Ira L. Savetsky and Daniel A. Del Vecchio

Abstract
Gluteal fat grafting is the most rapidly growing cosmetic surgery procedure in the current era and is the most controversial in terms of safety. Simultaneous separation tumescence (SST) and expansion vibration lipofilling (EVL), combined with proper training in aesthetics and in technique, empower the properly trained plastic surgeon to perform buttock augmentation effectively and safely.

Keywords: Gluteal fat grafting, Brazilian butt lift, simultaneous separation tumescence, expansion vibration lipofilling

Key Points

- Fat can be safely placed in the subcutaneous space without inadvertent injury to the gluteus maximus muscle fascia.
- Sufficient and reliable intraoperative expansion of the subcutaneous recipient site allows for adequate domal projection and aesthetics without the need to place fat into muscle.

87.1 Background

- Simultaneous separation tumescence (SST) and expansion vibration lipofilling (EVL) are technically superior to obsolete Klein needle tumescence and syringe-based fat grafting techniques for large volume fat grafting on the basis of multiple attributes:
  - Vibration allows ease of navigation in the recipient site, less fatigue, and better dispersion of fat.
  - Roller pump eliminates thumb adduction to propel fat flow, resulting in less fatigue.
  - Reduced fatigue allows surgeon to focus on location of cannula tip with every stroke.
  - Canister versus syringe design makes volume documentation easier for staff.
  - Canister design eliminates syringe transfers and is less time-consuming.
  - Vibrating exploded cannulas disrupt fibroseptal network, allowing intraoperative subdermal manipulation of recipient site.

87.2 Setup

- It consists of a double-barrel stand holding two canisters, a 3-L flat canister with a lid (suction canister), and a 3-L ("slant") canister. The slant canister has a 1/4″ spigot at the bottom of the slant, completely eliminating all contents of the canister out of the spigot by simple gravity.
- The canister stand is placed on a Mayo stand at the foot of the operating room (OR) table, but not over the table itself.
- From the spigot of the slant canister 0.25-inch tubing is connected, and a loop of this tubing is passed off the sterile field to a roller pump, which is situated immediately adjacent to the Mayo stand. Returning to the sterile field, the end of the tubing is connected to a basket cannula on a Microaire PAL handle. This constitutes the vibratory inflow setup.
- The flat canister (Medela Corporation, Highland Park, IL) containing a lid has two sets of tubing connected to it. From the canister, one tubing goes from the lid to a vacuum source, while the other tubing goes from the lid to a liposuction cannula, typically a 4 mm or 5 mm × 50 cm, 12-hole cannula (Wells Johnson, Tucson AZ) (▶ Fig. 87.1).

87.3 Simultaneous Separation Tumescence

- During tumescence, solution is simply poured into the slant canister and simultaneous separation (basket) and tumescence (SST) is performed. The combination of blunt tipped basket cannulas, vibratory motion, and fluid head advancement results in minimal to no bleeding during this maneuver.
- Liposuction is immediately commenced using manual cannulas and is collected into the flat canister. As each aesthetic is treated, the canister is changed out to guarantee equal removal in each side.
- Once all fat is removed from a donor site aesthetic perspective, fat is allowed to separate from blood and crystalloid while equalization is performed to the donor site.
- The harvested fat may be washed with Poloxamer 188 if the operator wishes (SurClens, Convatec Inc.) or simply divided into two equal volumes, placed into the slant canister, and grafted using EVL.

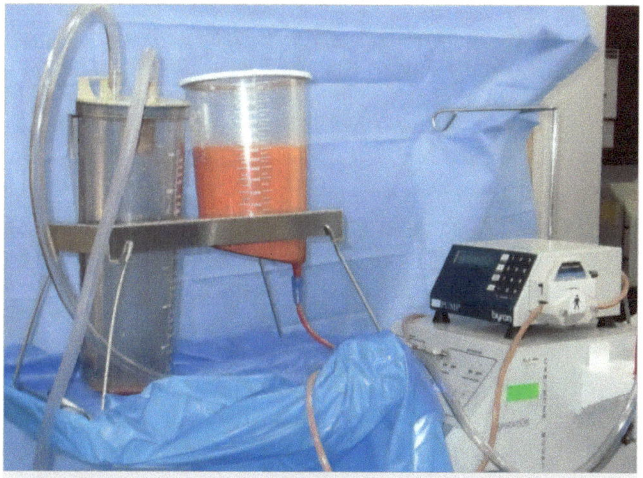

Fig. 87.1 Instrumentation setup for expansion vibration lipofilling. Canister spigot, tubing, and cannula size are all of equal diameter to avoid any one area of high resistance and shear.

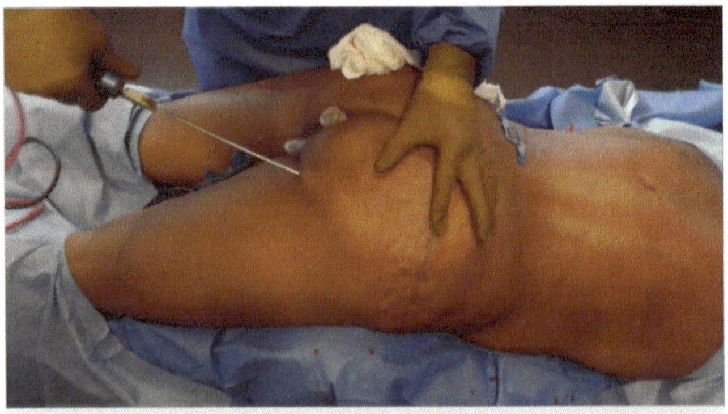

Fig. 87.2 Fat is placed in the subcutaneous position of the buttocks.

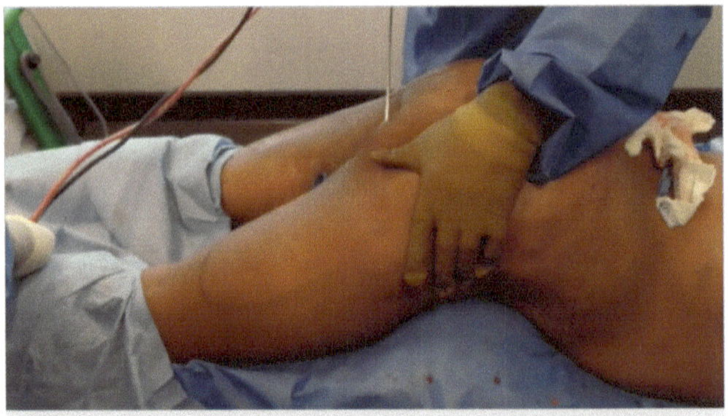

Fig. 87.3 Fat is placed in the subcutaneous position of the lateral thighs.

87.4 Expansion Vibration Lipofilling (EVL)

- With the patient in the prone position, three cannula access incisions are used for safe subcutaneous gluteal fat grafting: the natal cleft, the infragluteal crease, and the upper outer quadrant of the buttock.
- Using intermittent fat flow by means of a roller pump and vibration by means of a PAL device (Microaire, Charlottesville, VA), fat is placed in the subcutaneous position of the buttocks (▸ Fig. 87.2) and posterolateral thighs (▸ Fig. 87.3 and ▸ Fig. 87.4) to render a suitably aesthetic shape change and enlargement. Attention is paid to the establishment or preservation of symmetry.
- During grafting the surgeon is 100% focused on where the tip of the cannula is with every stroke. The surgeon should see the cannula tip beneath the skin or feel it with the nondominant hand; both sensory functions are considered easier, more efficient, and faster than staring at an ultrasound screen.

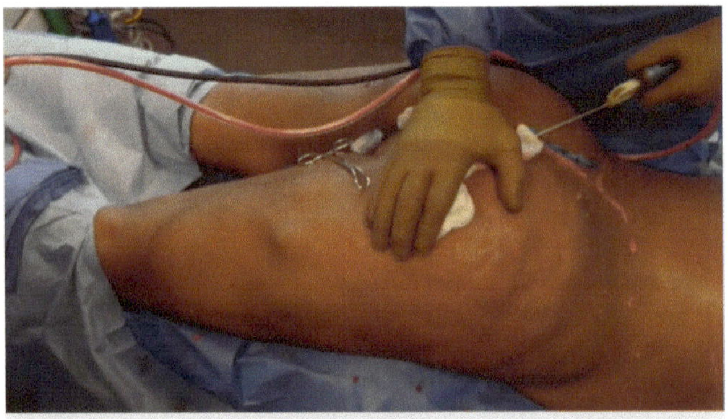

Fig. 87.4 Fat is placed in the subcutaneous position of the posterior thighs.

87.5 Case Examples

87.5.1 Case 1

This 34-year-old woman presented for Brazilian butt lift (BBL) evaluation. She complained of inadequate projection and excess fat in the waist, abdomen, and back. Her examination was notable for the presence of dense fat. The proportion of connective tissue to adipocytes varies by sex, race, and heredity; the higher the proportion, the more difficult it is to extract fat. The biggest mistake made in such cases is to end the liposuction too early, which will result in a more difficult redo, due the additional presence of scar tissue. The time to do dense fat cases correctly is the first time. Dense fat cases require an aggressive approach requiring effective separation of fat and a surgical strategy that requires stamina. After 1 year of lipo 360 and BBL, she demonstrates improved contours, buttock projection, and a snatched waist (▸ Fig. 87.5).

87.5.2 Case 2

This 26-year-old male presented for liposuction of his love handles. At the time of consultation, he mentioned he wanted a fuller buttock. Males presenting for BBL can be separated into two subtypes: (1) males who want a more athletic butt, with upper pole fullness (gluteus medius hypertrophy) while retaining the lateral hollowness of the gluteus maximus (hip dips), or (2) male patients who want a more feminine look with wider hips and filling of the hip dips. This patient desired the latter. After liposuction and BBL with 1,200 cc of fat in each buttock using EVL, he demonstrates a rounder, fuller buttock (bubble butt) and was very happy at 1 year postoperative (▸ Fig. 87.6).

87.6 Conclusion

SST and EVL, combined with proper training in aesthetics and in technique, empower the properly trained plastic surgeon to perform buttock augmentation effectively and safely. Safe subcutaneous buttock augmentation (SSBA) will eventually be the standard of care in this procedure, resulting in better cosmetic results, more efficient operating times, and most importantly a reduction in mortality and better safety for our patients.

See **Video 87.1**.

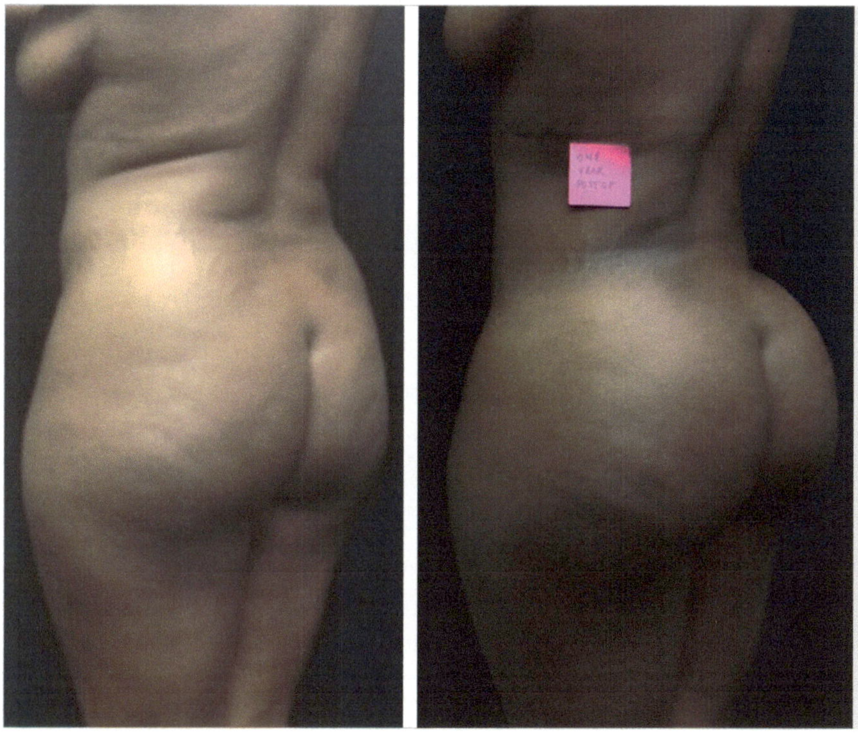

Fig. 87.5 Case 1. This 34-year-old woman presented for Brazilian butt lift (BBL) evaluation. She complained of inadequate projection and excess fat in the waist, abdomen, and back. Her examination was notable for the presence of dense fat. The proportion of connective tissue to adipocytes varies by sex, race, and heredity; the higher the proportion, the more difficult it is to extract fat. The biggest mistake made in such cases is to end the liposuction too early, which will result in a more difficult redo, due the additional presence of scar tissue. The time to do dense fat cases correctly is the first time. Dense fat cases require an aggressive approach requiring effective separation of fat and a surgical strategy that requires stamina. After 1 year of lipo 360 and BBL, she demonstrates improved contours, buttock projection, and a snatched waist.

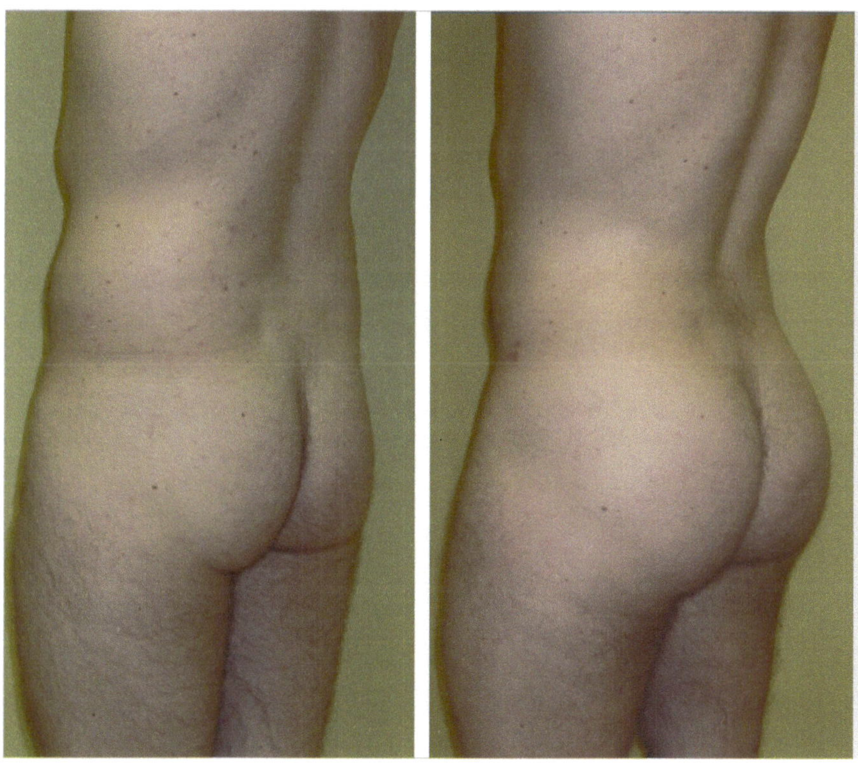

Fig. 87.6 Case 2. This 26-year-old male presented for liposuction of his love handles. At the time of consultation, he mentioned he wanted a fuller buttock. Males presenting for Brazilian butt lift (BBL) can be separated into two subtypes: (1) males who want a more athletic butt, with upper pole fullness (gluteus medius hypertrophy) while retaining the lateral hollowness of the gluteus maximus (hip dips), or (2) male patients who want a more feminine look with wider hips and filling of the hip dips. This patient desired the latter. After liposuction and BBL with 1,200 cc of fat in each buttock using expansion vibration lipofilling (EVL), he demonstrates a rounder, fuller buttock (bubble butt) and was very happy at 1 year postoperative.

Further Readings

Del Vecchio D. Common sense for the common good: staying subcutaneous during fat transplantation to the gluteal region. Plast Reconstr Surg. 2018; 142(1):286–288

Del Vecchio D, Wall S, Jr. Expansion vibration lipofilling: a new technique in large-volume fat transplantation. Plast Reconstr Surg. 2018; 141(5):639e–649e

Villanueva NL, Del Vecchio DA, Afrooz PN, Carboy JA, Rohrich RJ. Staying safe during gluteal fat transplantation. Plast Reconstr Surg. 2018; 141(1):79–86

Wall S, Jr, Delvecchio D, Teitelbaum S, et al. Subcutaneous migration: a dynamic anatomical study of gluteal fat grafting. Plast Reconstr Surg. 2019; 143(5): 1343–1351

Part XII

Vaginal Rejuvenation

XII

88 Extended Wedge Labiaplasty with Bipolar Radiofrequency Labia Majora Reduction (AVIVA)

Christine A. Hamori

Abstract

Aesthetic female genital surgery has been on the rise for several years. The popularity of Brazilian waxing and visibility of the vulva on the Internet contribute to the popularity of labia minora reduction or labiaplasty. Patients of all ages complain of labia minora excess causing embarrassment and physical discomfort. Safe and effective surgical procedures exist to reduce the bulk and protrusion of the labia minora and have been found to improve these patients' quality of life.

The education and evaluation of women presenting with aesthetic genital concerns require a unique skill set that may not be familiar to plastic surgeons. These women are usually embarrassed and somewhat ashamed of their genital appearance and hence need gentle encouragement to express their specific concerns. It is helpful to have patients fill out a questionnaire to help elicit their aesthetic and functional concerns.

The consultation with the patient should be in the presence of a female physician extender. It is helpful to educate patients regarding the anatomy of the vulva with digital or print media. Patients need to understand the great variability of the labia minora appearance and be assured that they are normal. It is helpful to show before and after photographs to the patients in order to determine their aesthetic goals. Some patients prefer a more natural appearance with the preservation of more labia minora where others prefer a very trim result.

Below are the step-by-step instructions for performing the wedge labiaplasty and radiofrequency treatment of the labia majora.

Keywords: Wedge labiaplasty, noninvasive labia majora reduction, preoperative labiaplasty assessment, postoperative care labiaplasty

Key Points

- Aesthetic vulvar surgery requires a thorough preoperative analysis of the anatomy as it pertains to meeting the aesthetic goals of the patient.
- Labia minora reduction or labiaplasty is the most common aesthetic genital procedure; patient selection and surgical planning provide the pathway to successful and reliable results.
- The minimally invasive labia majora radiofrequency (RF) treatment provides a "scarless" option for patients with mild to moderate labia majora skin laxity.

88.1 Preoperative Steps

- Female physician extender (physician assistant [PA], medical assistant [MA], nurse) sees the patient first to inquire about labial concerns (appearance, symptoms, and desires), any psychological issues, and a detailed sexual history. Written questionnaires given to the patients prior to the consultation are useful in determining aesthetic and functional vulvar complaints.
- Digital anatomic diagrams of the vulva are useful patient educational tools that demonstrate variations in anatomy, surgical techniques (animations), and scar location. The review of before and after photographs with patients at consultation aids in determining the patient's desired postoperative appearance.
- Patient examination (physician extender should be present in room) with the patient in the lithotomy and standing positions. A handheld mirror may be helpful for the patient to point out specific concerns.
- Assessment in the lithotomy position should include mons pubis and labia majora skin laxity and volume, clitoral hood redundancy in the sagittal and coronal planes, palpation of the clitoris to determine if any enlargement is present (clitoromegaly), labia minora skin excess, pigmentation, and connection at the posterior fourchette.
- Assessment in the standing position should include extent of labia minora visibility beyond the labia majora, width of the intervulvar commissure, projection of the clitoral hood, and the laxity of the labia majora.
- Informed consent with particular emphasis on the risks of dyspareunia, asymmetry, and cosmetic dissatisfaction due to existing anatomical limitations.

88.2 Intraoperative Steps

- Photograph patient in standing position.
- Oral or intravenous (IV) antibiotic.
- Topical anesthetic x 20 minutes if under local.
- Photograph patient in lithotomy position (pose labia in several positions).
- Mark wedge resection anteriorly just distal to junction of clitoral hood with labia minora and posteriorly so as to not cause excessive tension on approximation of wedge markings (▶ Fig. 88.1).
- Inject local 1% lidocaine with 1:100,000 epinephrine (30-gauge needle) subcutaneously and submucosally.
- Betadine prep and drape.

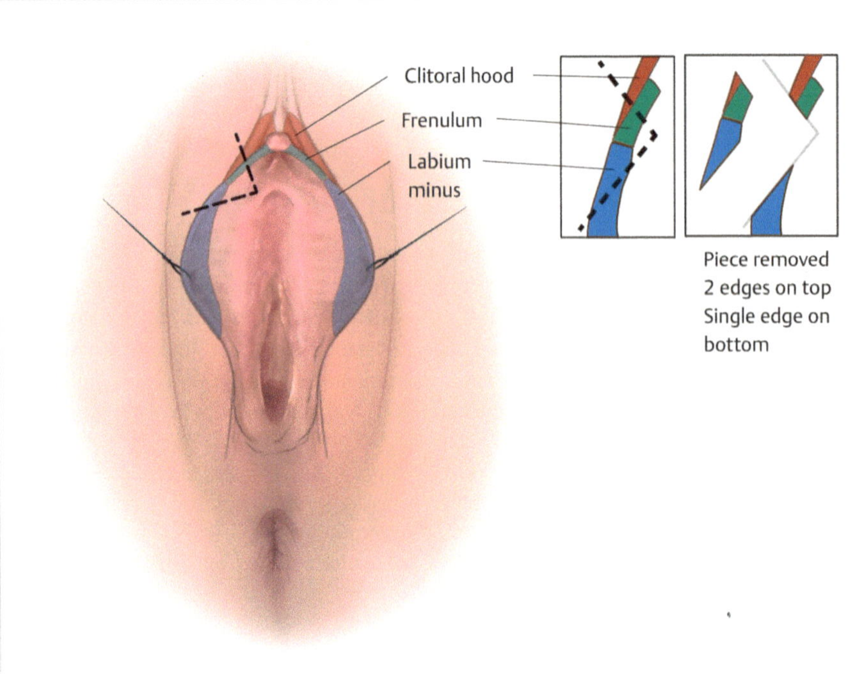

Fig. 88.1 The anatomy of wedge incision placement just posterior to the confluence to prevent closure of a W edge to a V edge. (Reproduced with permission from Hamori CA. Female Cosmetic Genital Surgery. Thieme; 2017.)

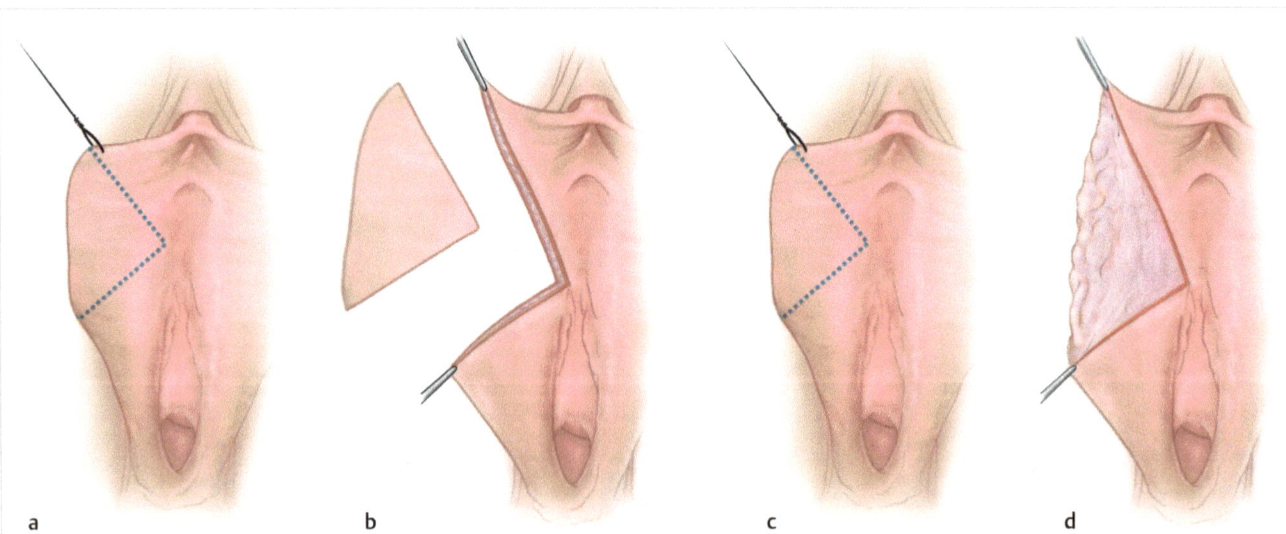

Fig. 88.2 (a–d) A full-thickness wedge resection for thick labia versus demucosalization for thin, atrophic labia. (Reproduced with permission from Hamori CA. Female Cosmetic Genital Surgery. Thieme; 2017.)

- Wedge resection:
  - #15 blade or low temperature RF device (needle tip Bovie or Peak Plasma blade on cutting mode).
  - Resect wedge superficially to maintain vascular pedicle (▶ Fig. 88.2a–d).
- Closure:
  - Buried suture of 4–0 Monocryl in dermis of leading edge of resection. Leave tail long and grasp with snap.
  - Close the wedge from medial to lateral with interrupted 4–0 or 5–0 buried Monocryl sutures.
  - Lateral closure:
    - Excise dog-ear (if present) superolaterally so scar falls near the sulcus of the labia majora.
    - If double fold is present (▶ Fig. 88.3) consider running dog-ear along the double fold.
  - Close leading edge with vertical mattress suture of 5–0 Monocryl. Edge eversion is important to prevent a notch.
  - Final layer closure with running 5–0 Vicryl Rapide.
  - Inject Marcaine 0.25% with 1:200,000 epinephrine.

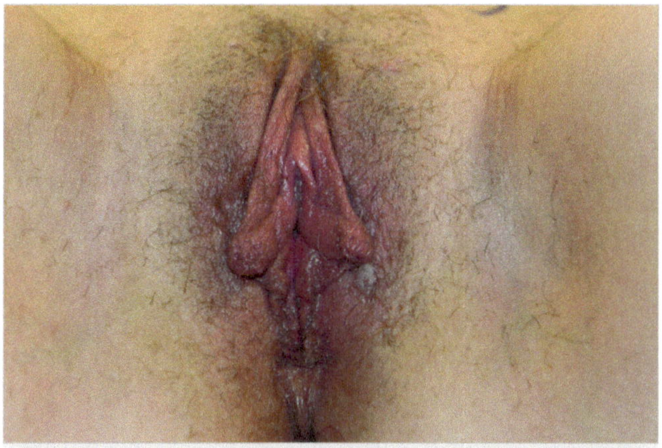

Fig. 88.3 This 50-year-old woman has a double-fold variant. (Reproduced with permission from Hamori CA. Female Cosmetic Genital Surgery. Thieme; 2017.)

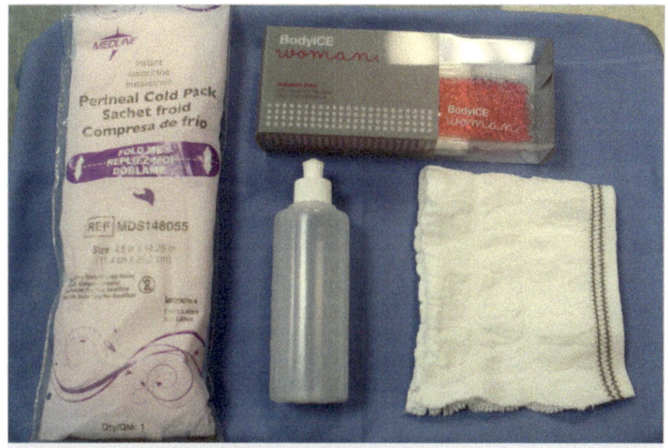

Fig. 88.4 Postoperative dressings.

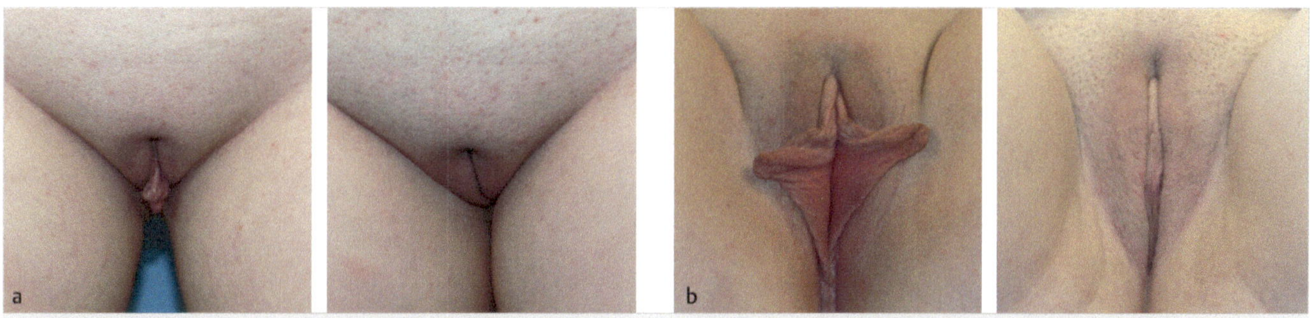

Fig. 88.5 (a, b) A 29-year-old patient standing and lithotomy position before and after wedge labiaplasty (result at 2 months).

88.3 AVIVA Radiofrequency Labia Majora Rejuvenation

88.3.1 Indication

- Mild to moderate skin laxity and fatty excess of labia majora in patients who do not require or are averse to surgical labia majora reduction.
- Tumescent injection (1 L lactated Ringer's [LR] + 1:1000 epinephrine + 50 cc 1% lidocaine) to right labia majora with small 14-gauge blunt cannula at 100 cc per minute with infusion pump.
- Apply sterile ultrasound gel.
- Insert AVIVA probe and treat right labia majora as per protocol (external temperature, 38 °C; internal temperature, 68 °C).
- Treat left labia majora next (tumescent injection…) and then mons pubis.
- Apply Neosporin to labia minora, Maxi pad, and mesh underwear (▶ Fig. 88.4).

88.4 Postoperative Care

- Rest and elevation of pelvis for 3 days.
- Peri bottle irrigation of area with lukewarm tap water three to four times per day.
- Narcotic medication may be necessary for 1 to 2 days.
- No exercise for 3 weeks.
- No sex or horseback riding or biking for 6 weeks.

88.5 Follow-up

- Postoperative visit at 2 weeks to evaluate incisions.
- Visit at 2 months for photographs in standing and lithotomy position.

88.6 Case Example

A 29-year-old patient standing and lithotomy position before and after wedge labiaplasty (result at 2 months) (▶ Fig. 88.5a, b).

88.7 Conclusion

Potential labiaplasty patients require a detailed sexual history. A review of normal vulvar anatomy with the assistance of diagrams and before and after photos help to determine the patient's aesthetic desires. The patient should be examined in the standing and lithotomy positions. Photographs are important in both positions to document asymmetries. It is important to mark wedges conservatively and maintain vascular pedicle in subcutaneous tissue. Layered closure with absorbable sutures is performed. No vigorous exercise for 3 weeks and no intercourse, biking, or horseback riding for 6 weeks postoperative.

See **Video 88.1**.

Further Readings

Alter GJ. Aesthetic labia minora and clitoral hood reduction using extended central wedge resection. Plast Reconstr Surg. 2008; 122(6):1780–1789

Gress S. Aesthetic and functional labiaplasty. Cham: Springer International Publishing; 2017

Hamori CA, Banwell P, Alinsod R. Female cosmetic genital surgery: concepts, classification, and techniques. New York: Thieme; 2017:41–58

Hamori CA, Banwell P, Alinsod R. Female Cosmetic Genital Surgery: Concepts, Classification, and Techniques. New York: Thieme; 2017:143–160

Sorice SC, Li AY, Canales FL, Furnas HJ. Why women request labiaplasty. Plast Reconstr Surg. 2017; 139(4):856–863

89 Radiofrequency-Assisted Vulvovaginal Rejuvenation

Erez Dayan

Abstract
Labiaplasty has increased in popularity over the past 10 years. Although traditional labiaplasty has a high satisfaction rate (>90%) many patients prefer minimally invasive approaches and downtime. The radiofrequency-assisted labiaplasty procedure uses thermal energy to contract labia majora and minora, avoiding traditional labiaplasty incisions and downtime.

Keywords: Labiaplasty, minimally invasive labiaplasty, radiofrequency, vulvovaginal rejuvenation

Key Points

- Traditional labiaplasty has been associated with potential complications such as dehiscence, hematoma, flap necrosis, narrowed introitus, pain, and asymmetry.
- Minimally invasive techniques such as radiofrequency (RF) have emerged as viable alternatives to traditional labiaplasty through a temperature controlled bipolar mechanism to heat tissues to target temperatures of 68 °C internally and 38 °C externally. This controlled energy delivery leads to an inflammatory cascade initiating neocollagenesis angiogenesis, and elastin remodeling over the subsequent 3 to 4 months.

89.1 Preoperative Steps

- A detailed medical history and physical is obtained on all patients prior to treatment. Exclusion criteria include: open wounds, active infection, dermatologic conditions, bleeding disorders, immunocompromised state.

89.2 Operative Steps

- Access points are injected at the caudal aspect of each labia (majora and minora) with 2.5 cc of local anesthesia (1% lidocaine with epinephrine). Next, an 18-gauge needle is used to create an access incision. In each treatment site 20 to 40 cc of tumescent solution is infiltrated (50 cc of 2% lidocaine, 1.5 mg epinephrine per liter of lactated Ringer's solution).
- Hydrosoluble lubricating gel is placed over the labia to improve transduction between the two ports of the RF device.
- The RF settings include a controlled internal temperature cutoff at 68 °C and 38 °C externally.
- The bipolar RF cannula is placed into the access port and moved in a radial cranio-caudal motion until the tissues reach target temperature (▸ Fig. 89.1).
- Fractional RF can contribute additively by producing a resurfacing and soft tissue tightening from the skin surface at adjustable depths (▸ Fig. 89.2).

89.3 Postoperative Care

- The usual post-op course involves some edema and ecchymosis. This typically resolves in 2 to 3 weeks.

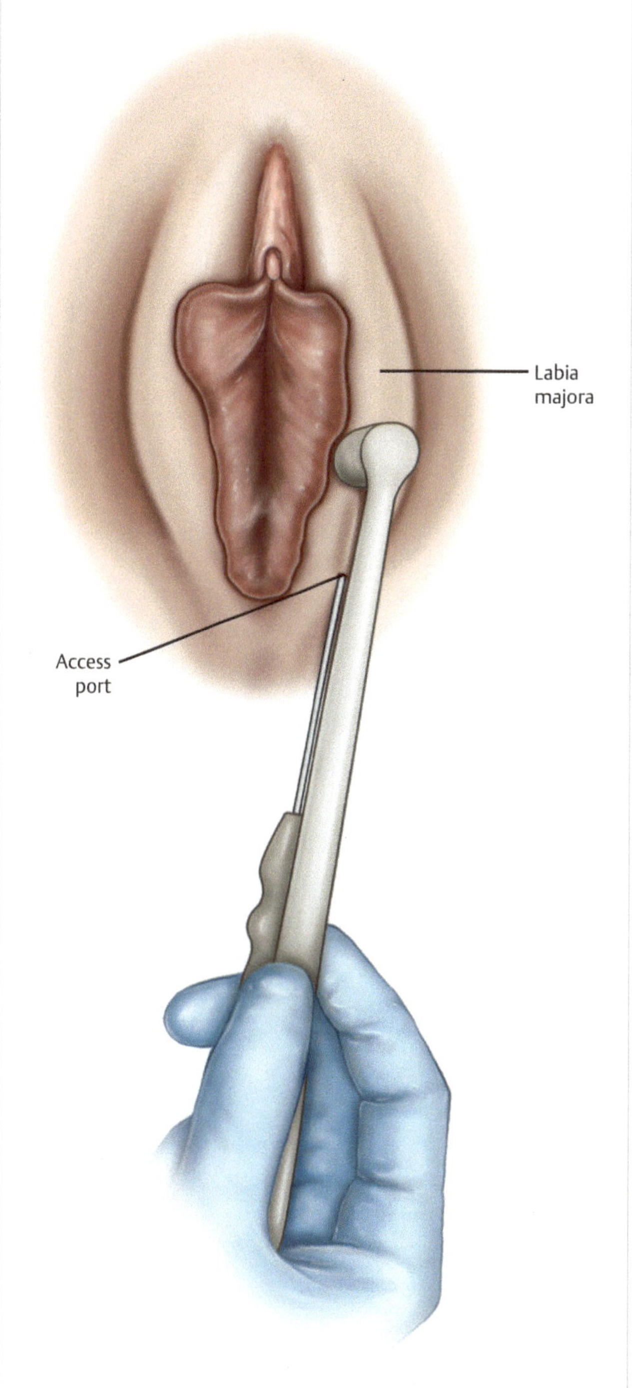

Fig. 89.1 Bipolar radiofrequency treatment of labia majora (AVIVA, Inmode, Lake Forrest, CA).

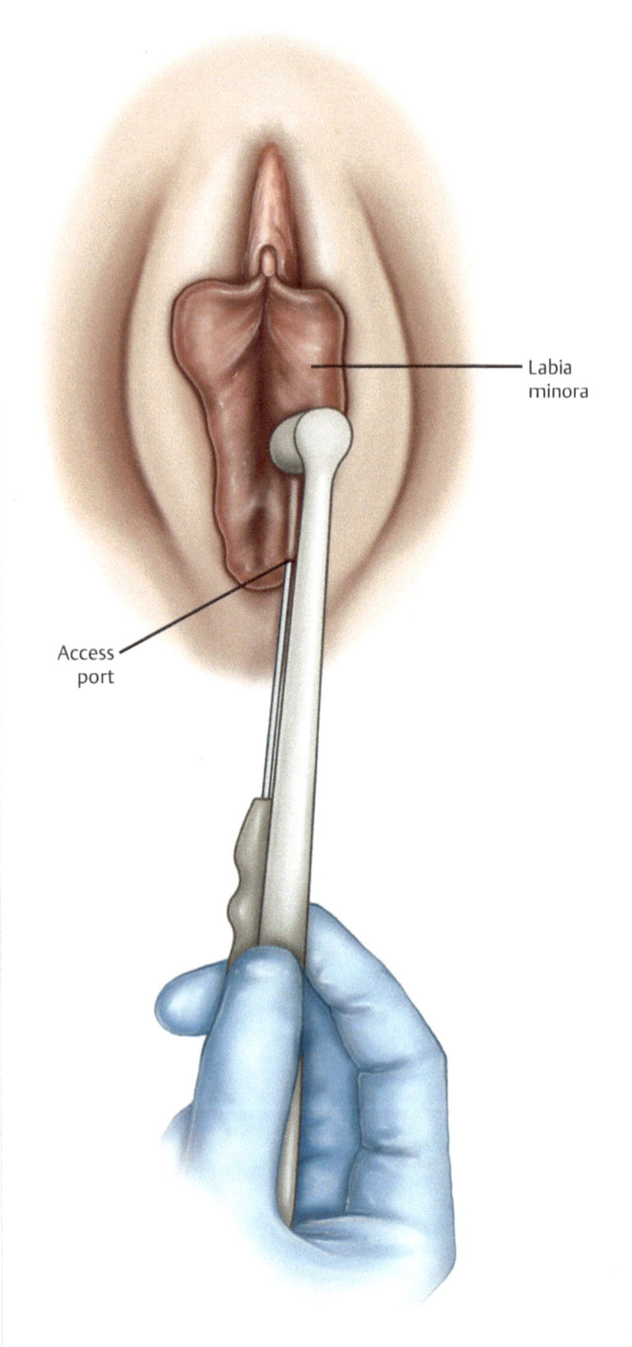

Fig. 89.2 Bipolar radiofrequency treatment of labia minora (AVIVA, Inmode, Lake Forrest, CA).

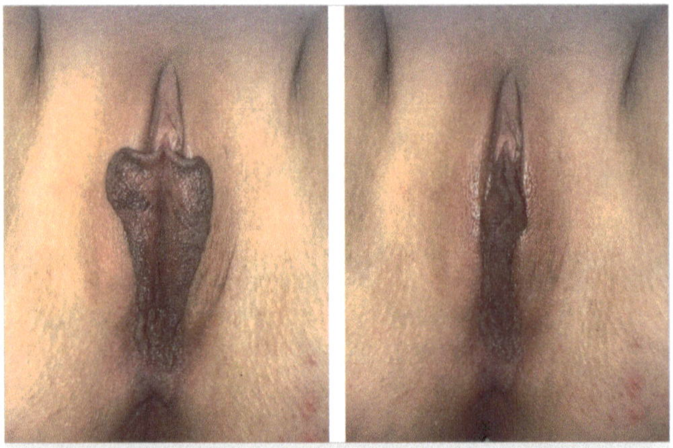

Fig. 89.3 Preprocedure and postprocedure result at 6 months after a combination of bipolar radiofrequency (AVIVA; InMode) and fractional radiofrequency are shown (Morpheus8; InMode).

- There is no need for an elaborate dressing as the incisions are 18-gauge needle access points that will seal on their own.
- Most patients return to work the next day.

89.4 Case Example

Preprocedure and postprocedure result at 6 months after a combination of bipolar RF (AVIVA; InMode) and fractional RF (Morpheus8; InMode) are shown (► Fig. 89.3).

89.5 Conclusion

Treatment of labia hyperplasia and laxity with bipolar RF may potentially fill a treatment gap of females seeking aesthetic and functional improvements without surgical labiaplasty. A powered prospective randomized double blinded study is needed to further elucidate the role of this technology.

See **Video 89.1** and **Video 89.2**.

Further Readings

Goodman MP. Female genital cosmetic and plastic surgery: a review. J Sex Med. 2011; 8(6):1813–1825

Hunter JG. Labia minora, labia majora, and clitoral hood alteration: experience-based recommendations. Aesthet Surg J. 2016; 36(1):71–79

Mayer HF. Vaginal labiaplasty: current practices and a simplified classification system for labial protrusion. Plast Reconstr Surg. 2015; 136(5):705e–706e

Sadick N, Rothaus KO. Aesthetic applications of radiofrequency devices. Clin Plast Surg. 2016; 43(3):557–565

Vanaman Wilson MJ, Bolton J, Jones IT, Wu DC, Calame A, Goldman MP. Histologic and clinical changes in vulvovaginal tissue after treatment with a transcutaneous temperature-controlled radiofrequency device. Dermatol Surg. 2018; 44(5):705–713

Part XIII

Non-Surgical Body Contouring

XIII

90 Cryolipolysis

Nathaniel L. Villanueva, Daniel J. Gould, Cory Felber, and W. Grant Stevens

Abstract

Cryolipolysis provides a nonsurgical modality to treat regional lipodystrophy in appropriately selected patients seeking to avoid surgical procedures and the downtime associated with liposuction. There are various treatment applicators, which have contour attachments to treat areas throughout the body. An important distinction in selecting applicators is whether or not the fat in the treatment area can be pinched. If so, applicators that have vacuum assistance can be used, whereas nonpinchable areas require flat applicators. Following the procedure, the treatment area should be massaged to improve the efficacy of treatment. Overall, cryolipolysis is a safe and effective treatment for nonsurgical subcutaneous fat reduction.

Keywords: Cryolipolysis, CoolSculpting, noninvasive, body contouring, paradoxical hyperplasia

Key Points

- Cryolipolysis is a safe and effective procedure for nonsurgical reduction of subcutaneous fat.
- Many areas on the body can be treated including submental, submandibular, arms, back, chest, flanks, abdomen, back, and thighs.
- Pinchable, subcutaneous fat can be treated with suction-assisted applicators, whereas nonpinchable fat (i.e., lateral thigh) can be treated with nonsuction, flat-panel applicators.
- Massage immediately following treatment of the treated areas improves efficacy of cryolipolysis.

90.1 Preoperative Steps

- Perform a standard history and physical including a whole-body assessment.
  - Contraindications include: Cryoglobulinemia, paroxysmal cold hemoglobinuria, cold agglutinin disease.
  - Relative contraindication: Cold intolerance and Raynaud's disease.
- It is important to establish realistic expectations for patients who will benefit from cryolipolysis and discuss the results attainable with this modality compared to surgical interventions.
- Create a treatment plan with the patient explaining that although there are recommended numbers of treatment cycles, the total number of treatments to obtain results may vary with each patient (▶ Table 90.1).
- Identify areas with pinchable fat and nonpinchable fat as this will dictate what applicators should be used (▶ Table 90.2).
- Mark the patient using the templates for the applicators which will be used. The templates will also help determine which applicators and corresponding contour attachments should be used depending on the convexity of the lipodystrophic area being treated.
- The risks and benefits of the procedure should be discussed with the patients and they should also be aware of paradoxical hyperplasia, which may occur 2 to 5 months after treatment and requires surgical excision.

90.2 Operative Steps

- The CoolSculpting device (Zeltiq Aesthetics, Pleasanton, CA) consists of a control unit and various applicators, which are selected based on the size of the treatment site and whether or not the subcutaneous fat can be pinched away from the body (▶ Fig. 90.1).
- The patient's skin is cleansed and covered with a protective gel pad and the applicator is applied. Foam borders (flat panel applicator only) and/or Velcro straps may be used to help secure the applicators in place.
- The suction-assisted applicator is used in most areas unless the fat cannot be pinched away from the body, as in the lateral thigh or saddlebag area.
- Treatment duration is dependent on the applicator used and the area treated.
  - Suction-assisted applicator treatment times vary from 35 minutes to 1 hour, depending on if the applicators are the latest generation of applicators.
  - Nonsuction-assisted applicators require up to 2 hours of treatment times.

Table 90.1 Typical numbers of treatments per site

Treatment site	Number of treatments Per site
Flanks	1 to 3
Abdomen	1 to 3
Inner thigh	1 to 2
Outer thigh	1 to 2
Submental area	1 to 2
Upper arm	1 to 2

Table 90.2 Applicators, contours, and treatment sites

Applicators	Contours	Treatment areas
CoolMini™ 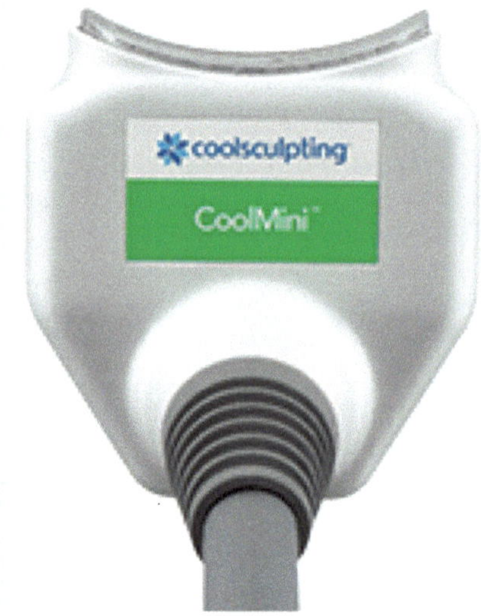 	N/A	Submental Submandibular Bra fat
Cool Advantage Petite™ 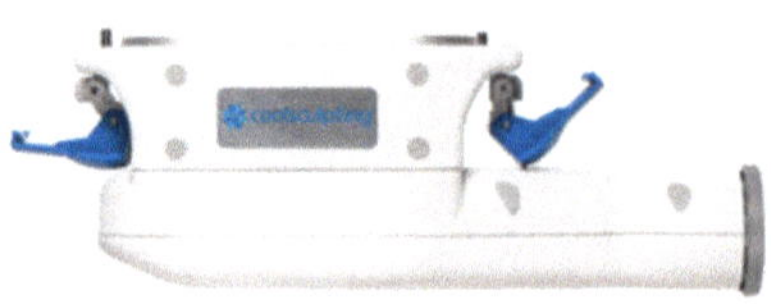	CoolFit™ 	Upper arms Flanks Abdomen Thighs
	CoolCore™ 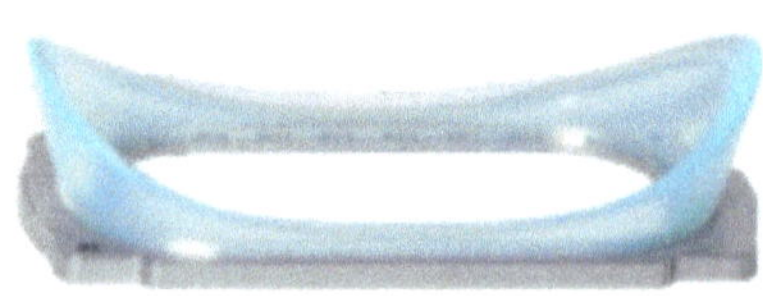	
	CoolCurve™ 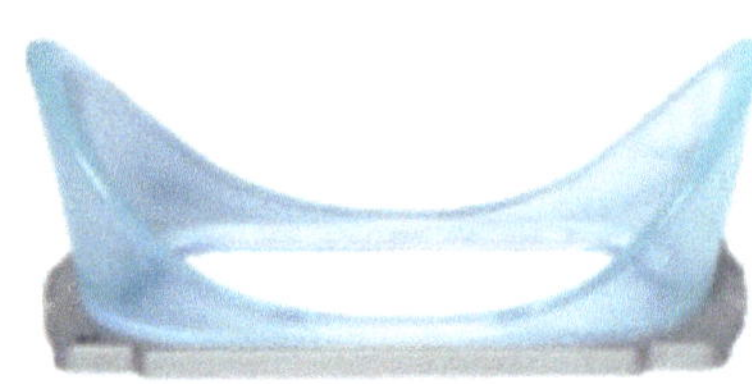	
Cool Advantage™ 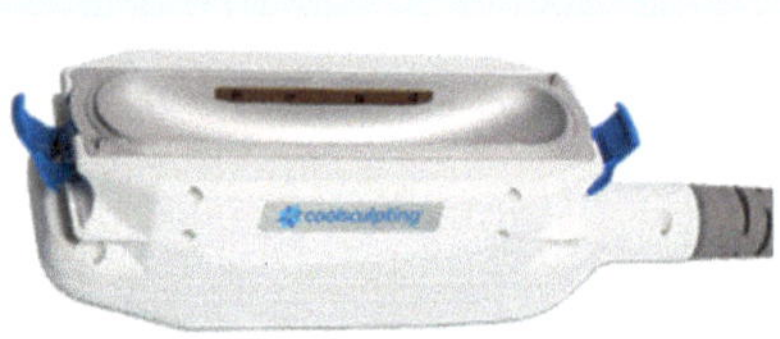	CoolFit™ 	Upper arms Flanks Abdomen Thighs
	CoolCore™ 	

(Continued)

Table 90.2 *(Continued)* Applicators, contours, and treatment sites

Applicators	Contours	Treatment areas
	Cool Curve™ 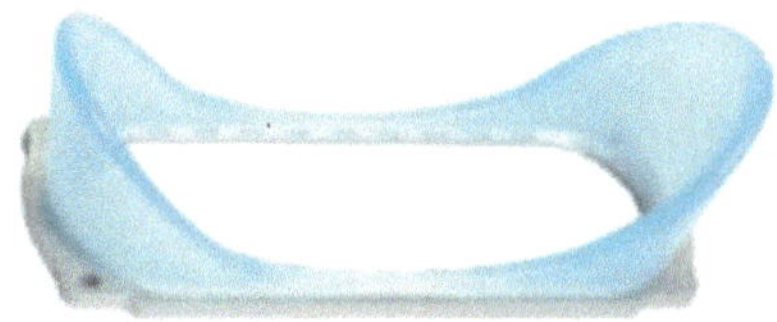	
Cool Advantage Plus™ 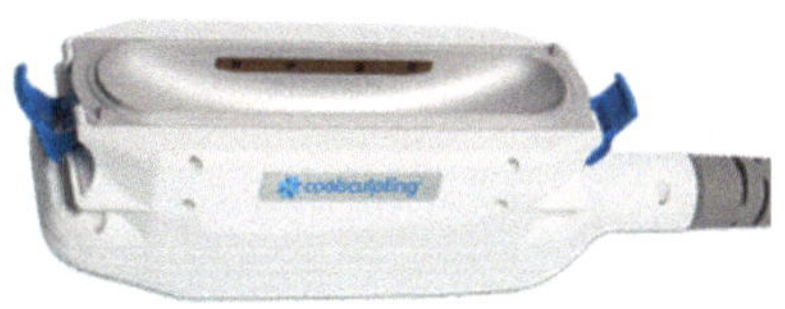	CoolCore™  CoolCurve™ 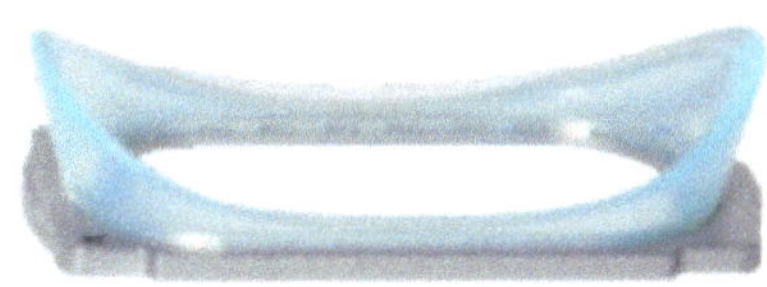	Flanks Abdomen Thighs
Cool Smooth™ 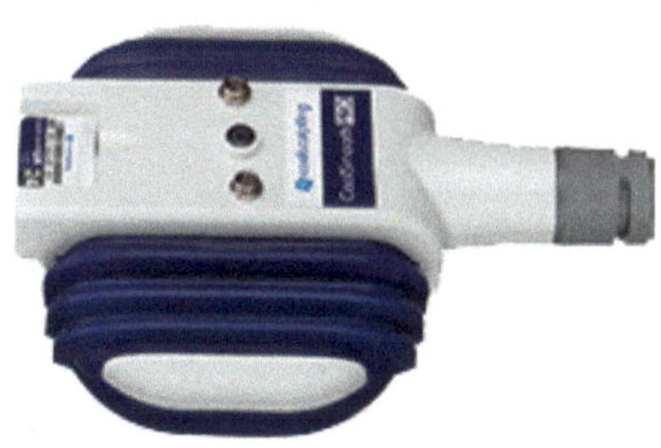	N/A	Lateral thighs Upper abdomen

90.3 Postoperative Care

- After removal of the applicator, 2 minutes of massage should be performed to maximize the efficacy of the treatment. We prefer to use the Z-wave (Zimmer Aesthetics, Irvine, CA), which is a radial pulse device for post-treatment massage.
- Patients should be reminded of the transient side effects of treatment which include:
  - Redness, bruising, swelling, tenderness, numbness, tingling, changes in skin sensation, late onset pain, subcutaneous induration, hyperpigmentation.
- Waiting 8 weeks between treatments is recommended.

90.4 Case Example

This female patient underwent two treatments 2 months apart. Her abdomen and flanks were treated on both visits for 35 minutes (▶ Fig. 90.2). The patient had maintained a significant improvement in her silhouette and abdominal contour at 1 year post treatment (▶ Fig. 90.3).

90.5 Conclusion

Cryolipolysis is a safe and effective treatment of subcutaneous fat in appropriately selected patients. Patients have variable responses to treatments and depending on the site they may require multiple treatments.

See **Video 90.1**.

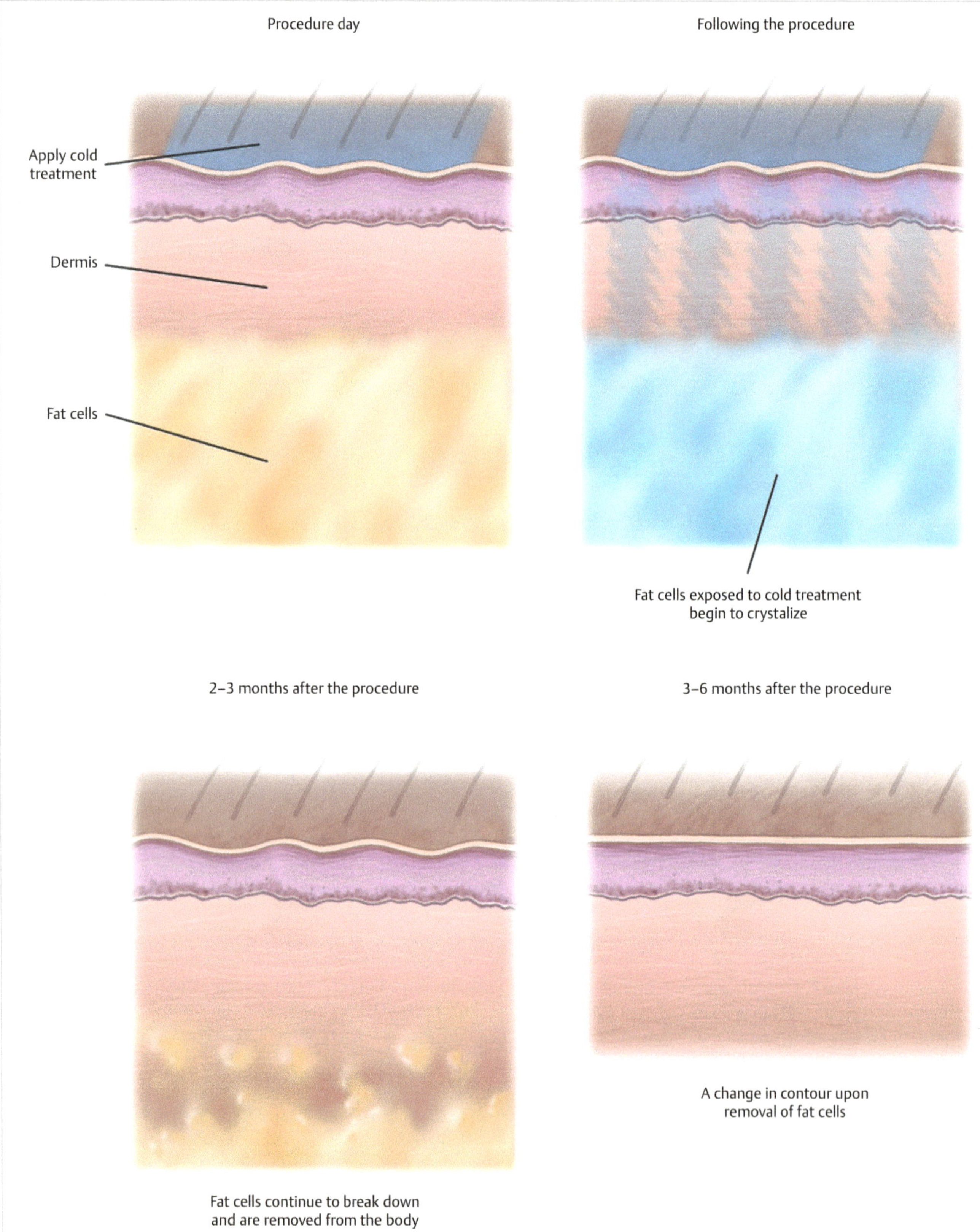

Fig. 90.1 Effect of cryolipolysis on adipose tissue.

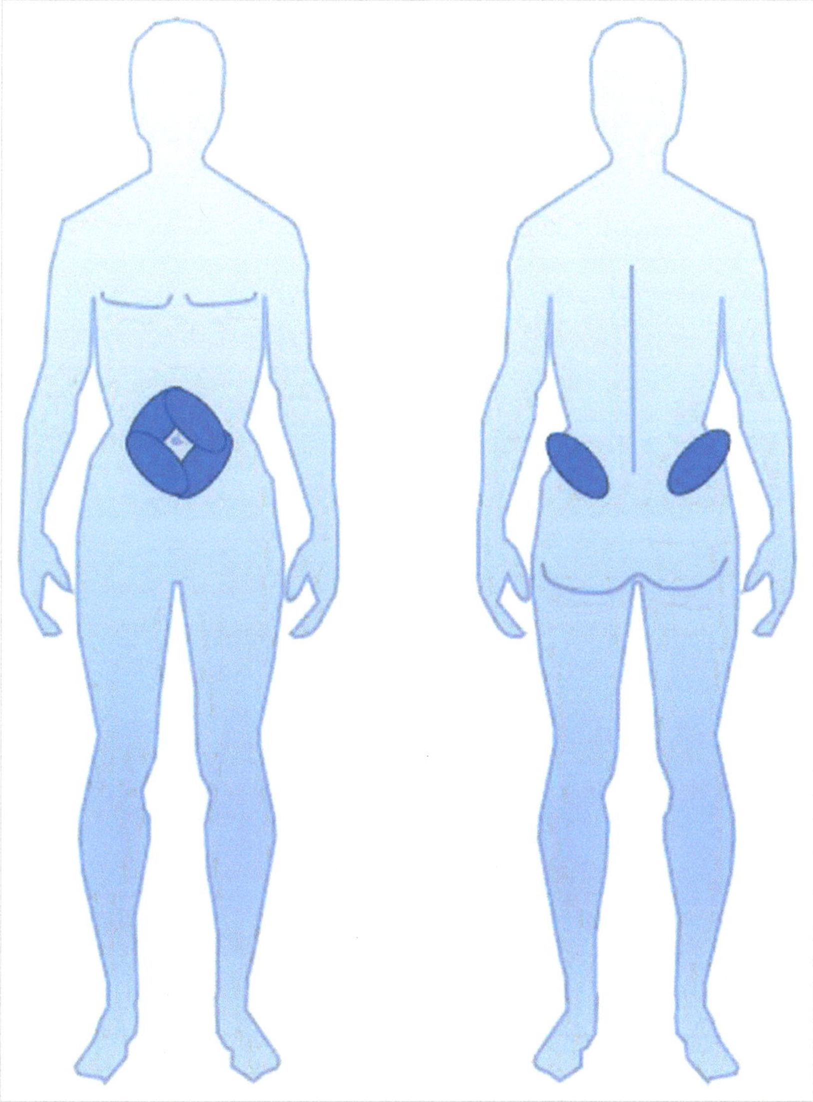

Fig. 90.2 Case example treatment areas. The diamond pattern was used on the abdomen and applicators were also placed on the flanks for 35 minutes per site.

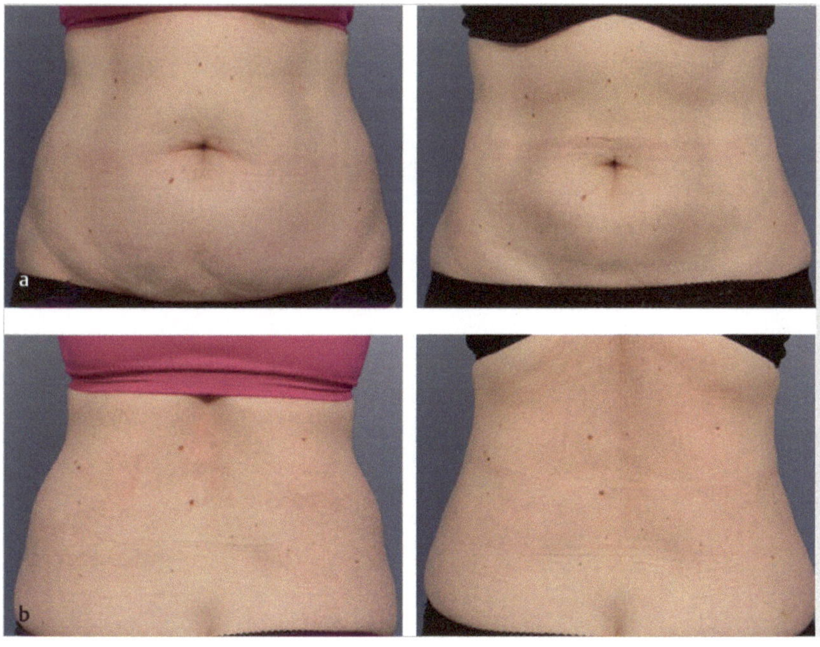

Fig. 90.3 (a, b) Treatment outcomes. Preprocedure (left), and postprocedure (right) at 1 year follow-up after two treatments.

Further Readings

Boey GE, Wasilenchuk JL. Enhanced clinical outcome with manual massage following cryolipolysis treatment: a 4-month study of safety and efficacy. Lasers Surg Med. 2014; 46(1):20–26

Carruthers J, Stevens WG, Carruthers A, Humphrey S. Cryolipolysis and skin tightening. Dermatol Surg. 2014; 40 Suppl 12:S184–S189

Ingargiola MJ, Motakef S, Chung MT, Vasconez HC, Sasaki GH. Cryolipolysis for fat reduction and body contouring: safety and efficacy of current treatment paradigms. Plast Reconstr Surg. 2015; 135(6):1581–1590

Stevens WG, Bachelor EP. Cryolipolysis conformable-surface applicator for nonsurgical fat reduction in lateral thighs. Aesthet Surg J. 2015; 35(1):66–71

Stevens WG, Pietrzak LK, Spring MA. Broad overview of a clinical and commercial experience with CoolSculpting. Aesthet Surg J. 2013; 33(6):835–846

91 Facial Radiofrequency Skin Tightening and Fractional Radiofrequency Technology

Erez Dayan, Joshua M. Cohen, and Spero J. Theodorou

Abstract

A treatment gap exists among patients who are not candidates for or prefer to not undergo traditional facelift and/or necklift. In these cases, radiofrequency skin tightening has been shown to achieve approximately 30% skin contraction through thermal injury to the dermis and tightening of underlaying fibroseptal networks. Subsequent collagen remodeling angiogenesis as well as elastin reorganization functions to visibly improve soft tissue laxity in these cases.

Keywords: Radiofrequency skin tightening, radiofrequency, FaceTite, bipolar radiofrequency

Key Points

- Radiofrequency (RF) technology has steadily gained popularity since the early 2000s with consecutive increases annually of 10% or more.
- Through impedance of electromagnetic current, RF waves lead to differential heating across distinct tissue types consistent with Ohm's law (energy = current^0 × impedance × time). For example, adipose tissue is less conductive than water (higher impedance), and leads to generation of higher temperatures than muscle. Once soft tissue temperatures reach 50 °C and skin surface reaches 40 to 42 °C there is a trigger to induce neocollagenesis, angiogenesis, and elastogenesis. Through different applications of RF energy (i.e., monopolar, bipolar, multipolar, microneedling), subdermal adipose remodeling (SAR) and long-term soft tissue contraction can be safely and consistently achieved.

91.1 Preoperative Steps

- A detailed medical history and physical is obtained on all patients prior to treatment. Exclusion criteria include: pregnancy, open wounds, active infection, dermatologic conditions, bleeding disorders, immunocompromised state.
- Patients are marked by first identifying the mandibular border and jowls bilaterally. The jowls are subdivided into Zone 1 (above mandibular border) and Zone 2 (below mandibular border). Areas of localized adiposity in the lower face and neck region are marked. Nontreatment zones are identified by carrying a line inferiorly perpendicular to the lip commissures (i.e., marionette lines) (▶ Fig. 91.1). The area medial to these lines are avoided to preserve marginal mandibular innervation to the depressor anguli oris, mentalis, and depressor labii inferioris. Five access points are identified: (1) the submental midline, (2) 1 to 2 cm inferior to the mandibular parasymphyseal/body junction, and (3) post auricular (▶ Fig. 91.2).
- Depending on clinical circumstances and patient desires, cases were performed either under general or local anesthesia. In cases of local anesthesia, patients were premedicated with oxycodone (5 mg) and/or benzodiazepine (5 mg).

91.2 Operative Steps

- Access sites are each injected with 2 to 4 cc of 2% lidocaine with epinephrine. A 14-gauge needle is then used to make access ports that are slightly dilated with Stevens scissors. A spinal needle is used to slowly infiltrate tumescent solution (1 g lidocaine per liter of lactated Ringer's solution) from deep

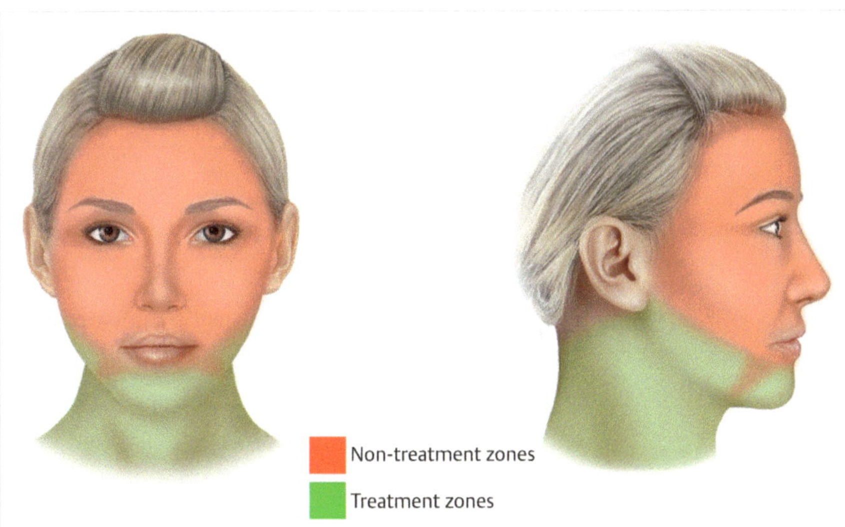

Fig. 91.1 Treatment and nontreatment radiofrequency zones. (Reproduced with permission from Rohrich R, Stuzin J, Dayan E, et al. Facial Danger Zones: Staying Safe with Surgery, Fillers and Non-invasive Devices. 1st ed. Thieme; 2019.)

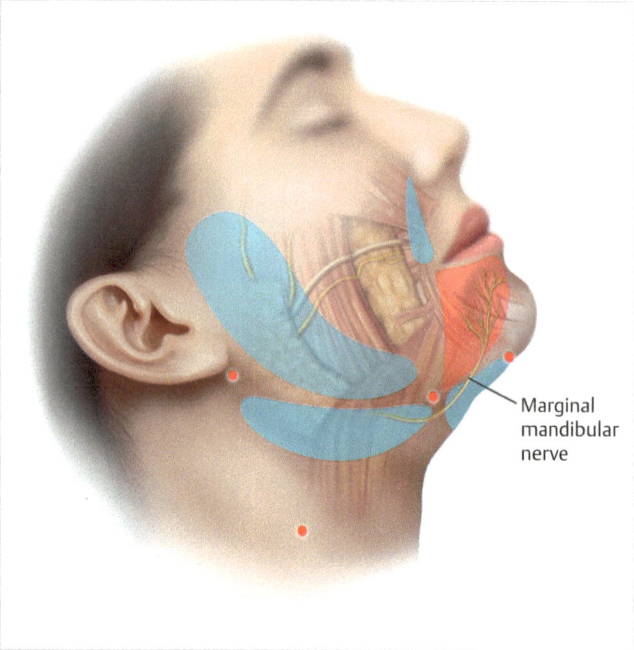

Fig. 91.2 Access ports placement to avoid marginal mandibular and mental nerve injury. (Reproduced with permission from Rohrich R, Stuzin J, Dayan E, et al. Facial Danger Zones: Staying Safe with Surgery, Fillers and Non-invasive Devices. 1st ed. Thieme; 2019.)

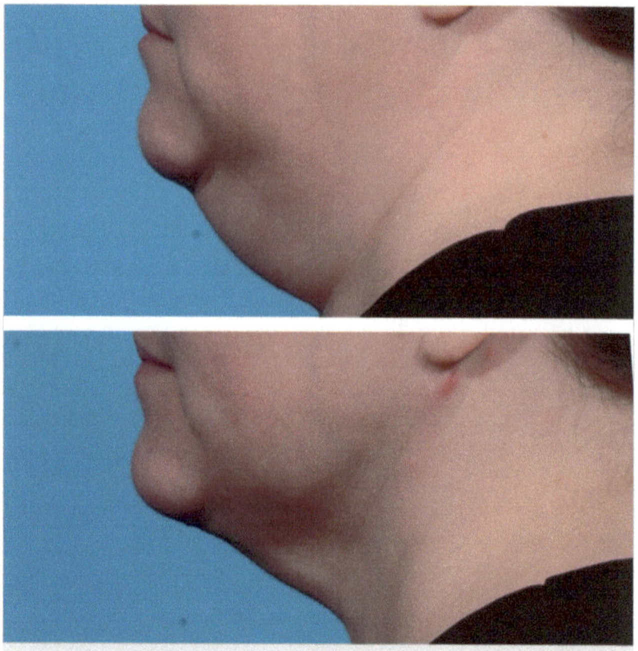

Fig. 91.3 Images showing before and 2 weeks after radiofrequency-assisted liposuction of lower face and neck using FaceTite (InMode; Lake Forest, CA).

to superficial, starting in the preplatysmal plane and moving to the subdermal plane (approximately 100–150 cc of tumescent in total). At the conclusion of tumescent infiltration, the cannula is passed through the subdermal plane to confirm adequate analgesia.

- Bipolar RF is performed first. The RF settings included an internal temperature cutoff of 68 °C and external temperature cutoff of 38 °C. The RF cannula is used to pretunnel treatment areas for ease of treatment. The predetermined treatment areas are systematically heated to avoid heat loss when treating wide areas. RF application is applied on retrograde movement of the cannula and stopped within 1 cm of the access port to prevent overheating this area. Audible and visual cues from the RF console are used to assess temperature of tissues and treatment is stopped after 1 minute of reaching target internal and external temperatures.
- RF microneedling (Fractora modified to Morpheus8, InMode) is subsequently used at a depth of 2 mm and energy of 35 with 50% overlap. The hand-piece is applied firmly and perpendicular to the treatment area prior to delivery of RF energy pulses. In patients with thinner skin or darker Fitzpatrick types, energy settings are reduced by 20%.
- Fractional RF is performed at the same stage with the Morpheus8 device (InMode). This device achieves subdermal adipose tissue remodeling in addition to bipolar thermal injury leading to reorganization of the reticular dermis.

91.3 Postoperative Care

- Patients are seen at 1 week, 1 month, 3 months, and 6 months intervals.
- Patient are instructed to not use any skin products for the first 3 to 4 days after fractional RF treatment.
- The usual postoperative course involves some edema and ecchymosis. This typically resolves in 1 week.
- A facelift type head wrap with moderate compression is applied for 3 to 4 days.
- Patients are instructed to not use cold compresses.
- Most patients return to work the following day.

91.4 Case Example

This patient is seen before and 2 weeks after RF-assisted liposuction of the lower face and neck using FaceTite (InMode; Lake Forest, CA) (▸ Fig. 91.3).

91.5 Conclusion

Internal and external generation of heat via combined bipolar RF and fractional RF serves to initiate neocollagenesis, elastogenesis, and subdermal adipose remodeling. This in combination with fibroseptal network tightening allows for safe and consistent soft tissue contraction to improve lower face and neck soft tissue laxity. This particularly benefits patients who previously may have fallen into a treatment gap.

See **Video 91.1**, **Video 91.2**, and **Video 91.3**.

Further Readings

Brightman L, Weiss E, Chapas AM, et al. Improvement in arm and post-partum abdominal and flank subcutaneous fat deposits and skin laxity using a bipolar radiofrequency, infrared, vacuum and mechanical massage device. Lasers Surg Med. 2009; 41(10):791–798

Chia CT, Theodorou SJ, Hoyos AE, Pitman GH. Radiofrequency-assisted liposuction compared with aggressive superficial, subdermal liposuction of the arms: a bilateral quantitative comparison. Plast Reconstr Surg Glob Open. 2015; 3(7):e459

Fritz K, Salavastru C. Ways of noninvasive facial skin tightening and fat reduction. Facial Plast Surg. 2016; 32(3):276–282

Sadick NS, Makino Y. Selective electro-thermolysis in aesthetic medicine: a review. Lasers Surg Med. 2004; 34(2):91–97

Sadick N, Rothaus KO. Minimally invasive radiofrequency devices. Clin Plast Surg. 2016; 43(3):567–575

92 Body Radiofrequency Fat Removal/Skin Tightening

Erez Dayan, Christopher T. Chia, and Spero J. Theodorou

Abstract

Radiofrequency (RF) technology has been used in different medical specialties for nearly 100 years (i.e., surgical electrocautery, cardiac ablation, joint tightening). However, aesthetic applications of RF first began in the early 2000s with monopolar modalities (i.e., Thermage). One historic challenge with RF has been the balance between efficacy and safety. Precedent devices lacked temperature control, which led to inconsistent results and potential thermal complications. This chapter discusses use of the latest bipolar RF modalities, which allow for volumetric heating of soft tissues with continuous temperature monitoring. This technology has been shown to successfully treat the "treatment gap" patients, demonstrating approximately 30% soft tissue tightening in properly selected patients.

Keywords: Radiofrequency, bipolar radiofrequency, minimally invasive, aesthetic technology, soft tissue tightening, soft tissue remodeling

Key Points

- Significant advancements in minimally invasive body contouring have been made over the past 10 years.
- Increasingly, patients are seeking minimally invasive methods to tighten skin and remodel adipose tissue. A large treatment gap exists among three types of patients: (1) the younger demographic, who desire soft tissue tightening without traditional operations, scars, and downtime; (2) patients with soft tissue laxity who are not "severe enough" to justify an excisional procedure, but not "mild enough" to rely on liposuction with soft tissue contraction alone; and (3) those with recurrent laxity who have already underwent traditional excisional procedure. In these populations, plastic surgeons risk under- or overtreating with traditional methods.
- Through impedance of electromagnetic current, radiofrequency (RF) waves lead to differential heating across distinct tissue types consistent with Ohm's law (energy = current × impedance × time). For example, adipose tissue is less conductive than water (higher impedance), and leads to generation of higher temperatures than muscle. Once soft tissue temperatures reach 50 °C and skin surface reaches 40 to 42 °C there is a trigger to induce neocollagenesis, angiogenesis, and elastogenesis. Through different applications of RF energy (i.e., monopolar, bipolar, multipolar, microneedling), subdermal adipose remodeling (SAR) and long-term soft tissue contraction can be safely and consistently achieved.
- The procedure may be performed safely and effectively under local anesthesia with an excellent safety profile and return to daily activities within 24 to 36 hours.

92.1 Preoperative Steps

92.1.1 Analysis

- A thorough history and physical examination with a focus on previous procedures, significant weight changes, pregnancy status, and a preoperative analysis to identify areas of subcutaneous excess, dermal striae, and tissue laxity.
- Areas of volume excess and areas of significant laxity are marked preoperatively with the patient in the standing position with the target areas in the dependent position to facilitate intraoperative accuracy.
- For upper extremities, the forearm is flexed at 90 degrees and the humerus parallel to the floor to demonstrate areas of maximal laxity in the upper posterior arm.
- Preoperative photography is essential for postprocedural analysis.
- When indicated, laboratory values including complete blood count (CBC), chemistry profile, coagulation tests, and urine pregnancy tests in women of child-bearing age are obtained.
- The patient is given oral medications including an antibiotic, sedative, and pain reliever 30 to 45 minutes preoperatively.

92.2 Operative Steps

See **Video 92.1**.

92.2.1 Tumescent Infiltration

- Following standard prep and drape, the previously identified access points are injected with 1% lidocaine with epinephrine.
- Access incision is made with either 14-gauge needle or #11 blade scalpel.
- Standard infiltration cannula is used to deliver the tumescent fluid (▸ Table 92.1) into the deep subcutaneous space at a low speed.
- Once the deep and intermediate subcutaneous fat spaces are adequately infiltrated, the cannula is placed into the superficial fat space in order to obtain complete analgesia of all layers with the most densely innervated subdermal space injected last.
- It is important to tumesce at least 1 to 2 cm beyond the marked areas to achieve full analgesia in the treatment zone.
- In the awake patient, slow infiltration speed will achieve a comfortable state for the patient because the rate of distension correlates with discomfort.

Table 92.1 Modified tumescent fluid (0.1% lidocaine concentration)

Modified tumescent fluid (0.1% lidocaine concentration)
1,000 mL normal saline
1000 mg lidocaine (50 mL of 2% plain lidocaine)
10 mL sodium bicarbonate
1.5 mL 1:1,000 concentration epinephrine

- Infiltrate “low and slow”: Begin with the tumescent injected into the less richly innervated deep subcutaneous fat space at low speed.
- Only progress to the next step once complete analgesia is achieved.

92.2.2 Application of Radiofrequency Energy

- Same access incisions are used that were made for tumescent infiltration.
- Zones of heating are identified for maximally efficient tissue heating.
- External and internal temperature maximum values are entered on the RF (RF) generator (typically 65–68 °C internally and 35–38 °C externally).
- Sterile ultrasound gel is used to maintain good conduction between the external electrode and the surface of the skin.
- The internal electrode is carefully placed into the subcutaneous fat space at the desired depth (i.e., intermediate layer) while maintaining at least 5 mm distance between the electrode tip and the underside of the dermis.
- A fan pattern of heating from the access point is made as both the internal and external temperatures of the soft tissues in between the two electrodes are gradually heated toward their respective maximum temperature goals.
- To avoid overheating and creating “hot spots,” there is no heating within 1 to 2 cm of the access point.
- Keeping the internal electrode parallel to the skin is important when treating areas where anatomic prominences can cause unintended superficial treatment resulting in “end hits” where the electrode abuts directly against the dermis.
- Adjust the speed of the heat application and/or the amplitude of the strokes when heating the tissues in order to gradually increase the temperatures of both the internal and external tissues.
- In general, the more quickly the hand-piece is moved and the longer the distance of the strokes, the more quickly the external temperature will rise.
- Conversely, the more slowly the hand-piece is moved and the shorter the amplitude of the strokes, the more quickly the internal temperature will rise.
- Once the proper cadence is found specific for the patient area treated, the more efficiently the heat can be transferred without the generator’s safety features defeating the delivery of the energy.
- Once the therapeutic temperatures both internally and externally are achieved, maintain the maximum temperatures for the clinically appropriate amount of time (typically 30–60 seconds).
- For large volumes of fat that are subjected to the heating (i.e., abdomen in large patients), it is recommended that aspiration of the emulsified fats that are liberated by the heat is performed in order to remove excess oil and fatty acids that can slightly increase the rate of seroma formation and fat necrosis if left for too long.
- Fractional bipolar RF is commonly performed at the same stage with the Morpheus8 device (InMode, Lake Forest, CA). This device achieves subdermal adipose tissue remodeling in addition to bipolar thermal injury leading to reorganization of the reticular dermis.
- Fractional RF is subsequently used at a depth of 4 mm (double-stacked) and energy of 35 with 50% overlap. The hand-piece is applied firmly and perpendicular to the treatment area prior to delivery of RF energy pulses. In patients with thinner skin or darker Fitzpatrick types, energy settings are reduced by 20%.

92.2.3 Liposuction Contouring

- Following application of RF energy, suction-assisted lipectomy may be performed.
- Manual or power-assisted liposuction may be used.
- Some practitioners may wish to perform liposuction in larger patients with substantial subcutaneous fat prior to application of the RF energy in order to save time in heating the soft tissues.
- If fat is to be harvested for transfer, liposuction must be done prior to RF heating which will cause lipolysis.
- If the fat aspirate portion of any single anatomic area treated exceeds on 1,000 mL, consider placement of a closed suction drain to reduce the risk of seroma formation.

92.3 Postoperative Care

- Standard compression garments following liposuction are routinely worn by the patient for 10 to 14 days.
- Patient are instructed to not use any skin products for the first 3 to 4 days after fractional RF treatment.
- Except for avoidance of high salt foods, there are no dietary restrictions.
- Patients are encouraged to walk as soon as possible.
- Heavy lifting and exercise are held off for 2 to 3 weeks.
- Sutures are removed between 7 and 10 days.

92.4 Case Example

A 39-year-old female presented for nonsurgical RF skin tightening to her abdomen. The patient had a total of two treatments spanning over a period of 8 weeks. Settings were as follows: First pass (Body, Power 30); second pass (Face, Power 25). Subsequent treatments increased power by 5 (▸ Fig. 92.1).

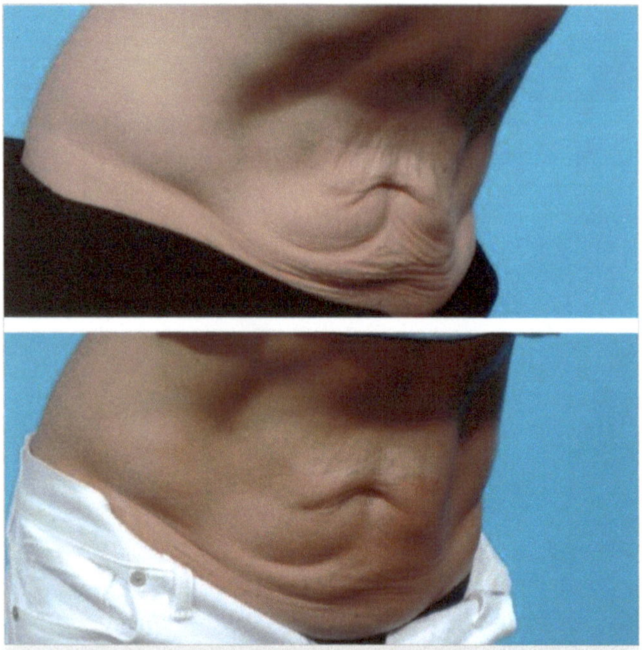

Fig. 92.1 A 39-year-old female presented for nonsurgical radiofrequency skin tightening to her abdomen. The patient had a total of two treatments spanning over a period of 8 weeks. Settings were as follows: First pass (Body, Power 30); second pass (Face, Power 25). Subsequent treatments increased power by 5.

92.5 Conclusion

Significant and reproducible soft tissue tightening may be achieved with the application of RF to the skin and underlying fibroseptal network. This allows inclusion of patients for minimally invasive contouring with liposuction who may otherwise be deemed as noncandidates due to the risk of unacceptable laxity postoperatively. In patients with good elasticity, it allows more aggressive and detailed liposuction to be performed. The procedure may be applied to nearly limitless areas of the body in addition to the trunk and extremities, to include the face, neck, upper and lower eyelids, forehead, and any other areas of soft tissue laxity where conventional excisional operations may not be indicated or wanted by the patient at the time.

Further Readings

Brightman L, Weiss E, Chapas AM, et al. Improvement in arm and post-partum abdominal and flank subcutaneous fat deposits and skin laxity using a bipolar radiofrequency, infrared, vacuum and mechanical massage device. Lasers Surg Med. 2009; 41(10):791–798

Chia CT, Theodorou SJ, Hoyos AE, Pitman GH. Radiofrequency-assisted liposuction compared with aggressive superficial, subdermal liposuction of the arms: a bilateral quantitative comparison. Plast Reconstr Surg Glob Open. 2015; 3(7):e459

Fritz K, Salavastru C. Ways of noninvasive facial skin tightening and fat reduction. Facial Plast Surg. 2016; 32(3):276–282

Sadick NS, Makino Y. Selective electro-thermolysis in aesthetic medicine: a review. Lasers Surg Med. 2004; 34(2):91–97

Sadick N, Rothaus KO. Minimally invasive radiofrequency devices. Clin Plast Surg. 2016; 43(3):567–575

93 Deoxycholic Acid Role in Fat Reduction

Sachin M. Shridharani and Grace M. Tisch

Abstract

Deoxycholic acid (DCA) is an injectable adipocytolytic agent that is FDA-approved for the reduction of convexity or fullness associated with submental fat. When injected into the subcutaneous tissue, DCA induces adipocytolysis by irreversibly disrupting the cell membrane. Most standard markings for submental DCA injections target only a small central area of the submentum to avoid complications. This approach, however, often undertreats patients with adipose deposition outside the central region. The expanded safe zone (ESZ) system was developed based on cadaveric dye studies of submental fat compartments and describes a method for safely expanding the standard centralized treatment area. This technique provides topographical landmarks that correlate to discrete fat compartments within the preplatysmal fat and presents an anatomical basis for individualized treatment of submental convexity. By using the ESZ system to identify the zone of treatment, clinicians are able to: customize treatment strategy, improve jawline definition and cervicomental angle, and optimize the outcome of submental DCA injection.

Keywords: Deoxycholic acid, submental fat, expanded safe zone, facial contouring, Kybella

Key Points

- Deoxycholic acid (DCA) is an injectable adipocytolytic agent approved for the reduction of convexity or fullness associated with submental fat.
- Most standard markings for DCA injections target a small central area of submental fullness to avoid complications, namely, marginal mandibular nerve paresis; this standardized treatment approach undertreats patients with adipose deposition outside the central region.
- The expanded safe zone (ESZ) system describes a method for safely expanding the standard treatment region based on anatomical studies of submental fat compartments.
- This technique provides topographical landmarks that correlate to discrete fat compartments within the preplatysmal fat and allows for targeted, patient-customized treatment of submental fullness.

93.1 Preoperative Steps

93.1.1 Analysis

- DCA injection to the submental region begins with a thorough analysis to assess the extent of fat deposition and identify the zone of treatment (▶ Fig. 93.1).
- Before proceeding with treatment, patients should be screened for other potential causes of submental fullness (e.g., low hyoid position, enlarged or ptotic submandibular glands, thyromegaly, and/or cervical lymphadenopathy).

93.1.2 Expanded Safe Zone (ESZ) System: Submental Markings

- All six regions of the ESZ system should be assessed to identify the target treatment area.
- The six regions of the ESZ system are marked (▶ Fig. 93.2a) preoperatively in the seated and upright position based on the following anatomic boundaries:
  - *No Treatment Zone (NTZ):* Region 4.5 cm cephalad to the gonion and approximately 2 cm caudal to the inferior border of the mandible (corresponding to location of the marginal mandibular nerve) (▶ Fig. 93.2b, c)
  - *Safe Zone 1:* Submental crease (superior border), thyroid cartilage (inferior border), caudal continuation of bilateral oral commissures (lateral borders) (▶ Fig. 93.2b, c)
  - *Safe Zone 2 (Bilateral):* Inferior edge of the *No Treatment Zone* (superior border), lateral extension of thyroid cartilage (inferior border), caudal continuation of oral commissure (medial border), and antegonial notch (lateral border) (▶ Fig. 93.2b, c)
  - *Safe Zone 3 (Bilateral):* Inferior edge of the *No Treatment Zone* (superior border), lateral extension of thyroid cartilage (inferior border), caudal continuation of antegonial notch (medial border), and anterior border of unilateral sternocleidomastoid muscle (lateral border) (▶ Fig. 93.2b, c)
  - *Safe Zone 4:* Thyroid cartilage (superior border), neck crease (inferior border), anterior border of bilateral sternocleidomastoid muscles (lateral borders) (▶ Fig. 93.2b, c)

93.1.3 Treatment Area and Injection Pattern

- Outline the planned treatment area with a surgical pen, particularly avoiding the *No Treatment Zone* (▶ Fig. 93.2b, c).
- Planned treatment area is confirmed by palpation to ensure the presence of sufficient subcutaneous fat.
- Prep treatment area with hypochlorous acid and apply a 1-cm injection grid to mark the injection sites.

93.1.4 Pretreatment Considerations

- Caution should be practiced in patients with prior surgical or cosmetic treatment in the submental area as anatomical changes or scar tissue may impact safe administration of DCA.
- Patients should be counseled on the likelihood of needing two to four treatments (at 6-week intervals) for optimal results.

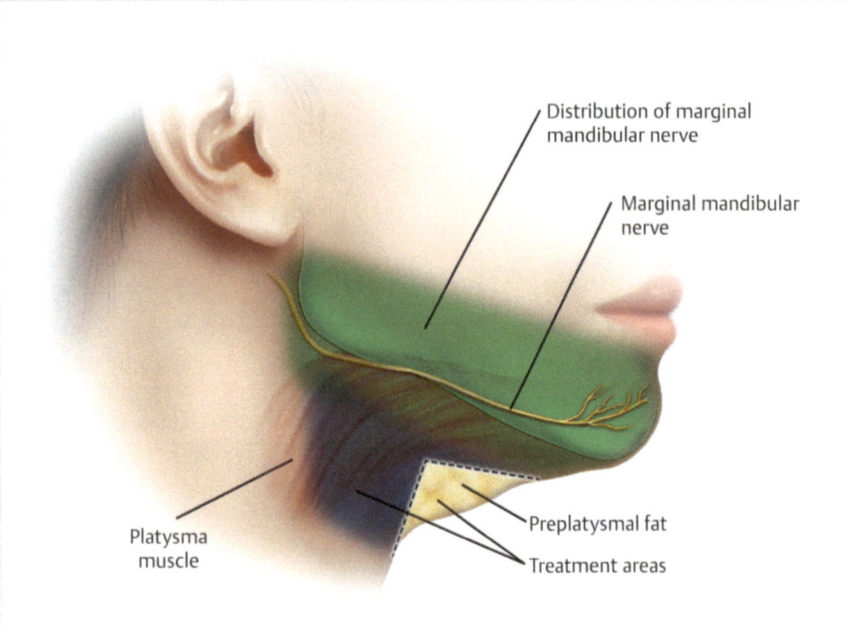

Fig. 93.1 Location of marginal mandibular nerve (MMN) and area of submental fat distribution. Distribution of MMN is shaded in *green*. Lateral aspect of submental fat is shaded in *blue*, and centralized preplatysmal fat is shaded in *yellow*.

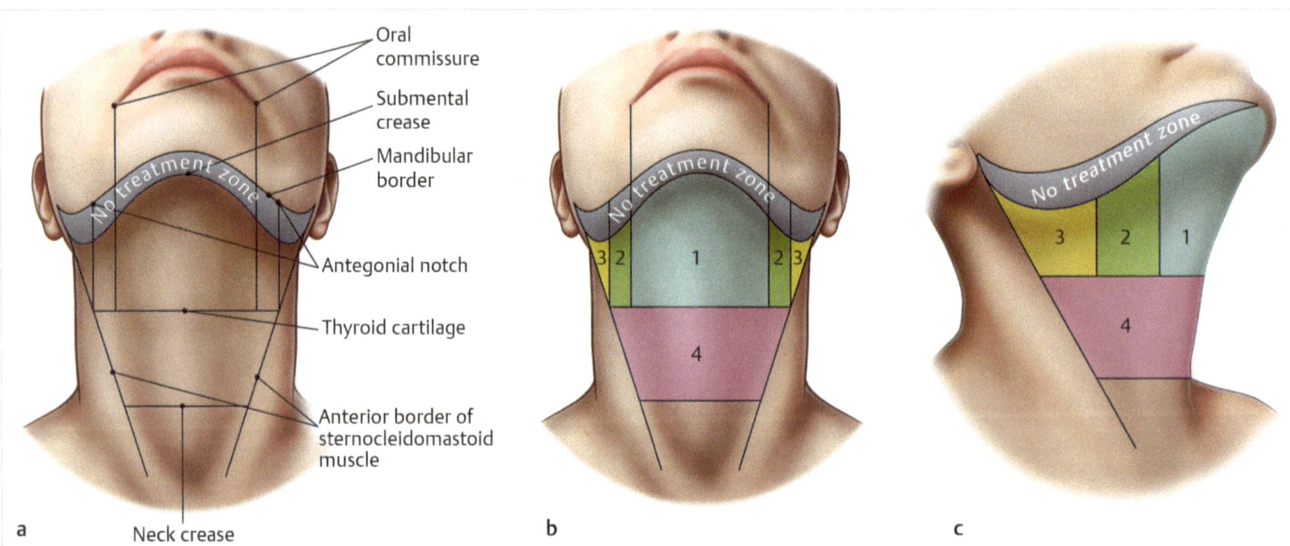

Fig. 93.2 **(a)** Key external anatomic landmarks of the expanded safe zone system and illustration of pretreatment markings. Shaded region represents the *No Treatment Zone* (corresponding to the location of the marginal mandibular nerve). **(b)** Anterior and **(c)** oblique views of the neck. Safe Zones 1, 2, 3, and 4 are delineated in *blue*, *green*, *yellow*, and *pink*, respectively. The *No Treatment Zone* is delineated in *gray*.

93.2 Operative Steps

See **Video 93.1**.

93.2.1 Local Anesthetic Administration

- To enhance patient comfort, the treatment area is injected with lidocaine (1 or 2%) with epinephrine 1:100,000. Volume of local anesthetic injection ranges from 3 to 6 cc depending on patient sensitivity and surface area being treated.
- Ice packs are applied to treatment area and 10 minutes are allotted for the local anesthetic to take effect.

93.2.2 Deoxycholic Acid Dosage and Administration

- DCA (10 mg/mL solution) is injected into the preplatysmal subcutaneous fat using an area-adjusted dose of 2 mg/cm^2.
- Throughout the treatment zone, 0.2 mL DCA injections spaced 1 cm apart are administered; do not taper DCA dosage laterally.
- A maximum of 50 injections (up to 10 mL DCA) may be injected in a single treatment and a maximum of 6 single treatments may be administered (at intervals no less than 4 weeks apart).

- The number of injections per treatment and the number of treatment sessions depend on the individual patient's submental fat distribution, cervicomental anatomy, and treatment goals.

93.2.3 Deoxycholic Acid Injection Technique

- Draw 1 mL of DCA into a sterile 1-mL syringe.

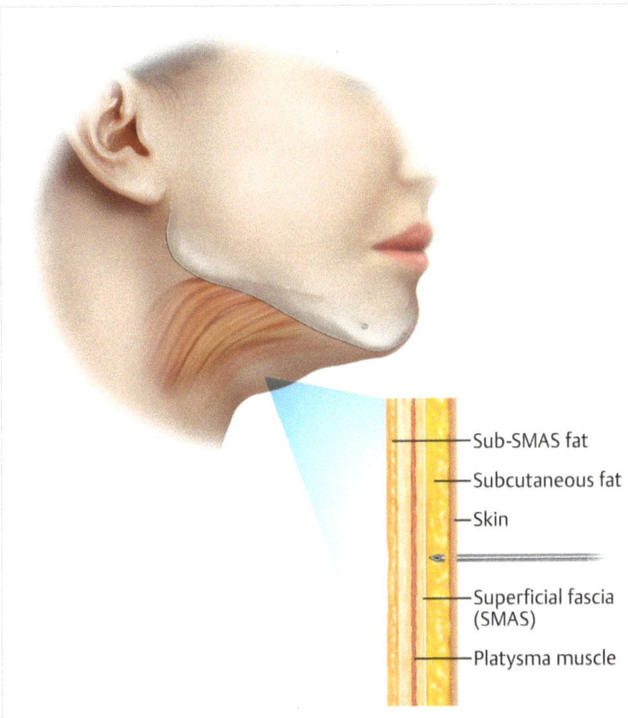

Fig. 93.3 Schematic illustration of sagittal neck area with position of needle in preplatysmal fat.

- Using a 32-gauge, 0.5-inch needle, inject 0.2 mL of DCA into the preplatysmal fat immediately adjacent to each 1-cm grid mark.
- Injections are administered perpendicular to the skin surface with the needle advanced midway into the subcutaneous fat (▶ Fig. 93.3).
- Do not withdraw the needle during injection as superficial (intradermal) DCA injection can result in dermal necrosis.
- Needle resistance indicates possible contact with nonadipose tissue and the needle must be repositioned to an appropriate depth before injection.
- To avoid injury to the marginal mandibular nerve do not inject within the region 4.5 cm anterior to the gonion and approximately 2 cm below the inferior border of the mandible.
- Immediately following treatment, an ice pack is applied to the injected area.

93.3 Postoperative Care

- Patients are instructed to avoid lying down for a minimum of 4 to 5 hours following treatment.
- Cold compresses are applied to the treatment area intermittently for the first 24 hours.
- Exercise, strenuous activity, alcohol, and salty foods are to be avoided for 48 hours.
- Patients rest with head elevated for 48 hours.
- Patients are encouraged to avoid unnecessary exposure to heat, excessive cold, and excessive sun for 1 to 2 weeks.

93.4 Case Example

Anterior, oblique, and lateral pre- and post-treatment photos of a patient 7 weeks following a single treatment session with submental DCA injections (▶ Fig. 93.4a–c).

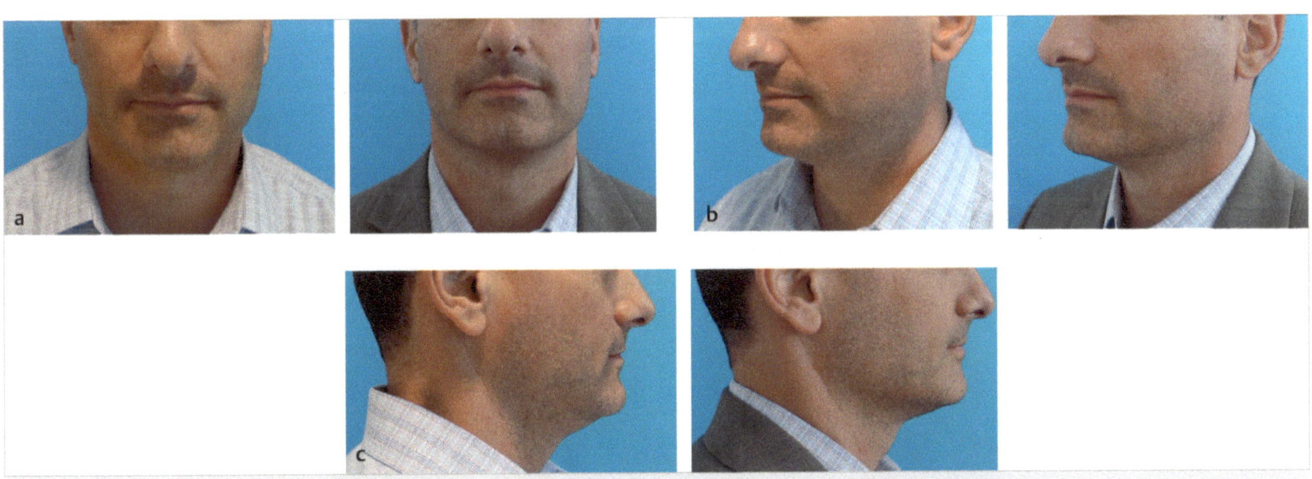

Fig. 93.4 **(a)** Anterior, **(b)** oblique, and **(c)** lateral pre- and post-treatment photos of a patient 7 weeks following a single treatment session with submental deoxycholic acid (DCA) injections.

93.5 Conclusion

Prior to administration of DCA injections, clinicians must consider the etiology of submental fullness and a thorough assessment of the cervicomental region should be performed. By using the ESZ system to identify the treatment area, clinicians are able to: customize treatment strategy, achieve better neck and jawline definition, and optimize the outcome of submental DCA injection. The six regions of the ESZ system are identified using surface anatomic landmarks, and all six regions should be evaluated for preplatysmal fat. To minimize the risk of adverse events, injections should be avoided in areas with insufficient subcutaneous fat and in regions near the marginal mandibular nerve.

Further Readings

Dayan SH, Humphrey S, Jones DH, et al. Overview of ATX-101 (deoxycholic acid injection): a nonsurgical approach for reduction of submental fat. Dermatol Surg. 2016; 42 Suppl 1:S263–S270

Dover JS, Shridharani SM, Bloom JD, Somogyi C, Gallagher CJ. Reduction of submental fat continues beyond 28 days after ATX-101 treatment: results from a post hoc analysis. Dermatol Surg. 2018; 44(11):1477–1479

Jones DH, Carruthers J, Joseph JH, et al. REFINE-1, a multicenter, randomized, double-blind, placebo-controlled, phase 3 trial with ATX-101, an injectable drug for submental fat reduction. Dermatol Surg. 2016; 42(1): 38–49

Kythera Biopharmaceuticals, Inc. KYBELLA (deoxycholic acid) injection [prescribing information]. https://www.allergan.com/assets/pdf/kybella_pi. Accessed July 10, 2019

Shridharani SM. Injection of an adipocytolytic agent for reduction of excess periaxillary fat. Aesthet Surg J. 2019; 39(12):NP495–NP503

Shridharani SM. Real-world experience with 100 consecutive patients undergoing neck contouring with ATX-101 (deoxycholic acid): an updated report with a 2-year analysis. Dermatol Surg. 2019; 45(10):1285–1293

Shridharani SM, Behr KL. ATX-101 (deoxycholic acid injection) treatment in men: insights from our clinical experience. Dermatol Surg. 2017; 43(11) Suppl 2: S225–S230

Shridharani SM. Early experience in 100 consecutive patients with injection adipocytolysis for neck contouring with ATX-101 (deoxycholic acid). Dermatol Surg. 2017; 43(7):950–958

Yang HM, Kim HJ, Park HW, et al. Revisiting the topographic anatomy of the marginal mandibular branch of facial nerve relating to the surgical approach. Aesthet Surg J. 2016; 36(9):977–982

Index

Note: Page numbers set **bold** or *italic* indicate headings or figures, respectively.